The MassGeneral Hospital for Children Handbook of Pediatric Global Health

Nupur Gupta • Brett D. Nelson
Jennifer Kasper • Patricia L. Hibberd
Editors

The MassGeneral Hospital for Children Handbook of Pediatric Global Health

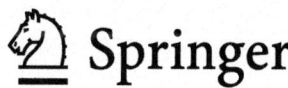

Editors
Nupur Gupta, M.D., M.P.H.
MassGeneral Hospital
 for Children
Harvard Medical School
Boston, MA, USA

Jennifer Kasper, M.D., M.P.H.
MassGeneral Hospital
 for Children
Harvard Medical School
Boston, MA, USA

Brett D. Nelson, M.D., M.P.H., D.T.M.&H.
MassGeneral Hospital
 for Children
Harvard Medical School
Boston, MA, USA

Patricia L. Hibberd, M.D., Ph.D.
MassGeneral Hospital
 for Children
Harvard Medical School
Boston, MA, USA

ISBN 978-1-4614-7917-8   ISBN 978-1-4614-7918-5 (eBook)
DOI 10.1007/978-1-4614-7918-5
Springer New York Heidelberg Dordrecht London

Library of Congress Control Number: 2013948913

© Springer Science+Business Media New York 2014
This work is subject to copyright. All rights are reserved by the Publisher, whether the whole or part of the material is concerned, specifically the rights of translation, reprinting, reuse of illustrations, recitation, broadcasting, reproduction on microfilms or in any other physical way, and transmission or information storage and retrieval, electronic adaptation, computer software, or by similar or dissimilar methodology now known or hereafter developed. Exempted from this legal reservation are brief excerpts in connection with reviews or scholarly analysis or material supplied specifically for the purpose of being entered and executed on a computer system, for exclusive use by the purchaser of the work. Duplication of this publication or parts thereof is permitted only under the provisions of the Copyright Law of the Publisher's location, in its current version, and permission for use must always be obtained from Springer. Permissions for use may be obtained through RightsLink at the Copyright Clearance Center. Violations are liable to prosecution under the respective Copyright Law.

The use of general descriptive names, registered names, trademarks, service marks, etc. in this publication does not imply, even in the absence of a specific statement, that such names are exempt from the relevant protective laws and regulations and therefore free for general use.

While the advice and information in this book are believed to be true and accurate at the date of publication, neither the authors nor the editors nor the publisher can accept any legal responsibility for any errors or omissions that may be made. The publisher makes no warranty, express or implied, with respect to the material contained herein.

Printed on acid-free paper

Springer is part of Springer Science+Business Media (www.springer.com)

To Ravi and Chandra Bhandari, my parents, for always being an inspiration to me and making me who I am today; Radha Krishna and Raj Kumari Gupta, my in-laws who have always supported me in all my endeavors; Dr. Gopal Gupta, my husband and best friend, for always being there for me; Jaya and Siddharth, my children, for always believing in me; Dr. Arun Bordia and Manjula Bordia, my uncle and aunt, without whom I would never have been a doctor; and last but not the least to my patients around the world, who bring love, wisdom, and humility into my life every day.

I would also like to thank our department chair, Dr. Ron Kleinman, Dr. Mark Goldstein and all the authors for sharing their time and expertise to make this handbook a reality.

Nupur Gupta

Brett would like to thank all of our colleagues who spent countless hours in preparing thoughtful and useful contributions to this handbook. He is also grateful for the many inspiring and deeply committed health care workers he has had the honor of working alongside and learning from in resource-limited settings.

Brett D. Nelson

I dedicate this handbook to the following people:

Dr Barry Zuckerman, who allowed me to use my call-free elective during my third year of pediatric residency at Boston City Hospital to work in Hospital Infantil in Mexico City (my life has not been the same since, for all the right reasons).

Dr Lanny Smith, Dr Maruca Figueroa, and the campesinos of Estancia, El Salvador, who taught me accompaniment, liberation medicine ("the conscious and conscientious use of health to promote human dignity and social justice"), human rights, and how to amplify the voices of the marginalized, underserved, and unheard.

To the board of directors and members of Doctors for Global Health who remind me to "promote health and other human rights with those most in need, while educating and inspiring others to action."

My parents, Bill and Kay Kasper, who gave me the confidence and latitude to work overseas.

My wife, Dr. MaryCatherine Arbour, who is my greatest inspiration. She is my staunchest supporter and reminds me to advocate for equity and social justice everywhere.

Jennifer Kasper

I would like to save a very special thank-you to all our authors and supporters who worked tirelessly to make their contributions to this handbook so relevant and important to a shared vision of health for children and adolescents around the world.

Patricia L. Hibberd

Preface

Welcome to the *MassGeneral Hospital for Children Handbook of Pediatric Global Health*. This *Handbook* is intended for the ever-increasing number of health professionals who are becoming involved in global health and spending a few weeks to months or even years providing medical care in resource-poor countries. Clinicians trained in the United States, Europe, Australia, and other resource-rich countries may take for granted ready access to tools for diagnosing and treating illness. Insufficient diagnostic services, treatment options, and health care infrastructure in resource-limited settings may prove challenging. This *Handbook* provides practical, evidence-based, hands-on guidance for managing and preventing childhood illnesses when resources are limited. It is not meant solely for pediatricians; it is designed for generalists, specialists, doctors, nurses, other health care workers, and those in training. The reality in many resource-limited settings is that the majority of the patients needing care will be young infants and children. Therefore, all providers need to be prepared to provide quality, evidence-based, compassionate pediatric care. The *Handbook* may also be a useful addition and resource for academic centers and universities in developed countries that are creating courses for trainees who will do clinical electives abroad during their training.

A focus on prevention and treatment of childhood illness for everyone providing care in developing countries remains highly relevant today. The United Nations' Millennium Development Goal 4 is to reduce the under-age-five mortality rate by two-thirds between 1990 and 2015. We are quickly approaching this target date. Overall there has been some progress: several countries in South America and China will achieve the 2015 goal. However, progress has been slower than desired in many countries in sub-Saharan Africa and parts of South Asia: they are not projected to reach the 2015 goal until after 2040. In 2013, nearly seven million children under age five will die, and almost half will be neonates (less than 1 month old), and the most common causes of death in those greater than 2 months of age will be pneumonia and diarrhea.

This *Handbook* provides setting-specific understanding and management approaches to the major causes of childhood mortality, including pneumonia, diarrhea, birth asphyxia, complications of preterm birth, and neonatal sepsis.

The first part of the *Handbook* provides an overview of childhood mortality, health systems, and the various stakeholders that play a role in the global health arena. The *Handbook* also contains chapters on adolescent health, which is increasingly recognized as important as focus shifts towards health preconception in order to improve health of neonates and young infants. Also targeting the unique health concerns of this age group will maintain gains made in childhood and help prevent the onset of adult illnesses. Finally, key topics in non-communicable diseases are covered, including trauma and injuries, pediatric mental health, child and adolescent rights, and oral health.

The *Handbook* is a collaborative effort of residents, fellows, and faculty from MassGeneral Hospital for Children, paired with internationally recognized content experts from all over the globe. The *Handbook* focuses on the equipment, laboratory resources, and medicines that are likely to be available in developing settings and deliberately does not include options that are not typically available. It provides practical, field-based suggestions for utilizing local resources for optimal clinical care.

For many of the authors, working in developing countries during both short- and long-term assignments has changed their lives and career goals. Global health providers will experience exhilarating moments when a baby's life is saved, as well as tragedies when simple, cheap, life-saving equipment or medicines are just not available. The goal of global health experiences is to help serve communities around the world. They also provide an opportunity for us to learn from our overseas colleagues and are a tremendous way to expand our own clinical understanding. Our hope is that respect for cultural issues, gratitude towards the people and providers from whom we learn, as well as the knowledge we bring will help all of us become competent and compassionate global health providers. This is the essence of the *Handbook*.

Boston, MA

Patricia L. Hibberd, M.D., Ph.D.
Nupur Gupta, M.D., M.P.H.
Brett D. Nelson, M.D., M.P.H., D.T.M.&H.
Jennifer Kasper, M.D., M.P.H.

Contents

Part I   Overview of Pediatric Global Health

1. **Child Mortality in Developing Countries** 3
   Norman Miles Farr and Brett D. Nelson

2. **Stakeholders and Approaches to Address Pediatric Global Health** 13
   Jennifer Kasper and Nancy Ringel

3. **Global Health Systems** 25
   Matthew Tobey and Patrick T. Lee

4. **Vulnerability of Children in Developing Countries and Disrupted Settings** 35
   Sylvia Veronica Romm, Iyah K. Romm, and Brett D. Nelson

5. **Fundamentals of Pediatric Care in Resource-Limited Settings** 43
   Julia Elisabeth von Oettingen, Roseda E. Marshall, and Jennifer Kasper

Part II   Newborn Health

6. **Maternal Health** 73
   Ariel Wagner, Veronica Maria Pimentel, and Melody J. Eckardt

7. **Preventive Newborn Care** 87
   Rebecca Cook and Gopal K. Gupta

8. **Newborn Resuscitation** 95
   Jonathan Reisman, Jonathan M. Spector, and Linda L. Wright

9. **Neonatal Infections** 105
   Hasan S. Merali, Anita K.M. Zaidi, and Brett D. Nelson

Part III Adolescent Health

10 Adolescent Global Health 121
Karen Sadler and Nupur Gupta

11 Adolescent Preventative and Clinical Care: A Checklist 139
Nupur Gupta and Karen Sadler

12 Sexually Transmitted Infections in Adolescents 151
Mark A. Goldstein and Nupur Gupta

13 Contraceptive Options for Adolescents 179
Nupur Gupta

Part IV Communicable Diseases

14 Acute Respiratory Infections 193
David A. Lyczkowski, Peter P. Moschovis, and Shamim Qazi

15 Diarrheal Illnesses 205
A. Kaytee Welsh and Archana Patel

16 Malaria 217
Paul J. Krezanoski and Davidson H. Hamer

17 Measles 243
Elizabeth R. Wolf and Elisa Margolis

18 HIV/AIDS 251
Kathleen M. Powis and Aura M. Obando

19 Tuberculosis 279
Rinn Song and Kristian R. Olson

20 Parasitic Diseases 287
Amanda P. Garcia and LeAnne M. Fox

21 Vaccine-Preventable Diseases 303
Michele S. Duke and Vandana L. Madhavan

Part V Non-Communicable Diseases

22 Malnutrition 321
Pornthep Tanpowpong, Sarah Messmer, Jennifer Kasper, and Ronald E. Kleinman

23 Micronutrient Deficiencies 337
Jyoti Ramakrishna and Jay Thiagarajah

24	Emergency Pediatric Care in Resource-Limited Settings............	347
	Sylvia Veronica Romm, Daniel P. Ryan, and Linda T. Wang	
25	Child and Adolescent Mental Health	361
	Giuseppe Raviola and Sarabeth Broder-Fingert	
26	Child and Adolescent Health and Human Rights..	381
	Ashkon Shaahinfar and Theresa S. Betancourt	
27	Pediatric Preventive and Clinical Oral Health Care	389
	Brittany Seymour, Michele Martin, and Grace Kim	
28	Neurological Issues and Epilepsy in Children and Adolescents in the Developing World	409
	Amy C. Lee	
29	Care of the Child Immigrant	419
	Jennifer Kasper, Nupur Gupta, Andrea J. Hunter, and Brett D. Nelson	

Appendix A: WHO Integrated Management of Childhood Illness for High HIV Settings 427

Appendix B: WHO Growth Charts Head Circumference Boys 493

Appendix C: WHO Growth Charts Head Circumference for Girls 495

Appendix D: WHO Growth Charts Weight for Age Boys 0–5 497

Appendix E: WHO Growth Charts Weight for Age Girls 0–5 499

Appendix F: WHO Growth Charts Weight for Height Boys 2–5 501

Appendix G: WHO Growth Charts Weight for Height Girls 0–5 503

Appendix H: WHO Growth Charts Weight for Length Boys 0–2 505

Appendix I: WHO Growth Charts Weight for Length Girls 0–2 507

Appendix J: Essential Medications for RLS................................ 509

Appendix K: GAPS Monograph... 513

Appendix L: GAPS Periodic Questionnaire 525

Appendix M: WHO Immunization Routine LifeSpan Vaccinations 529

Appendix N: WHO Routine Immunization Children........................ 539

Appendix O: WHO Delayed Routine Immunization 549

Index... 559

Contributors

Theresa S. Betancourt, Sc.D., M.A. Department of Global Health and Population, Francois-Xavier Bagnoud Center for Health and Human Rights, Harvard School of Public Health, Boston, MA, USA

Sarabeth Broder-Fingert, M.D., M.A. Department of Pediatrics, Center for Child and Adolescent Health Research and Policy, Massachusetts General Hospital, Boston, MA, USA

Department of Pediatrics, Harvard Medical School, Boston, MA, USA

Rebecca Cook, M.D., M.Sc. Medicine Department, Harvard University, Boston, MA, USA

MassGeneral Hospital for Children, Boston, MA, USA

Michele S. Duke, M.D. Division of Global Health, MassGeneral Hospital for Children, Boston, MA, USA

Melody J. Eckardt, M.D., M.P.H. Emergency Medicine, Global Health and Human Rights, Obstetrics and Gynecology, Boston Medical Center, Massachusetts General Hospital, Boston, MA, USA

Norman Miles Farr, M.D., M.P.H. Medicine-Pediatrics Department, MassGeneral Hospital for Children, Boston, MA, USA

LeAnne M. Fox, M.D., M.P.H., D.T.M.&H. Division of Parasitic Diseases and Malaria, Center for Global Health, Centers for Disease Control and Prevention, Atlanta, GA, USA

Amanda P. Garcia, M.P.H. Division of Parasitic Diseases and Malaria, Center for Global Health, Centers for Disease Control and Prevention, Atlanta, GA, USA

Mark A. Goldstein, M.D. Division of Adolescent and Young Adult Medicine, MassGeneral Hospital for Children, Harvard Medical School, Boston, MA, USA

Gopal K. Gupta, M.D. Boston Children's Hospital; Harvard Medical School, Boston, MA, USA

Nupur Gupta, M.D., M.P.H. MassGeneral Hospital for Children, Harvard Medical School, Boston, MA, USA

Davidson H. Hamer, M.D. Center for Global Health and Development, Boston University, Boston, MA, USA

Department of International Health, Boston University School of Public Health, Boston, MA, USA

Section of Infectious Diseases, Department of MedicineBoston University School of Medicine, Boston, MA, USA

Zambia Centre for Applied Health Research and Development, Lusaka, Zambia

Andrea J. Hunter, M.D., F.R.C.P.C., F.A.A.P., D.T.M.&H. Division of General Pediatrics, Pediatrics Department, McMaster Children's Hospital, McMaster University, Hamilton, ON, Canada

Jennifer Kasper, M.D., M.P.H. Division of Global Health, MassGeneral Hospital for Children, Boston, MA, USA

Grace J. Kim, D.M.D. Harvard School of Dental Medicine, Boston, MA, USA

Ronald E. Kleinman, M.D. Division of Pediatric Gastroenterology and Nutrition, Department of Paediatrics, MassGeneral Hospital for Children, Boston, MA, USA

Paul J. Krezanoski, M.D. Department of Pediatrics, Massachusetts General Hospital, Boston, MA, USA

Department of Internal Medicine, Massachusetts General Hospital, Boston, MA, USA

Amy C. Lee, M.D., M.P.H. Neurology Department, Palo Alto Medical Foundation, Mountain View, CA, USA

Patrick T. Lee, M.D., D.T.M.&H. General Medicine Division, Medicine Department, Massachusetts General Hospital, Boston, MA, USA

David A. Lyczkowski, M.D. Harvard MGH Medicine-Pediatrics Residency Program Massachusetts General Hospital, Boston, MA, USA

Department of Medicine, Massachusetts General Hospital, Boston, MA, USA

Vandana L. Madhavan, M.D., M.P.H. Pediatric Infectious Disease, MassGeneral Hospital for Children, Boston, MA, USA

Elisa Margolis, M.D., Ph.D. Infectious Disease Division, Pediatrics Department, Seattle Children's Hospital, Seattle, WA, USA

Roseda E. Marshall, M.D., M.P.H., M.A. (Parasitology) University of Liberia, Liberia, West Coast of Africa

Contributors

Michele Nations Martin, D.D.S., D.M.D. Harvard School of Dental Medicine, Boston, MA, USA

Hasan S. Merali, M.D. MassGeneral Hospital for Children, Harvard Medical School, Boston, MA, USA

Sarah Messmer, M.S4. Harvard Medical School, Boston, MA, USA

Peter P. Moschovis, M.D., M.P.H. Division of Pulmonary and Critical Care, Department of Medicine, Massachusetts General Hospital, Boston, MA, USA

Department of Pediatrics, Division of Global Health, Massachusetts General Hospital, Boston, MA, USA

Brett D. Nelson, M.D., M.P.H., D.T.M.&H. Division of Global Health, MassGeneral Hospital for Children, Harvard Medical School, Boston, MA, USA

Aura M. Obando, M.D. Internal Medicine/Pediatrics, Massachusetts General Hospital, Boston, MA, USA

Kristian R. Olson, M.D., M.P.H., D.T.M.&H. Department of Pediatrics, Mass General Center for Global Health, Massachusetts General Hospital, Boston, MA, USA

Internal Medicine, Inpatient Clinician Educator Service, Massachusetts General Hospital, Boston, MA, USA

Archana Patel, M.D., Ph.D., D.N.B. Clinical Epidemiology Unit, Department of Pediatrics, Indira Gandhi Government Medical College, Nagpur, India

Veronica Maria Pimentel, M.D., M.S. Department of Obstetrics and Gynecology, Boston University Medical Center, Boston, MA, USA

Kathleen M. Powis, M.D., M.P.H., M.B.A. Internal Medicine and Pediatrics, Pediatric Global Health, Massachusetts General Hospital, Boston, MA, USA

Department of Immunology and Infectious Diseases, Harvard School of Public Health, Boston, MA, USA

Shamim Qazi, M.B.B.S., M.Sc., M.D. Department of Maternal, Newborn, Child and Adolescent Health, World Health Organization, Geneva, Switzerland

Jyoti Ramakrishna, M.B.B.S., M.D. Division of Global Health, MassGeneral Hospital for Children, Harvard University, Boston, MA, USA

Giuseppe Raviola, M.D., M.P.H Psychiatry Quality Program, Department of Psychiatry, Boston Children's Hospital, Boston, MA, USA

Department of Psychiatry, Harvard Medical School, Boston, MA, USA

Program in Global Mental Health and Social Change, Department of Global Health and Social Medicine, Harvard Medical School, Boston, MA, USA

Jonathan Reisman, M.D. Harvard-MGH Medicine Pediatrics Program, Boston, MA, USA

Nancy Ringel, B.A. Harvard Medical School, Boston, MA, USA

Iyah K. Romm, B.S. Massachusetts Department of Public Health, Bureau of Healthcare Safety and Quality, Boston, MA, USA

Sylvia Veronica Romm, M.D., M.P.H. Department of Pediatrics, MassGeneral Hospital for Children, Boston, MA, USA

Daniel P. Ryan, M.D. Pediatric Surgery Division, Department of Surgery, Massachusetts General Hospital, Boston, MA, USA

Harvard Medical School, Harvard University, Boston, MA, USA

Karen Sadler, M.D. Pediatrics Department, Newton-Wellesley Hospital, Newton, MA, USA

MassGeneral Hospital for Children, Boston, MA, USA

Brittany Seymour, D.D.S., M.P.H. Harvard School of Dental Medicine, Boston, MA, USA

Ashkon Shaahinfar, M.D., M.P.H. Pediatrics Department, MassGeneral Hospital for Children, Boston, MA, USA

Rinn Song, M.D., Dr.Med., M.P.H. Division of Infectious Diseases, Children's Hospital Boston, Boston, MA, USA

Jonathan M. Spector, M.D., M.P.H. Division of Newborn Services, Massachusetts General Hospital, Boston, MA, USA

Pornthep Tanpowpong, M.D., M.P.H. Pediatric Gastroenterology, Hepatology and Nutrition, Department of Pediatrics, Harvard Medical School, MassGeneral Hospital for Children, Boston, MA, USA

Jay Thiagarajah, M.B.B.S., Ph.D. Department of Pediatrics, MassGeneral Hospital for Children, Boston, MA, USA

Matthew Tobey, M.D. Global Primary Care Program, Massachusetts General Hospital, Boston, MA, USA

Julia Elisabeth von Oettingen, M.D. Medicine Department, Pediatric Endocrinology, Boston Children's Hospital, Boston, MA, USA

Ariel Wagner, B.A., M.D./M.M.Sc. (candidate) Harvard Medical School, Boston, MA, USA

Linda T. Wang, M.D. Pediatric Emergency Medicine, Division of Global Health, MassGeneral Hospital for Children, Boston, MA, USA

Harvard Medical School, Harvard University, Boston, MA, USA

A. Kaytee Welsh, M.D. Massachusetts General Hospital, Boston, MA, USA

Elizabeth R. Wolf, M.D., D.T.M.&H. Pediatrics Department, Center for Child Health, Behavior and Development, University of Washington, Seattle, WA, USA

Linda L. Wright, M.D. Eunice Kennedy Shriver National Institute of Child Health and Human Development, National Institutes of Health, Rockville, MD, USA

Global Network for Women's and Children's Health Research, Center for Research for Women and Children, Rockville, MD, USA

Anita K.M. Zaidi, M.B.B.S., S.M. Department of Paediatrics and Child Health, Aga Khan University, Karachi, Pakistan

Part I
Overview of Pediatric Global Health

Chapter 1
Child Mortality in Developing Countries

Norman Miles Farr and Brett D. Nelson

Keywords Child mortality • Neonatal mortality • Infant mortality • Under-five mortality • Millennium Development Goal 4 • Child survival • Child health • Developing countries

Overview

- In recent decades, substantial progress has been made towards improving child health worldwide, including an accelerating rate of decline in under-five mortality.
- Nevertheless, Millennium Development Goal (MDG) 4—to reduce child mortality rate by two-thirds between 1990 and 2015—is the most offtrack of any of the eight MDGs.
- Of the 6.9 million childhood deaths each year, the large majority occur in sub-Saharan Africa and Southern Asia.
- Worldwide, the top five causes of child mortality include pneumonia (18 %), preterm birth complications (14 %), diarrheal illness (11 %), intrapartum-related complications (9 %), and malaria (7 %).
- Simple, cost-effective interventions currently exist to prevent the vast majority of these deaths.

N.M. Farr, M.D., M.P.H. (✉)
Medicine-Pediatrics Department, MassGeneral Hospital for Children,
5th Floor, 175 Cambridge St., Boston, MA 02114, USA
e-mail: nfarr@partners.org

B.D. Nelson, M.D., M.P.H., D.T.M.&H.
Division of Global Health, MassGeneral Hospital for Children, 100 Cambridge St.,
15th Floor, Boston, MA 02114, USA
e-mail: brett.d.nelson@gmail.com

Introduction to Child Mortality

Millennium Development Goal 4 (MDG4) calls for reducing the under-five mortality rate by two-thirds between 1990 (87 per 1,000 live births) and 2015 (29 per 1,000 live births). In recent decades, substantial progress has been made towards improving child health worldwide, including an accelerating rate of decline of under-five mortality (Fig. 1.1). Overall, despite population growth, between 1990 and 2011, the total number of annual under-five deaths was reduced by 4.4 million from 12 to 6.9 million—a 41 % decline in the mortality rate (Table 1.1). Nevertheless, the mortality rate in 2011 remains 51 per 1,000 live births, which is 19,000 under-five deaths per day or 13 under-five deaths per minute, a level not sufficient to meet MDG4 in many countries. Also of significant concern are the remaining health disparities between and within countries. For example, in 2011, the under-five mortality rate in sub-Saharan Africa was 1.8 times higher than in Southern Asia, 5.7 times higher than in Latin America and the Caribbean, 7.4 times higher than in Eastern Asia, and 16.5 times higher than in developed regions. In both high- and low-income countries, children from income-poor and rural households have a disproportionately high mortality rate.

Where Childhood Deaths Are Occurring

There has been an improvement in child survival in every region of the globe, with each developing region seeing at least a net 30 % reduction since 1990. In the period between 1990 and 2011, five of nine developing regions have had a reduction in the child mortality rate by more than 50 %; developed regions had a reduction of 55 % and developing regions by 41 % (Table 1.1). In this same time period, the number

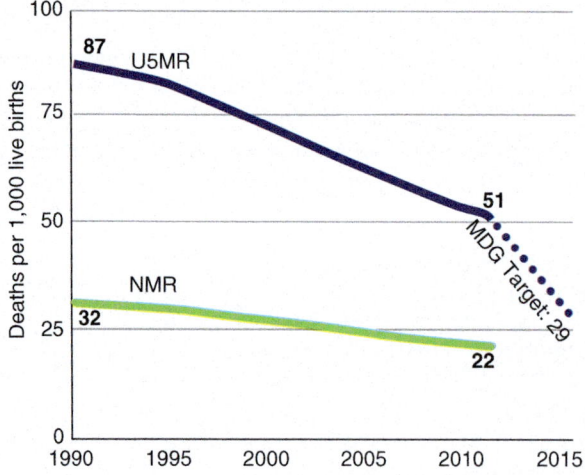

Fig. 1.1 Global under-five mortality rate (U5MR) and neonatal mortality rate (NMR), 1990–2011. (Reproduced with permission from UNICEF's Division of Policy and Strategy. Committing to child survival: a promise renewed progress report 2012. 2012; p. 1–44)

Table 1.1 Levels and trends in under-five mortality

Region	# (000s)			% decline	% of under-five deaths		Under-five mortality rate (per 1,000 births)			MDG target 2015	% decline	Annual % reduction	
	1990	2000	2011	1990–2011	1990	2011	1990	2000	2011		1990–2011	1990–2000	2000–2011
Developed	228	127	96	58	1.9	1.4	15	10	7	5	55	4.2	3.5
Developing	11,740	9,435	6,818	42	98.1	98.6	97	80	57	32	41	1.9	3.1
Northern Africa	284	146	87	69	2.4	1.3	77	45	25	26	68	5.4	5.5
Sub-Saharan Africa	3,821	3,988	3,370	12	31.9	48.7	178	154	109	59	39	1.5	3.1
Latin America and the Caribbean	610	390	203	67	5.1	2.9	53	34	19	18	64	4.4	5.2
Caucasus and Central Asia	152	85	72	52	1.3	1	76	61	42	25	44	2.2	3.3
Eastern Asia	1,325	746	265	80	11.1	3.8	48	35	15	16	70	3.3	7.8
Excluding China	29	30	17	42	0.2	0.2	28	30	17	9	38	−0.7	5
Southern Asia	4,454	3,366	2,341	47	37.2	33.9	116	88	61	39	47	2.8	3.3
Excluding India	1,393	1,010	686	51	11.6	9.9	119	87	60	40	50	3.2	3.4
Southeastern Asia	826	514	312	62	6.9	4.5	69	47	29	23	58	3.9	4.4
Western Asia	255	187	155	39	2.1	2.2	63	42	30	21	52	4.1	3
Oceania	14	15	13	7	0.1	0.2	74	61	50	25	33	1.8	1.9
World	11,968	9,562	6,914	42	100	100	87	73	51	29	41	1.8	3.2

Data from UN Inter-agency Group for Child Mortality Estimation. Levels and trends in child mortality report 2011/2012. 2011;1–24
On track is defined as either less than 40 deaths per 1,000 live births or the annual rate of reduction is at least 4 % over 1990–2011
Green = on track to meet MDG4, *Red* = not on track to meet MDG4

of countries with death rates above 100 per 1,000 live births has been reduced by more than half from 53 to 24. While in 1990 there were 13 countries with a rate above 200 deaths, since 2010, there is no country with a rate above 200 (Fig. 1.2). Despite this across-the-board improvement, a major reason for the limited progress in meeting MDG4 is the increasingly disproportionate share of under-five deaths that occur in sub-Saharan Africa and Southern Asia, which accounted for 83 % of under-five deaths in the world in 2011, up from 67 % in 1990 (Fig. 1.3). Twenty-three of the 24 countries with under-five mortality rates above 100 are in sub-Saharan Africa. Tackling the high mortality rate in sub-Saharan Africa is critical as it is estimated that by 2050 almost a third of all children under five will live in sub-Saharan Africa (Fig. 1.4).

More than 10 % of children in sub-Saharan Africa and over 6 % in South Asia die before the age of 5, compared to approximately 0.5 % in industrialized countries. Five countries—India, Nigeria, Democratic Republic of Congo (DRC), Pakistan, and China—account for about half of under-five mortality (Fig. 1.5). All of these countries, with the exception of the DRC, are populous middle-income countries.

Neonatal and Infant Mortality

In 2011, almost 72 % of children dying under the age of 5 died in the first year of life (37 deaths per 1,000 live births), the majority of those in the first 30 days of life (22 deaths per 1,000 live births). The world has made less progress in reducing neonatal mortality than overall under-five mortality. As a consequence, neonatal deaths account for greater than 43 % of all under-five deaths in 2011, a 17 % rise since 1990. Almost three million newborns died in 2011. There are a similar number of stillbirths each year, with many of these stillbirths being preventable. The distinction between these perinatal deaths and other childhood deaths is especially important as the causes and interventions to combat deaths in the perinatal period are frequently unique relative to general under-five mortality. Additionally, designing effective interventions for the two major perinatal killers—preterm birth complications and intrapartum-related complications—will frequently improve both child and maternal health.

Causes of Childhood Death

Approximately 64 % (4.9 million) of under-five deaths worldwide can be attributed to infectious causes; in Africa, 73 % of under-five deaths are due to infections. Pneumonia (including newborn pneumonia) is the leading cause of under-five deaths (Table 1.2). The second and fourth leading causes of childhood death, which account for one-quarter of childhood deaths, occur at or near the time of birth:

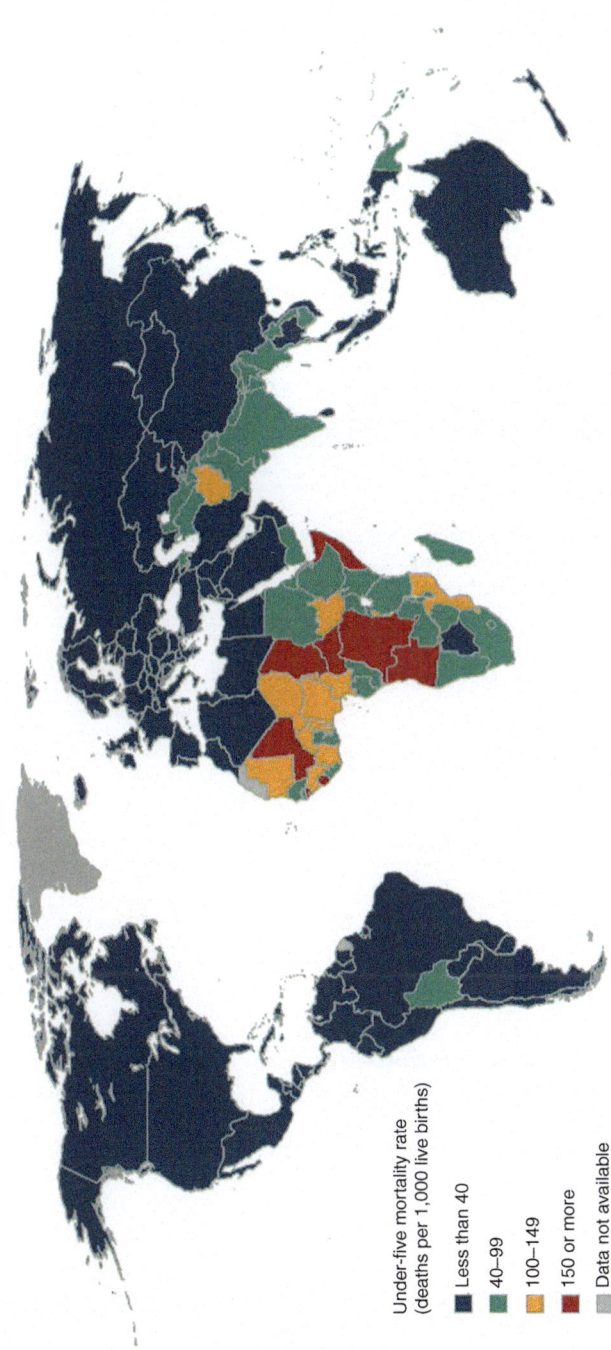

Fig. 1.2 Disproportionate mortality rates affect children in sub-Saharan Africa and Southern Asia. (Reproduced with permission from UN Inter-agency Group for Child Mortality Estimation. Levels and trends in child mortality report 2011/2012. 2011:p. 1–24)

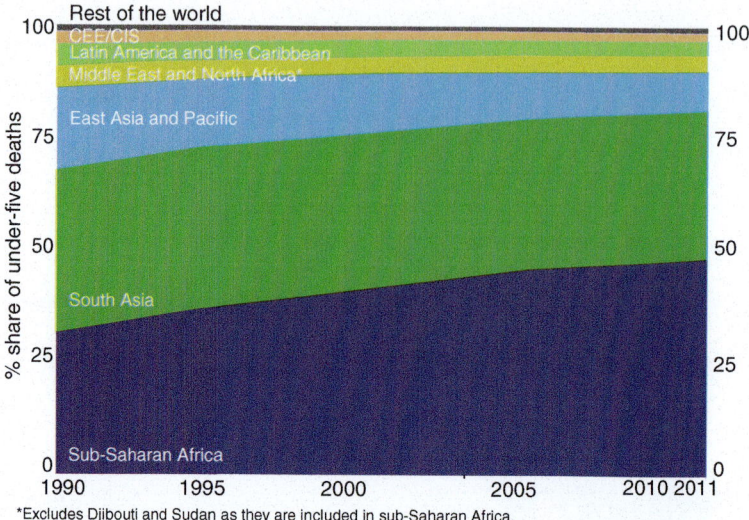

Fig. 1.3 Global burden of under-five death is increasingly concentrated in sub-Saharan Africa and Southern Asia. (Reproduced with permission from UNICEF's Division of Policy and Strategy. Committing to child survival: a promise renewed progress report 2012. 2012;p. 1–44)

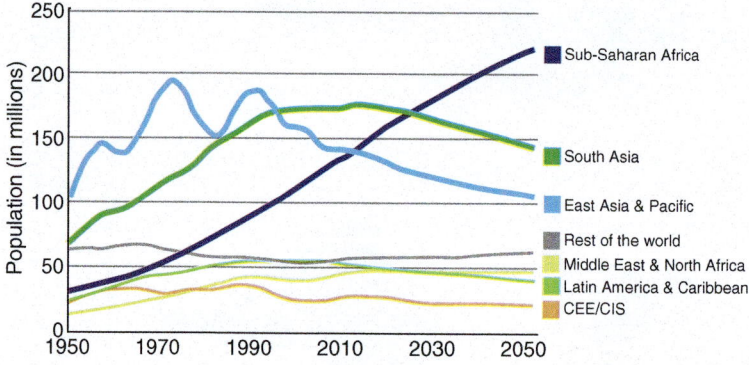

Fig. 1.4 Sub-Saharan Africa under-five population is projected to become the largest in the world, number of under-five by region, 1950–2050. (Reproduced with permission from UNICEF's Division of Policy and Strategy. Committing to child survival: a promise renewed progress report 2012. 2012;p. 1–44)

preterm birth complications and intrapartum-related complications (e.g., birth asphyxia). Malaria remains a leading cause of death and a striking example of disparity; while it is the fifth leading cause of death overall, 96 % (564,000) of total malarial deaths occur in Africa. Undernutrition is thought to contribute to a third of all deaths, while poor sanitation and poor water quality are contributing factors in about a fifth of all deaths. From 2000 to 2010, the total number of under-five deaths

1 Child Mortality in Developing Countries

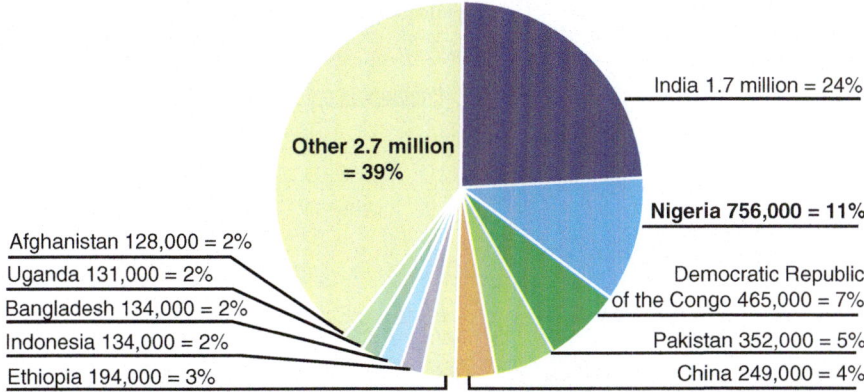

Fig. 1.5 Half of all under-five deaths occur in just five countries. (Reproduced with permission from UNICEF's Division of Policy and Strategy. Committing to child survival: a promise renewed progress report 2012. 2012;p. 1–44)

Table 1.2 Causes of childhood deaths, 2010

Cause	Neonatal (0–27 days)	Children (1–59 months)	Total under-five	% of decline from 2000 to 2010
Pneumonia	325,000 (4 %)	1,071,000 (14 %)	1,396,000 (18 %)	24 %
Preterm birth complications	1,078,000 (14 %)	NA	1,078,000 (14 %)	16 %
Diarrhea	50,000 (1 %)	751,000 (10 %)	801,000 (11 %)	31 %
Intrapartum-related complications	717,000 (9 %)	NA	717,000 (9 %)	19 %
Malaria	NA	564,000 (7 %)	564,000 (7 %)	11 %
Sepsis or meningitis	393,000 (5 %)	180,000 (2 %)	573,000 (7 %)	NA[a]
Injury	NA	354,000 (5 %)	354,000 (5 %)	3 %
Congenital abnormalities	270,000 (4 %)	NA	270,000 (4 %)	5 %
AIDS	NA	159,000 (2 %)	159,000 (2 %)	36 %
Measles	NA	114,000 (1 %)	114,000 (1 %)	76 %
Tetanus	58,000 (1 %)	NA	58,000 (1 %)	NA[a]
Other disorders	181,000 (2 %)	1,356,000 (18 %)	1,537,000 (20 %)	7 %
Total	3,072,000 (40 %)	4,549,000 (60 %)	7,621,000	21 %

Data from The Child Health Epidemiology Reference Group. http://cherg.org/main.html
Red = <20 % decline, *Yellow* = 20–30 % decline, *Green* = >30 % decline
[a]NA—Data on tetanus, sepsis, and meningitis aggregated into one number so that separate categories could not be analyzed

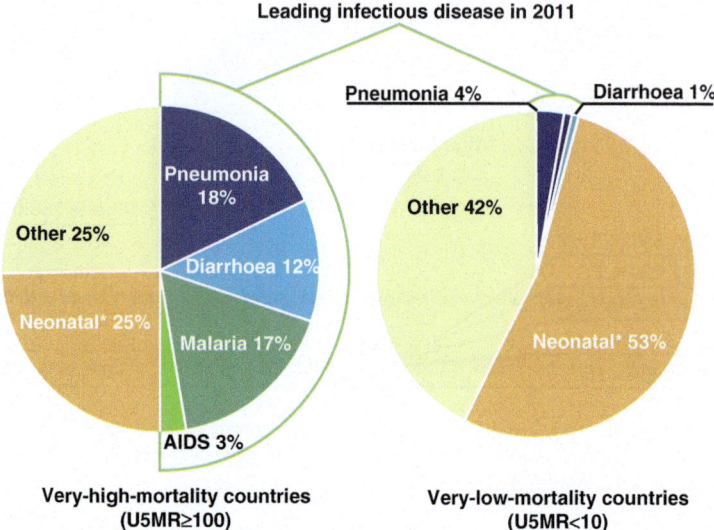

Fig. 1.6 Preventable infectious diseases are still the main causes of under-five deaths in very-high-mortality countries. (Reproduced with permission from UNICEF's Division of Policy and Strategy. Committing to child survival: a promise renewed progress report 2012. 2012;p. 1–44)

decreased by approximately two million (26 % decrease) despite an increase in both the number of births and under-five living children. Approximately 80 % of the reduction is attributable to a reduction in infectious causes—over half coming from the reduction in pneumonia, measles, and diarrhea. Death from preventable infectious diseases disproportionately affects children born in very-high-mortality countries (Fig. 1.6).

Disparities

The mortality rate gap between income-rich and income-poor households continues to rise despite a decrease in the overall under-five mortality rate. Children in the poorest 20 % of households are two times more likely to die before age 5 than those in the richest 20 % of households. Additional significant mortality risk factors include living in a rural area and less maternal education (Fig. 1.7).

1 Child Mortality in Developing Countries

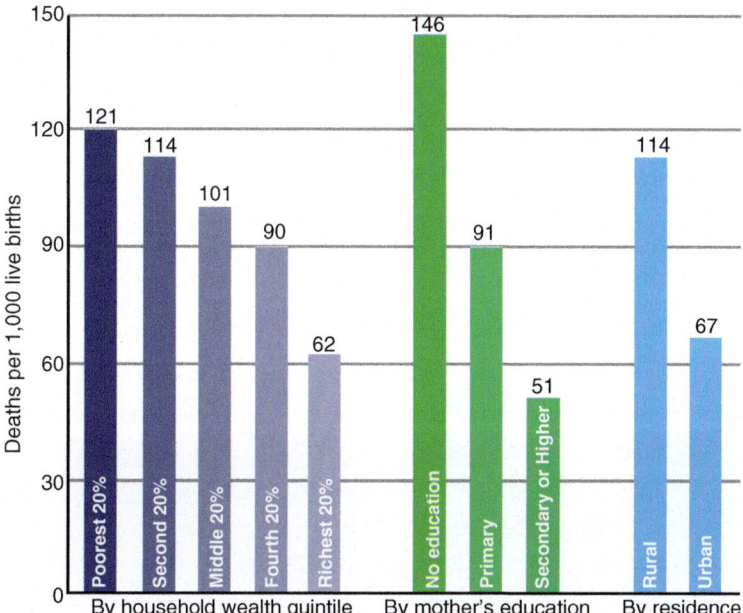

Calculation is based on 39 countries with most recent Demographics and health Surveys (DHS) conducted after 2005 with further analyses by UNCEF for under-five mortality rates by wealth quintile, 40 countries for rates by mother's education and 45 countries for rates by residence. The average was calculated based on weighted under-five mortality rates. Number of births was used as the weight. The country-specific estimates obtained from DHS refer to a ten-year period prior to the survey. Because levels or trends may have changed since then, caution should be used in interpreting these results.

Fig. 1.7 Children who live in poorer households, in rural areas, or whose mother has less education are at a higher risk of dying before age 5. (Reproduced with permission from UNICEF's Division of Policy and Strategy. Committing to child survival: a promise renewed progress report 2012. 2012;p. 1–44)

Survival Improvement

Significant progress has been made in reducing child mortality in the last 20 years. Large disparities still exist in both the mortality rates and causes of childhood deaths between various regions of the world, and the world remains far from achieving MDG4. Nevertheless, there is evidence that additional progress is obtainable even in the hardest hit regions of the world, including sub-Saharan Africa. Low-cost, evidence-based interventions can significantly reduce under-five mortality. Examples of these interventions include childhood vaccination, micronutrient supplementation, oral rehydration solution (ORS), insecticide-treated bed nets, exclusive breastfeeding, and prenatal and antenatal care through community health programs.

In the following chapters, the specific causes of child morbidity and mortality and descriptions of evidence-based, cost-effective interventions for reducing these deaths in resource-limited settings will be discussed in greater detail.

Recommended Reading

1. UN Inter-agency Group for Child Mortality Estimation. Levels and trends in child mortality report 2011/2012. p. 1–24. 2011. http://www.childinfo.org/mortality.html. Accessed 15 Sept 2011.
2. UNICEF's Division of Policy and Strategy. Committing to child survival: a promise renewed progress report 2012. p. 1–44. http://www.apromiserenewed.org/files/APR_Progress_Report_2012_final_web.pdf. Accessed Sep 2012.
3. Liu L, Johnson HL, Cousens S, Perin J, Scott S, Lawn JE, et al. Global, regional, and national causes of child mortality an updated systematic analysis for 2010 with time trends since 2000. Lancet. 2012;379(9832):2151–61.
4. The Child Health Epidemiology Reference Group (CHERG). http://cherg.org/main.html.
5. UNICEF. Millennium development goals: goal4, reduce child mortality. http://www.unicef.org/mdg/childmortality.html.

Chapter 2
Stakeholders and Approaches to Address Pediatric Global Health

Jennifer Kasper and Nancy Ringel

Keywords Global health • Child health • Global pediatrics • Stakeholders • NGOs • Official development assistance • Development • Funding • Aid • IMCI

Overview

- Many factors (e.g., country GDP and debt, human resource constraints, outside stakeholders, international and supranational financial institutions) affect the prioritization, design, and implementation of appropriate child health programs.
- Numerous stakeholders (e.g., multinational and supranational organizations, bilateral aid agencies, international NGOs, individual donors and foundations, financial institutions) play diverse roles in pediatric global health.
- The top three funders of global health are the US President's Emergency Plan for AIDS Relief (PEPFAR), the Bill and Melinda Gates Foundation, and the Organization for Economic Cooperation and Development—Official Development Assistance.
- The Integrated Management of Child Illness (IMCI) is a set of algorithms used by allied health professionals in more than 100 countries to guide diagnosis and treatment of the most common childhood illnesses in resource-limited settings.

J. Kasper, M.D., M.P.H. (✉)
Division of Global Health, MassGeneral Hospital for Children,
100 Cambridge St., 15th Floor, Boston, MA 02114, USA
e-mail: jkasper1@partners.org

N. Ringel, B.A.
Harvard Medical School, Boston, MA, USA

Introduction

Global child health is a complex field. It not only comprises the health care providers, medicines, interventions, health centers, and systems that help deliver essential health services to children around the world; agencies, stakeholders, funders, and global approaches influence how programs and funding translate into service delivery. As a global health practitioner, it is important to have an understanding of this landscape and know some of the factors that affect the selection, prioritization, design, and delivery of child health programs. Just as it is important to investigate the local epidemiology of disease, so too it is important to research which agencies work in a specific country or region or content area of interest.

Factors Affecting Appropriate Delivery of Child Health Programs

Before tackling the details of how stakeholders and approaches affect global child health, it is important to understand factors outside of these agencies and donors that affect the appropriate delivery of child health programs. A country's financial constraints have a significant impact on the success and scalability of programs; it is critical to assess these constraints and implement programs with the local environment in mind. In the 1970s, low-income countries sought loans from the World Bank (WB) and International Monetary Fund (IMF); these loans were predicated on privatizing many social programs (e.g., health, education) as a cost-saving strategy. Many resource-limited countries became heavily burdened by debt from these loans. Debt repayments outweigh their annual export earnings. Since 1980, countries' debts rose 7.4 %, but their economies grew only 1.1 %. In response, in 1996 the WB and IMF instituted the Heavily Indebted Poor Countries (HIPC) Initiative; 39 countries qualified for debt relief based on high poverty rates and unsustainable debt burden, and by 2005 significant amounts of debt were cancelled. Between 2000 and 2010 another 32 countries qualified for loans to pay off debt. Fifteen low- and middle-income countries that don't qualify for debt relief spend more than 10 % of their government budget (and some spend as much as 25 %) on debt relief. By default, these countries have less money to spend on vital social programs like health care and education, water, and sanitation and are unlikely to reach the MDGs.

The World Trade Organization (WTO), founded in 1995, is an important organization that impacts this interplay of global financing and resources for health. Its focus on trade, investment, and deregulation can run counter to public health. It is also a key player in shaping policies that affect health program implementation, as trade regulations not only govern countries' economic situations but also determine the availability of resources (e.g., production of inexpensive generic pharmaceuticals is threatened by trade agreements that argue for patent protections).

The WHO Commission on Macroeconomics and Health determined that countries need to invest a minimum of $34 USD per capita directed at basic health services to reach the health-specific MDGs. Currently, 25 countries spend less than this US$34 minimum, and have significantly worse maternal mortality and under-five mortality rates than countries that spend more than 34 USD. They are headed in the opposite direction from MDGs. This implies that there is a relationship between how much a country invests in health and its ability to achieve targeted outcomes.

Human resource constraints are also an issue, as resource-limited settings often have a disproportionately high disease burden in conjunction with a disproportionately low percentage of the health care workforce. The WHO estimates that countries need a minimum of 23 health care workers (doctors, nurses, and midwives) per 10,000 population to provide adequate primary care and reach Millennium Development Goals 4 and 5. Fifty-seven countries worldwide do not meet this minimum standard, including 32 of the 46 countries in sub-Saharan Africa. Also, when few health care workers are available, they tend to be overworked and have difficulty taking on additional responsibilities. Limited human resources inequitably distributed (i.e., concentrated in urban settings) also means large portions of populations, who typically live in rural areas, may not have access to health care workers at all, which limits the scope and impact of the interventions.

Less predictable issues, such as natural disasters and civil unrest, also play a role in the appropriate delivery of child health programs. When uncontrolled tragedies deplete a region's resources and infrastructure, systems no longer exist to effectively implement health interventions, and existing programs and new strategies suffer when these situations are not properly considered. Currently, there are >40 countries and territories experiencing armed conflicts or civil unrest and >15 countries that have required specific natural disaster-related assistance in the last 15 years. These two issues present unique challenges, and require specialized efforts from international agencies and national governments to address them.

A global health practitioner needs to consider this multitude of factors when designing and implementing global health programs. Agencies and organizations may dictate the terms, but a country's financial and political status may very well determine whether or not these terms will be realistic or successful.

Types of Agencies

There are many types of agencies that contribute to global child health, and they all play very different roles in the effective design and implementation of child health programs. Below we provide definitions of the major types of organizations, along with a summary of their major roles and contributions.

Official Development Assistance

Official Development Assistance (ODA) is not a specific agency, but rather a term describing the sum of contributions that resource-rich countries make to resource-poor countries, with the goal of improving the economic development and welfare

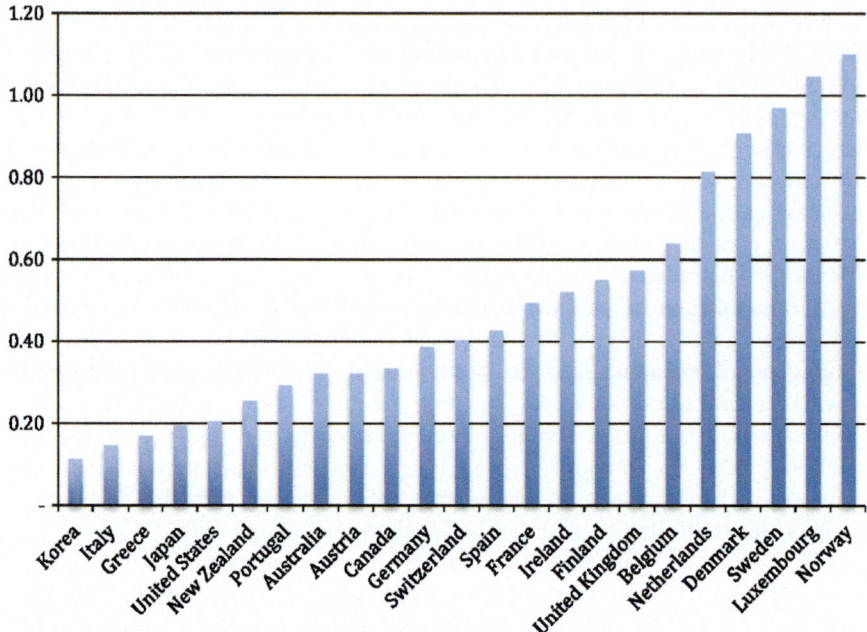

Fig. 2.1 2010 Net official development aid (ODA/GNI) by rich countries to poor countries (goal is 0.7 % GDP)

of developing countries. While these contributions are substantial, almost all rich countries are falling short of contributing 0.7 % of their GDP for ODA emphasized in the UN Millennium Development Goals. Figure 2.1 demonstrates the persistent gap between funding necessary to adequately finance global health and development efforts and the amount of ODA contributed by country.

Multinational Agencies

Multinational and supranational organizations (e.g., the United Nations, the World Health Organization (WHO), the United Nations Children's Fund (UNICEF), and the World Bank) are international groups with globally focused missions who play critical roles in pediatric global health. An important example is the United Nations (UN), which was founded after World War II with a commitment to maintain international peace and security. The UN encompasses agencies such as the WHO, UNICEF, the World Food Program (WFP), and the UN High Commissioner for Refugees (UNHCR), which oversee numerous child health projects worldwide. The UN's mandate is to develop friendly relations among nations and promote social progress, better living standards, and human rights worldwide. While UN agencies are well respected and widely regarded, they operate within a fixed budget made up of required contributions by member countries (based on GDP) and voluntary donations; hence, they lack some of the financial leverage that other major donors possess in driving implementation strategies. Their main functions are to set policies and create guidelines for evidence-based, practical practices for low-resource settings.

Multinational organizations have a stated mission to seek the attainment of all people to the highest possible level of health. While they often set standards and recommendations for methods of health care delivery and practice, they lack power of implementation or enforcement; it is up to individual countries to accept or implement these guidelines as their human, material, financial capacities, political will, and policies allow.

The WHO is the multinational agency most specifically dedicated to health. Some of the major functions of the WHO include the following:

- Assist governments in strengthening health systems and emergency aid
- Promote improvement of nutrition, housing, sanitation, recreation, economy, environment, and working conditions
- Develop international standards regarding diagnostic procedures, biologicals, and pharmaceuticals
- Promote campaigns with specific health goals, e.g., smallpox eradication (1967), the Expanded Program on Immunization (1974), and the Essential Drugs Program (1977)

The World Bank is also an important multinational player, as its financial role in global health and development has rapidly expanded in recent years. The Bank's original mandate was to reconstruct Europe after World War II, but its current mandate emphasizes a focus on development economics. The World Bank became the world's largest external funder of health (US$1 billion) in the mid 1990s, and it still plays a large role in shaping the policies and funding practices of numerous health and development initiatives. The Bank's policies overlap with those of the IMF, and include funding various national and international programs, providing development assistance in the form of grants or loans to countries, and determining countries' qualifications for things like bankruptcy and loan forgiveness.

While the Bank considers itself a democratic organization, the number of votes per member country is determined by the member's financial contribution to the Bank. The US holds the highest percentage of votes of any country, and the "Group of 7/G7" (the US, Japan, Germany, the United Kingdom, France, Canada, and Italy) holds >40 % of votes; sub-Saharan Africa has approximately 7 % of votes. Thus, the largest financial contributors hold the greatest power, and are more likely to vote on policies that directly benefit them. The Bank's role in effectively addressing global health issues is controversial; it has been criticized for supporting projects that worsen a country's economic situation and have detrimental public health effects (e.g., Kariba Dam, Chixoy Dam, Lesotho Highlands Water Project, Nam Theun 2 Dam).

Bilateral Aid and Development Organizations Based in Industrialized Countries

These types of organizations (e.g., the United States Agency for International Development (USAID), the Canadian International Development Agency (CIDA), and the European Commission for Humanitarian Aid Office (ECHO)) operate from within the donor country's government and work directly with local governments or indirectly via consulting agencies, contractors, or international NGOs (discussed below). These agencies offer technical expertise in program development, policy work, monitoring and evaluation, and disease surveillance and control, which can help local governments use funds to effectively implement public health interventions. These organizations are very prevalent in the global health sector, and often support a large proportion of programs and interventions in a region. USAID, with 283 unique projects in nearly 12,000 sites in more than 100 countries around the world, has the largest global presence of any of the bilateral agencies.

International Nongovernmental Organizations (INGOs)

International NGOs (INGOs) are the global equivalent of US nonprofit organizations. INGOs vary in mission, size, scope of work, geographic coverage, and political influence. They are engaged in all aspects of global health, including program design, implementation, direct service delivery, monitoring and evaluation, and capacity-building, although many INGOs have a primary focus on one issue. Some of the most well-known INGOs, grouped by their primary areas of concern, are:

- Amnesty International and Physicians for Human Rights (human rights)
- Oxfam (food security)
- Care and Save the Children (poverty)
- Medicines Sans Frontiers (complex humanitarian emergencies)
- World Vision and Catholic Relief Services (faith-based/missionary)

As INGOs receive their funding from donations and grants, which are obtained based on a combination of reputation and demonstrated results, there is often an unspoken sense of competitiveness among INGOs and groups with similar missions. It is important to recognize this and remember that collaboration and open communication are nonetheless vital for successful program implementation and ultimately positive child health outcomes. In response to the rising number of stakeholders in global health, a coalition of advocacy and service delivery organizations drafted the NGO Code of Conduct; the Code is a set of guidelines for local hiring and capacity-building, minimizing NGO burden and improving coordination with the Ministry of Health, and advocating for policies that support the public health sector. The Paris Declaration on Aid Effectiveness is a set of guidelines focused on donor and recipient country collaboration, alignment of development aid with recipient country's priorities, avoiding duplication of services, and mutual accountability for the donor and recipient country for more effective distribution and use of aid.

Foundations and Businesses

Mega-donors (e.g., Gates Foundation) are relatively new to the global health scene, largely arising within the last two decades; they represent a social phenomenon of some of the world's wealthiest people and companies striving to make positive and charitable contributions to the world. These mega-donors create large foundations, whose investments frequently influence global health priorities and can have a significant impact on health. The result has been an unprecedented rise in available funding for global health interventions. However, many argue that even the presence of mega-donors has not met the full financial need of poorer countries, and debates are ongoing about the best ways to fill the remaining gaps.

Global Financial Assistance

There are multiple funding streams for global health programming, each with specific goals, regulations, and reporting mechanisms. The total and relative contribution of each source of funding and geographic distribution can influence child health priorities, programs, and interventions that may or may not be in proportion to or commensurate with the disease entities that cause the greatest burden of disease in a particular country or region of the world. Table 2.1 illustrates the eight largest funders of global health; all make large contributions to child health specifically.

With this understanding of the different types of agencies and funders involved in global child health the authors will describe how these groups and efforts translate into actionable programs. Below is a brief discussion of some of the major child health programs, and how they have evolved in structure and form over the years.

Major Child Health Programs

As previously discussed, programmatic endeavors to improve global child health have been present for many decades. The formation of the United Nations and WHO marked the beginning of organized global health efforts, but the first concrete, targeted intervention was the campaign for smallpox eradication in the 1970s. This successful program demonstrated that a cooperative global effort could result in widespread, meaningful success, which paved the way for future collaboration towards improved global health. In child health specifically, numerous projects have developed over the years, which have had varying degrees of meaningful success.

The Global Access to Vaccines Initiative (GAVI) is one example of an effective global child health program. It is a public–private partnership to increase access to childhood immunization in 77 low-income countries by cofinancing essential vaccines with recipient countries and supporting implementation of vaccination programs. The use of oral rehydration solution (ORS), a simple solution of water,

Table 2.1 Largest funders of global health

Funding agency	Contribution
President's Emergency Plan for AIDS Relief in Africa (PEPFAR)	US$52 billion (US$15 billion in 2003–2008, US$37 billion in 2009–2013)
Bill and Melinda Gates Foundation	US$39 billion endowment
Organization for Economic Cooperation and Development, Official Development Assistance (OECD ODA)	US$12.4 billion (from 22 countries)
Global Fund to fight AIDS, TB, Malaria	US$11.3 billion
Global Access to Vaccines Initiative (GAVI)	US$5.9 billion ($US3.7 billion pledged by Gates, US$2.2 billion from Governments, NGOs, business)
World Health Organization (WHO)	US$4.2 billion
World Bank	US$2.8 billion
European Union (EU)	US$1.3 billion

salt, and sugar to prevent dehydration and death from diarrheal illnesses, is a low-cost, highly utilized intervention that has reduced deaths. In the realm of programmatic interventions, Helping Babies Breathe, an updated neonatal resuscitation curriculum for resource-limited settings that focuses on rapid assessment and simple but critical interventions to improve survival in the first minutes of life, holds great promise as another cost-effective strategy for reducing neonatal mortality.

While many of these programs have been quite successful, they are largely single interventions that address one aspect of the larger picture of global child health. In recent years, we have been moving towards a broader approach, focusing on health system strengthening rather than vertical interventions.

Integrated Management of Childhood Illnesses

Diagnosing pediatric illnesses in resource-limited settings is fraught with difficulties: most sick children have signs and symptoms associated with more than one illness; a single diagnosis may not be possible or appropriate; there are limited tools at your disposal to assist in diagnosis; and treatment for multiple illnesses can be complex. Also, as many countries worldwide have severe human resource constraints, including insufficient number of pediatricians, allied health professionals (medical officers, nurses, community health workers) provide basic health care.

In response to this reality, in 1996, the Pan American Health Organization (PAHO), WHO, and UNICEF devised the IMCI, guidelines for health care workers who work in the most basic and resource-limited health care settings with high child health burdens. IMCI is a series of algorithms that focus on the most serious child illnesses and serve as a tool to diagnose and treat the most common and serious illnesses that children face.

The IMCI guidelines were developed with the following objectives:

- Reduce mortality of children <5 years of age
- Decrease incidence and/or severity of cases of infectious diseases, especially pneumonia, diarrhea, intestinal parasites, meningitis, tuberculosis, malaria, measles, and nutritional disorders.
- Strengthen health promotion and preventive measures in infancy

The guidelines have been adopted by more than 100 countries and are used as a job aid for health care workers in first-level health settings. IMCI algorithms address the following:

- Clinical practice guidelines for countries that have a high burden of childhood mortality
- Curative and preventive strategies for addressing child health
- Disease prevention and health promotion elements, such as nutrition and immunizations
- Specific illnesses and approaches in infants 0–2 months of age and children 2 months–5 years of age

IMCI addresses these issues with three main components. First, it promotes improvements in the case management skills of health staff through the provision of locally adapted guidelines, and through activities to promote their use. Second, it encourages improvements in health systems required for effective management of childhood illness. Lastly, it endorses improvements in family and community practice. Although IMCI shows great promise in effecting widespread improvements in global child health care, studies have shown that its implementation must take into account the local context and encourage community participation.

See Appendix A for the *WHO Integrated Management of Childhood Illness for High HIV Settings*. If Internet is accessible, other useful WHO guidelines include the *Integrated Management of Childhood Illnesses: Caring for Newborns and Children in the Community* and *Recommendations for Management of Common Childhood Illnesses*.

Global Child Health and the Millennium Development Goals

As children make up one of the world's most vulnerable populations, a concerted and evolving effort to address issues affecting their health and well-being has been a global concern for many decades. From vaccination programs to individual child sponsorship, various parts of the world have engaged in global child health long before more structured efforts gained the visibility and popularity that they enjoy today. However, as global disparities in health care and health outcomes between rich and poor countries have become a greater international focus, the architecture of global child health has evolved from smaller fundraisers to a broader, global effort directed by international bodies and stakeholders. Currently, one of the most important driving forces behind these efforts is the Millennium Development Goals, which are shaping and directing global health efforts across all sectors.

Table 2.2 Millennium development goals

1. Eradicate extreme poverty and hunger
    (a) Halve, between 1990 and 2015, the proportion of people whose income is less than US$1 a day
    (b) Achieve full and productive employment and decent work for all, including women and young people
    (c) Halve, between 1990 and 2015, the proportion of people who suffer from hunger
2. Achieve universal primary education
    (a) Ensure that, by 2015, children everywhere, boys and girls alike, will be able to complete a full course of primary schooling
3. Promote gender equality and empower women
    (a) Eliminate gender disparity in primary and secondary education, preferably by 2005, and in all levels of education no later than 2015
4. Reduce under-five child mortality rate by two-thirds, between 1990 and 2015
5. Improve maternal health by reducing maternal mortality by ¾ and achieve universal access to reproductive services
6. Combat HIV/AIDS, malaria, and other diseases
    (a) Have halted by 2015 and begun to reverse the spread of HIV/AIDS
    (b) Achieve, by 2010, universal access to treatment for HIV/AIDS for all those who need it
    (c) Have halted by 2015 and begun to reverse the incidence of malaria and other major diseases
7. Ensure environmental sustainability
    (a) Integrate the principles of sustainable development into country policies and programs and reverse the loss of environmental resources
    (b) Reduce biodiversity loss, achieving, by 2010, a significant reduction in the rate of loss
    (c) Halve, by 2015, the proportion of the population without sustainable access to safe drinking water and basic sanitation
    (d) By 2020, to have achieved a significant improvement in the lives of at least 100 million slum dwellers
8. Develop a global partnership for development
    (a) Develop further an open, rule-based, predictable, nondiscriminatory trading and financial system
    (b) Address the special needs of least developed countries
    (c) Address the special needs of landlocked developing countries and small island developing states
    (d) Deal comprehensively with the debt problems of developing countries
    (e) In cooperation with pharmaceutical companies, provide access to affordable essential drugs in developing countries
    (f) In cooperation with the private sector, make available benefits of new technologies, especially information and communications

The Millennium Development Goals ("MDGs"), built upon a decade of major United Nations conferences and summits focusing on the need to reduce extreme poverty and alleviate global suffering, are a set of eight international priorities established in September 2000 to address these concerns. By adopting the United Nations Millennium Declaration, world leaders committed their nations to a new global partnership to act on a series of time-bound objectives, with a deadline of 2015. The eight goals are listed in Table 2.2.

Each goal has specific targets that guide concrete actions and measureable outcomes, and have influenced many institutions to create focused efforts towards achieving these goals. Due to the time limit and widespread buy-in of the MDGs, much of the culture of global health (including global child health) has centered on these goals in recent years.

Conclusion

After this review of the various players and approaches in global child health, it will be important to fill in this framework with more details. The subsequent chapters will address specific topics that describe health systems, health care delivery, and best practices in child health.

Recommended Reading

1. US Official Development Assistance Database. http://usoda.eads.usaidallnet.gov/.
2. Fuhrer H. The story of official development assistance. A history of the Development Assistance Committee and the Development Co-operation Directorate in dates, names and figures. Paris: OECD; 1994.
3. Piva P, Dodd R. Where did all the aid go? An in-depth analysis of increased health aid flows over the past 10 years. Bull World Health Organ. 2009;87(12):930–9.
4. Pitt C, Greco G, Powell-Jackson T, Mills A. Countdown to 2015: assessment of official development assistance to maternal, newborn, and child health, 2003–08. Lancet. 2010;376(9751):1485–96.
5. Bryce J, Victora CG, Habicht JP, Black RE, Scherpbier RW. Programmatic pathways to child survival: results of a multi-country evaluation of integrated management of childhood illness. Health Policy Plan. 2005;20 Suppl 1:i5–17.

Chapter 3
Global Health Systems

Matthew Tobey and Patrick T. Lee

Keywords Primary • Health • Care • Global • Systems • International • Engagement • Training

Overview

- Sustainable, ethical engagement begins with careful listening, cultural sensitivity, and responsiveness to local preferences and conditions.
- Few, if any, health systems provide ideal care; there are useful frameworks for improvement.
- Health systems built upon economic, social, public health, and primary care-based interventions at the community level have been the most consistently successful.
- Some outside efforts to buoy health systems have caused harm.
- There is growing access to information on health systems and understanding of routes to successful reform.

M. Tobey, M.D. (✉)
Global Primary Care Program, Massachusetts General Hospital,
86A W. Cedar St., Boston, MA 02114, USA
e-mail: mltobey@partners.org

P.T. Lee, M.D., D.T.M.&H.
General Medicine Division, Medicine Department,
Massachusetts General Hospital, Boston, MA, USA

Introduction

Sociologists have placed health systems—the groups, institutions, and resources devoted to health—into a small group of society's most confounding problems. They are poorly defined, difficult to fully conceptualize, and open to a wide range of interpretations.

Yet engaging with health systems is vital. Much of the world's population suffers from a lack of access to proven health interventions, and many interventions are delivered in inefficient, unsafe, or impoverishing ways. This chapter offers a first look at health systems in a global context, beginning with their common failings. It goes on to introduce several recognized frameworks that may be useful to trainees and practitioners in global health as they explore health systems' problems and seek solutions.

While conceptual frameworks are useful, humble listening, careful attention to local understandings and expectations, and flexibility are the most critical skills when exploring a new health system.

Five Common Health System Failures

Most health systems fail to provide ideal care. Their weaknesses generally lead to five ways in which care for individuals falls short:

Inverse care: When health resources do not reach the people who need them most. Examples include financing systems that do not sufficiently subsidize those with need, or rural populations unable to access care.

Impoverishing care: When health care costs result in significant economic burden. Countries that fail to protect their citizens from catastrophic health costs are vulnerable to this failure. In the United States, medical expenses contribute to more than 60 % of bankruptcies. Worldwide, approximately 100 million individuals are impoverished annually due to the costs of health care.

Fragmented care: When care is inefficient and fractured. For example, systems with insufficient primary care infrastructure or an imbalance of disease-specific initiatives tend to suffer from ineffective care transitions, suboptimal distribution of health workers, and a range of gaps and duplications in care.

Unsafe care: When health system design propagates avoidable errors. This often stems from a lack of investment in quality improvement, poor integration across the spectrum of care, or lack of standardization of care.

Misdirected care: When a system does not target the greatest health needs, leading to inefficiency and waste. For example, 96 % of US health spending is allocated to clinical services despite evidence that 70 % of the disease burden results from social determinants best addressed through public health measures. This "upside-down" biomedical model has been disseminated widely around the world.

Six Building Blocks of a Health System

What constitutes and drives a health system? The WHO describes a framework that includes six building blocks, four reforms, and four desired results (Fig. 3.1):

First, consider the six building blocks:

Service delivery: Selecting which services to provide and how to provide them is a complex task. Establishing a "package of care" defines the outer bounds of the public health system, and drives financing, purchasing, and staffing decisions, among others. In many countries, the package of care described in the national health policy and the set of services actually available are divergent, with a gradient of access and quality that tends to follow—and perpetuate—the social gradient. Yet innovative strategies, often emerging from partnerships between governmental and nongovernmental actors, can help bridge this gap. A notable example is Partners In Health's work in Rwanda, where a community health worker model demonstrated success and became the blueprint for national implementation of similar services.

Health workforce: Building and maintaining a sufficient health workforce may be the toughest global obstacle to ensuring decent health care. The WHO estimates that a health worker density of more than 2.3 workers per 1,000 individuals significantly increases the likelihood of sufficient measles vaccination or skilled birth attendance. Fifty-seven countries, comprising over 2.5 billion people, fall below this basic threshold. Part of the problem is "brain drain," or the migration of nurses and doctors within a country or to richer countries. Well-funded disease-specific initiatives, such as the US-sponsored President's Plan for Emergency AIDS Relief (PEPFAR), have resulted in "internal" brain drain, bolstering local HIV/AIDS care while enfeebling the public health system. Some countries have responded to the problem by developing innovative professional paths; for example a national

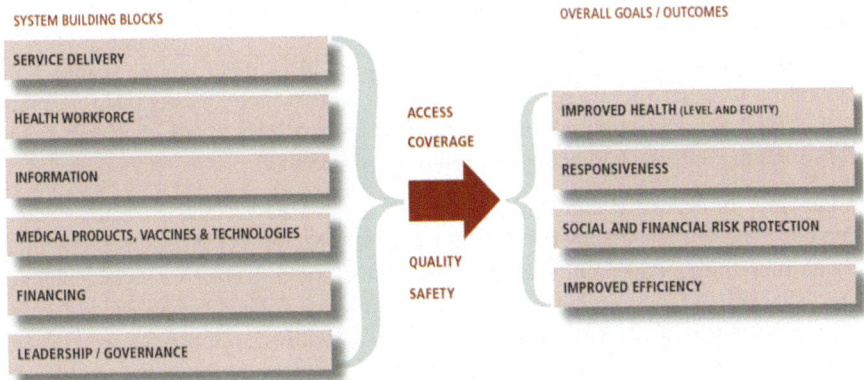

Fig. 3.1 Health system building blocks, reforms, and results. From WHO. Everybody's business. Strengthening health systems to improve health outcomes. 2007. http://www.who.int/healthsystems/strategy/en/. Reprinted with permission

system of mid-level obstetric and orthopedic clinicians in Malawi has helped bring cesarean section and trauma management capacity to far-flung areas of the country. These mid-level providers' certification is recognized within Malawi, but not in other countries, resulting in sustainable workforce development while minimizing brain drain.

Information: Managing the flow of patient and public health data in health systems can help set priorities and make care safer. Many places have far to go: in 60 countries, less than a quarter of deaths are officially reported. This results in a social gradient of health information, leaving much of the disease burden in poorer settings invisible. Given the influence of aggregate statistics, these large blind spots are particularly troubling. In Liberia, for example, WHO massively underestimated the prevalence of severe mental health problems. A subsequent study showed adult prevalence rates of major depression at 40 %, post-traumatic stress disorder at 44 %, and suicidal ideation at 10 %, with 6 % of adults reporting a suicide attempt in the previous year. As a result, Liberia's Minister of Health vetoed a proposal for Liberia's national health policy, insisting that mental health be incorporated as one of the six focus areas. Liberia subsequently formulated a National Mental Health Policy and is training a new cadre of mid-level mental health professionals.

Medical products, vaccines, and technologies: Selecting, purchasing, and ensuring the availability of health products can be challenging. Consider national "essential drug lists." Policy and advocacy initiatives, such as Universities Allied for Essential Medicines, have successfully lobbied for the inclusion of drugs such as generic simvastatin (a lipid-lowering agent) on the WHO Essential Medicines List. This list describes "minimal medicine needs" and "essential medicines for priority diseases." The presence of a medicine on either list opens the door for advocacy to increase access to the medicine.

Countries around the world have added simvastatin to their national essential drug lists, opening the door for improved cardiovascular care. Getting the medicines into the country is only a partial solution: stock outs, irregular delivery to rural areas, and other barriers often arise. Measures to help ensure adequate supply of medical products may involve strengthening basic infrastructure (e.g., roads), collaboration of other sectors (e.g., transportation and finance), and outside partners (e.g., China, which has built thousands of miles of roads in Africa in exchange for construction contracts and access to valuable resources).

Financing: In order for care to be delivered, it must be financed. Health system financing is often plagued by conflicting incentives. Ministries of health and finance have different mandates, cultures, and procedures, making collaboration challenging. The WHO Commission on Macroeconomics and Health estimated that an annual budget of US$40 per person is required to deliver a minimum package of basic health services, but noted that many of the poorest countries in the world only spend US$10 per person per year. Foreign aid, while viewed by many as a humanitarian necessity, is also problematic. Rich countries use aid in many ways, including as a tool to advance economic and strategic interests. Negative unintended consequences have occurred. For example, disease-specific funding on a scale that dwarfs available national health budgets—for example, the President's Plan for Emergency AIDS Relief (PEPFAR) or the Global Fund to fight AIDS, Tuberculosis, and Malaria—has resulted in strong "vertical" care programs alongside struggling public clinics. Patients in these settings have tried to fake HIV status—or even acquired HIV—in order to gain access to life-saving health care. A better approach has been called "diagonal" health financing: addressing the primary sources of disease burden while explicitly investing in the broader health infrastructure and workforce.

Leadership/governance: As addressed in more detail below, effective and transparent leadership can be pivotal in improving and maintaining a well-functioning health system.

A Brief History of "Primary Health Care"

In 1978, the recognition of common health system failures around the world prompted the landmark Declaration of Alma-Ata, affirmed by 134 countries and many International organizations. Alma-Ata declared:

- Health—"a state of complete physical, mental and social wellbeing, and not merely the absence of disease or infirmity"—is a fundamental human right.
- "Primary health care" should be the primary vehicle for achieving health for all by the year 2000.

Alma-Ata's definition of primary health care remains resonant today:
"Practical, scientifically sound and socially acceptable methods and technology made universally accessible through people's full participation and at a cost that the community and country can afford. It is the central function of the health system and its first level of contact, bringing health care as close as possible to where people live and work."

Unfortunately, the aspiration of democratically determined, equitable care that was united with public health measures was lost quickly in the midst of the Cold War and a global oil crisis. The concept became watered down to packages of "best buy" interventions such as GOBI-FFF (growth monitoring, oral rehydration solution, breast feeding, immunizations, family planning, female education, vitamin [food] supplementation) targeting maternal, child, and neonatal health. Thirty years of this fragmented strategy yielded little progress in advancing the promise of health for all.

A Modern Primary Health Care Approach to Health System Strengthening

In 2008, WHO reaffirmed Primary Health Care as the centerpiece of its approach to health system strengthening, advocating four interdependent sets of reforms, described below (Fig. 3.2):

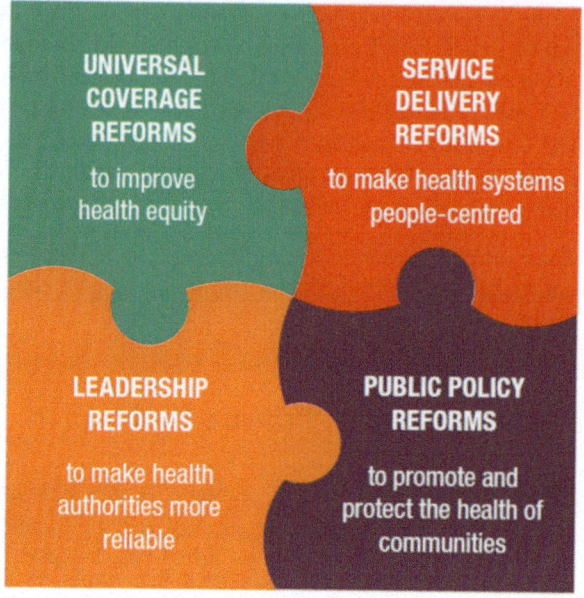

Fig. 3.2 Primary health care: an approach to health systems strengthening. From WHO. World report—primary health care: now more than ever. 2007. http://www.who.int/whr/2008/en/. Reprinted with permission

Universal Coverage Reforms: To Improve Health Equity

Access to care is defined by not only who is insured but also the costs they share and the set of services available to them (Fig. 3.3).

There are other determinants of access to care, including patients' understanding of the disease state; the apparent acuity; the quality of whatever care is available; the alternatives to conventional care (e.g., traditional cures); the direct costs (e.g., copay, transportation costs); and the indirect costs (e.g., lost work time, social stigma) of seeking care.

Examples of universal coverage reforms include the following:

- Mexico, in response to its significant social and health inequalities, in 2006 put forth a national health insurance system that guaranteed a comprehensive set of basic services in primary care, emergency care, and general surgery, greatly increasing the health care available to all of its citizens. The rollout shifted health reimbursement from one driven by political interests to one driven by public enrollment and need. Mexico's reform increased total funding for health to be more in line with international standards, addressed all three dimensions of access illustrated in Fig. 3.3, and prefaced the movement with a constitutional amendment guaranteeing the right to health. It has been hailed as a large success and an international model. One of its champions described three "pillars" of successful policy change: technical (evidence to argue for the change), ethical (to ground the change in moral need), and political (to facilitate its adoption).

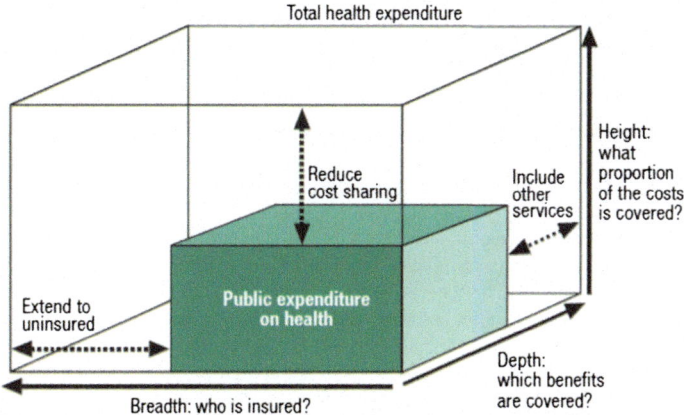

Fig. 3.3 Three dimensions of funding for access to care. From WHO. World report—primary health care: now more than ever. 2007. http://www.who.int/whr/2008/en/. Reprinted with permission

- Alaskan Natives' South Central Foundation is a patient-centered system revolutionary for deep integration of the societal and medical aspects of care. It extended previously inadequate and less-than-universal coverage to isolated rural areas over an area of >100,000 square miles (larger than the United Kingdom). Reliance on innovative uses of health workers and cultivating widespread patient engagement were critical to its success.

Service Delivery Reforms: To Make Health Systems More People Centered

All health systems struggle to optimize service delivery. Such issues are difficult to capture as a whole. These examples illustrate a few common themes:

The United States is struggling under the weight of its cost of care. Iora Health, a small start-up company, has offered one solution. Its community health worker primary care model in New Jersey (made possible through a doubling of the usual investment in primary care) saved 25 % of total health costs while eliminating health disparities between black and white patients after a single year of operation. Iora Health inverts the pyramid of high-acuity, high-cost care and replaces it with a broad base of preventive care, wellness promotion, and patient-centered services.

BRAC, a Bangladeshi nonprofit, has revolutionized its nation's health. For example, by using simple sessions to educate local women, it pioneered a large rollout of oral rehydration therapy in 1980; child mortality decreased more than 50 % nationally. By innovating in microfinance, tuberculosis care, and many other initiatives, it continues as an internationally hailed leader in social and health interventions.

Public Policy Reforms: To Promote and Protect the Health of Communities

Public policy reforms stand to improve the social determinants of health. As mentioned above, these account for a large portion of the burden of disease, and are defined by WHO as:

> The conditions in which people are born, grow, live, work and age, including the health system. These circumstances are shaped by the distribution of money, power and resources at global, national and local levels. The social determinants of health are mostly responsible for health inequities—the unfair and avoidable differences in health status seen within and between countries.

The WHO suggests that reforms focus on:

1. Improving daily living conditions
2. Tackling the inequitable distribution of power, money, and resources
3. Measuring and understanding socioeconomic problems and assessing the impact of action

A popular refrain is "all Ministers should be Health Ministers," since health is implicated in all decisions affecting the distribution of power, money, and resources.

Leadership Reforms: To Make Health Authorities More Reliable

Deregulation of health care has been seen as detrimental to health systems: deregulation worsened health outcomes in China in the 1980s; and the largely privatized system in the United States is plagued by high-cost care. Effective national leadership involves fair engagement of stakeholders, focus on meaningful reform, and the maintenance of the health data network necessary to make a case for change. In developing nations, lobbying for funding of local priorities and infrastructure is an essential function of government. Whereas a rigid hierarchy describes many Ministries of Health around the world, the WHO advocates for an evolution toward more egalitarian learning organizations that are able to respond promptly and flexibly to changing needs and conditions.

Ethical Engagement

It is the duty of all international trainees to engage ethically. We advocate three basic behavioral guidelines:

- Devote oneself to listening and observation above all else.
- Explore the local understanding of health and the expectations that surround it.

- Actively investigate the expectations of local groups regarding one's personal and professional behavior, and apologize in advance for shortcomings.

We offer these as suggestions for professional work:

- Only set expectations that are certain to be met.
- Recognize that solutions in one setting will work differently in another, and must be tailored to local needs and preferences.
- Engage stakeholders at all levels, with a focus on the community.

Conclusion

Health systems are dynamic, complex, and fraught with challenges. Trainees and practitioners, whether working in health systems overseas or actively engaged in health system strengthening overseas, should empower themselves with accepted frameworks and best practice examples, and engage with humility and tact.

Recommended Reading

1. WHO. World health report 2008: primary health care: now more than ever. http://www.who.int/whr/2008/en/.
2. WHO. Everybody's business: strengthening health systems to improve health outcomes. http://www.who.int/healthsystems/strategy/everybodys_business.pdf.
3. WHO. Global health observatory data repository. http://apps.who.int/ghodata/?vid=18900&theme=country.
4. Lee PT, et al. The Massachusetts general hospital global primary care curriculum. https://hub.partners.org/globalprimarycare/Programs/Curriculum.
5. The Institute for Healthcare Improvement. Knowledge center. http://www.ihi.org/knowledge/Pages/default.aspx.

Chapter 4
Vulnerability of Children in Developing Countries and Disrupted Settings

Sylvia Veronica Romm, Iyah K. Romm, and Brett D. Nelson

Keywords Child abuse prevention • Child development • Vulnerable populations • Hypervulnerable populations • Hunger • Poverty • Psychological stress

Overview

- Children are among the most vulnerable populations in developing countries.
- In adverse circumstances, children often are likely to have increased morbidity and mortality relative to adults.
- Early identification of vulnerable children has been demonstrated to significantly improve child health and psychosocial outcomes.
- Integrating multiple aspects of a child's environment into a security and protection model further enhances outcomes.
- One framework that addresses security and protection for children holistically is the SAFE model: *S*afety/protection; *A*ccess to health care and basic physiological needs; *F*amily/connection to others; and *E*ducation/livelihoods.

S.V. Romm, M.D., M.P.H. (✉)
Pediatrics Department, MassGeneral Hospital for Children,
5 Vinal Ave., #1, Somerville, Boston, MA 02143, USA
e-mail: svromm@partners.org

I.K. Romm, B.S.
Massachusetts Department of Public Health, Bureau of Healthcare Safety
and Quality, Boston, MA, USA

B.D. Nelson, M.D., M.P.H., D.T.M.&H.
Division of Global Health, MassGeneral Hospital for Children, 100 Cambridge St.,
15th Floor, Boston, MA 02114, USA
e-mail: brett.d.nelson@gmail.com

Introduction

Children are among the most vulnerable populations in developing countries. Due to both physiologic and environmental fragility, children are disproportionately affected by poverty, malnutrition, disease, and conflict. In disaster settings, young people have disproportionately high morbidity and mortality. As many more life years are at risk in children than adults, disease burden as measured through disability-adjusted life years (DALYs) and quality-adjusted life years (QALYs) is also substantially higher.

Children's vulnerability primarily stems from the co-occurring challenges of being young and lacking influence in society. Children are dependent on older persons for their economic and physical security, including food and shelter. As children are physiologically and psychologically immature, they are more susceptible to physical and mental damage. Finally, inherent power imbalances between adults and children found in many cultures, such as those where children are viewed as property, confer a dynamic in which the health and survival of youth is not the first priority. Instead, in cultures where children are treated and traded as goods and services, youth lack the autonomy and resources to make decisions in their own best interests.

Protective programs that identify and engage vulnerable children significantly improve their long-term outcomes for health and well-being. These interventions are most effective when centered in a framework that simultaneously addresses the diverse key drivers of wellness, including safety and protection, health, family engagement, education, and employment.

Burden of Child Vulnerability Worldwide and Reasons for Increased Vulnerability in Humanitarian Crisis Settings

At baseline, in developing countries, infants and children have increased morbidity and mortality relative to adults. Each year, more than 6.9 million children under the age of 5 die (the under 5 mortality rate—U5MR). Deprivation of children's rights and protections results in higher rates of mortality and decreased developmental outcomes. In fact, child mortality and malnutrition are nearly double among poor populations than among the rich. In every country worldwide, and across demographic groups, infants and children are abused, exploited, neglected, discriminated against, and victims of interpersonal violence. The true burden of this vulnerability is underreported.

Disasters greatly increase child vulnerability to neglect, abuse, exploitation, and trafficking. Armed conflict, other humanitarian crises, and displacement are not only responsible directly for mortality but also have widespread indirect and long-lasting impacts on health. Crisis increases vulnerability to communicable and non-communicable diseases, fosters malnutrition due to limited access to clean water and insufficient food supplies, and results in disrupted infrastructure (e.g., housing, schools, medical facilities), as well as limited access to health care and educational services. Displacement, disrupted social structures, interruption of parental livelihoods, and fragmented family systems increase vulnerability to abuse, abduction, and exploitation through loss of security. Interruption of education and livelihoods has rippling effects across generations. Without sufficient cognitive ability, developmental maturity, and social support to process these complex experiences, children suffer lifelong negative mental health effects from being witness to the horrors of conflict or natural disaster.

Children have higher mortality than adults in conflict settings. More than one billion children live in areas affected by conflict and other disasters each year. Since 1990, more than 3.6 million people have been killed in conflict worldwide, and at any given moment there are approximately 30–40 open armed conflicts. More than 45 % of the casualties in these conflicts are children, of whom 200,000 have been killed and 600,000 wounded as armed combatants. The average U5MR in conflict-affected countries is 81 per 1,000 live births, significantly higher than the global average of 51 deaths per 1,000 live births. Over six million children are in forced/bonded labor, one million in slavery, two million in prostitution and pornography, with 600,000 more involved in drug trafficking. Many more suffer from sexual violence, exploitation, and lifelong psychological trauma. Many become refugees or internally displaced persons (IDPs), of whom 70–80 % are women and children. Meanwhile, according to UNICEF, there are an estimated 210 million children worldwide who are orphans.

The children who survive a crisis are vulnerable to being in situations that put their health and well-being at peril. Children suffer disproportionately from impoverishment, medical and psychosocial issues, malnourishment, lack of family cohesion, personal insecurity, and geopolitical disruption. A recent Rand study describes a significantly increased risk of diarrheal illness, fever, and acute respiratory illness in the first month after a natural disaster. Disaster can have lasting health impacts, such as growth stunting and malnutrition. One study showed that exposure to a disaster in the past year reduced height-for-age and weight-for-age z-scores by 0.12–0.15 standard deviations. Moreover, a recent disaster reduced preventative health significantly, with an 18 % reduced likelihood of having received age-appropriate immunizations. Among Kurdish refugees at the Turkey–Iraq border in 1991, for example, U5MR represented 63 % of all deaths, even though these children only represented 18 % of the total population. Of all Rwandan and Burundian refugee deaths in the Democratic Republic of Congo in 1996, 54 % of deaths were in this age group. Consistently, the highest mortality rates in refugee and IDP populations were the U5MR. During the 1992 famine in Somalia, the U5MR was 74 % in IDP camps. In post-earthquake El Salvador, children with the highest exposure to disaster were 5.3 % less likely to be enrolled in school. In Mexico, natural disasters were shown to result in a regression on the Human Development Index by 2 years, and to increase poverty by up to 3.6 %.

Hypervulnerability

In settings of great need and limited response capacity, the global health community can stratify relief efforts by directing additional resources towards populations with greatest vulnerability, the hypervulnerable. The specific definition of vulnerability and hypervulnerability is situation specific and varies with population demographics and the sociopolitical environment. Illustrative categories of vulnerability, examples of specific vulnerable populations, and situations in which populations may become compromised to the point of hypervulnerability are given in Table 4.1.

Distinguishing between these vulnerable populations and hypervulnerable populations is not simply an academic exercise; hypervulnerability requires different planning and managing than vulnerability. Recognizing the existence of hypervulnerable populations, then, is a critical step in allowing the global health community to develop aligned philosophies, strategies, and priorities. Clearly defining the hypervulnerable in each setting can help guide effective programming, and giving priority to the most vulnerable can lead to cost-effective allocation of limited resources. Although such definitions do not encompass all those that require aid, identifying hypervulnerable populations facilitates communication and enhances focused coordination of relief efforts towards those with critical and uniquely complex needs. Adequately addressing the needs of the hypervulnerable should not compromise efforts directed towards the general pediatric population.

Practical Steps to Ensure Protection for Vulnerable Children

Each resource-limited setting and humanitarian crisis is a unique confluence of societal, cultural, structural, and environmental factors. Having a toolkit to ensure that the clinical services or public health programming you are developing and/or delivering address the integrated, complex needs of the children you are serving is essential. In creating or adopting your toolkit, you should use an evidence-based framework to ensure accounting for all of the potential needs of your patients. The SAFE model is a rights-based theoretical framework for examining key domains of children's security.

SAFE, and its applied tool, the SAFE Child Impact Assessment (SCIA), has been field-tested in India, Rwanda, and Haiti. The SCIA was developed to evaluate integrated systems of care, associated social structures, and protections for children and their families to ensure that the integrated needs of children are met.

While no standardized tools yet exist for implementation of the SAFE model across settings, clinicians should consider the following factors, adapted from Betancourt et al. (2012), when developing setting-appropriate interventions for addressing the needs of children.

Table 4.1 Illustrative categories of vulnerability and sample populations

Social stigma and discrimination	Lack of capital resources	Lack of political voice	Low health status	Limited self-sufficiency
Survivors of sexual and gender-based violence (SGBV)	Impoverished individuals	Women and children	Acutely ill	Children or elderly
Individuals living with HIV/AIDS	Unemployed	Ethnic minorities	Chronically ill	Physically or developmentally disabled
Lesbian, gay, bisexual, and transgender (LGBT)	Land tenure	Prisoners	Terminally ill	Child-headed households
Hypervulnerable populations (multiple, synergistic vulnerabilities)				
Female survivors of SGBV in non-supportive cultures	Children born of sexual violence in conflict settings	Child soldiers (poverty, limited self-sufficiency, and psychological trauma)	Unaccompanied minors and separated children in the setting of natural disasters	

Dimension 1: Safety/protection

- *Assess the risk of sexual abuse and exploitation, including sexually transmitted infections, regardless of age*
- *Assess exposure to and risk of physical violence*
- *Assess exposure to armed conflict (active participants in war, regional violence, gang violence)*
- *Assess exposure to and risk of hazardous child labor or other forms of enforced servitude*
- *Assess potential social stigmas, including but not limited to LGBT, SGBV, children of SGBV, discrimination against ethnic minorities, etc.*
- *Assess exposure to environmental hazards (unsafe roads, toxins, landmines)*
- *Assess access to trusted individuals who can provide care/protection (law enforcement, security guard, friends)*

Dimension 2: Access to health care and basic physiological needs

- *Assess access to nutritious food and history of hunger/malnutrition*
- *Assess access to affordable health care services (including immunization status), including physical, mental, reproductive, and sexual health*
- *Assess access to clean drinking water and sanitation*
- *Assess access to services for individuals with disabilities*
- *Assess access to services for substance abuse (drug and alcohol addiction)*
- *History of substance abuse, exposure to violence/conflict, presence of grief and loss, etc.*

Dimension 3: Family/connection to others

- *Assess the presence (or absence) of caregivers, the home environment, and existing familial relationships*
- *Assess the quality of institutional life/care where pertinent*
- *Assess the incidence and factors surrounding child-headed households, including access to resources under all domains*
- *Assess the status of street and/or abandoned children*

Dimension 4: Education/economic security

- *Assess access to early intervention services, as well as capacity of caregivers to provide appropriate early childhood engagement*
- *Assess history of and/or access to affordable primary and secondary education*
- *Assess head of household's economic and employment status*

Conclusions

In crises and indeed in noncrisis settings in many developing countries, the identification of vulnerable and hypervulnerable youth should not simply serve as a tool of acute response. The identification of these populations must be complemented by holistic, integrated approaches that fundamentally enhance the structures of basic security and health that are needed to mitigate the existence of child vulnerability and hypervulnerability. Societal recovery from humanitarian crises cannot happen overnight, but individual patients need not suffer disproportionately from problems that are amenable to intervention.

Screening for vulnerability and hypervulnerability should be integrated into all clinical encounters and global health initiatives. Once these populations are identified, appropriate responses to the most vulnerable individuals and communities should be developed as a core tenet of any global health initiative. Many of the complex challenges faced by individual patients in these settings can be addressed by an integrated approach that supports their social and health care needs. A focus on the hypervulnerable may be a nexus of focused, high-yield intervention. However, all global health clinicians engaged in program development or health care provision should consider the multifactorial needs of their patients, and apply screening tools guided by integrated models such as SAFE, to enhance the health of the children receiving their services.

Recommended Reading

1. Betancourt TS, Williams TP, Kellner SE, Gebre-Medhin J, Hann K, Kayiteshonga Y. Interrelatedness of child health, protection and well-being: an application of the SAFE model in Rwanda. Soc Sci Med. 2012;74(10):1504–11.
2. Datar A, Liu J, Linnemayr S, Stecher C. The impact of natural disasters on child health and investments in rural India. Rand Working Paper WR-886. 2011.
3. Moss W, Ramakrishnan M, Storms D, Siegle AH, Weiss WM, Lejnev I, Muhe L. Child health in complex emergencies. Bull World Health Organ. 2006;84:58–64.
4. Tamashiro T. Impact of conflict on children's health and disability. Education for all global monitoring report. 2010.
5. Tarazona M, Gallegos J. Recent trends in disaster impacts on child welfare and development 1999–2009. UNICEF. 2010.

Chapter 5
Fundamentals of Pediatric Care in Resource-Limited Settings

Julia Elisabeth von Oettingen, Roseda E. Marshall, and Jennifer Kasper

Keywords Global child health • Pediatrics resource-limited setting • Well child visit • Pediatric evaluation • Emergency pediatric care • Pediatric diagnostics • Pediatric treatment • Pediatric ultrasound • Microscopy resource-limited setting

Overview

- The health of any pediatric patient is strongly influenced by their family and home environment, socioeconomic status, cultural practices, disease epidemiology, and availability of medical resources.
- Lay medical personnel and mid-level providers play an important role in global pediatric care.
- Globally, medical providers must be familiar with the environment they work in, aware of resources available to them, and prepared for lack thereof. Setting-appropriate approaches to diagnosis and treatment must be used.

J.E. von Oettingen, M.D.
Medicine Department, Pediatric Endocrinology,
Boston Children's Hospital, Boston, MA, USA
e-mail: julia.v.oettingen@gmail.com

R.E. Marshall, M.D., M.P.H., M.A. (Parasitology) (✉)
University of Liberia, 1000 Monrovia, 10, PO Box 1061, Liberia, West Coast of Africa
e-mail: roseda.marshall@gmail.com

J. Kasper, M.D., M.P.H.
Division of Global Health, MassGeneral Hospital for Children,
100 Cambridge St., 15th Floor, Boston, MA 02114, USA
e-mail: jkasper1@partners.org

- The well child assessment is a major component of pediatric preventive care and includes regular developmental assessments, routine screenings, and immunizations.
- Priorities of emergency pediatric care focus on recognition of emergency and priority signs, stabilization of the child's airway, breathing, and maintenance of circulation. Caution should be paid to alter the approach to fluid resuscitation in any child with severe malnutrition.

General Considerations in Resource-Poor Settings

Developing countries struggle with extremely limited financial resources, lack of health care infrastructure, a significant shortage of health care providers, and limited opportunities for medical training. Lack of access to care frequently affects the most vulnerable population, children.

Whether a local clinic or a tertiary referral center, the medical provider must be familiar with limitations in medical resources and should be aware of the resulting unique ethical dilemmas they may face. In addition to local disease epidemiology, the patient's culture, local customs, and psychosocial environment influence approach and management.

Patient, Family, and Their Country

Children are often brought to health care facilities late in the course of their illness or with complications. Home remedies or native herbs given by a local healer have frequently been tried, or patients may have been partially treated for common diseases (e.g., malaria). Coupled with challenges in communication (e.g., language barriers or cultural misconceptions), the underlying problem may be challenging to uncover. In many instances, someone other than the mother or the father may bring the child to the health facility, thereby leading to erratic or nonexistent histories. Interpreters or local colleagues who can help with interpretation and understanding the local cultures will be invaluable to the expatriate working abroad. Ingenuity coupled with sound medical knowledge is a valuable tool in these situations.

Combining the Practical with Evidence-Based Medicine

Medical providers are faced with major limitations in resource-poor settings. Lack of ancillary tests (e.g., laboratory, imaging), unavailability of treatments (e.g., medications, procedures, surgery), or absence of specialty providers are amongst the daily challenges.

Often, the best clinical judgment must be relied on. For example, treating meningitis with chloramphenicol and penicillin instead of ceftriaxone may represent the best balance between drug availability, practicality, and clinical benefit. When deciding about whether or not to continue a treatment instituted by a local healer, it may be most beneficial to promote those treatments that are helpful, acknowledge those that neither help nor harm, and strongly discourage those that harm.

Simple medical equipment is frequently lacking and what might be considered outdated or not standard of care in the Western world might be life-saving in a resource-limited area. Urethra catheters for collection of sterile urine are usually unavailable, whereas suprapubic bladder aspiration using a 22- or 23-G needle may be available and, thus, the local standard.

Subspecialty care is often not available. Many clinics and hospitals have one skilled health care worker who may or may not be a physician. Textbooks and other resources can be scarce. However, as new technology is rapidly spreading to developing countries, mobile devices and the Internet are more commonly used resources, and e-mail consults have emerged as innovative ways to establish remote access to subspecialists.

For the medical provider, it is thus important to be familiar with the local availability of medical equipment, laboratory tests, imaging facilities, and surgical procedures, and to be prepared for creative approaches to diagnosis and treatment. It is helpful to seek out the local providers and learn local practices from them.

Health Care Workers

The number of doctors in many developing countries is greatly insufficient to meet the medical need of the populace; hence, a variety of other skilled and unskilled health care providers fill this gap. Nurses are frequently the primary and only medical providers. In addition to medical expertise, they usually have excellent knowledge of the local culture, practices, and remedies, as well as availability of medications, equipment, and other resources. Their role often exceeds that of a nurse in developed countries.

Paramedical practitioners (depending on the setting also referred to as medical officers, clinical officers, or physician assistants) provide medical services in a more limited scope, but frequently work autonomously with varying degrees of supervision by medical doctors. They frequently employ local treatment protocols (in many cases based on the World Health Organization's (WHO) Integrated Management of Childhood Illness (IMCI)) as guidelines for diagnosis and treatment.

Unskilled health care workers (i.e., lay people from the community who received minimal, if any, formal medical training) are frequently encountered in resource-limited settings. Examples include community health workers (also known as health promoters, village health workers, health volunteers, community aides) and traditional birth attendants (TBAs, also known as community or lay midwives).

They can be valuable members of the health care workforce and are often the first responders available to the community. A variety of models of community health care have been studied in developing countries and have demonstrated high success rates using lay workers for basic health supervision, vaccination, supervised drug administration, and care of patients with chronic conditions. In some settings, use of TBAs has contributed to important reductions in perinatal and neonatal deaths but, unfortunately, has not significantly reduced maternal mortality.

In most developing countries, demands on physicians are broad and may frequently exceed their training. Learning from them while offering targeted training that meets their requests and needs is often a mutually beneficial approach. Most academic centers' educational needs relate to specialty and subspecialty care. A health care worker—from the village health worker to the physician—must consider himself or herself a teacher at all times, teaching the parent, the child, and the coworker—but also learning from them in return. Care should be taken to familiarize oneself with the specific roles of each provider group in any given setting.

Assessment of the Well Child in Resource-Limited Settings

Well child assessment is a key component of basic pediatric primary care; however, it is frequently overlooked because of the overwhelming burden of acutely sick children.

History

In general, a complete history—including birth history, past medical history, review of systems, and psychosocial history—should be obtained at each well child visit.
Birth history should focus on the following:

- Mother's prenatal history including gravida/para status and age and cause of death of any previous children, prenatal screens (if any), complications, and/or medications during pregnancy.
- Place of delivery (home or health facility); what level of healthcare provider attended the delivery, if any; and complications during labor.
- Whether vitamin K, antibiotic eye ointment, and any vaccines were given at birth.

A feeding history in infancy is crucial in settings where death from malnutrition and diarrheal and respiratory illnesses is common and should include:

- Breast milk vs. formula, length of breastfeeding, and introduction of liquids and solids.
- Drinking water source and foods eaten.
- Ages of other children (spacing).

Psychosocial Health

Especially in low-income countries, living conditions such as the type of housing (material), location, and number of family members living in the household should be assessed. Inquire about parental age, education and work, and marital status and whether parents are living together. Depending on the setting and cultural practices, the primary caregiver may be distinct from the parents (e.g., grandmother, other family member, family friend). School attendance and performance should be assessed at least yearly.

Immunization history should be obtained. The parent may have an immunization card, or there may be physical exam findings such as an upper arm scar from BCG vaccine or a dark discoloration of the fifth fingernail marked as a sign of polio vaccine receipt. Providers should be familiar with the WHO and the locally recommended vaccine schedules. The WHO vaccination schedule is available in the appendix.

Developmental Assessment

Age-appropriate developmental milestones (Table 5.1) should be assessed at every visit and appropriate referrals made when available. Due to higher rates of hypoxic ischemic birth injury, cerebral palsy is a significant problem.

Physical Exam

Next to the history, the physical examination is usually the most important piece of information that the provider can obtain. The following should always be part of the complete examination:

1. Anthropometric measurements.
    - Height, weight, body mass index (BMI).
        - Plot on WHO growth charts and compare to standard deviation (SD) tables (see Appendix 2–9).
    - Mid-upper arm circumference (MUAC): Use a flexible tape and measure the upper arm circumference at a point half way between the shoulder and the elbow.
        - Use for children 6–59 months.
        - <11.5 cm = severe malnutrition.

Table 5.1 Major milestones in infants and toddlers

Age	Motor	Verbal	Social	Red Flags
2 months	Lifts head and shoulders while prone	Coos	Social smile	Lack of visual attention or fixation
4–5 months	Good head control, starts to roll over	Squeals and laughs ("ah-goo")	Imitates social interaction	Lack of visual tracking, lack of steady head control
6–7 months	Sits independently	Babbles	Feeds self finger food	Failure to turn to voice/sound
9–10 months	Crawls, pulls to stand	Mama/dada nonspecific	Stranger anxiety	Inability to sit. No babbling
12–15 months	Takes first steps	1–5 specific words	Initiates play	Inability to walk independently, no words
2 years	Walks well, kicks ball	Two-word sentences, ½ speech intelligible, 50 words	Parallel play, follows two-step command	No phrases
3 years	Runs, alternates steps when walking stairs	Three-word sentences, ¾ speech intelligible, 250 words	Group play, shares toy	Not speaking in three-word sentences, unintelligible speech

2. Routine assessment
   - Complete physical examination of all systems
3. Specific examination helpful in resource-limited settings
   - Anemia:
     - Conjunctival pallor
     - Palmar/plantar pallor (compare child's palms and soles to the parents')
     - Tachycardia, soft systolic ejection murmur/flow murmur
   - Malnutrition:
     - Severe wasting (marasmus) or edema and puffiness (kwashiorkor).
     - Brittle hair that falls out easily when stroking the head.
     - Rusty brown discoloration of the hair (in African children).
     - Bitot spots (conjunctival xerosis), sign of vitamin A deficiency.
     - Skin hypo- or hyperpigmentation, desquamation, ulceration.

- Hydration status:
  - Dry lips and mucous membranes
  - Sunken eyes
  - Tenting of the skin

Routine Screenings

Laboratory	Malaria smear or rapid diagnostic test (RDT) and hemoglobin at age 6 and 12 months
Vision	Clinical assessment at all visits; Snellen chart (E) at age 4 years (see Appendix)
Hearing	Clinical exam at all visits, assess by observing behavioral responses to sound:
	0–4 months — Startles
	9–12 months — Localization to sound in any plane
	15–18 months — Can point to an unexpected sound, person, or thing when asked
	24 months — Can point to body parts (tied to educational level of parents)
	48 months — Can use Play Audiometry (hearing test with playful methods where child is conditioned to place toy in a container when hearing a sound)

Anticipatory Guidance

Vaccine visits are a great opportunity to provide anticipatory guidance.

Every visit	Growth evaluation, developmental assessment, vaccines as indicated, mosquito net use reminder
Birth	Cord care, sleeping position, exclusive breastfeeding (EBF), family planning
2 months	EBF support, symptoms of acute illnesses, sleeping position
4 months	EBF support, infant stimulation techniques (IST, Table 5.2)
6 months	Introducing mixed solids (nutritional counseling, use local food), IST, hygiene
9 months	Accident prevention (AP), trauma, ingestion
12 months	Nutrition, IST, hygiene, AP, prevention of common diseases
18 months	IST, AP
2 years	Nutrition, hygiene, AP
3 years	Preschool readiness, prevention of common illnesses

Table 5.2 Infant stimulation techniques

	Newborn	1–6 months	6–9 months	9–12 months	12–24 months
Play	Provide ways for baby to see, hear, move arms and legs freely, and touch you. Gently soothe, stroke, hold child	In addition to newborn stimulation, slowly move colorful things for baby to see and reach for (e.g., rattle, big ring on string)	Give child clean, safe household things to handle, bang, and drop (e.g., container with lid, metal pot, and spoon)	Hide child's favorite toy under cloth/box and see if the child finds it. Play peek-a-boo	Give child things to stack up and to put into containers and take back out
Communicate	Look into baby's eyes and talk to him or her. A newborn sees your face and hears your voice	Smile and laugh with child. Talk to child. Get a conversation going by copying child's sounds or gestures	Respond to child's sounds and interests. Call child's name and see your child respond	Tell child names of things and people. Show child how to say things with hands (bye bye)	Ask child simple questions. Respond to his or her attempts to talk. Show and talk about nature, pictures, and things

Data from World Health Organization. Integrating Early Childhood Development (ECD) activities into Nutrition Programmes in Emergencies. Why, What and How. Recommendations for Care for Child Development. http://www.who.int/mental_health/emergencies/ecd_note.pdf

WHO Essential Drug List

The WHO essential drug lists for both adults and children, currently in their 17th and 3rd editions, respectively, are what most countries use for prescribing medications. The lists can be found online at http://www.who.int/medicines/publications/essentialmedicines/en/. They each comprises a core list and a complementary list—the former focusing on the "most efficacious, safe, and cost-effective medicines for priority conditions," whereas the latter expands to "medicines for priority diseases, for which specialized diagnostic, or monitoring facilities and/or specialist medical care and/or specialist training are needed." It is crucial to be familiar with the local drug list, which may vary frequently based on financial limitations, drug donations, and storage capacity, amongst others. See Appendix 10.

Assessment of the Sick Child in Resource-Limited Settings

Triage

Triaging is a vital skill to evaluate a child who is ill and rapidly decompensating. The younger the child, the higher the risk of rapid decompensation, morbidity, and mortality. Triage should begin with a rapid general assessment of the child's vital signs (Table 5.3). The WHO has defined *emergency signs* that need to be recognized and treated immediately (and possibly referred to higher level of care) and *priority signs* that should lead to rapid assessment and treatment.

WHO Danger Signs (Treat Immediately)

- *Airway and Breathing*: Obstructed breathing, central cyanosis, severe respiratory distress
- *Circulation*: Cold hands with capillary refill >3 s, weak and fast pulse
- *Coma or Convulsion*
- *Severe Dehydration*: Diarrhea with lethargy, sunken eyes, and/or slow skin pinch

WHO Priority Signs (Assess Rapidly and Treat)

- Infant <2 months
- High fever
- Trauma or other urgent surgical conditions

Table 5.3 Normal range of pediatric vital signs

Age	HR	BP	RR
Premature	120–170	55–75/35–45	40–70
0–3 months	100–150	68–85/45–55	35–55
3–6 months	90–120	70–90/50–65	30–45
6–12 months	80–120	80–100/55–65	25–40
1–3 years	70–110	90–105/55–70	20–30
3–6 years	65–110	95–110/60–75	20–25
6–12 years	60–95	100–120/60–75	14–22
>12 years	55–85	110–135/65–85	12–18

- Severe pallor
- History of poisoning
- Severe pain
- Respiratory distress
- Restlessness, continuous irritability, or lethargy
- Urgent referral from another health facility
- Malnutrition: Visible severe wasting
- Edema of both feet
- Major burns

History

A thorough medical history, especially in settings where few diagnostic tools are available, is crucial in helping to make a correct diagnosis. The specifics of each setting—language, level of education, cultural norms, and traditional medical practices—strongly influence how questions on history are perceived and answered. Taking an accurate history can be challenging, and cross-cultural sensitivity and local knowledge are indispensable. It is useful to be familiar with the common local treatments (herbs or drugs) for common illnesses and to learn the local terms for body parts, for describing certain illnesses, and for common diseases in the area.

Questions specific to tropical/communicable/infectious diseases include the following:

- Sick contacts
- Use of bed nets and whether they are chemically impregnated
- Living conditions (e.g., housing, near open water sources)
- Mother's health, including symptoms suggestive of HIV/AIDS or death of unknown cause

Questions particularly relevant in resource-limited settings include the following:

- Detailed feeding history, including details on breastfeeding (exclusive vs. partial)
- Access to food for the family and the child
- History of previous treatment by local healer, priest, or other lay person
- History of ingestion of herbs or other medicines, including antibiotics

Management of the Sick Child in Resource-Limited Settings

Many children in resource-limited settings arrive ill or in critical condition on first evaluation. Providers and patients benefit from a clear approach to medical management. The WHO has developed IMCI guidelines, which can be used in any setting for an organized, well-structured approach to the sick child. The goal of IMCI is to triage effectively, provide prompt attention to the most critically ill young patients, and deliver an integrated approach to all children undergoing evaluation.

The IMCI structured approach is outlined below. For each specific symptom and management plan, refer to the respective chapters in this book.

I. ASSESS
  1. Check for general danger signs:
     a. If present, child needs urgent attention and immediate treatment
  2. Ask about main symptoms:
     a. Does the child have cough or difficulty breathing?
     b. Does the child have diarrhea?
     c. Does the child have fever?
     d. Does the child have an ear problem?
  3. Check for malnutrition and anemia.
  4. Check the child's immunization status.
  5. Assess other problems.

II. CLASSIFY
  1. Classify the child condition according to findings on assessment: red = urgent/severely ill, yellow = moderately ill, or green = mildly ill.

III. TREAT
  1. Provide treatment, guided by the color-coded category.

IV. FOLLOW-UP
  1. Arrange for follow-up as indicated by the child's condition and treatment plan. Guidelines for major conditions and diagnoses are provided in the IMCI manual.

V. COUNSEL
  1. Provide illness-appropriate counseling to the mother and/or primary guardian. These are outlined for common problems and conditions in the IMCI manual.

Diagnostic Evaluation of the Sick Child in Resource-Limited Settings

Laboratory Investigations

Availability of laboratory testing is highly variable, and some tests may be unavailable. Bedside tests, rapid diagnostic tests, and microscopy are commonly used and can be very helpful ancillary tools if performed with the appropriate reagents and controls.

Table 5.4 Rapid diagnostic tests

	Test method	Sensitivity	Specificity	Example
Malaria[a]	Parasite antigen detection of one or more plasmodium species	Can reach >95 %	Often low, 40–70 %	Paracheck
HIV[b]	ELISA based, detects HIV antibodies	99–100 %	98–100 %	HIV ½ StatPak
Hepatitis B[c]	Agglutination or lateral-flow based, detects qualitative HBsAg	100 %	98–100 %	EQUIPAR HBsAg One Test
Hepatitis C[d]	Immunochromatography, immunofiltration, particle agglutination, or ELISA for qualitative detection of HCV Ab	98–100 %	80–100 % (SeroCard: 98–100 %)	SeroCard HCV
Tuberculosis[e]	Nucleic amplification assay under global rollout (likely available 2013–2015)	Uncertain	Uncertain	Xpert MTB/RIF

[a]WHO Malaria treatment guidelines recommend RDT or microscopy before initiating treatment for malaria
[b]http://www.who.int/diagnostics_laboratory/publications/Report16_final.pdf
[c]http://www.who.int/diagnostics_laboratory/evaluations/en/hep_B_rep2.pdf
[d]http://www.who.int/diagnostics_laboratory/evaluations/en/hcv_rep1.pdf
[e]http://www.who.int/tb/laboratory/mtbrifrollout/en/index.html

Bedside tests may include hemoglobin, HgbA1C, glucose, PPD and rapid diagnostic tests (RDT). Rapid diagnostic tests can be obtained at the bedside via pricking the finger for whole blood. Most RDT take less than 15 minutes to obtain a result. RDTs for malaria, HIV, and Hepatitis B and C are widely commercially available. See table 5.4 for more information on these RDTs.

Initial Diagnosis, Stabilization, and Treatment

Airway/Breathing

1. Upper airway obstruction

    a. *Foreign body*

- *Child ≤1 year*: Lay infant over arm or thigh head down and give five blows to the back with the heel of hand
- *Child ≥1 year*: Give five blows to the child's back with child sitting, kneeling, or lying. If unsuccessful, perform Heimlich maneuver

b. *Infection (croup)*

- *Mild*: Administer cool mist, hydration, and antipyretics, and give dexamethasone 0.6 mg/kg PO or IM × 1 (alternative: prednisolone 1–2 mg/kg)
- *Moderate–severe*: If stridor at rest, give racemic epinephrine (2.25 %) 0.05 ml/kg/dose in 3 ml NS (max 0.5 ml) every 15 min up to three times. Administer mist or humidified oxygen close to child's face. Give dexamethasone 0.6 mg/kg PO or IM

c. *Epiglottitis*

- If highly suspected, requires immediate intubation in controlled environment if possible. If unable to intubate, bag-mask ventilation with high pressures (may need to remove valve)
- Avoid manipulating child, administer oxygen as tolerated
- If moderately suspected, obtain lateral neck X-ray (look for thumbprint sign)
- Start antibiotic therapy (e.g., ceftriaxone 50 mg/kg) to cover *H. influenzae*, *S. pneumoniae*, Group A Strep

2. Lower airway obstruction

   a. *Asthma*

- Administer oxygen
- Give albuterol (also known as Salbutamol) (2.5 mg)/Ipratropium (0.5 mg) via nebulizer if available, repeat ×3
- If no nebulizer available, can use metered dose inhaler (MDI) with spacer 2-4 puffs as often as every 20 minutes depending on the severity of respiratory distress. An MDI can be made using a 500ml plastic bottle: cut a hole on the bottom of the bottle to hold the MDI and use the original bottle opening as the mouth piece
- Consider systemic steroids for moderate–severe exacerbations: Prednisone or Prednisolone 1–2 mg/kg/day divided twice daily (max dose 60 mg)
- Further options for severe asthma or if no response to initial nebulizers:
  - Continuous albuterol at 10–20 mg/h
  - SQ Epinephrine: 0.01 ml/kg of 1:1,000 dilution ×1, repeat PRN
  - Aminophylline: 6 mg/kg IV load, then 0.6–1.5 mg/kg/h
  - Magnesium: 25–75 mg/kg IV (max 2 g) ×1, repeat PRN
  - Terbutaline: 10 mcg/kg IV load, then 0.1–10 mcg/kg/min (Table 5.5)

  Albulterol, SQ Epinephrine, Aminophyllline, Magnesium, Terbutaline and their doses: Patients who require this level of medical intervention should be monitored very closely, preferably in a tertiary care setting

Circulation

There are specific clinical entities that result in unique derangements in circulation, blood volume and perfusion of vital organs and lead to shock. These require urgent management and resuscitation to avoid death. They are described in detail in Table 5.5.

Table 5.5 Circulation/shock

Type of shock	History	Exam	Management
Hypovolemic	Diarrhea, vomiting, inability to drink, blood loss, polyuria	HR↑, SVR↑ Dry lips and mucous membranes, sunken eyes, reduced skin turgor, cool extremities	Place IV (or IO or central line if needed) Bolus with NS: 20 ml/kg, repeat ×3 If blood loss give 15–20 ml/kg PRBC CAREFUL in severe malnutrition: – Give 10 % dextrose 5 ml/kg FIRST – THEN give 5 % dextrose in LR or ½ NS 15 ml/kg over 1 h
Septic	Infection, high fever	HR↑, SVR↓ Warm to touch, warm extremities, flash capillary refill	Place IV (or IO or central line if needed) Bolus with NS 20 ml/kg, repeat ×3 Start antibiotics promptly Start vasopressive therapy if needed and available (need central access for this) – Dopamine 5–15 mcg/kg/min – Norepinephrine 0.05–1 mcg/kg/min – Epinephrine (adrenaline) 0.1–0.5 mcg/kg/min
Cardiogenic	Previous symptoms of heart failure, congenital heart disease, course suggestive of rheumatic heart disease, endocarditis, pericardial effusion	HR↑, SVR↑ Murmur, muffled heart sounds (if effusion present), respiratory distress, hepatomegaly, elevated JVP, edema, cold extremities	Rule out pulmonary edema before giving volume If possible, obtain echocardiogram and consult with cardiologist (although rarely available) If effusion present, perform pericardiocentesis Begin inotrope therapy (rarely available) – Dobutamine 2–40 mcg/kg/min – Milrinone 50–75 mcg/kg IV load, then 0.5–0.75 mcg/kg/min – Epinephrine 0.1–0.5 mcg/kg/min
Anaphylactic	History of exposure to antigen, concurrent rash, wheeze, vomiting/diarrhea	HR↑, SVR↓ Warm to touch, angioedema, urticarial rash, wheezing, warm extremities	Epinephrine 0.01 ml/kg of 1:1,000 dilution IM ×1, repeat PRN Place IV (or IO or central line if needed) Bolus with NS 20 ml/kg, repeat ×3

HR heart rate, *SVR* systemic vascular resistance, *JVP* jugular venous pressure

Seizure, Unconsciousness, or Coma

The differential diagnosis of seizures, unconsciousness, and coma needs to be broad in most resource-limited settings (Table 5.6). Symptomatic treatment should be prompt, and investigation of the underlying etiology should follow.

Symptomatic treatment should include the following:

- Administer oxygen, and apply jaw thrust as necessary to maintain an open airway.
- Place patient on the side to reduce aspiration risk.

Seizures (active) should be treated as follows:

- Antiepileptic therapy in children <1 month
    - Phenobarbital 15–20 mg/kg IV/IM, can repeat in 30 min PRN. Then start maintenance at 3–5 mg/kg/24 h divided once or twice daily
- Antiepileptic therapy in children >1 month
    - First line: Lorazepam 0.05–0.1 mg/kg IV ×1, repeat ×1 PRN
    - Diazepam 0.2–0.5 mg/kg PR, IV, or IM ×1, repeat ×1 PRN
    - Fosphenytoin or phenytoin 20 mg/kg IV ×1 (max 1,250 mg)
    - Phenobarbital 10–20 mg/kg IV ×1 (max 300 mg)

Dehydration and Fluid Management

For any child who is dehydrated but not in shock, rehydration orally or via nasogastric tube is preferable to parenteral hydration whenever possible. Fluid management is divided into two phases: acute resuscitation/fluid replacement and maintenance fluids. But in order to determine what amount of fluid should be given in the acute resuscitation phase, one must estimate the degree of dehydration. Clinicians tend to overestimate the degree of dehydration, which can be especially harmful in severely malnourished children who need much slower rehydration to avoid cardiovascular compromise. Table 5.7 is a useful tool for estimating the degree of dehydration.

Recipes for oral rehydration solution (ORS):

Both non-malnourished and malnourished children with mild dehydration should be rehydrated using oral rehydration solution (ORS). If the WHO pre-packaged oral rehydration powder is unavailable for oral/nasogastric rehydration, one of the following two recipes are equally effective:

Recipe using household ingredients: 1 L water + 6 heaped teaspoons of sugar + 1 heaped teaspoon of salt. Banana and fruit juice can be added for taste and to provide extra potassium.

Recipe using cereal: 50 g of cereal (maize, millet, sorghum, or rice cereal) boiled in 1 L water for 6–7 min + 1 heaped teaspoon of salt. Banana and fruit juice can be added for taste and to provide extra potassium.

Table 5.6 Common causes of seizure, unconsciousness, or coma and management

Etiology	Suggestive history	Management
Infection		
Meningitis	High fevers, irritability, stiff neck, in young infants bulging fontanelle, vomiting, petechial rash (meningococcemia)	Obtain malaria test to rule out cerebral malaria, consider treating empirically for malaria CSF cell count, protein, glucose, CSF culture, CBC, and blood culture Administer broad-spectrum antibiotics as soon as possible Neonate <2 kg: – Ampicillin 50 mg/kg every 12 h + Gentamicin 3 mg/kg/24–48 h Neonate >2 kg: – Ampicillin 100 mg/kg every 12 h + Gentamicin 4 mg/kg/24–48 h Child: – Ceftriaxone: 100 mg/kg IV/IM every 24 h OR – Chloramphenicol 25 mg/kg IV/IM every 6 h + ampicillin 50 mg/kg IV/IM every 6 h OR + benzyl-penicillin 60 mg/kg IV/IM every 6 h *Treat for 14–21 days depending on lab results or clinical judgment, but gentamicin for only 5–7 days
Encephalitis	Low-grade fevers, upper respiratory infection symptoms, previous gastroenteritis	Supportive care If herpes encephalitis is suspected: – Acyclovir: 20 mg/kg IV every 8 h
Cerebral malaria	Endemic area for *P. falciparum*, jaundice, anemia, respiratory distress, diarrhea, high fevers	Obtain malaria blood smear Obtain blood glucose to rule out hypoglycemia; if unavailable, treat empirically with 5 ml/kg of dextrose 10 %, repeat PRN Treat with locally recommended antimalarials Consider treating empirically for bacterial meningitis
Neurocysticercosis	Afebrile, often seizure is the only symptom	Manage with anticonvulsive therapy DO NOT treat active disease, as inflammatory response may be lethal Consider praziquantel or albendazole for inactive or mild CNS disease

Neonatal tetanus	Age 3–14 days, inability to breast-feed, trismus, muscle spasm, characteristic opisthotonus, seizures	Tetanus immune globulin (TIG) IM 500–6,000 U (debated) and metronidazole 30 mg/kg/day PO or IV × 10–14 days. Equine tetanus antitoxin or IVIG (200–400 mg/kg) are alternatives if TIG is not available. Penicillin 100,000 U/kg/day is an alternative antibiotic. Non-pharmacologic: Appropriate wound cleaning/debridement. Adequate pain control and sedation as needed. Low-light and low-stimuli environment. Ventilatory support may be required
Febrile seizure	Prior episode of seizure with fever, regains consciousness, age 6 months–6 years, malaria smear negative	Rule out malaria (with smear or RDT) Observation
Noninfectious		
Hypoglycemia	Malnutrition, severe malaria	Obtain bedside glucose in all seizing or unconscious children. If low, treat with 5 ml/kg of 10 % dextrose IV, repeat blood sugar 15–30 min later, repeat dextrose dose PRN. If no glucometer available, treat empirically if suspicious
Hypoxic-ischemic injury	Neonate, first 3 days of life, history of complicated delivery	Anticonvulsive therapy with phenobarbital
Intracranial hemorrhage	History of trauma, or premature infant in first 3 days of life	Ultrasound if fontanelle is open CT scan if available Treat with anticonvulsant if >1 seizure
Diabetic ketoacidosis (DKA)	Polyuria, polydipsia, weight loss. Urinating despite dehydration. Respiratory distress but clear lungs	Obtain blood glucose level, urine ketones Obtain serum electrolytes and venous blood gas if available Treat according to DKA guidelines
Poisoning	History of poison ingestion or medication overdose	If possible, treat with antidote Activated charcoal 1 g/kg PO or via nasogastric tube
Electrolyte abnormalities	History of free water intake with gastroenteritis, iatrogenic, diuretic therapy	Measure serum electrolytes and correct as indicated

Table 5.7 Estimation of dehydration

Degree of dehydration	Percent loss of body weight (%)	Signs and symptoms
Mild	<5	Awake, alert
Moderate	5–10	Restless, irritable, sunken eyes, dry lips, tacky mucous membranes, drinks eagerly, thirsty, reduced skin turgor
Severe	>10	Lethargic, unconscious, sunken eyes, dry mucous membranes, unable to drink or drinks poorly, significantly reduced skin turgor

Non-malnourished Child

1. Moderate dehydration:

- Oral rehydration with ORS, approximately 20 ml/kg/h × 4 h
- Frequent small sips should be given from a cup or a syringe
- If breastfeeding, continue ad lib
- Give an extra 50–100 ml for each loose stool
- If the child vomits, wait for 10 min before restarting
- Once hydration status is improved, instruct offering extra fluids as needed

2. Severe dehydration:

- Place IV, IO, or central line. If unable to obtain IV, place nasogastric tube
- Give 20 ml/kg NS or LR IV over 1 h if < 12 months, over 30 min if >12 months, and more rapidly if hemodynamically unstable or hydration status not improving (assess every 15–30 min). Continue with 80 ml/kg over 5 h (<12 months) or over 2.5 h (>12 months)
- If nasogastric tube was placed, give 20 ml/kg of ORS, and slow down if abdomen gets distended or if repeatedly vomiting
- Give ORS 5 ml/kg/h PO as soon as the child can drink
- After 4–6 h, reassess hydration status, and continue rehydration as per moderate or severe dehydration guidelines

Malnourished Child

DO NOT use IV fluids for rehydration except in case of shock. WHO ReSoMal rehydration solution is more appropriate than ORS as the latter has high sodium but low potassium content, which is suboptimal for malnourished children.

ReSoMal is prepared in the following way: 2L water + 1 packet ORS + 50 g sucrose + 40ml electrolyte/mineral solution, or, if unavailable, use 45ml of KCL solution (i.e. 100g KCL in 1L water).

Moderate or severe dehydration

- Give 5 ml/kg of ReSoMal every 30 min for the first two hours.
- Give 5–10 ml/kg/h for the following for hours 3–10
- Introduce F-75 formula at hours 6 and 10 at the same volume if rehydration is still ongoing at that time

Maintenance Fluids

Once the acute phase of rehydration is complete, maintenance fluids should be calculated as follows:

- 4 ml/kg/h for the first 10 kg body weight
- 2 ml/kg/h for the subsequent 10 kg body weight
- 1 ml/kg/h for every kg thereafter

Examples: A 5 kg infant requires $5 \times 4 = 20$ ml/h. A 12 kg infant requires $10 \times 4 + 2 \times 2 = 44$ ml/h. A 25 kg child requires $10 \times 4 + 10 \times 2 + 5 \times 1 = 65$ ml/h.

If a child is unable to tolerate PO or nasogastric tube fluid resuscitation, then the best forms of fluid delivery are in the following list in order of preference (see Table 5.8 for instructions on how to give subcutaneous or intraosseous fluids):

1. *Intravenous*.
2. *Intraosseous*: Use same bolus and maintenance fluids as for IV fluids.
3. *Subcutanous* (or hypodermoclysis): Use intermittent normal saline (NS) or lactated Ringer's (LR) boluses of 20 ml/kg (maximum hourly, or use several sites), and repeat until rehydrated or vascular access is obtainable. Do not use hypo- or hypertonic fluids.
4. *Rectal* (or proctoclysis): Administer NS, LR, or tap water in 20 ml/kg boluses.
5. *Intraperitoneal*: Obtain intraperitoneal access using a 23-G needle. Administer NS or LR fluid boluses directly into the peritoneal cavity.

Helpful Procedures, Microscopy, and Imaging

Following is a list of procedures that can be extremely helpful in any setting, but particularly in resource-limited areas. It is recommended to be familiar with these procedures prior to arrival.

Microscopy

Learning techniques of simple slide preparation can be useful, especially in situations where little laboratory testing is available. See appendix for slide preparation instructions.

Table 5.8 Procedures

Intramuscular (IM) injection
- Site: Lateral thigh, deltoid muscle
- Needle: 23–25 G
- Technique: Hold skin between thumb and index finger of one hand, insert needle at 45° (thigh) or at 90° (deltoid) into muscle. Draw back, if no blood → inject, if blood → withdraw and try again. Briefly hold pressure with clean cotton/gauze

Subcutaneous (SQ) injection
- Site: Thighs, upper arm, abdomen
- Needle: 23–25 G
- Technique: Similar to IM injection, always insert needle at 45°, do not penetrate muscular tissue

Intradermal (ID) injection
- Site: Any, for PPD usually left volar forearm
- Needle: 25 G
- Technique: Stretch skin over insertion site with two fingers. Insert needle by 2 mm bevel up, close to skin surface. Slowly inject; you should feel resistance and see a blanching bullae develop within the dermis

Intraosseus (IO) access
- Site: Proximal tibial tubercle (antero-medial surface), distal femur (2 cm above lateral condyle)
- Needle: IO or bone marrow needle, if unavailable use 18- or 21-G needle
- Technique: Attach needle to 5 ml empty syringe. Position leg in 30° knee flexion, stabilize leg with free hand but DO NOT place hand under calf to hold (avoid penetration injury). Insert needle in 90° angle, apply steady pressure while twisting needle until you feel a sudden decrease in resistance. You should see bone marrow (thick red fluid) upon drawing back. Secure needle. Attach syringe for injection or tubing for infusion

UVC insertion

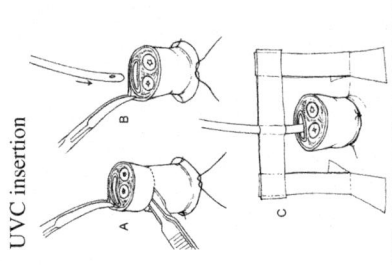

NG-tube insertion

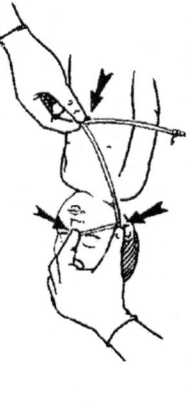

bladder aspiration

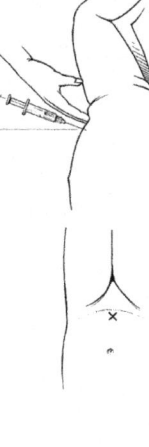

Umbilical venous catheter (UVC) insertion
- Site/use: Umbilicus in newborns 0–5 days old
- Catheter: 5F, attached to 3-way stopcock, filled with NS
- Technique: Use sterile technique. Tie suture around the umbilical stump—tight enough to prevent bleeding, loose enough to let catheter pass. Hold on to Warton's jelly using forceps. Cut umbilical stump 1 cm above skin line. Insert catheter into umbilical vein (larger, thin-walled structure towards head). Withdraw while inserting until blood is visible (usually 4–5 cm for low UVC, advance to 8–9 cm for high UVC). Secure to cord with two sutures. Fix to skin as demonstrated in image. If high UVC, take abdominal X-ray to ensure that line is in the vena cava and not in the hepatic vein

NG-tube insertion
- Tube size: Infant 5F, toddler 8F, adult 12–16F
- Technique: Measure the tube length=distance nose-ear-epigastrium. Lubricate tube with gel, or water if unavailable. Pass tube directly through one nostril, aiming downward and slightly medially. Tube should pass easily. Fix once measured distance is reached. Aspirate to make sure that the tube is in stomach. If no stomach content aspirated, inject air down the tube and listen over stomach. If unsure, remove and try again

Suprapubic bladder aspiration
- Needle: 23 G, attached to 5 or 10 ml syringe
- Technique: Use sterile technique. Find proximal skin crease in suprapubic area. Palpate/percuss bladder to assure that it is full. Hold barrel of syringe with four fingers, place thumb on plunger. Insert needle in 20° angle in rapid but controlled motion and aspirate using thumb while inserting. Do not insert slowly as bladder may move and not be penetrated. Remove needle quickly once urine is obtained. Apply pressure. TIP: Have urine jar available in case child urinates during procedure

(continued)

Table 5.8 (continued)

Lumbar puncture

Lumbar puncture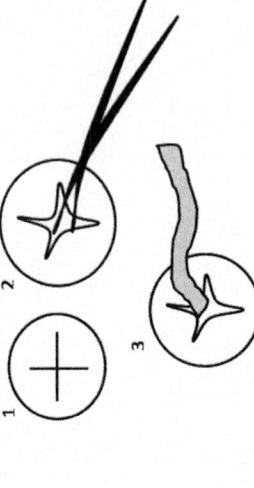

- Needle: 20- or 22-G spinal needle, if unavailable use regular needle
- Technique: Place child on left side or sitting and flex back anteriorly as shown in picture. Assistant should hold child. Find anatomical landmark for space between vertebrae 3–4 or 4–5: draw imaginary line between iliac crest, site is between spinous processes midline. Use sterile technique. Numb skin with topical or injected 1–2 % Lidocaine if available. Insert needle aiming towards umbilicus, advance slowly. You will encounter resistance at spinal ligament. Once penetrated, withdraw stylet; drops of CSF should pass through needle. Obtain 1 ml each for cell count, chemistry, culture. If no CSF visible, reinsert stylet and advance needle further. If advancing too far, venous plexus may be punctured, resulting in bloody "traumatic" tap. Withdraw needle and try again in different vertebral space. Once done, remove needle and apply pressure

Incision and drainage

Incision and drainage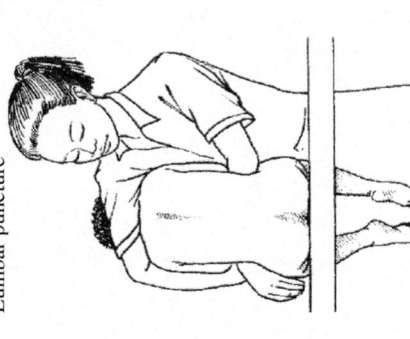

- Tools: Scalpel, hemostat, or dull scissors
- Technique: Use sterile technique. Numb skin with 1–2 % Lidocaine if available. Using scalpel, make cross incision over abscess (1), widen incision with hemostat (2). Drain abscess fluid. Pack incision with gauze to prevent skin closure and reaccumulation (3). Change gauze every 2 days until no further drainage. Skin will close spontaneously

Needle decompression of pneumothorax
− Tools: 16- or 18-G 2in needle
− Technique: Use sterile technique. Find anatomic location: feel for clavicle, second rib is below, feel for second IC space below second rib, go to mid-clavicular line (above nipple). Disinfect skin. Numb area with 1–2 % Lidocaine if available. Insert needle at a perpendicular angle at full length. If successful, gush of air should emerge and patient should improve quickly. Follow directions for chest tube, then remove needle

Chest tube insertion
− Tools: 16-G chest tube, forceps, needle, suture
− Technique: Use sterile technique. Find anatomic location: fifth IC space in mid-axillary line (just below nipples). Disinfect skin. Numb area with 1–2 % Lidocaine. Make 2 cm skin incision above superior edge of sixth rib (nerves and vessels are along inferior edge), use forceps to push through skin and puncture pleura. Dilate with gloved finger as possible. Introduce chest tube using forceps to advance, making sure that all holes of the tube are within the chest. Attach tube to bottle with underwater seal. Secure tube by suturing it to the skin

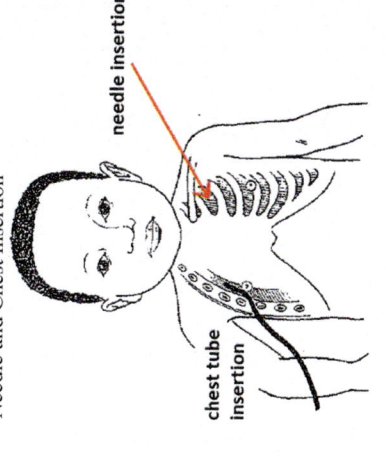

Needle and Chest insertion

1. Thick and thin blood smear
    a. Diagnosis of malaria and speciation of malaria-causing plasmodium species
2. Gram stain:
    a. Abscess fluid, CSF, urine, blood
3. Blood smear
    a. Complete blood count and differential
    b. Red blood cell morphology for detection of hemoglobinopathies
    c. Detection of anemia and its etiology
    d. Diagnosis of leukemic process
4. Urine sediment
    a. Bacteria, white blood cell, red blood cell for detection of urinary tract infection
    b. Cast morphology

Imaging Studies

Whereas plain film X-rays can be obtained in many resource-limited settings, advanced imaging technology such as CT and MRI is often limited or unavailable. Ultrasound can be a valuable tool and an alternative imaging technique in many circumstances.

Helpful ultrasound techniques include the following:

1. Newborn head ultrasound (through open anterior fontanelle):
    a. Diagnosis of hydrocephalus, brain malformation
    b. Intracranial hemorrhage
    c. Calcifications suggestive of TORCH infection
2. Abdominal ultrasound
    a. Focused assessment with sonography in trauma (FAST scan)
        - Rapid ultrasound method to detect peritoneal, thoracic, or pericardial fluid or blood after blunt trauma
    b. Evaluation of hepatosplenomegaly
    c. Evaluation of gallbladder, including duct dilation, lithiasis, and cholecystitis
    d. Gross overview of renal anatomy (e.g., detection of hydronephrosis, pyelonephritis)
    e. Detection of ascites fluid, ascites puncture under ultrasound guidance
    f. Screening for abdominal mass

3. Other uses:
   a. Detection and drainage of pericardial effusion
   b. Detection and drainage of pulmonary effusion
   c. Urine volume assessment and detection of obstructive uropathy
   d. Skin abscess if clinically unclear
   e. Detection and assessment of pregnancy

Child Protection

Awareness of, and policies and programs for child protection vary around the world. Political and social instability, familial economic hardship, and high burden of infectious diseases often result in a lack of attention paid to a child's mental and emotional health. Nevertheless, child protection is an important aspect of general pediatric care.

The WHO defines child maltreatment as "all types of physical and/or emotional ill-treatment, sexual abuse, neglect, negligence and commercial or other exploitation, which results in actual or potential harm to the child's health, survival, development or dignity in the context of a relationship of responsibility, trust or power." Examples of abuse include non-accidental trauma (e.g., shaken infant or battered child, sexual abuse, and child soldiers). Examples of neglect include failure to comply with medically necessary prevention or medical care, and failure to provide adequate nutrition, hygiene, housing, or child supervision. All forms of abuse, whether in developing or developed countries, have similar predisposing factors:

- Child: Younger age, gender, vulnerability (twin, premature infant, disabled)
- Caregiver: Young or single parent, poverty, unemployment, mental health issues, history of abuse or violence, stress and social isolation
- Societal factors: Cultural norms, gender inequalities, policies, conflicts, and civil war

History and Physical Exam Findings of Abuse

As in all abuse, obtaining a history needs to be done in a careful, thoughtful manner and ideally by personnel trained in this area. However, in most resource-limited settings, these trained personnel are few, if not nonexistent, and the health care provider must be prepared to fill this gap. Familiarity with the cultural environment, practices, and norms is indispensable. Usual guidelines for history taking should be followed while paying special attention to the caretaker and child's reactions and keeping a high level of suspicion. On physical exam, special attention should be paid to the behavior of the child, general appearance, skin, skeletal system, eyes, and external genital areas. All findings should be documented carefully. Specific findings that raise a suspicion of abuse include, but are not limited to, the following: bruises on uncommon sites (e.g. stomach and back); burn marks on arms or legs or immersion burns (e.g. on the buttocks); marks on hands and feet that may represent whipping; bite marks; injuries in different stages of healing; retinal hemorrhages; poor hygiene; unexplained failure to thrive; and parental apathy or lack of parental interest in responding to child's needs.

Diagnosis of Child Abuse

Diagnosis of abuse can be difficult, especially without ancillary testing and child protection specialist support. If possible, skeletal survey, CBC, vaginal and urethral swabs to test for STDs, urinalysis, and urine culture should be obtained based on clinical suspicion and availability. Medical and psychological support should be provided, social worker referral initiated as available, and police involved as indicated.

Globally, a variety of strategies for the prevention, recognition, and management of child abuse have been employed, and approaches have included family support, health services and therapeutic approaches (victim services), legal approaches (mandatory reporting, child protection services, arrest and prosecution policies), community-based efforts (school programs, prevention campaigns), and societal approaches (national policies and programs). Unfortunately, in many developing countries, there are no dedicated systems in place, and specialized child protection consultants are limited or nonexistent. The WHO has outlined specific recommendations in its most recent report on violence (http://whqlibdoc.who.int/publications/2002/9241545615_eng.pdf).

Conclusions

The health of any pediatric patient is strongly influenced by their environment, socioeconomic status, cultural practices, disease epidemiology, and availability of medical resources. Globally, medical providers must be familiar with the environment they work in, aware of resources available to them, and prepared for lack thereof. Setting-appropriate approaches to diagnosis and treatment must be used. In all settings, the well child assessment should be a major component of pediatric care and primary prevention, and includes regular developmental assessments, routine screenings, and immunizations. Providers are well advised to be familiar with priorities of emergency pediatric care focus on recognition of danger and priority signs, and an organized management approach. Physicians, mid-level providers, and lay medical personnel form the global pediatric health care team and must work together efficiently, offering productive mutual teaching and learning opportunities.

Recommended Reading

1. Spector JM, Gibson TE. Atlas of pediatrics in the tropics and resource-limited settings. IL: American Academy of Pediatrics; 2009.
2. World Health Organization. Hospital care for children, guidelines for the management of common illnesses with limited resources. Geneva: WHO Press; 2005.
3. Kliegman RM, Stanton BMD, St. Geme J, Schor N, Behrman RE. Nelson textbook of pediatrics. St. Louis: Elsevier Saunders; 2009.
4. Prasad P, editor. Pocket pediatrics: the Massachusetts General Hospital for children handbook of pediatrics. Philadelphia, PA: Lippinkoot Williams and Wilkins; 2010.
5. WHO, UNICEF. Integrated management of childhood illnesses. Geneva: WHO Press; 2005.
6. Rouhani S, Meloney L, Ahn R, Nelson BD, Burke TF. Systematic literature review of alternative rehydration methods: lessons for resource-limited care. Pediatrics. 2011;127(3):e748–57.
7. Child abuse and neglect by parents and other caregivers, Chapter 3, World report on violence and health. WHO 2002. http://whqlibdoc.who.int/publications/2002/9241545615_eng.pdf

Part II
Newborn Health

Chapter 6
Maternal Health

Ariel Wagner, Veronica Maria Pimentel, and Melody J. Eckardt

Keywords Maternal health • Antenatal care • Complications of pregnancy • Obstetrical care • Global health • Resource-poor settings • Contraindicated medications in pregnancy • Developing countries • Antenatal care • Birth plan • Child survival • Preventive treatments

Overview

- The health of the neonate and child is initiated during the antenatal period.
- Maternal health is essential for newborn and child survival.
- Antenatal care (ANC) is underutilized in much of the developing world.
- Interventions during pregnancy, including treatment of maternal health conditions, iron and folate supplementation, HIV screening, IPT for malaria, as well as vaccination, can be essential to newborn and child health.
- ANC visits provide opportunity for counseling regarding emergency planning and safe delivery as well as newborn care provisions, early vaccinations for children, and breastfeeding.

A. Wagner, B.A., M.D./M.M.Sc. (candidate) (✉)
Harvard Medical School, Boston, MA, USA

V.M. Pimentel, M.D., M.S.
Department of Obstetrics and Gynecology, Boston University
Medical Center, Boston, MA, USA

M.J. Eckardt, M.D., M.P.H.
Emergency Medicine, Global Health and Human Rights, Obstetrics and Gynecology,
Boston Medical Center, Massachusetts General Hospital, Boston, MA, USA

Antenatal Care Essentials

The purpose of ANC is to screen pregnant women for risk factors and early signs of disease and then to intervene as necessary to ensure the health of the woman and child. It also provides the opportunity for counseling and health education for pregnancy and parenting as well as administration of preventive treatments. Although ANC services can be useful to reduce maternal and perinatal morbidity and mortality, worldwide only 55 % of pregnant women, and only 36 % in the lowest income countries, complete four ANC visits. Many women still do not have access to ANC due to social, economic, cultural, and political factors. Ultimately, 785 women die every day as a result of complications during pregnancy and delivery; 99 % of these occur in the developing world. Maternal morbidity and mortality are associated with poor perinatal outcomes and overall child survival.

Visit Frequency

For surveillance of normal pregnancy, the World Health Organization recommends that all women should attend a minimum of four antenatal visits as outlined below:

- First ANC visit before 4 months
- Second ANC visit at 6 months
- Third ANC visit at 8 months
- Fourth ANC visit at 9 months

The frequency of visits should increase for women who have maternal health conditions or pregnancy complications, Table 6.1.

A. Basic assessment of pregnancy:

- Maternal weight check to help assess nutrition and fetal growth.
- Fetal growth monitoring.
- Evaluation of uterine size: 12 weeks—palpable at pubic symphysis, 16 weeks—palpable midway between pubic symphysis and umbilicus, 20 weeks—palpable at umbilicus. After 20 weeks, the fundal height in centimeters ±1 cm should be equal to the number of gestational weeks.
- A fundal height greater than expected may suggest multiple gestation, macrosomia, extra amniotic fluid, or the presence of uterine leiomyomata. A fundal height less than expected may signify fetal demise, a fetus with transverse lie, intrauterine growth retardation (IUGR), or false pregnancy. If the fundal height differs in either direction from what is expected, incorrect pregnancy dating may also be the cause. Referral for ultrasound is indicated, if available.
- Fetal heart rate (FHR) monitoring: If available, FHR may be detected with a Doppler ultrasound probe after 10 weeks or a fetoscope after approximately 18 weeks.

Table 6.1 Overview of ANC visits (superscripts denote sections in the text where each intervention is discussed)

	First visit	Second visit	Third visit	Fourth visit
General				
Complete physical and pelvic exam	x			
Basic assessment of pregnancy[A]	x	x	x	x
Determine estimated due date[B]	x			
Review past obstetric history	x			
Ask about signs and symptoms[C]	x	x	x	x
Prepare a birth and emergency plan[D]	x			
Review birth and emergency plan		x	x	x
Disease screening				
Check for preeclampsia[E]	x	x	x	x
Syphilis testing[F]	x			
Check for anemia[G]	x	x	x	x
HIV testing[H]	x			(x)
Preventive measures				
Tetanus toxoid immunization[I]	x	x		
Multivitamin or iron with folic acid[J]	x	x	x	x
Deworming[K]		x		
Intermittent preventive treatment (IPT) for malaria[L]		x	x	x
Encourage sleeping under an insecticide-treated bednet	x	x	x	x
Counseling				
Family planning counseling[M]			x	x
Counseling on cessation of smoking and alcohol and drug use (if applicable)	x	x	x	x
Counseling on nutrition and self-care[N]	x	x	x	x
Domestic violence screening	x	x	x	x

- From 12 to 18 weeks, the FHR is located in the midline of the woman's lower abdomen. After 28 weeks, it is best heard over the mother's back.
- The FHR is typically in the 160 s during early pregnancy, slowing to the 120–140 s close to term. The FHR should increase with fetal movement after 32–34 weeks of gestation.
- Fetal position (≥28 weeks): By abdominal palpation, identify fetal lie (longitudinal, transverse, oblique) and presentation (vertex, breech, shoulder).

B. *Estimation of due date*: First day of last menstrual period + 9 months + 7 days (Naegele's rule).
C. *Signs and symptoms*: Ask about vaginal bleeding, leaking of fluids, fetal movements (after 4 months), contractions, fever, and dysuria. Headache, visual changes, and nondependent swelling may be symptoms of preeclampsia. Ask other questions pertinent to individual health conditions or risk factors.

D. *Birth and emergency plan*: Includes where the woman will deliver, who will assist her, and a plan for transport in case of emergency.
- Determining where a woman should deliver: All women should deliver with a skilled birth attendant, ideally at a health facility. However, this may not always be possible. In high-risk pregnancies, delivering at a health facility or a hospital is essential to ensure access to medical and surgical interventions that may be necessary to save the life of the mother and/or child.
    - Recommend hospital-based delivery in the following cases: age <14 years, prior cesarean delivery, malpresentation within 1 month of expected delivery, multiple pregnancy, documented third-degree tear, history of vaginal bleeding or other complication during the current pregnancy, or tubal ligation or intrauterine device (IUD) desired immediately after delivery.
    - Recommend health center-based delivery in the following cases: age <16 years, >5 previous births, first birth, last baby stillborn or died in first day of life, prior delivery with heavy bleeding, prior delivery with forceps or vacuum, prior delivery with convulsions, or lack of an available skilled birth attendant.
- WHO's six "cleans" for safe birth: clean hands of the attendant, clean surface, clean blade, clean cord tie, clean towels to dry and then wrap the baby, and clean cloth to wrap the mother. A clean birth kit includes soap, a plastic sheet, a clean razor blade, and clean thread for cord tying.
- All pregnant women should be taught to recognize and seek medical care in the case of the following warning signs in labor:
    - Prolonged labor >12 h
    - Labor before the completion of the eighth month of pregnancy (37 weeks)
    - Fetus in an abnormal position (breech, transverse)
    - Heavy vaginal bleeding or vaginal bleeding preceding labor
    - Severe headache/visual disturbances/convulsions
    - Fever and/or foul-smelling vaginal discharge

E. *Check for preeclampsia*: Measure blood pressure (BP). If resting BP is $\geq 140/90$ mmHg, check for urine protein.
F. *Syphilis testing*: Test all pregnant women for syphilis at first ANC visit with rapid plasma reagin (RPR) test.
G. *Anemia*: Assess for risk factors and for conjunctival and palmar pallor. Anemia in pregnancy is defined by a hemoglobin ≤ 11 g/dl or hematocrit ≤ 33 %. If available, lab evaluation should be performed at the second or the third visit or if clinical signs are present.
H. *HIV testing*: Perform rapid HIV test at first ANC visit and again in the third trimester for high-risk women or highly endemic areas. If positive, begin appropriate maternal treatment and PMTCT protocols (see Chap. 18).

I. *Tetanus toxoid*: The goal is for all pregnant women to have received at least two doses of tetanus toxoid vaccine before delivery. If a woman received a tetanus immunization in childhood or adolescence, one dose in pregnancy is sufficient.[1] In any pregnant women with unknown tetanus immunization, give 0.5 ml tetanus toxoid (TT) IM in upper arm according to the following schedule:

TT1: First ANC visit
TT2: ≥4 weeks after TT1
TT3: ≥6 months after TT2
TT4: ≥1 year after TT3
TT5: ≥1 year after TT4

J. *Vitamin supplementation*: Facilitate daily intake of a multivitamin with ≥60 mg elemental iron and 400 μg folic acid during pregnancy and postpartum while breastfeeding. If a multivitamin is not available, you can use iron and folic acid alone in those doses.

K. *Deworming*: If hookworms are endemic (prevalence ≥20–30 %), give antihelminthic once in the second trimester. If hookworm prevalence is >50 %, give anti-helminthic once in the second trimester and once in the third trimester. Anti-helminthic treatment options (outside of the first trimester):

- Albendazole 400 mg × 1
- Mebendazole 500 mg × 1 or 100 mg twice daily × 3 days
- Levamisole 2.5 mg/kg × 1
- Pyrantel 10 mg/kg × 1

L. *Intermittent preventive treatment (IPT) for malaria*: In areas of moderate to high malarial transmission, give three tablets of sulfadoxine–pyrimethamine treatment in the second trimester and three tablets in the third trimester (1 tablet = 500 mg sulfadoxine + 25 mg pyrimethamine).

M. *Family planning*: Counsel on birth spacing and available contraceptive options.

N. *Nutrition and self-care*: Encourage a diverse array of healthy foods, good hygiene practices, and adequate rest.

Maternal Conditions and Risks to Child

Maternal health is essential for newborn and child survival. Maternal co-morbidities can have detrimental effects on the health of the child, including severe acute morbidity, long-term disability, and death of the baby. Therefore, careful treatment of maternal health conditions is essential (Tables 6.2 and 6.3).

---

[1] Two doses of tetanus toxoid will provide immunity in approximately 90 % of pregnant women.

Table 6.2 Maternal conditions, risks, and interventions

Condition	Fetal risks	Prevention	Treatment	Comments
Anemia	• Low birth weight • Preterm delivery • Prenatal mortality • Abnormal fetal oxygenation as a result of severe anemia may lead to: • Non-reassuring fetal heart rate patterns • Reduced amniotic fluid volume • Fetal cerebral vasodilation • Fetal death	• Iron and folate supplementation for all pregnant women • Malaria control • Helminth control • Exclusive breastfeeding • Delayed cord clamping • Family planning (reduction of total number of pregnancies, increase in the time between pregnancies)	• Women with severe anemia 120 mg iron + 400 µg folic acid for 3 months, then continue with preventive regimen • Iron transfusion • Maternal blood transfusion for fetal indication	• Severe anemia = maternal hemoglobin <7 g/dl
Asthma	• Mild to well-controlled moderate asthma: excellent perinatal outcomes • Severe and poorly controlled asthma: risk of prematurity, need for cesarean section, preeclampsia, growth restriction	• Peak expiratory flow rate monitoring • Avoid asthma triggers such as known allergens or use of biofuels without ventilation	• Medical management in pregnant women is the same as in the general adult population	
Malaria	• Neonatal death • Stillbirth • Low birth weight • Congenital infections		WHO guidelines for *Plasmodium falciparum* malaria: • First-trimester options: – Quinine + clindamycin × 7 days (if treatment failure, artesunate + clindamycin × 7 days – Quinine monotherapy if no clindamycin • Second- and third-trimester options: – Artesunate + clindamycin × 7 days – Quinine + clindamycin × 7 days – Artemisinin-based combination therapy (ACT) known to be effective in the country/region	• There is insufficient evidence to support the safety of ACTs in pregnancy, for which reason the US treatment guidelines recommend against their use in pregnant populations. Therefore, if safer regimens are available, they are preferred. • Quinine carries a risk of hypoglycemia • Mefloquine carries a risk of stillbirth

Chronic hypertension (HTN)	Premature birth, fetal growth restrictions, fetal demise, placental abruption, and risk of cesarean delivery	• Antihypertensive drug therapy for mild hypertension can decrease the risk of developing severe HTN, but has no other noticeable benefit
		• Surveillance for preeclampsia
		• Measure baseline proteinuria
			• Mild chronic HTN: No treatment recommended
			• Severe chronic hypertension
			  – No specific antihypertensive is superior
			  – WHO recommends hydralazine because it is effective, inexpensive, and safe
			• Calcium-channel blockers may be more effective but are more costly
				• Hypertension occurs in 6–8 % of pregnancies
				• Chronic HTN = hypertension present before the 20th week of gestation
				• Mild HTN: BP 140–159/90–109
				• Severe HTN: BP>159/109
				• BP must meet the criteria on more than one occasion, at least 4–6 h apart
				• Increased risk of preeclampsia (up to 20 % in mild HTN, but up to 50 % in severe HTN)
				• Do NOT use: ACE inhibitors and angiotensin-receptor blockers (ARB)
				• Caution with diuretics

(continued)

Table 6.2 (continued)

Condition	Fetal risks	Prevention	Treatment	Comments
Preeclampsia		• Controversial • No well-supported or established preventive treatment	• Severe preeclampsia: Magnesium sulfate (in lieu of other anticonvulsants) • Treat severely elevated BP to keep below 160/110 using IV hydralazine or labetalol • Termination of pregnancy or delivery of the fetus and placenta is the only definitive treatment	WHO definitions: • Preeclampsia: Diastolic BP ≥90 mmHg on two readings and 2+ proteinuria • Severe preeclampsia: Preeclampsia criteria + severe headache, blurry vision, epigastric or right upper quadrant pain, or 3+ proteinuria • If available, check complete blood count, liver function tests, urine protein/creatinine ratio, and/or 24-h urine protein to establish disease severity and identify the development of HELLP syndrome

Pregestational diabetes	- Major congenital anomalies, e.g., complex cardiac defects, central nervous system anomalies, and skeletal malformations - Intrauterine fetal death, large babies (>4,000 g), and shoulder dystocia - Hypoglycemia, respiratory distress syndrome at birth - Polycythemia, organomegaly, electrolyte disturbances, and hyperbilirubinemia - Long-term outcomes for Type 1 DM: Obesity and carbohydrate intolerance in the child - Hydramnios which may cause preterm labor - Preeclampsia: In 15–20 % of Type 1 DM without nephropathy and 50 % if nephropathy - Risk of cesarean delivery - Risks are improved with good pregestational and gestational glycemic control	- Type 2 DM: Healthy diet and exercise	- Maintain maternal glucose near physiologic levels before conception and throughout pregnancy - Insulin management during labor and delivery with glucose monitoring every 1–2 h and IV insulin or D5NS fluid titration as needed to maintain euglycemia	- Consider cesarean delivery if estimated fetal weight is >4,500 g in women with diabetes to prevent traumatic birth injury

(continued)

Table 6.2 (continued)

Condition	Fetal risks	Prevention	Treatment	Comments
Syphilis	• Perinatal death • Preterm birth • Low birth weight • Active congenital syphilis in neonate (blistering rash, hepatosplenomegaly, respiratory distress) • Congenital anomalies • Long-term sequelae (deafness, bone changes, neurologic impairment)	• Condoms • Routine screening (see ANC essentials)	• Give benzathine benzylpenicillin 2.4 million units IM once and consider repeat dose in 1 week[a] • Plan to treat newborn • Encourage testing and treatment of partner • Counsel on condom use	• In the case of penicillin allergy, WHO recommends erythromycin 250 mg, 2 tablets every 6 h × 15 days. However, its effectiveness is unclear, so desensitization is recommended where feasible. • Treatment of maternal syphilis reduces congenital infection rates to nearly zero • Risk of Jarisch–Herxheimer reaction within 24 h of maternal treatment, but typically resolves on its own

Tuberculosis (TB)	• Decreased birth weight of baby if mother is untreated • Infant can be born with TB in rare cases	• Initiate treatment in cases where TB probability is moderate to high • Follow adult TB treatment guidelines with consideration for MDR-TB, previous treatment, or concomitant HIV • Pyridoxine, 10 mg daily along with anti-TB regimen	• The tuberculin skin test is valid and safe throughout pregnancy • Contraindicated TB drugs: Streptomycin, kanamycin, amikacin, capreomycin, fluoroquinolones • If a pregnant woman is being treated with a second-line anti-TB drug, she should receive counseling concerning the risk to the fetus • HIV-positive pregnant women suspected of having TB should start TB treatment immediately
Malpresentation	• Obstructed labor leading to fetal asphyxia or death • Birth trauma		• Arm or shoulder presentation or face with chin down must be delivered by cesarean section • Breech twin A, vertex twin B, deliver via cesarean section for risk of locked twins • Improved fetal outcomes with cesarean delivery for breech in developed countries

(continued)

Table 6.2 (continued)

Condition	Fetal risks	Prevention	Treatment	Comments

Premature rupture of membranes (PROM)	• Perinatal infection
	• Umbilical cord compression
	• Placental abruption
	• Cord accident or cord prolapse
	• Preterm delivery
		• Smoking cessation
		• Treatment of pulmonary disease
		• Good nutritional status
			• Avoid digital cervical exams
			• ≥34 weeks gestation: Induction of labor, antibiotics for Group B Strep
			• Viable and <34 weeks and no intrauterine infection evident: Corticosteroids for fetal lung maturity and latency antibiotics consisting of:
			  – 48-h course of IV ampicillin and erythromycin followed by 5 days of amoxicillin and erythromycin
			  – Recommended to prolong pregnancy and reduce neonatal morbidity
				Most deliver within 1 week of premature PROM

[a]This is the recommendation of the WHO and CDC. However, some experts do recommend a second dose within 1 week of the first. Additionally, the CDC recommends three doses 1 week apart for pregnant women with late latent or tertiary syphilis, or those with syphilis of unknown duration

Table 6.3 Contraindicated medications in pregnancy: this is not a complete list but includes medications commonly used or well known for their teratogenic effects

Drug	Use	Adverse effect	Drug risk category[a]
Isotretinoin (accutane, retin-A)	Cystic acne	Miscarriage, microcephaly or hydrocephalus, anomalies of the great vessels, microtia (absence of external ears)	X
ACE inhibitors (lisinopril, captopril, others)	HTN, congestive heart failure	Oligohydramnios, fetal death, fetal skull hypoplasia, IUGR, and pulmonary hypoplasia	D
Tetracyclines (tetracycline, doxycycline, others)	Acne, respiratory infections	Tooth discoloration when taken after the fourth month of pregnancy	D
Streptomycin	TB	Reports of 8th cranial nerve damage and deafness	D
Warfarin (coumadin)	Blood thinner	Central nervous system defects, spontaneous abortion, stillbirth, prematurity, hemorrhage, and ocular defects	X
Lithium	Bipolar disorder	Cardiac malformations with first-trimester use; hypotonia, lethargy, cyanosis, if used near term	D
Methotrexate	Chemotherapy, arthritis	Fetal death, CNS, cardiac and skeletal anomalies	X
Thiouracil	Hyperthyroidism	Fetal and neonatal goiter and thyroid abnormalities	D
Methimazole	Hyperthyroidism	Esophageal atresia, choanal atresia, aplasia cutis, coloboma, neonatal thyroid disorders	D
Thalidomide	Leprosy	Limb deformities	X
Diethylstilbestrol (DES)	Hormone	Gynecologic cancers in female offspring	X
Androgens	Hormone for sexual function, prostate cancer	Female virulization	X
Phenytoin (dilatin)	Anticonvulsant	Fetal malformations, fetal hydantoin syndrome, neuroblastoma	D
Valproic acid (depakene, valprotate)	Anticonvulsant, bipolar disorder	Neural tube defects, dysmorphic features	D
Carbamazepine (tegretol)	Anticonvulsant, bipolar disorder	Spina bifida, craniofacial defects, cardiovascular malformations, hypospadias	D

[a]FDA pregnancy category definitions: Category D: There is positive evidence of human fetal risk based on adverse reaction data from investigational or marketing experience or studies in humans, but potential benefits may warrant use of the drug in pregnant women despite potential risks. Category X: Studies in animals or humans have demonstrated fetal abnormalities and/or that there is positive evidence of human fetal risk based on adverse reaction data from investigational or marketing experience, and that the risks involved in use of the drug in pregnant women clearly outweigh potential benefits

Recommended Reading

1. Aga Khan University, The Partnership for Maternal, Newborn & Child Health (PMNCH), World Health Organization. Essential interventions, commodities and guidelines for reproductive, maternal, newborn and child health: a global review of the key interventions related to reproductive, maternal, newborn and child health. Geneva: World Health Organization; 2011.
2. International Nutritional Anemia Consultative Group (INACG), World Health Organization (WHO), United Nations Children's Fund (UNICEF). Guidelines for the use of iron supplements to prevent and treat iron deficiency anemia. Geneva: World Health Organization; 1998.
3. World Health Organization. Pregnancy, childbirth, postpartum and newborn care—a guide for essential practice. Geneva: World Health Organization; 2006.
4. World Health Organization. World Health Organization antenatal care randomized trial: manual for the implementation of the new model. Geneva: World Health Organization; 2001.
5. World Health Organization. World Health Organization antenatal care randomized trial: manual for the implementation of the new model. Geneva: World Health Organization; 2001.
6. World Health Organization. World Health Organization guidelines for the treatment of malaria. 2nd ed. Geneva: World Health Organization; 2010.

Chapter 7
Preventive Newborn Care

Rebecca Cook and Gopal K. Gupta

Keywords Newborn • Neonatal mortality • Breastfeeding • Prenatal care • Asphyxia • Skin-to-skin care • Preventive • Birth weight • Immunization

Overview

- Most of the deaths in children under 5 years of age occur in the first month of life.
- Interventions to decrease neonatal mortality include essential newborn care for all newborns, emergency preparedness, and extra newborn care for high-risk infants.
- Preventive newborn care, such as presence of skilled birth attendant, umbilical cord care, home visits in the first days of life, early initiation of breastfeeding, skin-to-skin care, and newborn vaccinations, is underutilized in resource-limited settings.

R. Cook, M.D., M.Sc. (✉)
Medicine Department, Harvard University, 175 Cambridge St.,
5th Floor, Boston, MA 02114, USA

MassGeneral Hospital for Children,
Boston, MA 02114, USA
e-mail: rcook1@partners.org

G.K. Gupta, M.D.
Boston Children's Hospital, Harvard Medical School, Boston, MA, USA

Epidemiology of Newborn Deaths

An estimated three million babies (43 % of deaths under age 5) die in the first 4 weeks of life, and 25–45 % of neonatal deaths occur in the first 24 h of life. Up to two-thirds of the deaths can be prevented (Fig. 7.1). Neonatal deaths are a stark reflection of global health inequalities: 99 % occur in low- and middle-income countries. Even within wealthy nations, resource-limited settings such as the Mississippi delta and inner cities in the United States have neonatal mortality rates that approach those of developing countries. Yet the relationship between GDP and neonatal mortality is not linear, as several of the world's poorest countries have dramatically reduced neonatal mortality with simple interventions Table 7.1.

Interventions

Comprehensive newborn care involves three main areas of interventions:

- *Emergency preparedness* includes early recognition and response to complications during pregnancy, delivery, and the neonatal period to maximize survival
- *Essential newborn care* is the basic preventive care package for all newborns
- *Extra newborn care* involves the identification and additional support to infants with extra medical needs such as low-birth-weight infants and HIV-exposed infants

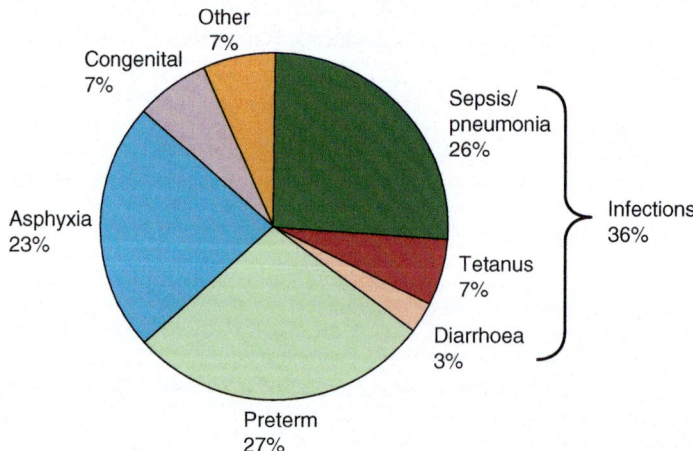

Fig. 7.1 Estimation of distribution of direct causes of neonatal deaths. From Lawn et al. 4 million neonatal deaths: When? Where? Why? Lancet 2005, 365:881–900. Reprinted with kind permission from Elsevier

Table 7.1 Interventions for newborn health

Intervention	Benefits to newborn
During pregnancy	
Treatment of sexually transmitted infections (STIs)	Reduced stillbirth, preterm birth, intrauterine growth restriction (IUGR), infections, death
Prevention/treatment of malaria	Reduced stillbirth, preterm birth, IUGR
Tetanus vaccination	Prevention of neonatal tetanus
Iron, folic acid, hookworm treatment	Reduced risk of low birth weight (LBW), asphyxia, stillbirth
Targeted protein supplements	Reduced risk of LBW, preterm, perinatal death
Vitamin A (if deficient)	Reduced neonatal and postnatal infections
Diagnosis and treatment of preeclampsia	Reduced LBW, asphyxia, stillbirth, neonatal death
Identification of major risk for obstructed labor	Reduced risk of birth asphyxia, trauma, death
During delivery	
Skilled attendant and access to emergency obstetric care	Reduced neonatal asphyxia, provision of neonatal resuscitation
Clean delivery	Reduced risk of tetanus, sepsis, death
Antibiotics for PROM	Reduced sepsis, death
Corticosteroids for preterm labor	Reduced risk (40–60 %) of respiratory distress
Immediate postpartum care	
Integrated maternal and newborn care	Reduced risk of neonatal death
Promotion of early breastfeeding	Prevention of early hypoglycemia and dehydration, reduced risk of early neonatal jaundice, sepsis, and acute respiratory infections
Appropriate cord, eye, and skin care	Reduced risk of sepsis, tetanus, and ophthalmia neonatorum
Promote skin-to-skin contact	Enhanced thermal regulation
High-dose vitamin A to mother	Possible reduction of neonatal mortality
Family planning counseling	Reduced risk of early malnutrition

Adapted from table 1 in Lawn J, McCarthy B, Ross S. The healthy newborn: A reference manual for program managers. CDC. 2002

Preventive newborn care begins in the antenatal period with care and anticipatory guidance for expectant mothers. Maternal vaccinations, particularly tetanus toxoid, are essential in preventing neonatal death. Appropriate screening and management of maternal malnutrition, anemia, STIs including HIV, and malaria (in endemic areas) during pregnancy have been shown to improve neonatal outcome. Identification and referral of high-risk pregnancies can further contribute towards this goal (see Chap. 6).

Having a skilled attendant at birth trained in newborn resuscitation has the potential to reduce asphyxia-related newborn deaths by up to 40 %. In high-risk resource-limited settings where infection is a significant contributor to neonatal mortality, several studies have shown morbidity and mortality gains with the application of 4 % chlorhexidine solution to the umbilical cord shortly after birth and for the first 7 days of life (although the World Health Organization still recommends that the cord should be kept clean and dry with no application of any substances). Immediate postpartum care including early breastfeeding, eye and cord care, and temperature regulation (such as skin-to-skin care) helps to prevent many common causes of morbidity and mortality in the first days of life. In addition, a postnatal visit in the first week of life by a community or a village health worker is a cost-effective strategy to reduce newborn deaths. In health programs in India, Pakistan, and Bangladesh, cluster-randomized control trials have shown that a community intervention with home visits reduces neonatal mortality by 30–61 %. At these visits, health workers can reinforce the pillars of preventive newborn care (Table 7.1) including early breastfeeding, hand hygiene and umbilical cord care, skin-to-skin care (which is particularly important for preterm and low-birth-weight infants), as well as routine newborn care. This also allows for earlier identification of newborn illnesses.

Guidelines for Preventive Newborn Care

To provide appropriate newborn care one should initially obtain a comprehensive maternal and birth history:

1. Maternal history: Take antenatal history if available and assess for maternal conditions that may pose a risk to the child and any medications used (see Chap. 6).
2. Intrapartum or birth history

    (a) Assess site of birth, home or health care center, and assess whether trained health care provider with basic skills in neonatal resuscitation was available at birth (see Chap. 8).
    (b) Assess whether there was a clean delivery—availability of clean environment for delivery with clean supplies (soap, gloves (if available)), clean/sterile cord clamp or tie, and clean/sterile (disposable) blade to cut the cord.
    (c) Did the mother have a fever or an indication of uterine infection during delivery or just after birth? Was there prolonged rupture of membranes for >18 h before birth?
    (d) Were there any complications during the delivery like breech presentation, shoulder dystocia, large baby, and application of forceps/vacuum, or was the baby delivered by lower segment C-section (LSCS)?
    (e) Did the baby require resuscitation at birth?

Preventive care begins immediately after birth and should extend through the neonatal period as mortality is highest in that period of time.

1. *Immediate postpartum*:

    (a) Maintain temperature by skin-to-skin contact, appropriate clothing for the baby, and use of a hat and blankets to prevent heat loss. Make sure that the baby is in the same room as mother and either in her bed or within easy reach. Early attempts at breastfeeding should be made. In situations where breastfeeding is not possible for maternal reasons, formula and in some cases where formula is not available humanized cow's milk can be used in resource-limited settings. This is prepared by diluting whole cow's milk with clean water and adding carbohydrate. Feeding should preferably be done with a clean, hygienic cup and spoon when bottle hygiene cannot be maintained.

(b) Delay first sponge bath until at least 6 h after birth to help maintain temperature, and a tub bath should be avoided until the cord falls off to prevent omphalitis.

(c) Keep the eyes clean and if available, provide erythromycin eye ointment to prevent ophthalmia neonatorum.

(d) Administer injectable vitamin K to prevent hemorrhagic disease of newborn (HDN). Oral vitamin K can be used as a substitute but is believed to be less effective.

(e) Conduct newborn examination to ascertain safe transition of baby from intrauterine to extrauterine life by checking color, tone, breathing (30–60 breaths per minute), and heart rate (100–180 beats per minute). Evaluate for any life-threatening congenital malformations such as cleft palate, imperforate anus, and meningomyelocele.

(f) Assess and treat for infection: Antibiotic treatment is indicated in cases of prolonged rupture of membranes (>18 h), signs of chorioamnionitis in mother, or maternal temperature >38 °C/100.4 °F (within 2 days of delivery) (see Chap. 9).

2. *Immediate newborn (first 7 days of life)*:

(a) Advise frequent hand-washing with soap and water before handling the baby, and avoid/limit visitors.

(b) Maintain temperature by proper clothing and infrequent bathing.

(c) Recommend and encourage exclusive breastfeeding. Educate care-givers about dangers of supplementing with honey, herbs, or sweetened water.

(d) Monitor for jaundice: For mild jaundice, limited sun exposure may be beneficial. If jaundice is noted within 24 h of birth, baby is sick or premature, or there is rapid progression, then refer to a higher center for further treatment.

(e) Umbilicus care: Advise hand-washing before and after cord care. Educate parents/caregivers about cord care and to avoid putting anything on the cord (unless otherwise advised, for example, in the case of chlorhexidine). If the umbilical stump appears soiled, then wash with soap and clean water and dry it with a clean cloth. Make sure that the diaper is folded below the stump. If the stump appears red, has a foul odor, and/or is draining pus, a health care provider needs to examine the baby and manage appropriately (see Chap. 9).

(f) Check skin for infection: If skin pustules, wash with boiled and cooled clean water and soap, dry area, and apply gentian violet. If baby appears sick then treat appropriately (see Chap. 9). Check back in 2 days, and if worse, refer to hospital.

(g) Check eyes: If infected, then wipe pus away using a clean cloth, soaked in boiled and cooled water. Apply 1 % tetracycline or 5 % erythromycin eye ointment three times daily. Check back in 2 days, and if worse, refer to hospital.
(h) Immunize: Oral polio vaccine, hepatitis B, and (in areas where tuberculosis is endemic) BCG in first week of life. However, if unimmunized child is first seen after first week of life, give BCG only (see Chap. 21 for details).
(i) Extra care for small baby (premature or small for gestational age):

- Encourage mom to breast-feed more frequently.
- Weigh daily, and if baby is not sucking effectively, alternative feeding methods may be needed, such as hand-expressing breast milk directly into baby's mouth.
- Maintain extra warmth for baby.
- Monitor for breathing difficulty and jaundice.

3. *Neonatal period (first 28 days of life)*:

(a) Reinforce breastfeeding emphasizing its advantages:

- Decreased risk of diarrhea, respiratory illness, otitis media, meningitis, and other infections.
- Provides complete, balanced nutrition for at least first 6 months of life.
- Includes many immunologic factors.
- Does not require costly formula, bottles, or water.
- Other possible benefits: increased bonding, higher IQ, and promotes pregnancy spacing.

(b) Monitor weight to make sure that feeding is adequate. Weight loss should not be more than 10 % in the first week. Weight gain should be about 15 g per day in the first 2–4 weeks or at least 300 g in the first month.
(c) Counsel about immunization, feeding, sleep hygiene, and encourage sleeping on back.
(d) Continue prenatal vitamins to mother.
(e) Vitamin D supplementation.
(f) Advise mother about newborn danger signs and when to seek care:

- Difficulty breathing.
- Not feeding.
- Has a fever or feels extra "hot or cold."
- Abnormal movements (convulsions).
- Bleeding.
- Diarrhea.
- Pus from eyes, umbilical stump, skin.
- Yellow skin or very dark urine.

(g) Treat appropriately when history of maternal TB, syphilis, or HIV:

- Maternal TB diagnosed and treatment started at less than 2 months before delivery:
  - Give 5 mg/kg of isoniazid (INH) once per day orally for 6 months.
  - Delay BCG until after treatment is complete or repeat BCG.
  - Continue breastfeeding.
  - Weigh child every 2 weeks to monitor adequate weight gain.
- If the mother is HIV positive, treat the baby as per guidelines (see Chap. 18).

Progress in Preventive Newborn Care

Progress towards Millennium Development Goal 4 of reducing childhood deaths by two-thirds by 2015 varies widely by country. Some evidence-based interventions such as childhood immunizations have reached 80–90 % coverage in much of the developing world, while other interventions, particularly those at birth and in the neonatal period, lag far behind (Fig 7.2).

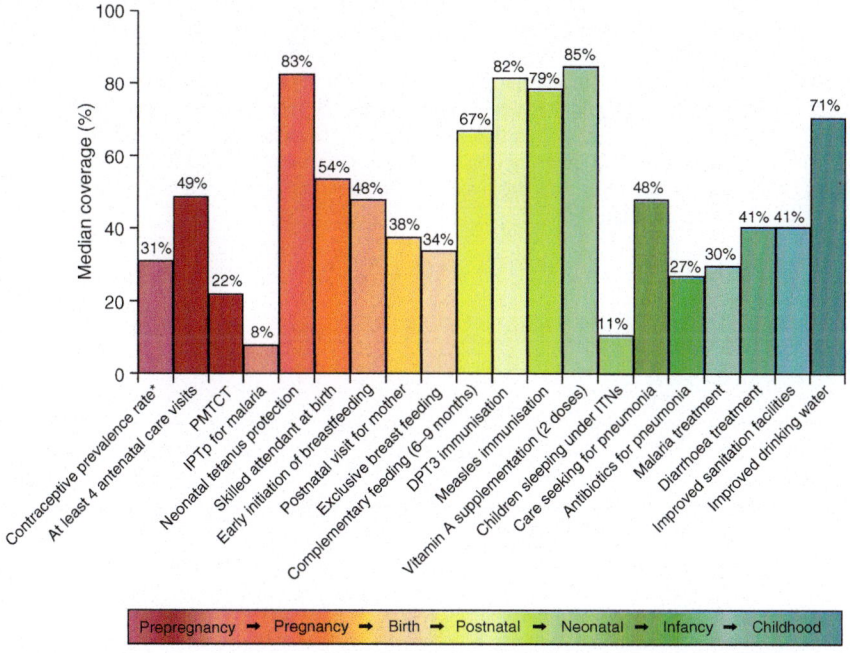

Fig 7.2 Median coverage for effective interventions in 68 countries. From Bhutta Z, Chopra M, Axelson H, Berman P, Boerma T, Bryce J, et al. Countdown to 2015 decade report (2000–10): taking stock of maternal, newborn, and child survival. Lancet 2010; 375S: 2032–44. Reprinted with kind permission from Elsevier

Interventions require involvement at every level, from the household to the hospital. For example, particularly in resource-limited settings, significant reductions in neonatal mortality have been achieved with community- and family-based care and education often delivered by community health workers or mother-to-mother programs. Health outreach by health professionals, such as vaccination campaigns in the community by nurses, can also complement these efforts. Finally, only integrated facility-based care that spans the continuum from preconception (provision of folic acid and family planning to women of reproductive age) to prenatal care (routine screening, vaccinations, anticipatory guidance) to delivery (hospital-based delivery with health professionals trained in basics of neonatal resuscitation) and neonatal care (newborn vaccinations, birth registration, and integrated management of neonatal illnesses) will help achieve our goals.

Recommended Reading

Darmstadt G, Bhutta Z, Cousens S, Adam T, Walker N, Bernis L, et al. Evidence-based, cost effective interventions: how many newborn babies can we save? Lancet. 2005;365(9463):977–88.

Lawn J, Zupan J, Lancet Neonatal Survivial Steering Team. 4 million neonatal deaths: when? Where? Why? Lancet. 2005;365:881–900.

Bhutta Z, Chopra M, Axelson H, Berman P, Boerma T, Bryce J, et al. Countdown to 2015 decade report (2000–2010): taking stock of maternal, newborn, and child survival. Lancet. 2010;375S:2032–44.

WHO, UNICEF. Integrated management of childhood illness chart booklet. Geneva: WHO/UNICEF Department of Child and Adolescent Health and Development; 2008.

WHO. Pregnancy, childbirth, postpartum and newborn care: a guide for essential practice. Integrated management of pregnancy and childbirth. Geneva: WHO; 2009.

Kinzie B, Gomez P, Chase R, editors. Basic maternal and newborn care: a guide for skilled providers. Baltimore, MD: Jhpiego; 2006.

Chapter 8
Newborn Resuscitation

Jonathan Reisman, Jonathan M. Spector, and Linda L. Wright

Keywords Newborn • Resuscitation • Asphyxia • Developing countries • Neonatal mortality

Overview

- An estimated 5–10 % of newborns need some form of assistance to successfully initiate regular and sustained breathing at birth.
- Preparation is essential for effective newborn resuscitation: a birth attendant skilled in newborn resuscitation should be present at each and every birth; resuscitation equipment must be clean, functioning, and immediately accessible at every delivery.
- Babies should breathe spontaneously or receive assisted ventilation with a bag-mask within 1 min after birth (the "Golden Minute" of life).
- Universal provision of neonatal resuscitation training, using validated curricula such as the Neonatal Resuscitation Program (NRP) or Helping Babies Breathe, is fundamental to improving neonatal outcomes throughout the world.

J. Reisman, M.D.
Harvard-MGH Medicine Pediatrics Program, Boston, MA, USA

J.M. Spector, M.D., M.P.H. (✉)
Division of Newborn Services, Massachusetts General Hospital,
55 Fruit Street, Founders 5-526A, Boston, MA 02114, USA
e-mail: jmspector@partners.org

L.L. Wright, M.D.
Eunice Kennedy Shriver National Institute of Child Health
and Human Development, National Institutes of Health, Rockville, MD, USA

Global Network for Women's and Children's Health Research, Center for Research
for Women and Children, Rockville, MD, USA

Background: Why Some Babies Fail to Breathe at Birth

An intrapartum-related hypoxic event in a newborn, previously referred to as birth asphyxia, results from insufficient oxygen delivery to the baby's brain during birth and/or immediately after delivery. In utero, a fetus relies entirely on the mother's placenta for oxygen. At birth the baby's oxygen source abruptly shifts when she cries, expands her lungs, and the umbilical cord is clamped. To achieve a healthy transition, the baby must immediately begin regular and sustained breathing or crying to take in oxygen from the atmosphere. This process occurs naturally and without complication in many babies but not all. In those that have difficulty transitioning, inadequate breathing can quickly (within minutes) cause hypoxemia, brain hypoxia, and ultimately death or disability.

Of the nearly 140 million babies born each year, an estimated 5–10 %, or ten million, need help taking the first breath of life. Intrapartum-related hypoxic events cause more than 800,000 newborn deaths annually, representing approximately one quarter of all neonatal deaths. Those babies that survive poorly managed intrapartum-related hypoxic events are at risk of permanent neuronal injury and long-term morbidities, including epilepsy, cerebral palsy, and other forms of neurodevelopmental impairment.

Any condition that disrupts normal intrapartum or delivery processes can increase the risk of adverse intrapartum-related events in newborns. These include depressed maternal neurologic status (due to sedative drugs or medications), prematurity, prolonged labor, difficult or precipitous delivery, placental abruption, and newborn conditions that obstruct gas exchange (e.g., pneumonia, meconium aspiration, and congenital anomalies).

Newborn Resuscitation Saves Lives

"Newborn resuscitation" describes the practice of helping to initiate breathing in babies that fail to breathe spontaneously at birth. It is a proven method for avoiding or mitigating harm from intrapartum-related hypoxic events. The vast majority (>90 %) of infants that require assistance at birth need only basic resuscitation measures such as stimulation. Fewer babies will require the more advanced resuscitation technique of positive-pressure ventilation in which air is manually pushed into the newborn's lungs using a bag-mask (though it is a life-saving procedure for those who need it). Very few babies (<1 %) require the highly advanced techniques of chest compressions, administration of resuscitation medications, or intubation and ventilation.

The "Golden Minute" is a term that was coined by the developers of the *Helping Babies Breathe* curriculum and refers to the first 60 seconds after birth. It is meant to emphasize the urgency of initiation of newborn breathing. If a baby fails to breathe spontaneously, immediate and appropriate action by a skilled birth attendant in the Golden Minute is crucial to maximize the likelihood of a good outcome.

Despite the fact that newborn resuscitation practice is well described and is dependent on few supplies and equipment that are relatively inexpensive and largely reusable, ensuring the universal delivery of effective newborn resuscitation for all babies continues to be a major global health challenge. Roughly half of the world's births, and a preponderance of those in the developing world, take place in the absence of trained birth attendants, which increases the risk of death or injury from intrapartum-related events. Fortunately, as described below, progress in this area has been encouraging.

Global Advances in Newborn Resuscitation

The most important development relating to newborn resuscitation in recent years has simply been the widespread acceptance of its efficacy in reducing avoidable harm. The World Health Organization endorses the presence of at least one birth attendant skilled in neonatal resuscitation at each and every birth. In recognition of this, and in order to address content deficiencies in training programs that were not designed for low-resource settings where most deaths occur, the American Academy of Pediatrics and partners developed an innovative neonatal resuscitation curriculum in 2010 that is intended for use "wherever a baby is born." *Helping Babies Breathe* is a hands-on, flipchart-based training program that focuses on the initial steps of resuscitation (including bag-mask ventilation) that will save most babies' lives. It is commonly taught using an inflatable, low-cost newborn manikin that can simulate breathing and a pulse. The new curriculum and training tools have sparked global enthusiasm for scaling up newborn resuscitation training. At the same time, a global public–private partnership has made the curriculum and tools widely available, revolutionizing the ability to provide effective training in settings where it is most needed.

The remainder of this chapter reviews the key steps involved in neonatal resuscitation practice.

Newborn Resuscitation: Essential Elements

Be Prepared Before the Birth Occurs

1. Environment
    (a) Ensure a warm temperature in the delivery room by closing windows, blocking drafts, and turning on heat sources as needed. Ensure there is adequate light to assess the newborn's skin color.
    (b) Prepare a clean, warm flat surface near the mother on which the newborn can be placed if resuscitation is required. Resuscitation can also occur on the mother's abdomen if no other surface is available.

(c) All birth attendants should wash their hands with soap and water (or alcohol-based hand rub) and wear gloves before attending to the woman or baby. Consider washing the mother's hands and chest as well.

2. Supplies and equipment
   (a) All equipment should be cleaned and sterilized before the birth, for example by using boiling water or chlorhexidine wash.
   (b) All equipment should be tested before each birth to be sure it functions properly.
   (c) The following supplies and equipment should be immediately accessible and ready-to-use at every birth:
   - Clean clothes or towels to catch and dry the baby
   - Two sterile umbilical cord clamps or ties
   - Sterile scissors or blade to cut the umbilical cord
   - Hat or head covering to keep the baby warm
   - Timer or clock
   - Suction device to clear the baby's airway if necessary
   - Self-inflating bag-mask to provide assisted ventilation if necessary
       Two masks of different sizes should be available to ensure that a good seal can be attained for term and preterm babies
       – Function of the bag-mask should be checked by forming a seal against the palm of your hand and delivering test breaths against your hand; you should feel pressure on your palm
           – Squeeze the bag hard enough for the escape (pop-off) valve to open; if the valve does not open appropriately, it may be necessary to obtain a new bag
   - Stethoscope, if available, to facilitate measurement of the newborn's heart rate and to auscultate the lungs

3. Skilled birth attendants
   (a) A birth attendant skilled in neonatal resuscitation should be present at each and every birth.
   (b) Identify a helper in case a crisis situation arises.
   (c) If the mother is high-risk but delivery is not imminent, consider transport to a referral center before birth.
   - Examples of high-risk mothers include the following: very old or very young, chronically ill, infections during pregnancy, bleeding during pregnancy or labor, high blood pressure, multiple gestations (twins or triplets), poor fetal movements, previous fetal or neonatal death, fever during labor, foul-smelling or meconium-stained amniotic fluid, premature labor, abnormal presentation, prolonged labor (>24 h), slow fetal heart rate, and prolapsed cord.
   (d) Have an emergency transport plan in place in case the mother or newborn requires referral after delivery.

Take Action I: Care for All Babies at Birth

1. When the baby is delivered, immediately dry the baby and remove wet cloths (however, if meconium is present, see note below).
   (a) The process of drying will naturally provide stimulation to the baby. Stimulation alone is usually all that is required to help most babies to breathe at birth.
   (b) Cover the baby with a warm, dry cloth and cover the head with a hat or other covering.
2. Treat babies that have meconium.
   (a) If meconium is noted and the baby is not breathing, crying, or active, then suction the meconium from the mouth and nose before drying and stimulating the baby.
3. If the baby is breathing or crying, give routine care.
   (a) Keep the baby warm.
      - Ideally the baby is kept warm by skin-to-skin contact with the mother's chest. This also facilitates successful initiation of breastfeeding.
      - The baby can also be kept warm by wrapping in a warm blanket if the mother is unable to have the baby on her chest.
   (b) Position the neck slightly extended to ensure an open airway.
   (c) Check the baby's breathing.
   (d) In a healthy baby, wait 1–2 min and then clamp or tie the cord and cut it.
      - Place the first clamp or tie on the cord 2 cm (or two fingerbreadths) from the baby's abdomen. Place the second clamp or tie 5 cm (or five fingerbreadths) from the baby's abdomen.
      - Cut between the two clamps or ties with sterile scissors or blade.
      - If the cord continues to bleed or ooze, place another clamp or tie between the first one and the baby's abdomen.
   (e) Consider the application of chlorhexidine or other antiseptic to the umbilical cord according to local guidelines.

Take Action II: Care for Babies that Need Help to Breathe

1. If the baby does not breathe or cry at birth, then neonatal resuscitation may be necessary to help the baby to breathe.
2. Remember the Golden Minute! Your aim is to help all babies to breathe by 1 min after birth.

Fig. 8.1 Sniffing position for best newborn airway position

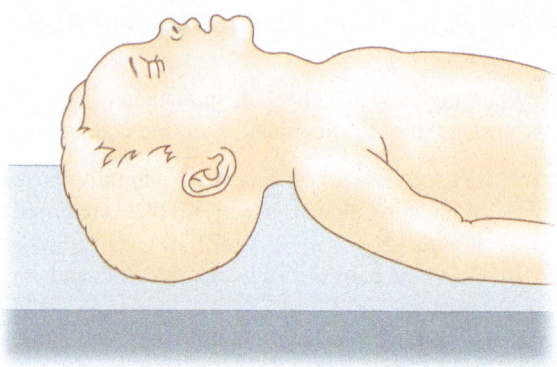

3. Position the baby's head in order to provide a clear passage through the baby's airway to make it easier for the baby to breathe.
   (a) Extend the neck slightly, without over- or under-extending it, to maximally open the airway. The nose should be as far forward as possible; this is called the "sniffing" position (Fig. 8.1).
4. Dry the baby, keep warm, and stimulate.
   (a) Simultaneously dry and stimulate the baby by gently rubbing the trunk, back, and limbs with a cloth or towel. Do not shake, slap, or squeeze the baby as this can cause the baby harm. Many babies will begin to breathe and cry when dried and stimulated.
5. Assess the baby's breathing.
   (a) A baby that is breathing regularly or crying has a *normal breathing pattern*.
   (b) A baby that gasps (a single deep breath followed by a long pause) or is not breathing at all (apnea) has an *abnormal breathing pattern*.
6. If the baby continues to have an abnormal breathing pattern, provide more stimulation and assess whether the baby's nares and/or oropharynx needs to be suctioned. Suction or wipe with a clean cloth if secretions obstruct the mouth or nose.
7. If the baby continues to have an abnormal breathing pattern after drying and stimulating (and suctioning if needed), then urgent assisted ventilation with a self-inflating bag-mask is required to help the baby initiate breathing.
   (a) Ventilation is the *most important* intervention for a newborn with abnormal breathing and should be initiated before the Golden Minute (1 min after birth) has elapsed.
   (b) Call for help. If assisted ventilation is required then it means that the baby is potentially very sick. It is important to have another person available to help you to resuscitate the baby and to provide additional help if needed.

(c) Cut the cord prior to ventilation and move the baby to a nearby flat surface for resuscitation.
(d) Position the baby so that you are standing over the baby's head. Your helper should be positioned to the side of the baby's trunk from where they can easily feel the umbilical pulse or auscultate the baby's lungs.
(e) Select a correct mask size to ensure a good seal and to achieve successful ventilation. The mask should be rolled up from the chin to cover the mouth and nose with the rim of the mask resting on the chin. The mask should not cover the eyes and should make a tight seal on the face with only light pressure. If the mask has a pointed side, the pointed side should fit over the bridge of the nose.
(f) Form an air-tight seal by pressing down lightly on the mask using the thumb and index finger. The middle, fourth, and fifth fingers should lift the jaw slightly without putting pressure on the soft tissue underneath the chin as this can occlude the airway and prevent ventilation. The baby's airway should now be in the "sniffing position". Do not firmly push the mask down onto the face. Avoid bruising the face or damaging the eyes with unnecessary and misplaced pressure.
(g) Squeeze the bag. Give 40–60 breaths per minute. Pace yourself by speaking out loud as you ventilate: "Breathe…two…three…Breathe…two…three."
(h) Signs of successful ventilation are as follows:

- Rise of the chest wall with each assisted breath
- Improving color
- Increasing heart rate
- Improving muscle tone
- Onset of spontaneous breathing or crying

(i) If the above signs of successful ventilation do not occur, the assisted ventilation is not effective and you must act immediately to improve your ventilation technique. NRP suggests the mnemonic *MR SOPA* to help remind you of the steps to take to achieve better ventilation: ensure a good seal between the *M*ask and the face so that air does not escape between the baby's face and the mask, *R*eposition the newborn's neck to ensure it is in the "sniffing" position so that the airway is maximally open, *S*uction the mouth, use a finger to make sure the newborn's mouth is slightly *O*pen to allow air movement, increase the *P*ressure of bagging, and consider an *A*lternative airway such as an endotracheal tube or laryngeal mask airway.

8. The vast majority of babies will respond to drying, stimulating, suctioning, and assisted ventilation. If the baby is still not improving, the most important action is to be absolutely sure that the assisted ventilation technique is adequate!
9. If the baby still does not improve despite adequate resuscitation technique, then the baby is very sick.

    (a) Contact a higher-level health facility to inform them you are providing prolonged ventilation and that the baby needs to be referred.
    (b) If equipment is available, proceed with the advanced newborn resuscitation practices outlined below.

Advanced Newborn Resuscitation Practices

1. If equipment is available for intubation (e.g., laryngoscope, endotracheal tubes of various sizes, and styles) then intubation should be considered in the following circumstances:

    (a) If the amniotic fluid or baby is stained with meconium and the baby is not breathing, crying, or active at birth.

    - Intubate and suction the trachea to remove as much meconium as possible, then remove the tube before drying and stimulating the baby.

    (b) If assisted ventilation with bag-mask is not effective.

    - Achieving effective assisted ventilation is the most important step of helping gasping or apneic babies to breathe at birth. If assisted ventilation with bag-mask is not adequate, then intubation and ventilation through an endotracheal tube can help to improve ventilation.

    (c) If prolonged assisted ventilation with bag-mask is required.

    - Intubation can help you to deliver more effective breaths without needing to maintain a proper seal between the mask and the baby's face. It also will deliver less air into the esophagus (which can lead to distension and aspiration).

2. Chest compressions are indicated if a baby's heart rate is less than 60 beats per minute despite adequate assisted ventilation with a bag-mask or endotracheal tube for 60 seconds.

    (a) One person must continue assisted ventilation, while a second person begins chest compressions. Chest compressions will be ineffective without continuing assisted ventilation!

    (b) Place two fingers on the bottom third of the baby's sternum or wrap both of your hands around the baby's torso with your thumbs on the lower third of the baby's sternum. Compress one-third of the anterior–posterior diameter of the chest.

    (c) The proper rate is 90 compressions per minute, coordinated with ventilation, which should occur after every third chest compression. Speak out loud as you perform chest compressions to make coordination with ventilation easier: "One…two…three…Breathe…one…two…three…Breathe."

    (d) Check the heart rate after 30 s of well-coordinated chest compressions and ventilation.

3. If available, supplemental oxygen should be given to babies who remain cyanotic despite adequate spontaneous breathing and heart rate.

4. If available, medication should be given to babies that are unable to be resuscitated using the above methods. Epinephrine (or adrenaline) is indicated if the baby's heart rate remains below 60 beats per minute after 30 s of effective

assisted ventilation and another 30 s of coordinated chest compressions and ventilation. Epinephrine is most effective if administered through an intravenous line placed in a peripheral vein or in the umbilical vein. The intravenous dose is 0.01–0.03 mg/kg or 0.1–0.3 mL/kg of a 1:10,000 solution, followed with a 0.5–1 mL flush of normal saline. If intravenous access cannot be obtained, epinephrine can be delivered directly into the endotracheal tube, usually at a higher dose of 0.05–0.1 mg/kg or 0.5–1 mL/kg. Endotracheal delivery of epinephrine should be followed by several positive-pressure breaths to ensure drug distribution into the lungs.
5. If any advanced newborn resuscitation practices are implemented, call for additional help immediately.

Summary

Newborn resuscitation saves lives and prevents avoidable morbidity. A skilled birth attendant who can deliver effective newborn resuscitation, and who has the supplies and equipment to do so, should be present at each of the 140 million births that take place around the world each year. Most babies that do not breathe at birth will begin to do so with simple drying and stimulation. For those babies that do not respond to these initial measures, assisted ventilation with a bag-mask is the single most important step in helping babies to breathe. Scaling up newborn resuscitation training in countries where most newborn deaths occur remains an urgent global health priority.

Recommended Reading

Lee AC, Cousens S, Wall SN, et al. Neonatal resuscitation and immediate newborn assessment and stimulation for the prevention of neonatal deaths: a systematic review, meta-analysis and Delphi estimation of mortality effect. BMC Public Health. 2011;11 Suppl 3:S12.

World Health Organization. Guidelines on basic newborn resuscitation. Geneva: World Health Organization; 2012.

American Academy of Pediatrics, American Heart Association. Textbook of neonatal resuscitation, 6th ed. American Academy of Pediatrics and American Heart Association; 2010.

Carlo WA, Wright LL, Chomba E, et al. Educational impact of the Neonatal Resuscitation Program in low-risk delivery centers in a developing country. J Pediatr. 2009;154(4):504–8.

American Academy of Pediatrics. Helping babies breathe. www.helpingbabiesbreathe.org.

Wall SN, Lee AC, Niermeyer S, et al. Neonatal resuscitation in low-resource settings: what, who, and how to overcome challenges to scale up? Int J Gynaecol Obstet. 2009;107 Suppl 1:S47–64.

Crofts JF, Winter C, Sowter MC. Practical simulation training for maternity care – where we are and where next. BJOG. Nov 2011;118 Suppl 3:11–6.

Chapter 9
Neonatal Infections

Hasan S. Merali, Anita K.M. Zaidi, and Brett D. Nelson

Keywords Neonatal infections • Developing countries • Early detection • Treatment • Prevention

Overview

- The majority of neonatal deaths worldwide occur in the developing world.
- Newborns are at particularly higher risk for infection and death from untreated infections.
- Several prevention strategies have been shown to significantly decrease the burden of neonatal infections.
- Most neonatal infections can be treated with prompt diagnosis but early detection can be challenging.
- Education regarding the importance of antenatal care, clean birth practices, and postnatal care can have a significant impact on decreasing the incidence of neonatal infections.

H.S. Merali, M.D.
MassGeneral Hospital for Children, Harvard Medical School,
Boston, MA, USA

A.K.M. Zaidi, M.B.B.S., S.M.
Department of Paediatrics and Child Health, Aga Khan University, Karachi, Pakistan

B.D. Nelson, M.D., M.P.H., D.T.M.&H. (✉)
Division of Global Health, MassGeneral Hospital for Children, 100 Cambridge St.,
15th Floor, Boston, MA 02114, USA
e-mail: brett.d.nelson@gmail.com

Epidemiology

Infection in the neonatal period (0–28 days of life) is one of the greatest problems facing newborns in the developing world. Globally, 43 % of deaths in children younger than 5 years occur in the newborn period. Of these three million neonatal deaths, 99 % occur in low- and middle-income countries. Sepsis, pneumonia, and meningitis account for about a third of these deaths. Newborns are at the highest risk for fatal infections due to several factors including immature immune systems and a poorly developed skin barrier. In the developing world, they are at even higher risk due to limited access to antenatal care for their mothers, high rates of home deliveries by unskilled providers, unhygienic practices during and after birth, delay in seeking care for ill newborns, and acquisition of nosocomial infections due to lack of hygienic practices in birthing clinics and hospitals.

The following is a discussion of the leading causes of neonatal infections, with additional treatment details outlined in Table 9.1.

Pneumonia

Neonatal pneumonia is responsible for significant mortality, with the incidence ranging from 0.4 to 12.6 per 1,000 live births in the developing world. WHO estimates that 10 % of all newborn deaths in developing countries are due to pneumonia. Neonatal pneumonia has a wide variety of causes including viruses, bacteria, and parasites. The infection can be acquired congenitally, transplacentally, at birth, or after birth. The most common bacteria responsible for neonatal pneumonia are Group B streptococcus, *Escherichia coli*, *Klebsiella* species, *Staphylococcus aureus*, and *Streptococcus pneumoniae*. Infants present with signs of respiratory distress including tachypnea, retractions, nasal flaring, grunting, cyanosis, rales, and decreased breath sounds. They may also develop fever, lethargy, or other signs of systemic illness. In the WHO Integrated Management of Childhood Illness (IMCI) algorithm (Appendix), respiratory rates of greater than 60 breaths per minute and chest retractions have been identified as indicators of possible bacterial pneumonia. Where available, a chest X-ray can also be useful, especially with severe or persistent illness or acute worsening. Pneumonia treatment involves antimicrobials, oxygen, and supportive therapy as needed. WHO currently recommends therapy with injectable penicillin/ampicillin and gentamicin. Prevention includes clean birth practices and early initiation of exclusive breastfeeding. Maternal influenza vaccination has also been shown to prevent neonatal respiratory illness in Bangladesh.

Table 9.1 Newborn infections and treatments

Infectious syndrome	Usual etiology	Specific prevention	Suggested empirical therapy	Suggested length of treatment
Pneumonia	Group B *Streptococcus*, *E. coli*, *Klebsiella* species, and *S. pneumoniae*		Ampicillin (25–50 mg/kg IV/IM every 6–12 h) and gentamicin (2.5 mg/kg IV/IM every 8–24 h; OR 5 mg/kg IV/IM once daily)	10–14 days
Bacterial sepsis and meningitis	Group B *Streptococcus*, *S. aureus*, *Escherichia coli*, *Listeria*, and *Klebsiella* species		Ampicillin (25–50 mg/kg IV/IM every 6–12 h) and gentamicin (2.5 mg/kg IV/IM every 8–24 h; OR 5 mg/kg IV/IM once daily). If available, consider adding acyclovir for HSV meningitis	Sepsis: 10 days Meningitis: 14–21 days
Tuberculosis	*M. tuberculosis*	Treatment of infected mothers. If mother started treatment <2 months before delivery, give infant isoniazid for 6 months and BCG vaccine when treatment complete	Isoniazid (10–15 mg/kg PO daily), rifampin (15–20 mg/kg PO daily), pyrazinamide (30–40 mg/kg PO daily), and an aminoglycoside (e.g., amikacin). Breastfed newborns should also receive pyridoxine	After the first 2 months, continue isoniazid and rifampin to complete 6–12 months of treatment and discontinue the other medications
Tetanus	*C. tetani*	Vaccination of mother	Spasms: diazepam or paraldehyde Give anti-tetanus immunoglobulin if available, tetanus vaccine and metronidazole	Metronidazole for 10–14 days
Eye infections (ophthalmia neonatorum)	*N. gonorrhoeae, C. trachomatis, S. aureus*	1 % silver nitrate drops or 2.5 % povidone–iodine drops or 1 % tetracycline ointment	Gonococcal: Ceftriaxone or kanamycin Chlamydia: oral erythromycin *S. aureus*: 1 % tetracycline ointment	Gonococcal: One-time dose Chlamydia: 14 days *S. aureus*: Until resolution
Skin infections	*S. aureus*		Cloxacillin (25–50 mg/kg/day PO/IV/IM divided every 6 h)	Until resolution
Umbilical infections (omphalitis)	*S. aureus*		Cloxacillin (25–50 mg/kg/day IV/IM/PO divided every 6 h)	10 days

(continued)

Table 9.1 (continued)

Infectious syndrome	Usual etiology	Specific prevention	Suggested empirical therapy	Suggested length of treatment
Syphilis	T. pallidum	Treatment of infected mothers. If mother RPR positive, give a single dose of benzathine penicillin to infant	Aqueous crystalline penicillin G (25,000–50,000 Units IV/IM every 6–12 h)	10 days
Hepatitis B	Hepatitis B virus	Vaccination of mother. If mother is positive, give first dose of vaccine to infant within 12 h of birth and give hepatitis immune globulin within 24 h of birth if available		
Toxoplasmosis	T. gondii		Limited treatment options in developing countries. Sulfadiazine (100 mg/kg/day divided every 6 h PO) and pyrimethamine (loading 2 mg/kg/day divided 12 hourly PO × 2 days, then 1 mg/kg PO daily × 2–6 months, then 1 mg/kg PO three times weekly for reminder of year) with supplemental leucovorin	1 year
Rubella	Rubella virus	Rubella vaccination of mothers	Limited treatment options. Immunoglobulin if available	
CMV	Cytomegalovirus		Limited treatment options in developing countries. Ganciclovir (6 mg/kg/dose IV every 12 h)	6 weeks
HSV	Herpes simplex virus		Acyclovir (20 mg/kg/dose IV every 8 h)	14 days for skin/eyes/mouth; 21 days for CNS involvement

Dosing in this table lists the general range of recommended doses. However, please consult local treatment guidelines for specific dosing, which can vary significantly depending on newborn age, weight, and condition

Bacterial Sepsis and Meningitis

Neonatal sepsis has traditionally been classified as early (within 7 days of life) and late (7–28 days of life). This classification, however, does not always apply in the developing world as newborns are also exposed to environmental pathogens at birth that are typically thought of as causing late-onset sepsis. In developing countries, clinical sepsis has been reported to affect 49–170 infants per 1,000 live births. A relatively common sequela of bacterial sepsis in the newborn is meningitis, with approximately 15 % of septic newborns having concomitant meningitis. However, as they regularly share a common etiology, bacterial sepsis and meningitis are frequently considered and managed together. The most common responsible pathogens are Group B *Streptococcus* (GBS), *Staphylococcus aureus*, *Escherichia coli*, and *Klebsiella* species. Infants can present with difficulty feeding, convulsions, increased respiratory rate, retractions, temperature instability including hyperthermia or hypothermia, and lethargy. Blood and CSF cultures are useful for diagnosis and to guide management; however, due to limited resources, the diagnosis is often clinical. Treatment for sepsis and meningitis is similar to that used for neonatal pneumonia, although the higher range of dosing is recommended when considering meningitis. Additionally, since distinguishing between viral and bacterial meningitis can be difficult, acyclovir is often added to the antibiotic coverage in resource-rich settings although less frequently available in resource-limited settings (see HSV below). Important prevention strategies include appropriate antenatal care, clean delivery and cord care, and exclusive breastfeeding. Chlorhexidine antiseptic application to the umbilical stumps of newborns born at home has been shown to decrease mortality. Furthermore, chlorhexidine skin washings have also been shown to decrease newborn skin flora, although evidence for any impact on newborn mortality or morbidity is not yet available. Among women whose newborns are at high risk for sepsis (e.g., premature rupture of membranes or Group B streptococcus colonization), intrapartum antibiotics are routinely used in many developed countries for prevention of neonatal infection, although data that intrapartum antibiotic prophylaxis prevents neonatal infection in developing countries are not available.

Tuberculosis

Tuberculosis, caused by *Mycobacterium tuberculosis*, affects approximately 1.3 million children younger than 15 years of age in the developing world. The infection of the neonate can be congenital, acquired via the placenta or amniotic fluid, or neonatal, acquired by infected droplets, infected milk, or by contamination of traumatized skin. Infants usually become symptomatic between the ages of

2–3 weeks. The most common signs and symptoms are hepatosplenomegaly, respiratory distress, and fever. Other common signs and symptoms include lymphadenopathy, abdominal distention, lethargy, and ear discharge. Diagnosis is made by chest radiograph, which most often demonstrates adenopathy and parenchymal infiltrates, and with a positive acid-fast bacilli smear, most often from a morning gastric aspirate. Neonates require combination therapy with isoniazid, rifampin, pyrazinamide, and an aminoglycoside. If possible, a repeat chest X-ray should be obtained 1–2 months after starting therapy. The current WHO recommendation is to vaccinate all infants with the BCG vaccine in countries with a high burden of TB. In infants with congenital TB, vaccination should be delayed. If an infected mother started treatment less than 2 months before delivery, the current recommendation is to give the infant isoniazid for 6 months and then vaccinate the child with BCG. Long-term follow-up is recommended for infants given the BCG vaccine and who were born to HIV-positive mothers due to the risk of disseminated BCG disease in infants who ultimately are found to be HIV positive.

Tetanus

Neonatal tetanus, caused by *Clostridium tetani*, is a rapidly progressing illness that is fatal in 85 % of untreated infants. It has been eliminated in the developed world with the tetanus toxoid vaccine, but neonatal tetanus still remains a problem in resource-limited countries. In 2008, it was estimated that 59,000 neonates died of neonatal tetanus. Typically, infants with neonatal tetanus present with poor sucking and inability to feed after 3–10 days of normal feeding and a strong sucking reflex. Poor ability to suck can be accompanied by spasms, stiffness (Fig. 9.1), and convulsions, eventually leading to death in most cases. The diagnosis is clinical and the treatment is multifold. First, the spasms should be controlled with diazepam or paraldehyde, and the infant should be kept in a quiet, dark room. If available, tetanus immune globulin and metronidazole should be given to the infant. If metronidazole is not available, penicillin can be used for antimicrobial therapy. The site of the presumed entry point (e.g., umbilical stump or wound) should be cleaned and debrided. Given the risk of aspiration, oral feeds should be avoided. Finally, infants with tetanus are at higher risk of airway obstruction and a tracheotomy may be needed. Neonatal tetanus is entirely preventable with three doses of tetanus toxoid vaccine provided to the mother. Less than three doses have also been shown to significantly reduce mortality. Finally, clean birth and cord care practices can also prevent tetanus.

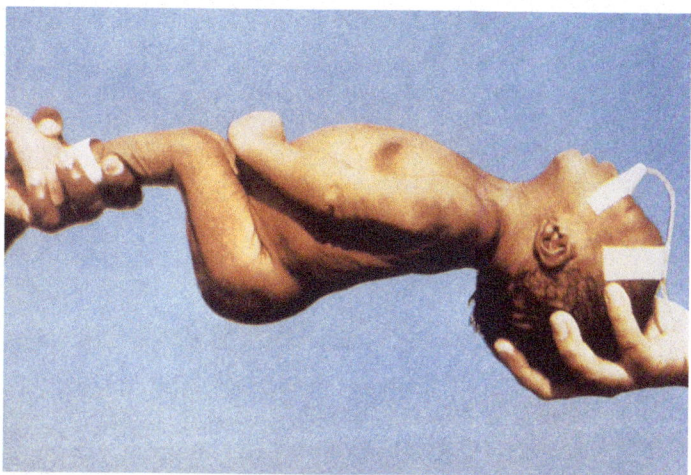

Fig. 9.1 Neonatal tetanus (*Source:* Centers for Disease Control. Public Health Image Library. Available at: http://phil.cdc.gov)

Eye Infections

Ophthalmia neonatorum is defined as purulent conjunctivitis in the first 28 days of life and the prevalence ranges from 1.6 to 12 %. The two most common causes are *Neisseria gonorrhoae* (Fig. 9.2) and *Chlamydia trachomatis*. Exposed neonates born to mothers with these infections develop an ophthalmic infection in 30–42 % with gonococcus and 30 % with *Chlamydia* if the infants do not receive prophylactic eye treatment. Gonococcal infection can lead to corneal ulceration, perforation, and blindness, while *Chlamydia* infection tends to be milder. Rarely, gonococcal infection can disseminate, leading to arthritis, sepsis, and meningitis. Clinically, disease caused by either organism is indistinguishable, although gonococcal infection usually presents earlier. A Gram stain of the purulent discharge can aid in the diagnosis. Treatment of gonococcal infection includes a single dose of ceftriaxone or cefotaxime, and *Chlamydia* conjunctivitis can be treated with oral erythromycin. Effective prevention strategies include primary prevention of STIs, antenatal screening and treatment of STIs, and provision of eye prophylaxis at birth: 1 % silver nitrate is highly effective and inexpensive, although it may cause chemical conjunctivitis; 1 % tetracycline and 0.5 % erythromycin are more expensive options that are equally effective and reduce the risk of chemical conjunctivitis. More recently, povidine–iodine, which is very inexpensive, has also been shown to be effective. It has not been tested enough, however, to recommend routine use.

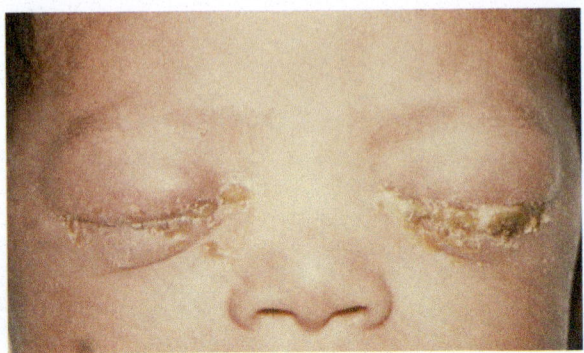

Fig. 9.2 Congenital gonococcal eye infection (*Source:* Centers for Disease Control/J. Pledger. Public Health Image Library. Available at: http://phil.cdc.gov)

Skin Infections

Newborns have many risk factors for skin infections, including absent microflora, a severed umbilical cord, possibly a circumcision site, and exposure to multiple pathogens. The most common microorganism that causes skin infections in the newborn period is *S. aureus*. These infections usually present with a rash consisting of vesicles and pustules, crusting, erythema, warmth, and drainage. If the pathogen invades deeper, the infant may develop bloodstream infection. Often the diagnosis can be made based on the appearance of the rash, but a wound culture can also be helpful. Superficial wounds should be cleaned with chlorhexidine or gentian violet. If cellulitis is present, then systemic antibiotics should be used with an antistaphylococcal agent such as cloxacillin (Table 9.1). Heating pads may be useful to induce spontaneous drainage, while abscesses that do not spontaneously drain will require incision and drainage. Skin infections can be prevented by frequent diaper changes and keeping the infant clean and bathed.

Umbilical Infections

Although many, highly effective strategies have been developed to reduce the incidence of umbilical infections, omphalitis continues to be a problem particularly for home births. There is limited data regarding the incidence of omphalitis. Hospital-based studies range from 2 to 77 infections per 1,000 infant births and the few community-based studies report rates of 55–197 infections per 1,000 births. Omphalitis is a local infection that presents with redness, pus, and foul odor. If not treated promptly, it can spread to the abdominal wall and then to the blood stream and liver. The diagnosis is clinical and treatment involves antimicrobial therapy.

Although the WHO current recommendation is to not apply anything to the umbilical cord, recent studies have shown that applying 4 % chlorhexidine to the umbilical stump daily in the first week of life has reduced mortality. Prevention is key in reducing omphalitis and includes avoiding application of possibly infectious substances (cow dung, mustard oil), hand washing, and the use of clean equipment to cut the cord. If there is evidence of infection, antibiotic therapy should be targeted against staphylococci as these are the most common infecting pathogens. Current recommendations are to use a combination of cloxacillin and gentamicin.

Syphilis

Syphilis is caused by *Treponema pallidum*, and transmission most often occurs prenatally. The chance that an infant will become infected depends on the maternal stage of syphilis. The transmission rate ranges from 8 % in late latent maternal infections to 60–100 % in untreated primary or secondary infections. Only about one-third of live-born infants with syphilis will manifest symptoms, while the other two-thirds will be asymptomatic at birth and later develop signs and symptoms. Early congenital syphilis has a wide range of effects on the newborn that can affect any organ system. Infants will often present in the first 8 weeks of life with pseudoparalysis, rhinitis, jaundice, hepatosplenomegaly, lymphadenopathy, and a maculopapular or papulosquamous rash, particularly in the diaper area, palms of the hands, or soles of the feet (Fig. 9.3). The diagnosis is usually made clinically and can be

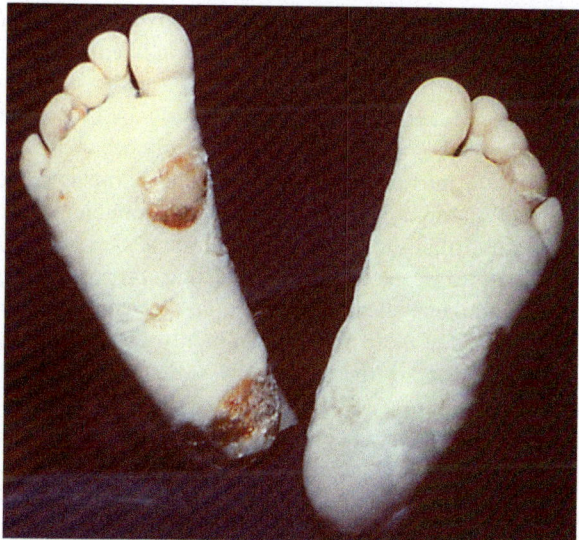

Fig. 9.3 Congenital syphilis rash on the soles of a newborn's feet (*Source:* Centers for Disease Control. Public Health Image Library. Available at: http://phil.cdc.gov)

supported by serologic findings if available (RPR, VDRL). Treatment of congenital syphilis is IV penicillin G for 10 days. Asymptomatic infants born to mothers who are RPR positive should be given a single dose of benzathine penicillin at birth. The most important aspect of prevention is testing and treating pregnant women.

Hepatitis B Virus (HBV)

It is estimated that more than 350 million people worldwide are currently infected with HBV. Mothers who are positive for Hepatitis B early antigen and who have high serum DNA levels are at high risk for passing the virus to their fetus. Even with active and passive immunization of newborns within the first 24 h of life, infants are still at risk. Six percent of infants born to mothers who are positive for Hepatitis B early antibody will develop fever, jaundice, and hepatic tenderness by 2 months of age. The rest, who do not develop acute hepatitis, will be asymptomatic. Hepatitis B immunoglobulin, although usually not available in developing countries, should ideally be given to neonates in conjunction with the HB vaccine within the first 24 h of life to infants born to mothers who are known HBV carriers. The HB vaccine alone, given in the first 24 h of life, is 70–95 % effective in preventing perinatal HBV infection. As part of a larger prevention strategy, the HB vaccine should be given to all children. Maternal Hepatitis B infection is not a contraindication to breastfeeding.

Toxoplasmosis

Congenital toxoplasmosis, caused by *Toxoplasma gondii*, causes serious problems for the newborn including blindness and deafness. Mothers who are infected by *T. gondii* often have mild symptoms or are asymptomatic, and the disease can go unrecognized. Higher transmission rates are observed as mothers acquire the infection later in pregnancy. Infection primarily occurs by consuming undercooked meat, or coming into contact with soil or drinking water contaminated by cat feces. Currently, there is no prevalence data for congenital toxoplasmosis from developing countries. Infants can have signs and symptoms at birth, during the first few months of life, or even later. The acute infectious process often manifests with chorioretinitis, anemia, convulsions, jaundice, hydrocephalus, fever, and hepatosplenomegaly. CSF studies of these patients commonly demonstrate xanthochromia, mononuclear pleocytosis, and increased protein level. In the blood, patients may have leukocytosis or leucopenia (e.g., WBC <5,000 or >30,000). Eosinophilia may also be present. IgM, IgA, or IgE antibodies in the blood stream, when not contaminated by maternal blood, are diagnostic but are unlikely to be available in resource-limited settings. Infants with congenital toxoplasmosis should be treated with pyrimethamine, sulfadiazine, and leucovorin. Prevention can be achieved through education, serologic testing, and treatment of pregnant women. Women should be educated to cook meat well done, practice frequent hand washing, and to avoid materials that could be contaminated by cat feces, such as raw unwashed vegetables. There are very limited testing and treatment options available in resource-limited settings.

Rubella

Since the introduction of the rubella vaccine, the incidence of congenital rubella syndrome (CRS) has dramatically decreased; however, it still remains a problem in the developing world. In 2003, the WHO estimated that CRS affected >100,000 infants worldwide. Mothers who acquire the infection earlier in pregnancy have an increased risk of having an infant with congenital anomalies. Although some infants will be symptomatic at birth, most will be asymptomatic with the majority of those patients presenting with symptoms before the age of 5 years. CRS affects multiple organ systems and commonly presents with adenopathy, encephalitis, pulmonary arterial hypoplasia, patent ductus arteriosus, hearing deficits, intra- and extrauterine growth restriction, hepatosplenomegaly, interstitial pneumonitis, neurologic deficits, and thrombocytopenia. The classic "blueberry muffin" rash (dermal erythropoiesis) is present in less than 20 % of cases (Fig. 9.4). The diagnosis should be suspected in any infant born to a mother with confirmed or suspected rubella anytime during the pregnancy. The diagnosis can be confirmed by the presence of IgM antibody in the cord serum, or IgG levels can be monitored over time in the infant to see if this persists. There are few treatment options available, and no specific medication has been shown to be effective for CRS. Immunoglobulin, if available, can be given to rubella susceptible women who have had an exposure. Management of an infant with CRS will require a multidisciplinary team. The best prevention against CRS is active immunization of children and adolescents.

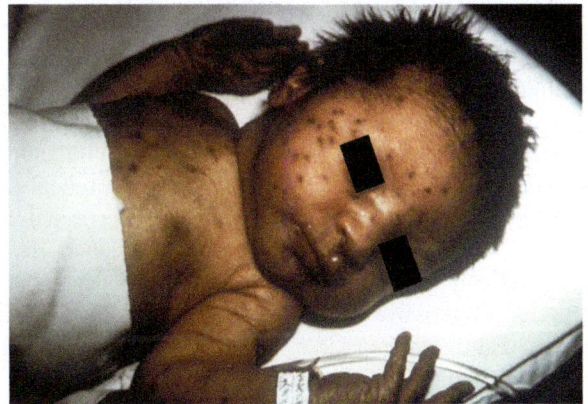

Fig. 9.4 "Blueberry muffin" rash of congenital rubella (*Source:* Centers for Disease Control. Public Health Image Library. Available at: http://phil.cdc.gov)

Cytomegalovirus (CMV)

CMV can be a devastating illness if acquired congenitally. CMV is commonly acquired early in childhood in developing countries, with preschool children in sub-Saharan Africa, South America, and Asia demonstrating 95–100 % seropositivity. Congenital CMV is a result of transplacental transmission, although it can also be transmitted via the genital tract and through breastmilk. Infants with congenital CMV most commonly present with petechiae, hepatosplenomegaly, and jaundice. Microcephaly is the most common neurologic finding. Diagnosis is mainly clinical, and simple laboratory findings such as elevated alanine aminotransferase and thrombocytopenia can be helpful. Other laboratory tests to confirm the diagnosis are expensive and likely not available in resource-limited settings (culture, shell vial assay, immunoflourescence, antigenemia). In infants who have life-threatening or sight-threatening disease, gancilovir or foscarnet can be considered as treatment options. There are currently no recommendations for prevention of CMV infection other than education. Women of childbearing age should be aware that the most common sources of CMV infection are sexual contacts and exposure to infected children.

Herpes Simplex Virus (HSV)

Congenital HSV remains a problem both in the developing and developed world. It can be acquired in utero, intrapartum, or postnatally; however, the vast majority of infections are acquired intrapartum. Women who have HSV-2 can shed the virus in genital secretions and infect their newborns. It is important to note that women who do not have active lesions can also shed the virus, as only 30 % of infants with neonatal herpes were born to mothers with symptomatic lesions or recognized contact with an HSV-positive partner. The disease usually presents at birth and affects multiple organ systems including the skin, eye, mouth, and CNS with approximately one-third experiencing encephalitis. Skin, eye, and mouth lesions typically appear within the first 7–10 days and can be either individual vesicles or clusters of vesicles (Fig. 9.5). Keratoconjunctivitis is the primary eye finding. Clinical diagnosis can be difficult as enteroviral and bacterial infections can present similarly. Viral cultures (e.g., from skin lesions, CSF, naso-oropharynx, rectum, urine) are diagnostic; however, since viral cultures are unlikely to be available, providers should be familiar with the clinical presentation and have a low threshold for treating if the diagnosis is suspected. The treatment of choice is acyclovir and has been shown to be safe in newborns. In terms of prevention, the current recommendation is that women at or beyond 36 weeks gestation should be offered suppressive therapy until delivery. A vaginal examination should be performed at the time of labor, and if active lesions are present, an elective cesarean section should be performed.

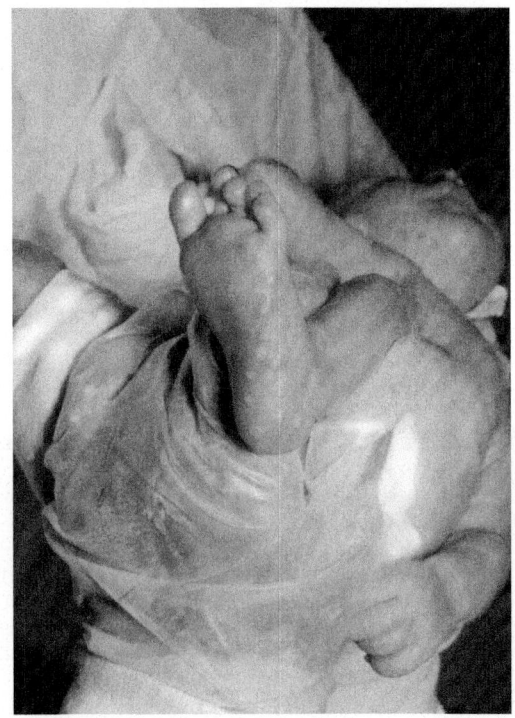

Fig. 9.5 Congenital herpes lesions on the soles of newborn's feet (*Source:* Centers for Disease Control/ Judith Faulk. Public Health Image Library. Available at: http://phil.cdc.gov)

Prevention

There are several interventions from periconceptional care to postnatal care that can have a dramatic impact on reducing neonatal infections. The chapter on maternal health describes in details peri-conceptual and antenatal interventions available to help ensure women are in good health. These interventions include good nutrition, iron and folic acid supplements, tetanus toxoid vaccinations, insecticide-treated bednets and intermittent presumptive treatment for malaria, and diagnosis and treatment of other infections, such as sexually transmitted infections, urinary tract infections, and tuberculosis.

During the intrapartum period, it is essential that all individuals involved in the delivery use hygienic practices. In particular, hands, instruments, and the delivery surface should be clean. It is also important to avoid unnecessary vaginal exams, keep the perineum clean, and prevent prolonged labor. Antibiotics should be provided to laboring mothers who have preterm/premature rupture of membranes, chorioamnionitis, or puerperal sepsis. Use of corticosteroids in women with preterm labor at less than 34 weeks gestation is routine practice to prevent respiratory distress syndrome and hyaline membrane disease in industrialized countries, but it is currently being evaluated for feasibility and effectiveness in resource-limited settings.

After delivery, mothers should be counseled on immediate and exclusive breastfeeding for 6 months, thermal care, hand washing, clean cord care, and skin-to-skin care. It is important to educate families on unsafe traditional practices, such as the application of cow dung on the umbilical stump. All of these simple preventive interventions can significantly decrease the risk of neonatal infections.

Recommended Reading

1. Remington JS, Klein JO, Wilson CB, Nizet V, Maldonado Y. Infectious disease of the fetus and newborn infant. Philadelphia, PA: Saunders; 2010.
2. Edmond K, Zaida A. New approaches to preventing, diagnosing, and treating neonatal sepsis. PLoS Med. 2010;7(3):e1000213.
3. Ganatra HA, Zaidi AK. Neonatal infections in the developing world. Semin Perinatol. 2010;34(6):416–25.
4. WHO. Save the children. Supplement on neonatal infection. Pediatr Infect Dis J. 2009;28(1):Supplement.
5. WHO. Integrated management of pregnancy and childbirth. Managing newborn problems: a guide for doctors, nurses, and midwives. Geneva: WHO; 2003.
6. WHO. Pregnancy, childbirth, postpartum and newborn care: a guide for essential practice. 2006. http://www.who.int/reproductivehealth/publications/maternal_perinatal_health/924159084X/en/.

Part III
Adolescent Health

Chapter 10
Adolescent Global Health

Karen Sadler and Nupur Gupta

Keywords Adolescent health • Social determinants of health • Risk and protective factors • Health promotion and prevention

Overview

- Adolescence is a critical, yet underserved, life phase with respect to global health
- Adolescence is a life phase that is both inconsistently defined and changing
- Health-related decisions made during adolescence and their effects track strongly into adulthood
- Social forces have strong inputs into adolescent health and well-being
- Data on the health of the world's adolescents are incomplete and few indicators are currently well measured

---

K. Sadler, M.D. (✉)
Pediatrics Department, Newton-Wellesley Hospital, 2014 Washington St., Newton, MA 02462, USA

MassGeneral Hospital for Children, Boston, MA, USA
e-mail: ksadler@partners.org

N. Gupta, M.D., M.P.H.
MassGeneral Hospital for Children, Harvard Medical School,
55 Fruit Street, Boston, MA 02114, USA
e-mail: ngupta3@partners.org

Adolescence from a Global Perspective

"Adolescence" as a life phase is a concept that has only existed in high-income societies for 100 years, and in others, for a much shorter time, if at all. It is traditionally defined as beginning with the onset of pubertal changes—which fell in many countries through the first half of the twentieth century from 12 to 10 years—and ending with the attainment of social maturity, defined as the completion of role transitions (marriage, employment, education, parenthood) to adult members of society. Though a useful construct, it is one that is both changing and inconsistent among countries. Earlier puberty and (a more recent trend) the later attainment of mature social roles has lengthened this life phase. Moreover, the formerly close sequence of marriage and childbirth, education, and employment is also increasingly spread out. The WHO defines adolescence as the period from 10 to 19 years, whereas "youth," as defined by the UN, spans the 15–24 year age range. Currently, the population group of 10–24 year olds is 1.8 billion, the largest in history, and accounts for one-fifth of the world's population (Figs. 10.1 and 10.2). Nine in ten adolescents live in low- or middle-income countries (Fig. 10.2). Demographically, they comprise a larger percentage of these countries, as opposed to higher-income nations, where their impact will expand as they become tomorrow's adults.

Adolescence is increasingly recognized, along with the very young, as a critical health period, but one that is still underserved. Indeed, there have been fewer gains in global adolescent health than in younger age groups. Health-related decisions made during adolescence track strongly into adulthood, creating (or alleviating) a social burden of illness. Alcohol use, unsafe sex, limited use of contraception and multiple partners, and risky transportation often begin during these years and are all leading risk factors for future disease and disability. The longer span from puberty to adult social roles translates into more time for exposure to sexually transmitted infections, alcohol and tobacco initiation, and other risky behaviors. Mental health issues, an important and largely neglected area, are thought to be a factor in 45 % of the 2.6 million yearly deaths in this age group. Early life experiences, from antenatal nutrition to the devastating effects of war and social unrest, can alter health trajectories. The age of child-bearing, though variable among countries, largely begins in this period. One-third of the world's adolescents enter into marriage, which is closely related to early childbirth in this subpopulation. In low-income countries, approximately 12 % of births are to mothers aged 15–19 years. Thus, the health and well-being of the next generation begins with our current youth.

Adolescent Development as a Social Determinant of Health

Research on the neurobiology and cognitive development of adolescence illuminates the biological basis for adolescent behavior, highlighting both strengths and vulnerabilities. Brain volume peaks in early adolescence, decreasing by early

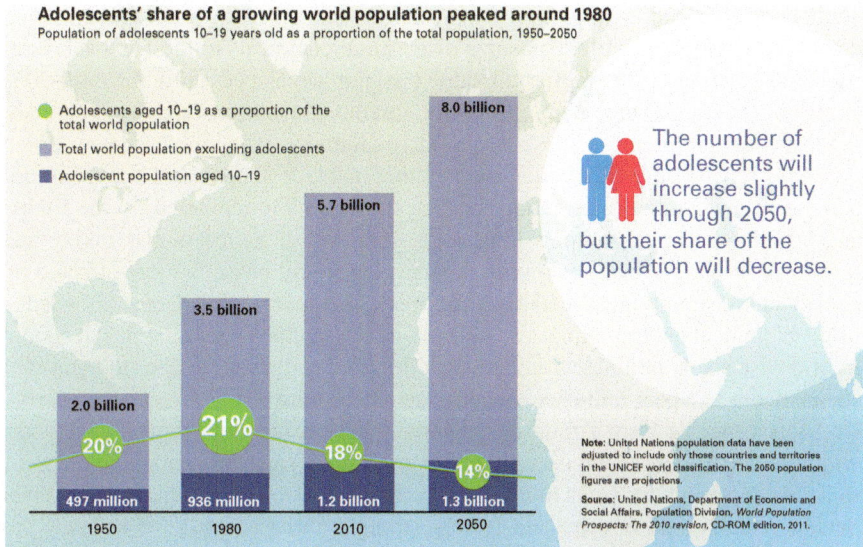

Fig. 10.1 Adolescent population: 1950–2050. From Progress for Children: a report card on adolescents. Number 10, April 2012 UNICEF Report. Reprinted with permission from UNICEF

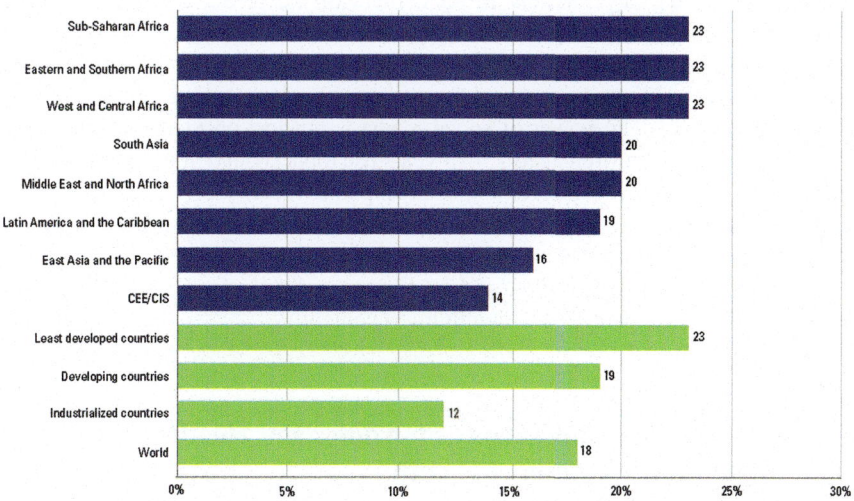

Fig. 10.2 Adolescents, 10–19 years old, as a proportion of the total population, by region, 2010. From Progress for Children: a report card on adolescents. Number 10, April 2012 UNICEF Report. Reprinted with permission from UNICEF

adulthood. This is thought to represent synaptic pruning, as the brain is shaped and modeled in response to life exposures, from illicit chemicals to the feedback from social interactions. The prefrontal cortex is not developed until the mid-20's, explaining the improvement in self-control, forethought, and rational decision-making that occurs from mid-adolescence to early adulthood. The limbic system, which processes reward and stimulation, on the other hand, develops earlier. It is in mid-adolescence when the differential between the behaviors regulated by the limbic and prefrontal cortical systems is greatest, resulting in a time of risk-taking and reward seeking. Decision-making in this developmental phase is more affected by stress and high emotion, as well as by the presence of peers. As a deeper knowledge of the biological underpinnings of "normal" adolescent behavior emerges, it should inform wise social policies: from the legal drinking and smoking ages to the use of social media as a peer influence on adolescent decisions.

Adolescence is also a time of potentially increasing involvement and voice within society. Many social movements, from the civil rights movement in the USA to the Arab Spring uprisings more recently, have been fomented among the young. Seeking change and novelty and feeling strongly about one side of an issue are hallmarks of adolescent behavior. While activism can bring empowerment and positive change, fostering active citizenship among the rising adult population, exposure to violence and the penal system can negatively impact health and development.

A final general consideration for adolescent global health is the sea change being brought by the digital age. As access to technology increases, the internet will bring the world's notable events, both good and bad, to a worldwide audience instantaneously, impacting development in all corners of the globe. Exposure to social media sites, coincident with the strong peer influence of normal early and mid-adolescence, can have both positive and negative consequences. Cyber-bullying, sexting, internet addictions, and social contagion phenomenon are new health morbidities of this era. The power of social media is not lost on the corporate world. Currently, 17 % of children aged 13–15 years use tobacco, and 90 % of adult smokers began before age 20 years. As tobacco companies reach young markets in lower-income countries, the disparity between male and female smoking rates is diminishing. On the other hand, this powerful technology, as witnessed by the current American. First Lady's "Let's Move Campaign," can also be marshaled as an agent for social engagement and health improvement.

Impact of Culture and Society on Adolescent Health: The Social Determinants of Health

Comparatively, adolescents and young adults are a healthy group, having survived early childhood and not yet afflicted with the morbidities of older generations. Much of what determines health and well-being in this group, therefore, are factors found in the larger social context. The pathways by which the social context impacts health are divided into two groups, called structural and proximal determinants.

Structural determinants operate on a global or national level and include how the world's wealth is distributed, how well nations provide access to wealth, employment, and education, and how social policies regulate transportation safety or access to substances known to harm health, through laws and taxes.

1. *Wealth*: The overall wealth of a nation correlates positively with its health, but the "GINI Index," which reflects income disparity within the nation, must also be considered. As the gap between rich and poor closes, national health increases—mediated in part through more robust employment, better mental health, access to medical care, and other cumulative factors.
2. *Education*: Access to education is a critical structural determinant, especially for girls. While only 4 % of American, Canadian, and Western Europeans girls are not in school in the early high school years, this number rises to 33 % in low- and middle-income countries. Better education is firmly linked to many improved health indices: fewer pregnancies, lower infant mortality, better health in both adolescents and their offspring, and a decrease in risky behaviors.
3. *War and conflict*: Violence, conflict, and social upheaval can have severe negative impacts on both physical and emotional health trajectories.
4. *Gender issues*: The inequalities between the sexes found within societies and ethnic groups also impact health. In low-income countries, greater sex inequalities correlate into poorer health indices for both sexes. For females in particular, cultural practices such as early marriage, or the demand to stay home and care for siblings, impacts education and income potential. Severe cultural practices such as female genital mutilation can lead to death or have signified long-term consequences. Access to contraception is often more difficult for the youngest ages. Though 44 % of married 15–19 year olds do not desire pregnancy, contraception is available to less than one-third. In sub-Saharan Africa, this age group accounts for 25 % of unsafe abortions. Early marriage is also a risk factor for HIV/AIDS in sub-Saharan Africa. It is the sixth leading cause of death among 10–24 year olds, and there are one million new infections in this age group yearly. In high-income countries, from early adolescence onward, there are differences in somatic complaints (more headaches in girls) and rates of injury and overweight (higher in boys). Overweight is burgeoning as a non-communicable disease worldwide, and one that tracks strongly from adolescence to adulthood. Furthermore, two-thirds of overweight adolescents have one or more risk factors for cardiovascular disease.

Proximal determinants work on a more local level, that of communities, families, peers, and individuals and are also called the "circumstances of daily life." Beyond educating children, schools perform an essential function for the world's youth: a strong school environment with engaged students and parents reduces risky behaviors, enhances healthy adolescent development, teaches leadership, and provides positive role models. Likewise for families: their strength, cohesiveness, and expectations correlate positively with health outcomes. Health-promoting parental behaviors serve as models for teens, and parental vigilance is a deterrent against negative peer pressures. Neighborhoods also factor in, promoting a sense of belonging, social cohesion (and acceptance), and a more involved citizenry.

Not surprisingly, for a population seeking identity through peer affiliation, teens also strongly influence each other with respect to health and wellness, largely through the adoption (or avoidance) or risky behaviors. Finally, decisions are ultimately made by individuals and can promote, or impair, future and present health. Individual temperament, self-esteem, risk-taking tendencies, intelligence, and resiliency can all effect health trajectories.

While no one determinant, on any level, provides the sole point of entry for health promotion efforts, each should be considered an opportunity. Interventions can thus be in the form of three crucial actions as proposed by Russell in an article entitled "Adolescence and the Social Determinants of Health" in *The Lancet*.

1. *Improvement in daily living*: These include interventions on a local level involving schools, neighborhoods, families, or individuals. Special note is made of safe driving initiatives and better employment and improved educational opportunities for girls in resource-poor settings.
2. *Structural changes*: Targeting youth poverty levels and better employment options, through loan programs, microfinance projects, and social policy and including improved road safety and gun control.
3. *Improvement of knowledge*: Efforts should be made to increase knowledge of the health of the young using health indices, and this knowledge should be shared and used to pave the way for consensus, awareness, and intervention.

Global Burden of Disease in Adolescence

The causes of mortality in the age group of 10–24 years depend greatly on the area of the world the individual resides in and whether they are male or female. Mortality rate rises by with age, irrespective of region, from 95 to 139 to 224 per 100,000, in the 10–14, 15–19 to 20–24 year groups, respectively (Fig. 10.3).

The World Health Organization classifies causes of mortality in young people into four groups: Group 1A, deaths related to maternal causes; Group 1B, those due to communicable diseases and nutritional disorders; Group II, due to non-communicable diseases; and Group III, deaths caused by injuries.

Patton, Coffey et al., in their study demonstrated that, although the main causes remained the same, the distribution of deaths varied widely from country to country with about half the mortality in adolescent women worldwide being accounted for by causes in the Group 1A and 1B with these being concentrated in the African regions. The deaths attributable to non-communicable diseases and injuries doubled from early to late adolescence in both males and females. In adolescent males, the majority (>50 %) of mortality was due to injuries globally and Group 1 and II contributed 28 and 21 %, respectively.

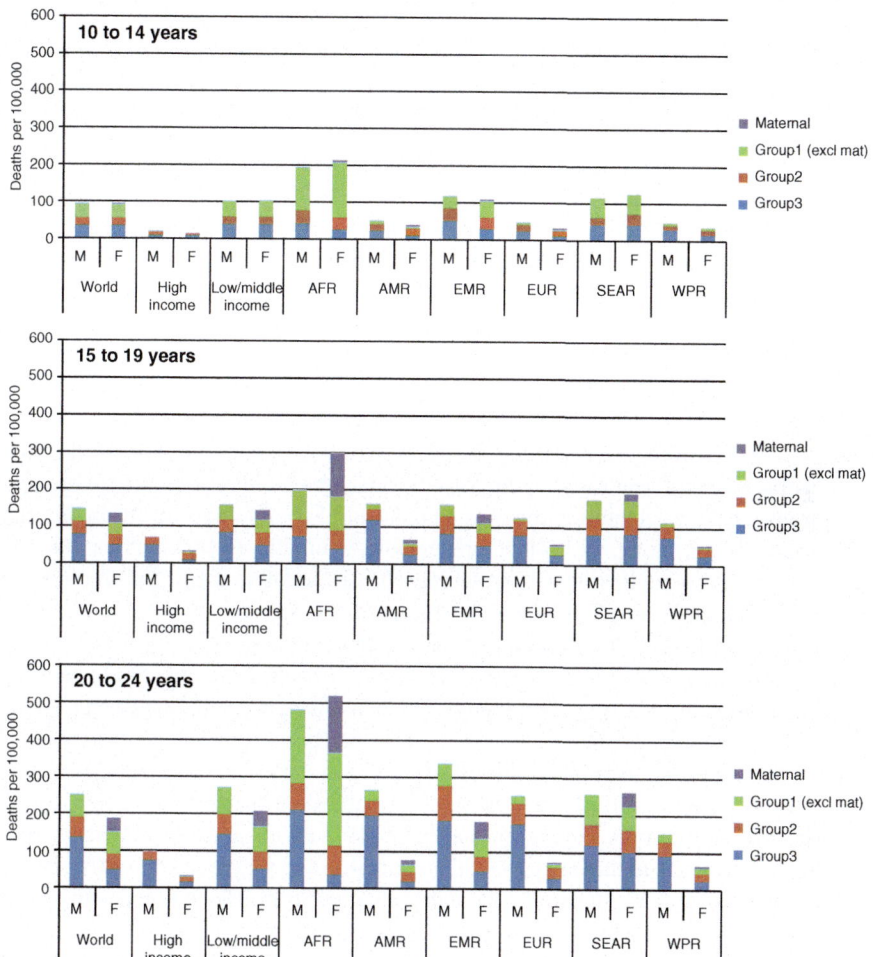

Fig. 10.3 Mortality rates (per 100,000) due to maternal, communicable, non-communicable, and injury causes. From Patton GC, Coffey C, Sawyer SM, Viner RM, Haller DM, Bose K, Vos T, Ferguson J, Mathers CD. Global patterns of mortality in young people: a systematic analysis of population health data. Lancet. 2009;374(9693):881–92. Reprinted with kind permission from Elsevier

The spectrum of disease also changes as this population becomes older with younger adolescents (10–15 years) being affected by both environmental and behavioral factors, while older ones are more likely to bear the consequences of risky behaviors like unsafe sex and drug use. Gender also plays a part with females more likely to suffer the effects of unsafe sex in developing countries as compared to their male counterparts. The burden of disease is measured by the sum of disability-adjusted life years (DALYs) for a region. It is conceptualized as the difference between the health situation of a region and an ideal one where everyone lives longer free of disease and disability. The burden of adolescent disease worldwide is concentrated in the following domains (Fig. 10.4):

1. *Neuropsychiatric disorders (including substance use)*: 20 % of the world's young people are affected by mental health issues in any given year, with 75 % of all serious mental illness presenting before the age of 24, making it a leading cause of disability in this age group. The prevalence varies across both developed and developing countries with the latter data being limited by the lack of mental health professionals who can provide diagnostic services. Therapeutic services are also scarce and the shame and stigma associated with such disorders further prevents young people from accessing available treatment. Six percent of all deaths in this age group can be attributed to suicide.
2. *Injuries*: Each year, 2.6 million people aged 10–24 years die worldwide. The leading cause of death is road traffic accidents, which kills 700 people in this age group each day accounting for 14 % of male and 5 % of female deaths in this age group. These, along with other preventable traumatic events such as suicide, homicide, war and violence, drowning and fire-related accidents account for 40 % of all deaths in this age group. Unintentional injuries also are a major cause of years of life lost due to disability (YLD) around the world.
3. *Pregnancy and childbirth*: Maternal deaths are greater in this age group because of the inherent risks related to pregnancy, which increase with decreasing age of the mother. Each year, 16 million adolescents become mothers, representing 11 % of all births worldwide (Fig. 10.5); in Latin America, Caribbean, and Sub-Saharan Africa approximately 20 % of all babies are born to girls aged 15–19. Maternal mortality is high in girls aged 15–19 with about 14 % of all maternal deaths occurring in this age group. Complications of pregnancy and delivery are a major cause of YLDs around the world ranging from 2 % in females in developed countries to about 20 % in low-income countries.
4. Communicable diseases including TB, parasitic diseases, and HIV: Adolescent HIV/AIDS affects about 2.2 million young people, with most of them being unaware of their status; 2,400 new infections occur daily (Fig. 10.6). HIV/AIDS and tuberculosis contribute to 11 % of deaths in this age group.
5. Tobacco and alcohol use are increasing global health concerns. Roughly 150 million young people use tobacco, and half of them will die prematurely because of this practice (Fig. 10.7).
6. Nutritional Issues: Poor nutrition (including under- and overweight) and anemia are also a major cause of morbidity and may contribute to early death in adolescent girls (Figs. 10.8 and 10.9).

Data on the health of adolescents in developing countries are sparse, with resultant huge knowledge gaps. What is available suggests that the major causes of death and disability are largely preventable and that a focus on this age group will

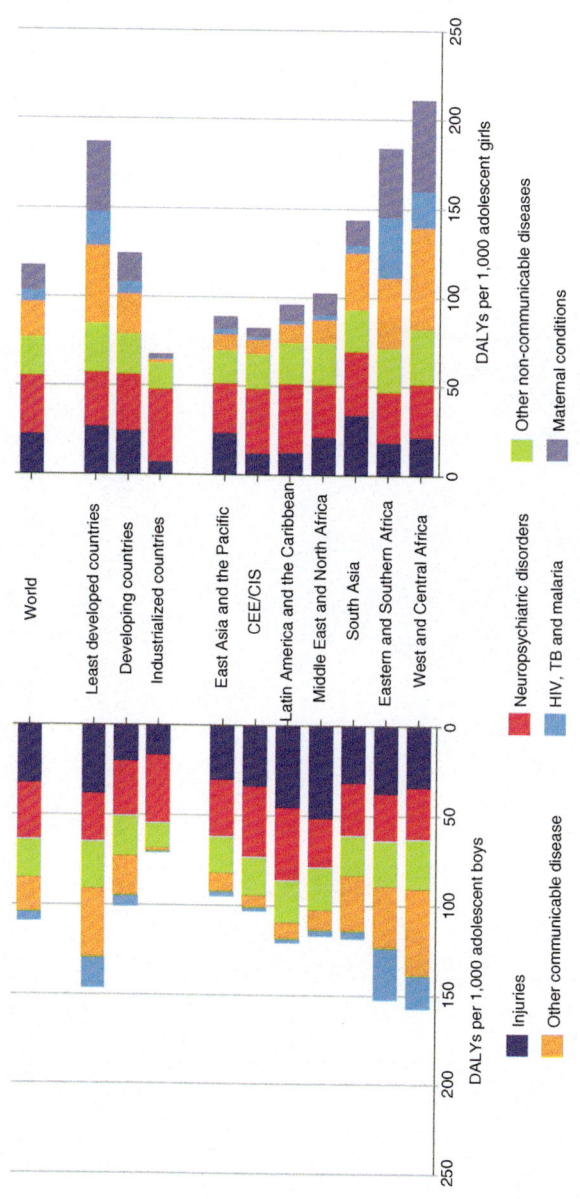

Fig. 10.4 Causes of disease burden in disability-adjusted life years per 1,000 adolescents by region and sex. From Progress for Children: a report card on adolescents. Number 10, April 2012 UNICEF Report. Reprinted with permission from UNICEF

Births among adolescent girls 15–19 years old as a percentage of total births, 2000-2010

Note: This map is stylized and not to scale. It does not reflect a position by UNICEF on the legal status of any country or territory or the delimitation of any frontiers. The dotted line represents approximately the Line of Control in Jammu and Kashmir agreed upon by India and Pakistan. The final status of Jammu and Kashmir has not yet been agreed upon by the Parties. The final boundary between the Republic of the Sudan and the Republic of South Sudan has not yet been determined. The final status of the Abyei area has not yet been determined.

Source: United Nations Department of Economic and Social Affairs, Population Division, *World Population Prospects: The 2010 revision,* CD-ROM edition, 2011, and '2011 Update for the MDG Database: Adolescent Birth Rate' (POP/DB/Fert/A/MDG2011), reanalysed by UNICEF.

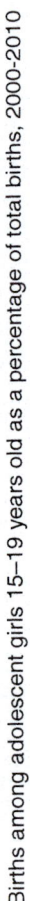

Fig. 10.5 Prevalence of births among adolescents aged 15–19 as a percentage of total births. From Progress for Children: a report card on adolescents. Number 10, April 2012 UNICEF Report. Reprinted with permission from UNICEF

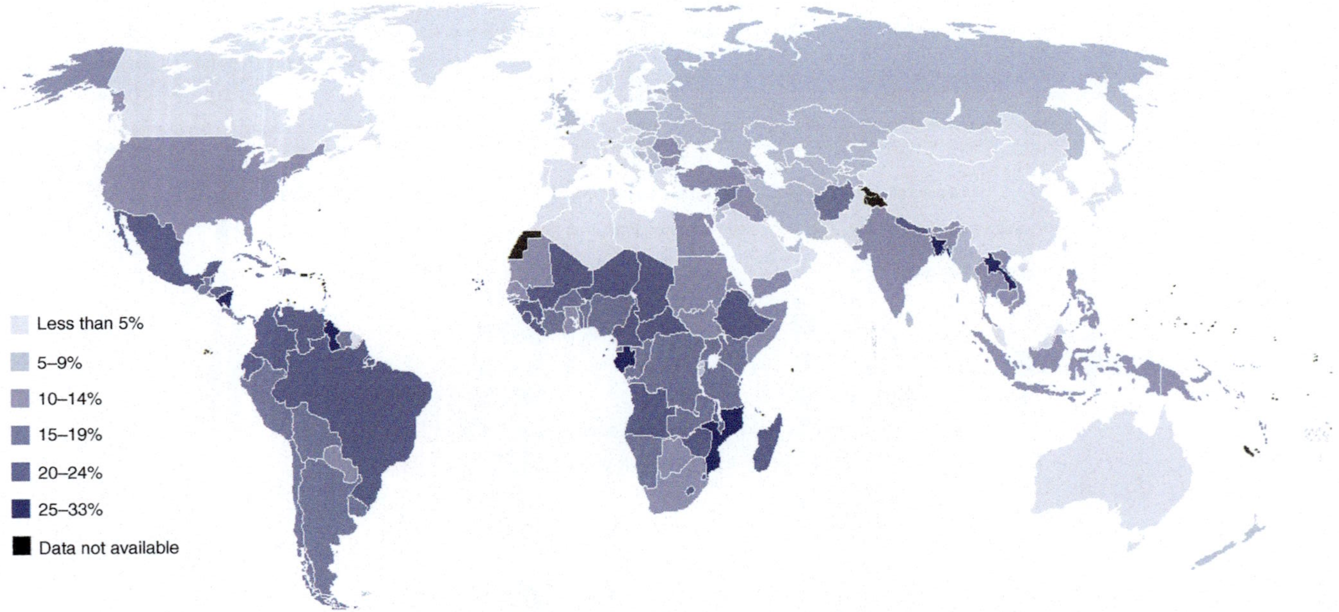

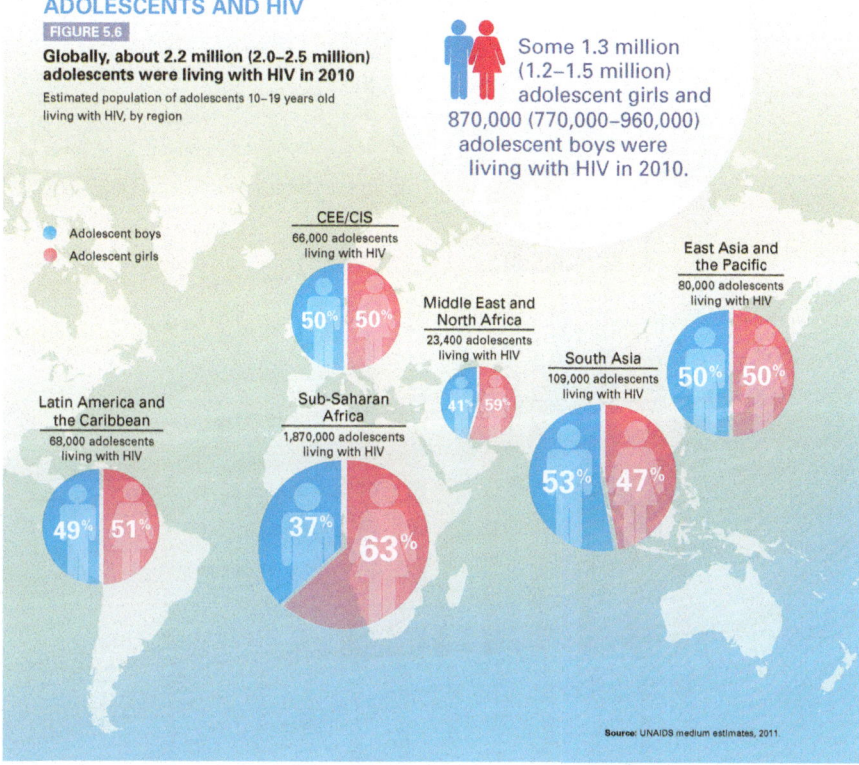

Fig. 10.6 Prevalence of HIV in adolescents globally. From Progress for Children: a report card on adolescents. Number 10, April 2012 UNICEF Report. Reprinted with permission from UNICEF

consolidate the gains made in childhood and improve adult health. Reduction in adolescent morbidity and mortality can have a significant impact on the achievement of the Millennium Development Goals (MDG), particularly MDG 5 and 6 (Table 10.1). However, other diseases like mental health disorders and substance abuse are being increasingly recognized to take root in the teenage years; injury and violence contribute significantly to mortality in this age group as well. Thus increased attention to health and disease in the younger population may prevent disability and death by early diagnosis and treatment. More comprehensive data collection on adolescent health parameters is needed, particularly from resource limited countries, to enhance our ability to channel services and resources where they are most needed.

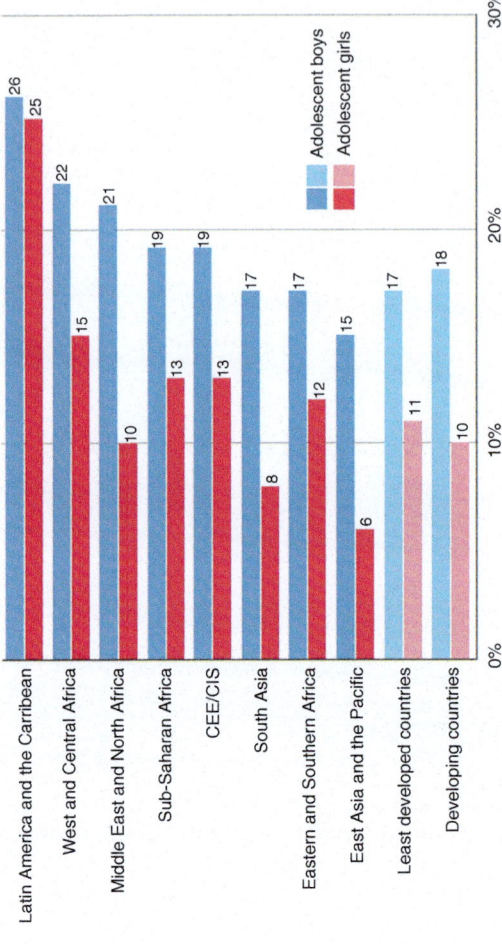

Fig. 10.7 Tobacco use among young adolescents (13–15 years). From Progress for Children: a report card on adolescents. Number 10, April 2012 UNICEF Report. Reprinted with permission from UNICEF

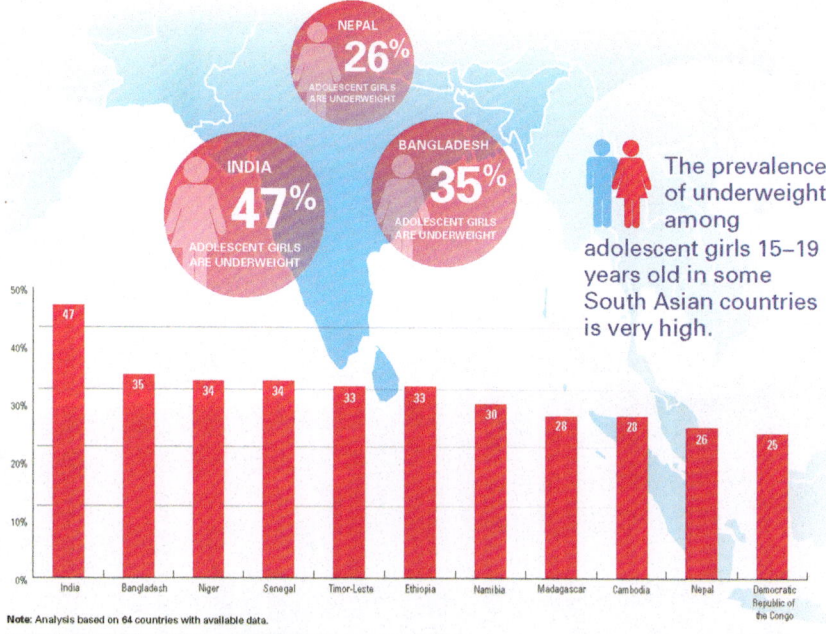

Fig. 10.8 Prevalence of underweight in adolescent girls 15–19 years. From Progress for Children: a report card on adolescents. Number 10, April 2012 UNICEF Report. Reprinted with permission from UNICEF

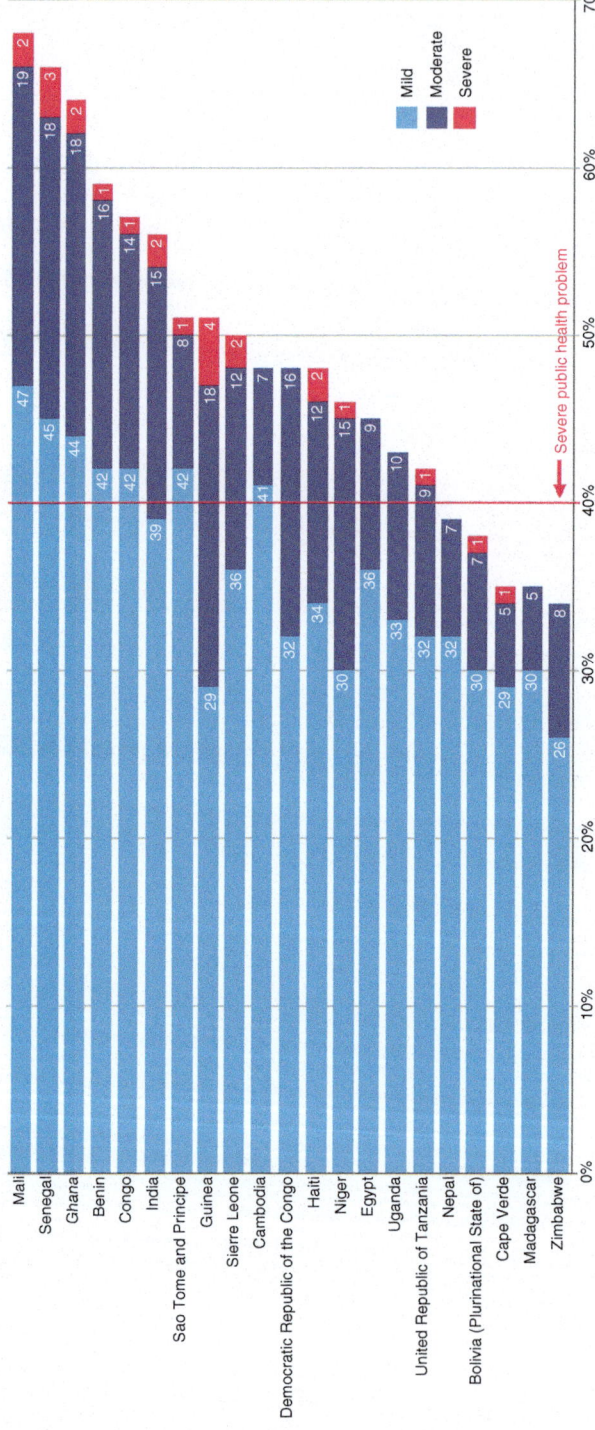

Fig. 10.9 Prevalence of anemia in adolescent girls 15–19 years. From Progress for Children: a report card on adolescents. Number 10, April 2012 UNICEF Report. Reprinted with permission from UNICEF

Table 10.1 Examples of global public health goals and the contribution of adolescence

Global health initiative	What is the problem?	Examples of the contribution made by adolescents
Improve maternal health (MDG 5)	– Only 23 countries are on track to achieve a 75 % reduction in maternal mortality ration by 2015 – Satisfying unmet need for contraception would cut maternal deaths by one-third – Nearly one in two of 42 million induced abortions annually are unsafe – Complications from induced abortions account for 13 % of maternal deaths	– About one in eight of all births in the developing world are to girls aged 15–19 – 44 % of married 15–19 year-old-girls in the developing world want to avoid pregnancy; less than one in three is using effective contraception – In Sub-Saharan Africa, 15–19-year-old females account for 25 % of all unsafe abortions
Reduce the spread of HIV (MDG 6)	– 33.3 million people were living with HIV at the end of 2009 – Over half of those with HIV live in sub-Saharan Africa; about 20 % live in the Asia Pacific region	– More than one million new HIV infections occur in the 15–24 age group each year, accounting for 41 % of new infections in those >15 years – HIV/AIDS is the sixth leading cause of death in 10–24 year olds and the second leading cause of death in 20–24 year olds – Early marriage is a risk factor for HIV/AIDS
Respond to the burden of mental disorders	– About half the population meets the criteria for one or more mental disorder in their lifetime	– The highest likelihood of first onset mental disorder is in the adolescent and young adult years: 75 % of adult mental disorder has its onset before 24 years of age, 50 % before 14 years – Anxiety and impulse control disorders have a median age range of onset in early adolescence (11–15 years), followed by substance use disorders (19–21 years) and mood disorders (24–30 years) – Neuropsychiatric disorders are the leading cause of global disability in 10–24 year olds – Self-inflicted injury is the second leading cause of death in 10–24 year olds

(continued)

Table 10.1 (continued)

Global health initiative	What is the problem?	Examples of the contribution made by adolescents
Respond to the burden of accidents and injuries	– In addition to 1.27 million annual deaths from road traffic accidents, there are 20–50 million nonfatal injuries – People from poor economic settings are disproportionately affected by road traffic accidents, even in high-income countries – The costs to governments of road traffic injuries is more than they receive in development assistance	– Road traffic accidents are the leading cause of death in 10–24 year olds – Road traffic accidents, suicide and homicide, violence and war, drownings, and fire-related incidents account for about 40 % of all 10–24-year-old deaths in comparison to older ages where injuries account for only 10 % – Road traffic accidents are the second leading cause of lost Disability-Adjusted Life Years in 10–24 year olds
Tobacco control	– Tobacco is the single largest preventable cause of premature death and disability – Up to half of the world's more than one billion smokers will die prematurely of a tobacco-related disease – Tobacco is responsible for about 8.4 million deaths each year, 70 % in developing countries	– The tobacco industry targets adolescents to generate nicotine addicted adults – 90 % of adult smokers are estimated to have started smoking before 20 years
Respond to the burden of NCDs	– Two out of three deaths each year are attributable to NCDs – Age-specific NCD deaths rates are nearly two times higher in LMIC than in HIC – Tobacco use accounts for one in six of all deaths from NCD	– Many risk factors for NCDs commonly start in adolescence, such as tobacco use, low physical activity, high blood pressure, and overweight and obesity – 70 % of premature deaths among adults are considered largely due to behaviors initiated during adolescence

Source: Adolescence: a foundation for future health. Lancet. 2012;379(9826):1630–40. doi: 10.1016/S0140-6736(12)60072-5, modified with permission

Recommended Reading

1. Sawyer SM, Afifi RA, Bearinger LH, Blakemore SJ, Dick B, Ezeh AC, Patton GC. Adolescence: a foundation for future health. Lancet. 2012;379(9826):1630–40.
2. Viner RM, Ozer EM, Denny S, Marmot M, Resnick M, Fatusi A, Currie C. Adolescence and the social determinants of health. Lancet. 2012;379(9826):1641–52.
3. Catalano R, Fagan AA, Gavin LE, Greenberg MT, Irwin CE, Ross D, Shek DT. Worldwide application of preventive science in adolescent health. Lancet. 2012;379(9826):1653–64.
4. World Health Organization. WHO Fact Sheet #345, Young people: health risks and solutions. Geneva: WHO; 2011.
5. Progress for Children: a report card on adolescents. Number 10, April 2012 UNICEF Report.
6. Patton GC, Coffey C, Sawyer SM, Viner RM, Haller DM, Bose K, Vos T, Ferguson J, Mathers CD. Global patterns of mortality in young people: a systematic analysis of population health data. Lancet. 2009;374(9693):881–92.

Chapter 11
Adolescent Preventative and Clinical Care: A Checklist

Nupur Gupta and Karen Sadler

Keywords Adolescents • Preventive care • Health promotion • High-risk behaviors

Overview

- Adolescents (10–19 year olds) constitute 18 % (1.2 billion) of the total world population and 90 % of them live in resource-poor countries.
- Focusing on adolescent health will help maintain the gains made in childhood through prevention and treatment of illnesses in the under-five age group.
- Two-thirds of premature deaths in adults and one-third of all illnesses presenting in adult life are linked to adolescent problem behaviors, such as substance use, unprotected sex, exposure to violence, and lack of physical activity.
- Maintaining the health of pregnant adolescents can have an intergenerational effect on the health of their offspring and thus future generations.
- Promoting health in adolescent populations around the world and providing services that prevent them from engaging in unhealthy behaviors can have far-reaching positive consequences.

N. Gupta, M.D., M.P.H. (✉)
MassGeneral Hospital for Children, Harvard Medical School,
55 Fruit Street, Boston, MA 02114, USA
e-mail: ngupta3@partners.org

K. Sadler, M.D.
Pediatrics Department, Newton-Wellesley Hospital, 2014 Washington St., Newton, MA 02462, USA

MassGeneral Hospital for Children, Boston, MA, USA
e-mail: ksadler@partners.org

Why Do Adolescents Require Special Attention?

Adolescents (10–19 year olds) constitute 18 % (1.2 billion) of the total world population and 90 % of them live in resource-poor countries. The significance of adolescent health is elaborated on in previous chapters and the importance of preventative care cannot be emphasized enough in the realm of health and disease particularly in the following three domains.

1. *Maintaining the gains made in child health*: Significant strides have been made in reducing childhood mortality in the neonatal and under-five age group, by public health investments in safe delivery, newborn care, and prevention of infectious disease by immunizations. Addressing causes of morbidity and mortality in adolescents will further strengthen these achievements.
2. *Effects on adult disease*: The World Health Organization reports that two-thirds of premature deaths in adults and one-third of all illnesses presenting in adult life are linked to adolescent problem behaviors, such as substance use, unprotected sex, exposure to violence, and lack of physical activity. Promoting health in this age group and providing services that prevent them from engaging in unhealthy behaviors can have far-reaching positive consequences. Furthermore, identification and enhancement of protective factors within the individual, family, and community has been shown to help increase resiliency and may mitigate the effect of risk factors in the creation of these behaviors.
3. *Effects on future generations*: The health of pregnant adolescents can affect the health of their fetuses and thus their offspring. These trans-generational effects occur when pregnant teens are exposed to infectious diseases like HIV, rubella, and hepatitis; suffer from malnutrition, micronutrient deficiencies, or diabetes; indulge in problems behaviors such as excessive use of tobacco, alcohol, and other drugs; or are exposed to violence. Preventive programs that target adolescents and young adults can thus influence the next generation.

Primary prevention is the mainstay of effecting change to keep adolescents healthy and disease free. In the 1980s, the American Medical Association developed the "Guidelines for Adolescent Preventative Services" (GAPS) (see Appendices K and L) to help providers screen for risky behaviors and intervene as necessary. In the US and other western countries such adolescent preventative services are usually provided at the time of the "annual physical." In low and middle–income countries a modified version of these could provide some guidance to doctors and health care worker who participate in the care of this population.

Research has shown that in young people problem behaviors can be prevented by modifying factors at the structural (societal or community), intermediate (family, school, peers), and individual levels. These can be "risk factors" that increase the probability of a disorder (e.g., abuse, neglect, violence exposure, poor health care), or "protective factors" that inhibit, reduce, or buffer the probability of a problem behavior (e.g., parental monitoring, problem-solving skills, and school connectedness).

However, in most of the world adolescents, who are otherwise a generally healthy population, rarely visit a hospital or a health care provider, and the concept of an "annual physical" does not exist. Thus, although it is evident that the majority of adult disease is preventable, that its inception is often in the teenage years, and that preventative measures are effective, the traditional model of screening and counseling cannot be utilized for most adolescents around the world.

Instead, adolescents can be targeted for intervention at times they present to providers for illness, pregnancy and delivery, accidents, etc., and in places where they are typically found, such as schools, places of work, on the streets, in shelters, and occasionally in prisons.

Providing Preventative Care

Preventative services for adolescents should thus focus on screening for, identifying and providing interventions for the following:

1. Nutritional Issues.
2. Infectious diseases including STIs and HIV.
3. Mental health Issues.
4. Substance use and abuse.
5. Violence and motor vehicle accidents.
6. Diseases related to pregnancy and delivery.

Providers should understand their own limitations and those of their patients as they attempt to engage the adolescent in discussion, screen for problems, provide counseling, seek interventions and reinforce follow-up. Screening tools could be utilized, keeping in mind that these may have not been validated in developing countries; in all cases, the cultural context must be considered.

A. *Screen* for:

1. *Nutritional issues*:
   History taking supplemented by anthropometric measurements plotted on WHO growth charts will help the provider assess for malnutrition, obesity, and for eating disorders. Assess for anemia and vitamin deficiencies utilizing clinical evaluation and lab testing where available.
2. *Infectious disease*:
   Obtain a comprehensive history for STIs, HIV, TB, parasitic infestations, and skin diseases.

   (a) STIs including chlamydia, gonorrhea, trichomonas, syphilis, and others can be identified and treated using syndromic diagnosis if more specific testing or lab facilities are not available (see Chap. 12). Elicit a complete sexual history and history of contacts/sexual partners so that treatment can be offered to them as well.

(b) Rapid HIV testing may be available in some clinics and must be offered to all adolescents. Counsel patients about HIV testing and treatment prior to performing the test.

(c) Testing for tuberculosis could include a tuberculin skin test (TST). Check for BCG vaccination as this could change the interpretation of the test. If the TST is positive a chest X-ray should be performed where possible and HIV testing offered. Treatment for TB should start immediately and contact tracing and treatment should be undertaken.

(d) Screen for parasites especially when associated with anemia. History and stool testing are useful in diagnosis, especially for hookworm. Some adolescents may be treated empirically by history alone if a stool specimen or lab testing is not available.

(e) Skin Disease: History and examination will help diagnose skin infections. Common infections and infestations include scabies, pediculosis, impetigo, and fungal infections. Counsel about basic hygiene, handwashing, and washing of linen in the house especially in cases of contagious diseases. Again reinforce that all contacts must be treated in these cases.

3. *Mental health Issues* (depression, anxiety, and major psychiatric issues):

(a) Depressive disorders often manifest as physical, somatic, emotional, or cognitive symptoms. Providers could use a screening questionnaire or the SIGECAPS screening tool. Presence of depressive symptoms (include irritability in children and adolescents) along with at least five of the following symptoms for more than 2 weeks suggests a major depressive disorder (DSM-IV) (Table 11.1).

(b) Screen for suicidal ideation.

(c) In many countries and cultures mental health diagnoses are not acceptable and psychiatric illness often will present with somatic complaints.

(d) Take a detailed history of psychiatric illness in the family and a history of attempted and completed suicide. For providers who can and choose to medicate, knowing what medications have been efficacious for other family members may help guide them in their choice of medication for their patients (see Chap. 25).

(e) Questions that could help:

- In the past few weeks have you often felt sad?
- Have you ever had thoughts about killing yourself, made a plan or attempted to kill yourself?
- Have you ever been so angry that you felt like hurting others?

Table 11.1 SIGECAPS screening tool

S	*S*leep—too little or too much
I	lose *I*nterest or pleasure
G	feelings of *G*uilt or worthlessness
E	decreased *E*nergy
C	decreased *C*oncentration
A	change in *A*ppetite or weight
P	*P*sychomotor agitation or retardation
S	*S*uicidal ideation

Data from Diagnostic and statistical manual of mental disorders, ed 4. Washington, DC: American Psychiatric Association; 1994
If five or more symptoms endorsed along with depressed mood or irritability for more than 2 weeks, consider a major depressive disorder

4. *Substance use*:

    (a) Take a detailed history including:

    - History of tobacco use in the patient and family. Also inquire about the use of chewing tobacco and snuff; alcohol use; illicit drug use, including marijuana, opium, cocaine, heroin, other hallucinogenic drugs, and inhalation of glue.
    - History of failing grades, aggressive or depressive behavior, stealing, excessive or inadequate sleep, isolating behaviors, or physical symptoms like staggering walk or clumsiness.
    - Take a complete history from the patient about drug use, psychological issues, mood changes, depression, and suicidal ideation, if possible without the parents in the room

    (b) Examine the patient:
    Conduct a thorough physical examination including a complete neurological examination. Check for signs of drug abuse (Table 11.2).

    (c) Test for:

    - Urine drug testing may be used if available.
    - HIV testing particularly in IV drug users.
    - Hepatitis B and C if possible in these patients.

    (d) Questions that could help:

    - Have you ever smoked a cigarette or marijuana, chewed tobacco, sniffed glue or inhalants, consumed alcohol, or used intravenous drugs?
    - In the past month have you ever smoked a cigarette or marijuana, chewed tobacco, sniffed glue or inhalants, consumed alcohol, or used intravenous drugs?

Table 11.2 Stigmata of drug use

Eyes	Red conjunctiva	Marijuana
	Occasionally watery	Inhalants
	Dilated pupils	Amphetamines, cocaine, crystal meth, LSD, PCP
	Constricted pupils	Heroin and other opioids, benzodiazepines
Skin	Track marks	Intravenous drugs
Nasal septum	Perforation	Cocaine use
Buccal mucosa	Staining, local irritation, leukoplakia	Chewing tobacco
Smell of substance on body, breath, and clothes	Associated odor	Alcohol, marijuana

Data from: Ali S, Mouton PC, Jabeen S et al. Early detection of illicit drug use in teenagers. Innov Clin Neurosci. 2011;8(12):24–28

- Do any of your friends smoke cigarettes or marijuana, chew tobacco, sniff glue or inhalants, drink alcohol, or use intravenous drugs?
- Have you ever been in trouble with the law or been in trouble for drug or alcohol use?

5. *Violence* (fights, gang membership, domestic, or dating): Screening for domestic and dating violence can also be a very sensitive issue. Exposure to violence, trauma and being part of organized crime, or being recruited as soldiers as adolescents can have long-term physical and mental health consequences. The safety of the patient must be kept in mind at all times. Legal recourse and counseling services may or may not be available. Providers can provide support and refer to local agencies if available or may have to seek the services of local nongovernmental organizations (NGOs). Questions that could help:

    (a) Do you or anyone in your family own a weapon?
    (b) Have you ever been worried about your safety?
    (c) Do you or have you ever carried a weapon to protect yourself?
    (d) Have you ever been in a physical fight in the past 3 months?

6. *Reproductive health needs*:
    Obtain a detailed sexual history, screen for pregnancy, and unmet contraceptive needs especially with young women who are more likely to be married or in union, sexually active, and less likely to seek care.

    (a) Sexual History should include:
    - Age of menarche, coitarche
    - Number of life time sexual partners, number of current sexual partners, and age of partners.

- History of survival sex (i.e., sex being sold for favors like food for the family or self, clothing, fees for school, etc.)
- History of sexual abuse and/or rape.
- Whether patient is married or betrothed.

(b) Screen for present and past pregnancies, miscarriages, and abortions. Adolescent pregnancies are more common in the developing world with 95 % of adolescent births occurring in low- and middle-income countries.

(c) Screen for contraceptive use and determine whether there is an unmet need for contraception. The unmet need for contraception remains high in adolescents especially in developing countries.

(d) Questions that could help:

- Have you ever been sexually active or are any of your friends?
- Do you use any method to prevent pregnancy?
- Have you ever been pregnant or had an abortion?
- Have you ever been told that you have a sexually transmitted infection?
- Do you and your partner always use condoms?
- Have you ever been forced to have sexual relations with a person or persons?

7. *Abuse* (physical, sexual, and emotional):
Screening for abuse especially in younger teenagers is important, but it again may be difficult to elicit. Resources for child protective services are few in most resource-limited settings. To help provide abused adolescents culturally competent counseling services, try to access the services of local social workers, if available, or agencies and NGOs that deal with these issues. Sometimes eliciting the support of the family and the extended family to ensure safety of the patient may be the only option available.

8. *Hypertension*:
Screen for hypertension at every visit. Most health centers have a manual blood pressure machine. If the systolic or diastolic blood pressure is greater than the 90th percentile for age and gender, repeat it at least three times in similar circumstances to confirm the accuracy of the result. A blood pressure reading that is between the 90th and 95th percentile is considered pre-hypertension, 95th–99th +5 mm of Hg is Stage I, and more than 99th +5 mm of Hg is considered Stage II hypertension. The guidelines recommend that the provider must initially offer non-pharmacologic treatment including counseling about a low fat and low sodium diet, regular exercise, weight loss, tobacco cessation, and abstinence from alcohol. If the hypertension does not respond to these measures, or if a patient with a blood pressure that is consistently over the 95th percentile is not responding to lifestyle management, or has evidence of end organ damage, then referral to a specialist, if available or pharmacologic treatment should be considered.

9. *Refractive errors*:
   These may be difficult to detect, but if suspected, use a Snellen's Chart to screen and then refer if possible for correction of refractive errors. Vision problems are an important cause of school failure and dropout. Adolescents rarely receive routine vision screening as there is often no routine care.
10. *TV and social media use (where relevant)*:
    With economic progress and with improved access to the internet, screening for internet addiction, cyber-bullying, addiction to video games and pornography is an important aspect of preventative services. These risks are magnified when combined with illiterate parents or those who are unfamiliar with the dangers of unmonitored media access.

B. *Assess* social determinants of health:

1. *Education*: Enquire about whether the adolescent is in school. Always ask about grade level, academic achievement, absenteeism, and tardiness. Never presume by age as often children and teenagers will drop in and out of school and may stay in the same grade for many years. Assess the risk involved in female adolescents in particular of dropping out of school. Girls are often forced to stay home to help with the care of younger siblings and household chores, or because of pregnancy. For those in school, ask about future educational and career aspirations.
2. *Family situation*: Enquire about living situations, relationships, marital status, pregnancies, and offspring.
3. *Economic status (income)*: This can often be determined by surrogate markers like living situations, type of house (brick, mud, thatched hut, etc.), method of transportation, and employment (of the patient and their parents).
4. *Food security*: Enquiring about the availability of food and distribution of food within the family is an important determinant of health. Also determining the nutritional quality of the diet and whether it includes all food groups may provide insight into the patient's health.
5. *Gender issues*: These can affect health in different ways in different countries and communities. Girls are more likely to drop out of school, be discriminated against, have less health seeking behavior, receive less attention paid to their health, and receive less food as compared to their male counterparts.
6. *Ethnicity and race*: These may also play an important part in determining health and well-being in different parts of the world. Discrimination because of race or ethnicity may result in mental health issues, physical violence, and food insecurity.
7. *Identify* risk and protective factors in individual, families, schools, and communities.

C. *Counsel* adolescents regarding:

1. *Provision of confidential care*: Confidentiality is often the premise of care in working with adolescents whether in developed or developing countries. Shame, stigma, and fear of consequences may prevent teenagers from seeking

care and allow disease to progress and spread within the community. Providers should try and engage their young patients, and reassure them, where possible, that their evaluation and treatment will not be disclosed to parents and caretakers. They should, however, remember to set limits of safety to this confidential care and make their patients aware of this from the outset. These include but are not limited to self-harm/suicidality or homicidality, sexual or physical abuse, and sometimes excessive drug use or indulging in other behaviors that may be life threatening. Often keeping this area "grey" is suggested and the comment "I would break confidentiality if I felt that the behaviors you are indulging in will put your life or that of another at risk," may help to keep the patient safe but at the same time win their confidence.

2. *Physical growth, psychosocial, and psychosexual development*: Discuss stages of adolescent development, puberty, menstrual issues, sexuality, positive body image, identity, independence, goal setting, and aspirations.
3. *Healthy diet and exercise*: Emphasize healthy eating; introduce simple concepts of food groups and having regular meals. Encourage exploring and challenging cultural beliefs about food and reinforce regular exercise.
4. *Prevention of injuries and safety issues*: Encourage use of seat belts in cars and helmets for both cycle and motorcycle travel. Ask about possession of a firearm and discuss firearm safety. Also, depending on country and circumstance, counsel about water safety (swimming in lakes, ponds, rivers) and fire safety measures especially where cooking is done over fire pits, kerosene stoves, or coal.
5. *Contraceptive methods, both hormonal and natural*: After assessing availability of different methods, advise about different methods of hormonal contraception (see Chap. 13). Natural family planning methods may be an option when other methods are not available or acceptable.
6. *Responsible sexual behavior*:
    (a) Reinforce condom use at all times, discuss risk of pregnancy, STIs, and HIV.
    (b) Also among female adolescents, increase awareness about antenatal care and options for safe abortions including the option of using emergency contraception (if locally available) if they become pregnant.
    (c) Whenever possible, include male partners in these discussions.
7. *Substance use*: Discuss dangers of tobacco, alcohol, and other drugs and consider using motivational interviewing techniques to help teenagers quit or reduce harm because of illicit drug use. Also increase awareness about clean needles and syringes for those who are IV drug users and at risk of HIV transmission.
8. *Mental health issues*: Counsel about how mental health can affect physical health and how often somatic symptoms may be a manifestation of depression, anxiety, or mood disorders. Educating health care providers, community health workers, and parents about mental health issues, and the effect these diseases can have on the health of adolescents is essential as this would facilitate early identification and quick access to treatment.

D. *Administer* immunization:

Providers should assess whether their teenage patient have received all required immunization and age-appropriate immunizations should be administered. The World Health Organization has no clear cut policies about adolescent immunization in developing countries. Most immunization programs in developing countries target infants and women of child-bearing age. Unimmunized teenagers can acquire and be affected by vaccine-preventable diseases and also serve as a source of infection to unimmunized infants with whom they are in contact; moreover adolescent mothers, if not adequately immunized, may be infected by diseases that have serious consequences for their unborn or infant child (e.g., rubella, pertussis, and Hepatitis B). Adolescent immunization also helps to boost the effects of childhood immunization and may contribute to the development of herd immunity.

Providers may use the WHO Delayed routine immunization schedule to help guide them with such teenage and young adult patients. (Appendix O: WHO Delayed routine immunization schedule)

In special circumstances, adolescent immunization may also be needed to:

1. Mitigate risk that may be related to travel (e.g., polio vaccination when individuals are travelling to endemic areas).
2. Protect adolescents engaging in activities that may endanger their health (e.g., Hepatitis B vaccination in drug users).
3. Confer protection related to residence (e.g., meningococcal vaccine for individuals who will live in close proximity, such as in college, prisons, and military training institutions).

Conclusion

Adolescent and adult mortality and morbidity is attributable to both communicable and non-communicable diseases often acquired in the adolescent years. Most of these diseases are related to adolescent high-risk behaviors such as violence, use of illicit or prescription drugs and alcohol, unprotected sex, unsafe driving, and mental health issues, all of which are largely preventable. This chapter outlines some of the ways adolescents can be screened and counseled for these risk factors and behaviors and is an attempt to create some guidelines for adolescent care in developing countries. Research in developed countries has shown that adolescent preventative programs that target risk and/or protective factors at the structural, intermediate and individual level can reduce problem behaviors and thus their effects on adolescent morbidity and mortality. However, more research data are needed on the prevalence of adolescent problem behaviors in developing countries so that preventative programs can be designed, taking into account the culture, and engaging the community, schools, family, and the teenagers themselves for effective and long-term gains in adolescent and young adult health.

Recommended Reading

1. Norman J, Montalto DO. Implementing the guidelines for adolescent preventive services. Am Fam Physician. 1998;57(9):2181–8.
2. Sawyer SM, Afifi RA, Bearinger LH, Blakemore SJ, Dick B, Ezeh AC, Patton GC. Adolescence: a foundation for future health. Lancet. 2012;379(9826):1630–40.
3. Catalano RF, Fagan AA, Gavin LE, Greenberg MT, Irwin Jr CE, Ross DA, Shek DT. Worldwide application of prevention science in adolescent health. Lancet. 2012;379(9826):1653–64.
4. WHO. Guidelines on preventing early pregnancy and poor reproductive outcomes among adolescents in developing countries. Geneva: WHO; 2011.
5. U.S. Department of Health and Human Services. The fourth report on the diagnosis, evaluation, and treatment of high blood pressure in children and adolescents. http://www.nhlbi.nih.gov/health/prof/heart/hbp/hbp_ped.pdf. Accessed May 2005.

Chapter 12
Sexually Transmitted Infections in Adolescents

Mark A. Goldstein and Nupur Gupta

Keywords Adolescents • Developing countries • Sexually transmitted infections • Disease prevention • Syndromic management

Overview

- Adolescents have a unique susceptibility to sexually transmitted infections (STIs).
- Early diagnosis and treatment of patients and their partners with STIs may help to prevent complications from the STI as well as transmission to others.
- There is an association between STIs and the acquisition and transmission of HIV infection.
- Syndromic management of STIs may be helpful in resource-limited settings where medical providers and laboratory facilities are scarce.

Prevalence of STIs Around the World and Burden of Disease

The World Health Organization estimates that 340 million new cases of curable bacterial and protozoal STIs (chlamydia, gonorrhea, syphilis, and trichomonas) occur every year worldwide. Although data about specific STIs are scarce,

---

M.A. Goldstein, M.D. (✉)
Division of Adolescent and Young Adult Medicine, MassGeneral Hospital for Children, Harvard Medical School, Room 508, 175 Cambridge St., Boston, MA 02114, USA
e-mail: mgoldstein@partners.org

N. Gupta, M.D., M.P.H.
MassGeneral Hospital for Children, Harvard Medical School, 55 Fruit Street, Boston, MA 02114, USA
e-mail: ngupta3@partners.org

especially in resource-limited settings, it is estimated that approximately 150 million occur in South and South-East Asia, 69 million in sub-Saharan Africa, 38 million in Latin America and the Caribbean, and 10 million in North Africa and the Middle East. Adolescents aged 15–24 have the highest reported prevalence: one in 20 acquires an STI, and one in four is diagnosed with such an infection each year.

Accurate data, especially in sexually active unmarried adolescents, are limited. What is available are survey data from family planning clinics; often the data are skewed as more studies are published in Africa than Asia and Latin America.

Chlamydia: Rates are highest in adolescent girls, with one-third of all cases worldwide occurring in this age group. Prevalence data can vary from 10 % in rural Nigeria to 40 % in sex workers in Senegal. Data in boys are limited.

Gonorrhea: Data on gonorrhea prevalence are limited, but estimates are well below 10 % in most studies from developing countries.

Syphilis: Not seen often in adolescence, but prevalence is estimated to be 5–8 % based on some studies done in Africa.

Herpes Simplex Virus 2: Prevalence varies by region: in sub-Saharan Africa, 30–80 % of women and 10–50 % of men are infected; in Central and South America, 20–40 % of women are infected; and in developing Asian countries, 10–30 % are infected.

Human Papilloma Virus: The prevalence of HPV infection around the world has been estimated epidemiologically to be between 9–13 % or about 630 million people. Of these infections 70 % are sub-clinical and the majority regress spontaneously. However some women have persistent pre-malignant intra-epithelial neoplasia and go on to develop cervical cancer. Globally there are 470,000 new cases of cervical cancer each year with about 240,000 deaths annually, mainly in developing countries.

Hepatitis B: 350 million cases of chronic hepatitis and one million deaths each year.

Adolescents' Unique Susceptibility to STIs and Barriers to Diagnosis and Treatment

Biological risk factors: Increased cervical ectopy, decreased cervical mucus, possible lower levels of secretory IgA, larger cervical transformation zone, increased trauma during intercourse, presence of other STI, douching, coitus during menses contribute towards making adolescents more at risk for STIs.

Behavioral risk factors: Use of licit and illicit substances during sex, multiple sexual partners, unprotected intercourse, early coitarche, coercive sex, having sex with partners who have had multiple partners, inconsistent use of condoms further increase the risk.

Cognitive risk factors: Lack of information about STIs and a sense of invulnerability may make adolescents more likely to suffer the consequences of unprotected sex.

Other Risk Factors:

- Lack of access to health care and/or confidential services.
- Many STIs are asymptomatic and so adolescents may not seek care.
- Poverty and homelessness, inability to afford treatment.
- Shame and fear of being examined (testing would require examination and this may not be acceptable to the teenage patient).

Early Diagnosis and Treatment of STIs

Tables 12.1, 12.2 and 12.3 elaborate the diagnosis and treatment of common STIs with varying presentations.

Secondary Syphilis

Symptoms: Generalized skin rash or mucocutaneous lesions or lymphadenopathy.
Signs: Macules, papules, or pustules on palms and soles, or as mucous patches on the oral mucosa or scaly or non-scaly lesions on other body areas. Multiple types of lesions may be present at any one time. Local or generalized lymphadenopathy may be present (Figs. 12.15 and 12.16).

Diagnosis:

1. Clinical
2. Serological:
   (a) Non-treponemal tests such as VDRL and RPR.
   (b) Treponemal tests: Fluorescent treponemal antibody absorbed [FTA-ABS] tests and the T. pallidum passive particle agglutination [TP-PA] assay.

Use of only one test is associated with a high degree of false positivity so a positive non-treponemal test should be confirmed by using a treponemal test.

Secondary Syphilis Treatment

Children and adolescents: Benzathine penicillin 50, 000 U/kg IM up to a maximum of 2.4 million units IM in a single dose.

Young adult: Benzathine penicillin 2.4 million units IM in a single dose.

In cases of penicillin allergy: Doxycycline 100 mg po twice per day or Tetracycline 500 mg po four times per day for 14 days may be considered.

Table 12.1 Vaginal/urethral/penile discharge

Disease	Symptoms	Signs	Diagnosis	Treatment	Management of partners/follow-up
Chlamydia (*Chlamydia trachomatis*) (Figs. 12.2 and 12.3)	Male: Scant to copious urethral discharge, stinging on urination, urinary frequency	Male: Scant clear, mucoid, or mucopurulent urethral discharge	Male: Gram stain of the urethral discharge that shows five or more white blood cells per oil field is consistent with urethritis. NAATs if available on first-catch urine (Fig. 12.5)	1 g Azithromycin orally or Doxycycline 100 mg orally two times a day for 7 days (Erythromycin base 500 mg orally four times a day for 7 days or Levofloxacin 500 mg once a day for 7 days or Ofloxacin 300 mg orally two times a day for 7 days)	All sexual partners for the past 60 days should be treated. If a patient last had intercourse more than 60 days before the symptoms began or diagnosis established, that partner should be referred for evaluation
	Female: None or vaginal discharge, dysuria, or some intermenstrual vaginal bleeding	Female: None or purulent cervical discharge, cervical motion tenderness, and/or increased friability of cervix (Figs. 12.2 and 12.3)	Female: NAATs (if available) on first-catch urine or cervical secretions		Follow up: Not needed unless symptoms persist or recur, pregnancy or a question of medication compliance
Gonorrhea (*Neisseria gonorrhoeae*) (Figs. 12.1 and 12.2)	Male: Dysuria, urethral discharge, increased urinary frequency	Male: Erythema and edema of urethral meatus	Male: NAATs on first-catch urine or urethral discharge	Ceftriaxone 250 mg IM + 1 g Azithromycin orally or Doxycycline 100 mg orally two times a day for 7 days	All sexual partners for the past 60 days should be treated. If a patient last had intercourse more than 60 days before the symptoms began or diagnosis established, that partner should be referred for evaluation
	Female: Vaginal discharge, vaginal bleeding, dysuria, pelvic pain, dyspareunia	Purulent vaginal/cervical discharge, tenderness and/or friability of the cervix, discharge from urethra, periurethral glands or Bartholin gland ducts or Bartholin gland abscess	Gram stain: gram negative intracellular diplococci (Fig. 12.4) Female: NAATs on cervical discharge or first-catch urine		Follow-up: Not needed unless symptoms persist or recur, pregnancy or a question of medication compliance
Rectal GC		Pruritus, anal discharge, bleeding	Gonorrhea culture*		
Pharyngeal GC		Asymptomatic	Gonorrhea culture*		

Trichomoniasis (*Trichomonas vaginalis*) (Fig. 12.5)	Male: Asymptomatic, urethral discharge, pruritus, dysuria, rarely prostatitis Female: Diffuse, malodorous, yellow–green vaginal discharge with vulvar irritation; asymptomatic	Male: None, urethral discharge Female: Greenish yellow vaginal discharge with frothy appearance; strawberry cervix (Fig. 12.5)	Clinical wet mounts are not sensitive for use in males but can be done on a spun urine. (NAATs have superior sensitivity for *T. vaginalis* infections in men) Wet prep of vaginal secretions for presence of trichomonads	Metronidazole 2 g orally in a single or Tinidazole 2 g orally in a single dose. Alternative treatment: Metronidazole 500 mg two times a day for 7 days	Sex partners should be treated to reduce transmission Follow-up: Not needed unless symptoms persist or recur, pregnancy or a question of medication compliance
Bacterial vaginosis (*Gardnerella vaginalis*) (Fig. 12.7)	Malodorous (fishy smell) vaginal discharge; >50 % of women are asymptomatic	Thin gray or white homogenous discharge coating the vaginal walls (Fig. 12.7)	Amsel criteria (three out of four): 1. Vaginal pH >4.5 2. Fishy odor of vaginal discharge 3. Gray or white vaginal discharge 4. Clue cells on vaginal wet prep (Fig. 12.6)	Metronidazole 500 mg orally two times a day for 7 days or Metronidazole gel 0.75 %, one full applicator (5 g) intravaginally once a day for 5 days or Clindamycin cream 2 %, one full applicator (5 g) intravaginally at bedtime for 7 days	Not recommended Follow-up: Not necessary if symptoms resolve

(continued)

Table 12.1 (continued)

Disease	Symptoms	Signs	Diagnosis	Treatment	Management of partners/follow-up
Candidiasis (*Candida albicans*) (Figs. 12.10 and 12.11)	Vulvar pruritus, vaginal discharge, vaginal soreness, dysuria, dyspareunia	Vulvar erythema, edema, excoriations or a thick curd like vaginal discharge (Fig. 12.11)	Clinical wet mount: (10 % KOH) pseudo-hyphae and budding yeast. Gram stain may also show yeast, hyphae, or pseudohyphae (Fig. 12.10)	Topical antifungal formulations in single dose or regimens of 1–3 days (Because some of the topical treatments are oil-based, latex condoms and diaphragms may be weakened) Butoconazole 2 % cream 5 g intravaginally for 3 days or Terconazole 80 mg vaginal suppository, intravaginally for 3 days or Clotrimazole 1 and 2 % cream or Miconazole 2 and 4 % cream or vaginal suppositories or Oral treatment: fluconazole 150 mg tablet orally ×1 dose	Not usually recommended
Nongonococcal urethritis (NGU) (Chlamydia and gonorrhea 15–40 % of cases, *Mycoplasma genitalium* 15–25 %)	Urethral discharge: purulent or mucopurulent; dysuria and urethral pruritus	Urethral discharge, periurethral inflammation (Fig. 12.9)	Test for Chlamydia and Gonorrhea. Gram stain showing five or more WBC per oil immersion field is highly sensitive and specific to document urethritis (Fig. 12.8)	Azithromycin 1 g orally in a single dose or Doxycycline 100 mg orally twice a day for 7 days (Alternative: Erythromycin base 500 mg orally four times a day for 7 days)	Recommended Follow-up: If symptoms persist

Table 12.2 Vaginal and penile ulcers

Disease	Symptoms	Signs	Diagnosis	Treatment	Management of partners/follow-up
Genital herpes (Herpes simplex type 1 or 2) (Fig. 12.12)	Local: painful genital ulcer or vesicular/ulcerative genital rash, dysuria, and pruritus Systemic: fever, malaise, headache, and myalgia	Painful ulcer localized genital swelling and inguinal adenopathy	Clinical: (PCR assays for HSV DNA or isolation of HSV in cell culture)	*First episode genital herpes:* Acyclovir 400 mg orally three times a day for 7–10 days or Acyclovir 200 mg five times a day for 7–10 days or Valacyclovir 1 g twice a day for 7–10 days *Recurrent genital herpes:* Acyclovir 400 mg orally three times a day for 5 days or Acyclovir 800 mg two times a day for 5 days or Acyclovir 800 mg three times a day for 2 days *Suppressive therapy* (can reduce genital herpes recurrences by up to 80 %): Acyclovir 400 mg two times a day or Famciclovir 250 mg two times a day or Valacyclovir 500 mg one time a day (this dose may be less effective for patients who have ten or more recurrences a year) or Valacyclovir 1,000 mg one time a day	Symptomatic partners should be evaluated and treated
Chancroid (*Hemophilus ducreyi*) (Fig. 12.13)	Tender papule that becomes pustular then a painful, friable ulcer	Ulcer (chancre) is 1–20 mm in size, with a purulent exudate and a granulomatous base. Edges are non-indurated ± tender inguinal adenopathy	Clinical: Culture for *H. Ducreyi* (not readily available)	Azithromycin 1 g orally in a single dose or Ceftriaxone 250 mg IM once or Ciprofloxacin 500 mg two times a day for 3 days or Erythromycin base 500 mg orally three times a day for 7 days	Partners who have had sexual contact with the patient in the 10 days prior to the patient's onset of symptoms should be examined and treated regardless of symptoms Follow-up: Patients should be reexamined 3–7 days after therapy begins

(continued)

Table 12.2 (continued)

Disease	Symptoms	Signs	Diagnosis	Treatment	Management of partners/follow-up
Syphilis (primary) (*Treponema pallidum*) (Fig. 12.14)	Painless ulcer(s) or chancre(s) at the site of inoculation	Chancre with a indurated generally painless perimeter; solitary or multiple at the inoculation site	Clinical: Darkfield microscopy or direct fluorescent antibody tests from lesion exudates for *T. pallidum* are definitive. Serological testing: Screening non-treponemal antibody test (RPR or VDRL) followed by a treponemal serologic test if the screening test is positive	Benzathine penicillin G 2.4 million units IM in a single dose	Sexual partners within the 90 days prior to diagnosis of primary, secondary, or early latent syphilis may be infected even if seronegative and should be treated presumptively
Lymphogranuloma venereum (LGV) (Serotypes of *Chlamydia trachomatis*) (Fig. 12.17)	Genital ulcer or papule at the site of inoculation, rectal exposure may cause tenesmus, mucoid/hemorrhagic rectal discharge, anal pain, and fever. Untreated LGV proctocolitis is an invasive systemic infection and can cause chronic colorectal strictures and fistulae	Painless ulcer followed by unilateral tender inguinal or femoral lymphadenopathy (often ulcer disappears by the time patient presents)	Clinical findings as well as the exclusion of other possible etiologies. A definitive diagnosis is best made by isolating the organism	Doxycycline 100 mg two times a day for 21 days or Erythromycin base 500 mg four times a day for 21 days. Buboes may require aspiration through intact skin or incision and drainage to prevent inguinal/femoral ulcers	Persons who have had contact for up to 60 days prior to onset of symptoms should be examined and tested for chlamydia and treated with a chlamydial regimen Follow-up: Follow clinically until signs and symptoms have improved

Granuloma inguinale (Donovanosis) (*Klebsiella granulomatis*) (Fig. 12.18)	Painless ulcer on genitals or perineum without regional lymphadenopathy ± subcutaneous granuloma or "pseudobuboes". The infection may disseminate to the abdomen, pelvis, bones, or the mouth. The lesions may also become infected secondarily	Beefy red, friable but painless ulcerative lesions on the genitals with subcutaneous granulomas	Visualization of Donovan bodies* on a tissue sample	Doxycycline 100 mg two times a day or Azithromycin 1 g orally each week or Ciprofloxacin 750 mg orally two times a day or Erythromycin base 500 mg four times a day or Trimethoprim–sulfamethoxazole one tablet (160 mg/800 mg) two times a day. All must be given for at least 21 days until all lesions have completely healed	Partners who have had contact up to 60 days before the onset of symptoms in the index case must be offered treatment Follow-up: Follow clinically until signs and symptoms have improved

Table 12.3 Genital warts and buboes

Disease	Symptoms	Signs	Diagnosis	Treatment	Management of Partners/follow-up
Genital warts (Human Papilloma Virus) (90 % caused by HPV strains 6 or 11) (Fig. 12.19)	Flat masses in genital and/or areas, painless but sometimes pruritic	Flat, papular or pedunculated growths around the introitus, under the foreskin in the uncircumcised penis or on the shaft of the circumcised penis. May also be intra-anal, in the cervix, or vaginal	Visual inspection, a hand lens may be helpful	*Provider applied*: (If untreated may resolve on their own, stay the same or grow in number) 1. Cryotherapy with liquid nitrogen or cryoprobe or 2. Podophyllin resin 10–25 % in a compound tincture of benzoin or 3. Trichloracetic acid or bichloracetic acid (80–90 %) May use vinegar if available Use the back of a cotton swab to apply to prevent damage to the surrounding skin Repeat every 1–2 weeks as needed 4. Surgical removal *Patient applied*: 1. Podofilox 0.5 % solution or gel or 2. Imiquimod 5 % cream or 3. Sinecatechins 15 % ointment	Persons with warts should inform their partner and refrain from sexual activity until the warts have resolved. It is unclear how long a patient stays contagious after warts have disappeared. Both partners should be tested for other STIs as well

		Visual diagnosis	
Bubo	A bubo is an inflamed, enlarged, tender lymph node that is usually found in the groin and may be associated with Chancroid, Syphilis, or Lymphogranuloma venereum. Buboes should not be confused with pseudobuboes which may feel like buboes but are caused by subcutaneous granulation (see Granuloma inguinale)	Enlarged lymph nodes in the groin (see symptoms)	Treatment is for Chancroid, syphilis, or LGV. If diagnosis is not clear then Syndromic diagnosis and treatment should be considered: Cipro 500 mg BID/3 days + Doxycycline 100 mg BID for 14 days or Erythromycin 500 mg po QID for 14 days. Buboes may require aspiration through intact skin or incision and drainage to prevent inguinal/femoral ulcers

Fig. 12.1 Gonococcal urethritis (*Source*: photo courtesy of the Centers for Disease Control)

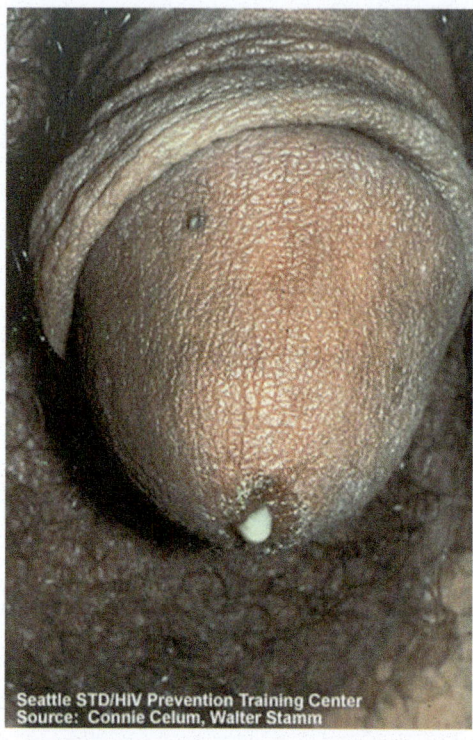

Fig. 12.2 Mucopurulent cervicitis (*Source*: photo courtesy of the Centers for Disease Control)

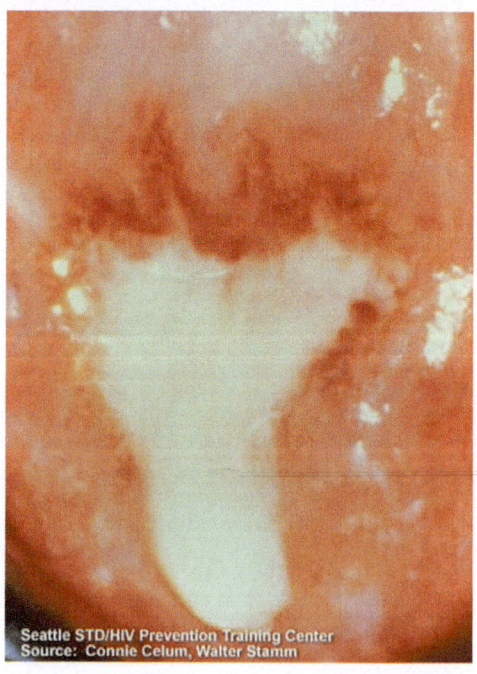

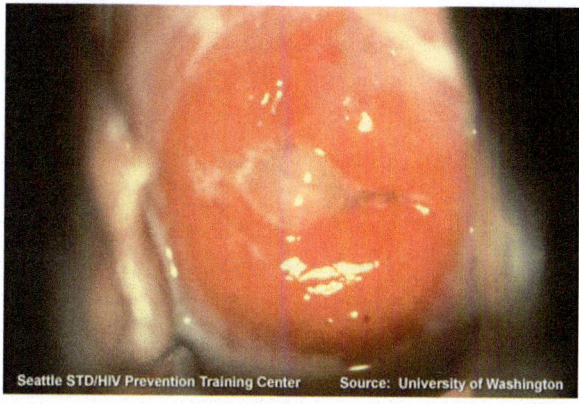

Fig. 12.3 Chlamydia cervicitis (*Source*: photo courtesy of the Centers for Disease Control)

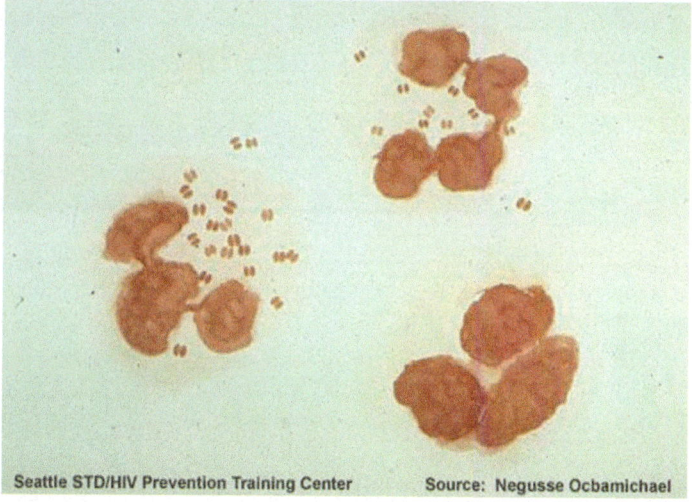

Fig. 12.4 Gram negative intracellular diplococci (*Source*: photo courtesy of the Centers for Disease Control)

Management of sex partners: Sexual partners within the 90 days prior to diagnosis of primary, secondary, or early latent syphilis may be infected even if seronegative and should be treated presumptively.

Fig. 12.5 Strawberry cervix (*Source*: photo courtesy of the Centers for Disease Control)

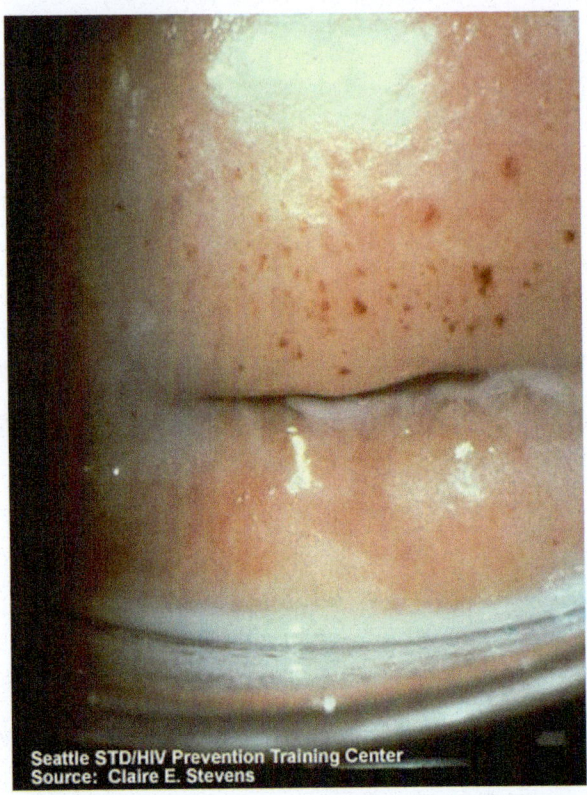

Fig. 12.6 Clue cells and Saline prep of vaginal fluids (*Source*: photo courtesy of the Centers for Disease Control)

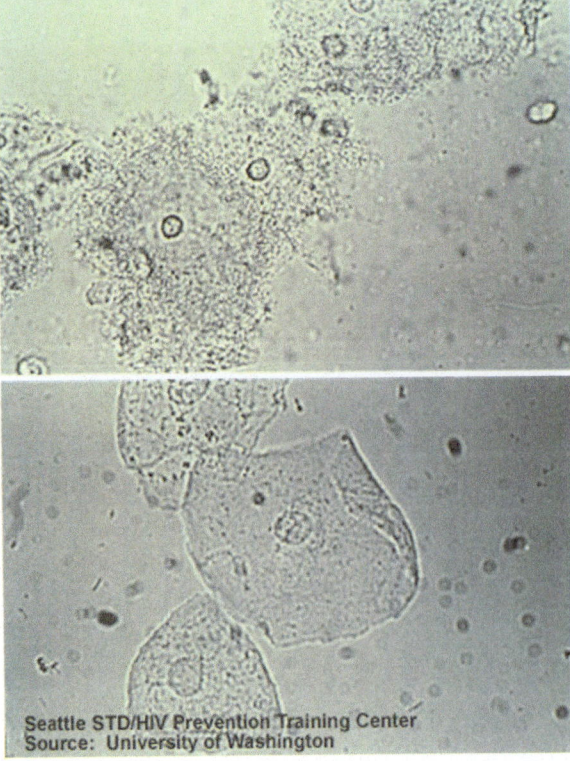

Fig. 12.7 Vagine Discharge in Bacterial Vaginosis (*Source*: photo courtesy of the Centers for Disease Control)

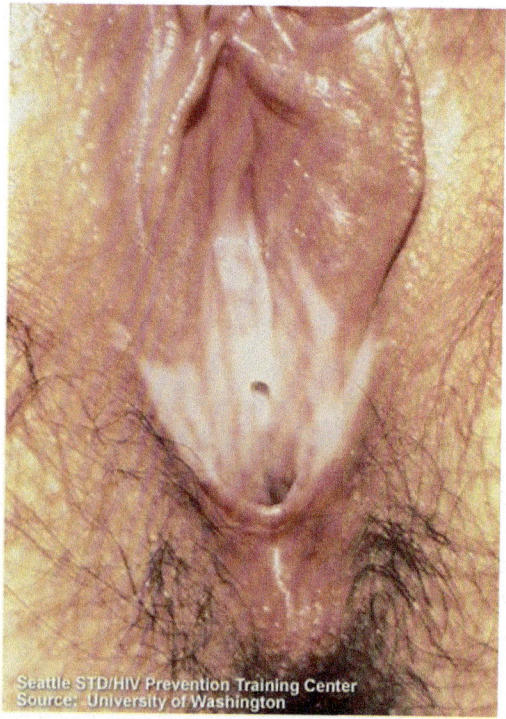

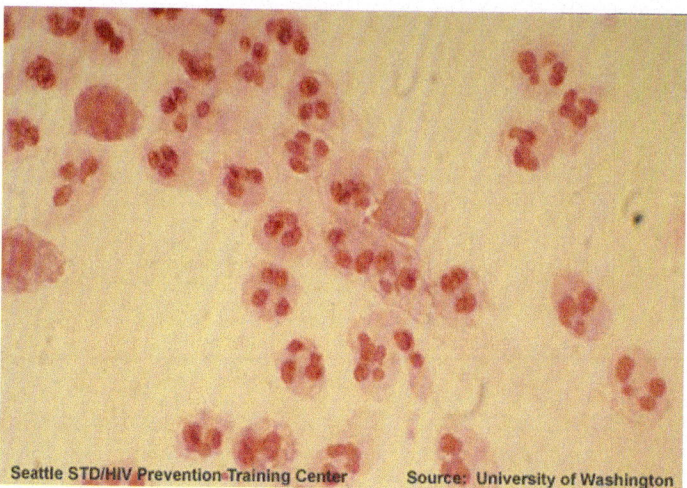

Fig. 12.8 Urethral gram stain as seen in non-gonococcal urethritis (*Source*: photo courtesy of the Centers for Disease Control)

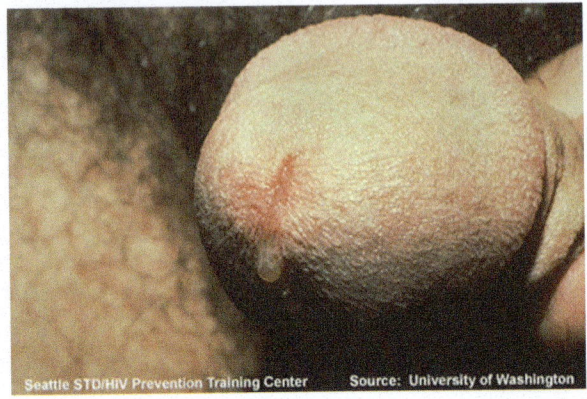

Fig. 12.9 Nongonococcal urethritis (*Source*: photo courtesy of the Centers for Disease Control)

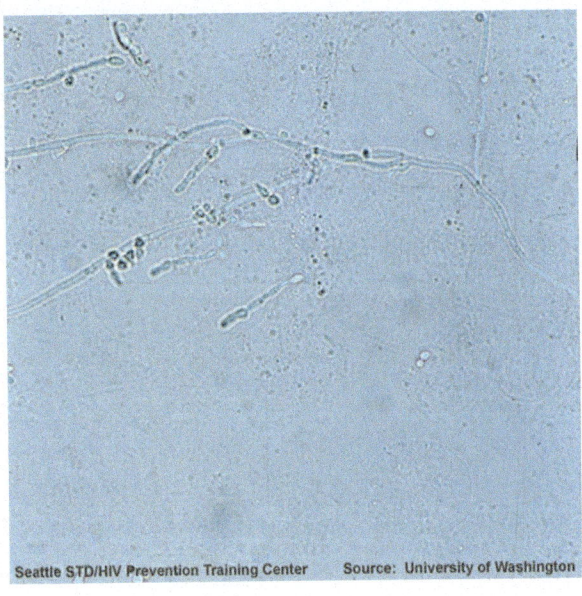

Fig. 12.10 Yeast KOH prep (*Source*: photo courtesy of the Centers for Disease Control)

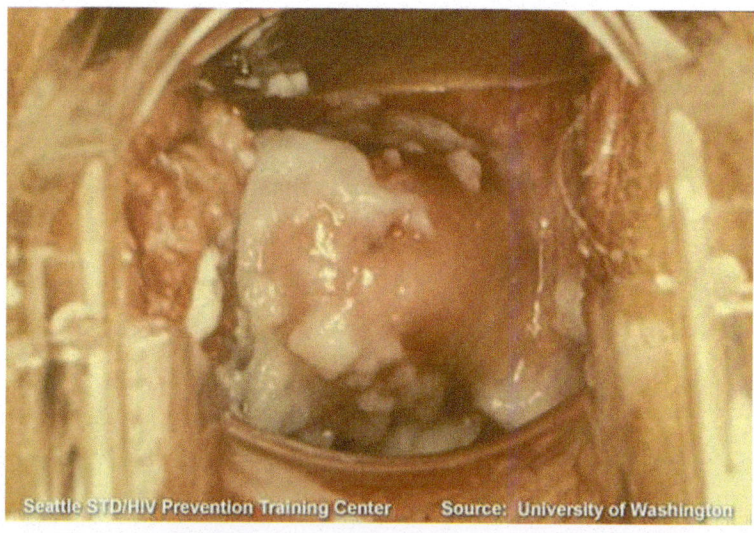

Fig. 12.11 Candida vaginal discharge (*Source*: photo courtesy of the Centers for Disease Control)

Fig. 12.12 Genital herpes lesions (photo courtesy of the Centers for Disease Control)

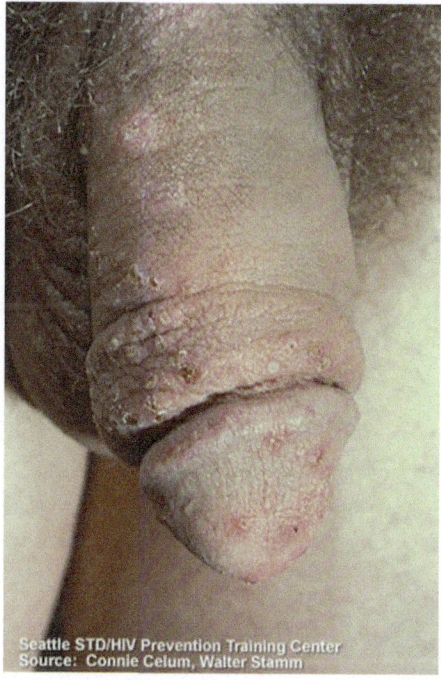

Fig. 12.13 Chancroid (photo courtesy of the Centers for Disease Control)

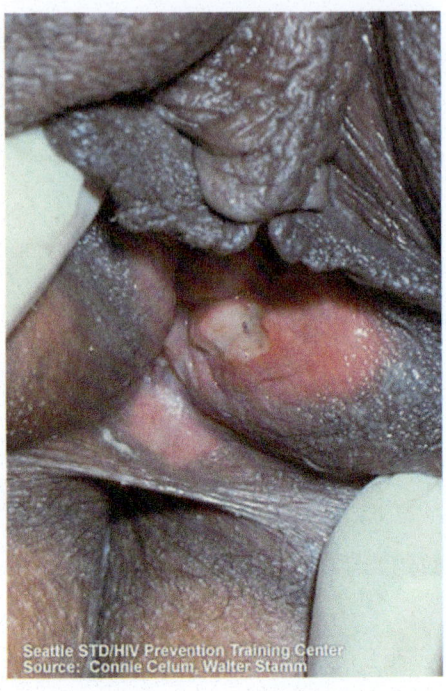

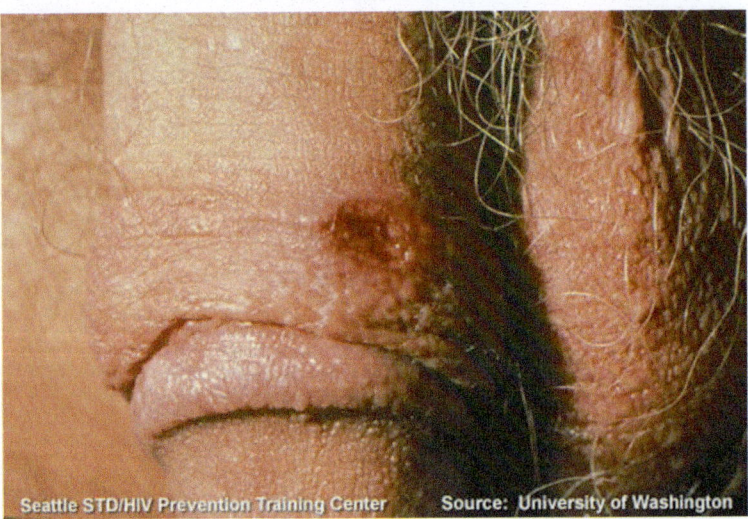

Fig. 12.14 Primary syphilis (photo courtesy of the Centers for Disease Control)

Fig. 12.15 Secondary syphilis (photo courtesy of the Centers for Disease Control)

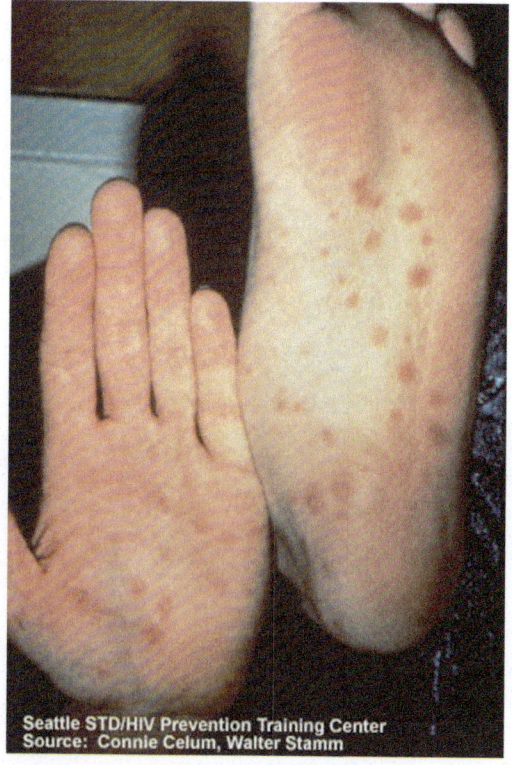

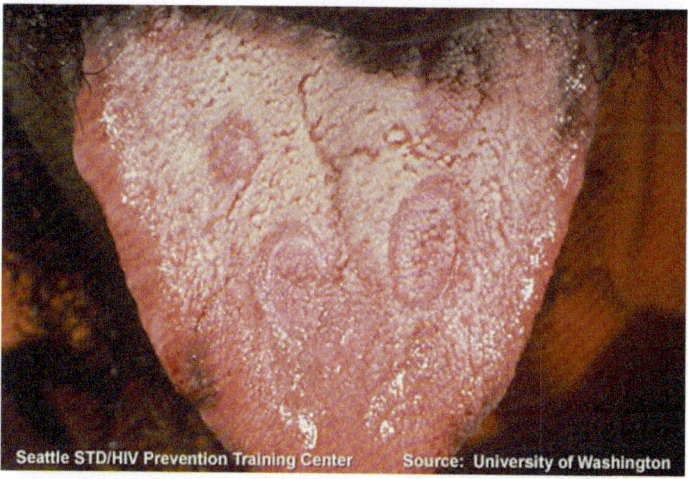

Fig. 12.16 Secondary syphilis (photo courtesy of the Centers for Disease Control)

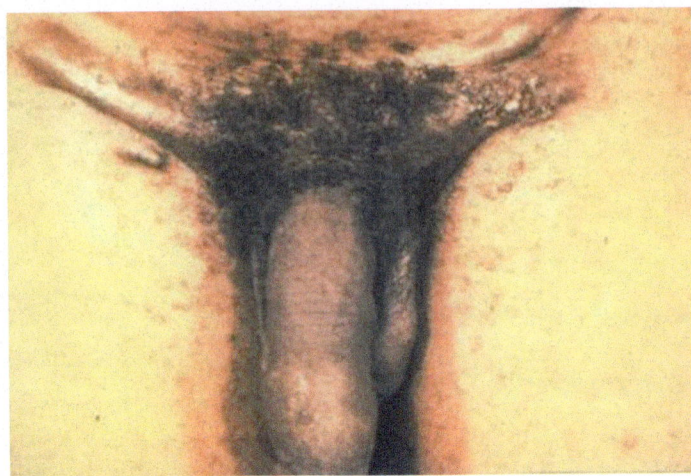

Fig. 12.17 Lymphogranuloma venereum (photo courtesy of the Centers for Disease Control)

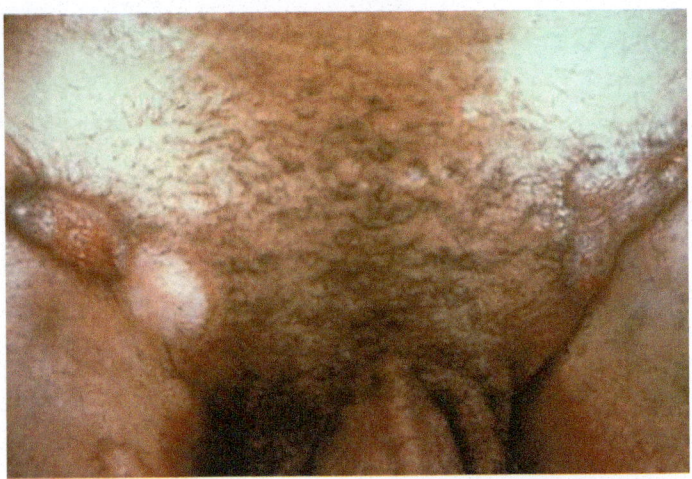

Fig. 12.18 Granuloma inguinale (photo courtesy of the Centers for Disease Control)

Fig. 12.19 Genital warts (photo courtesy of the Centers for Disease Control)

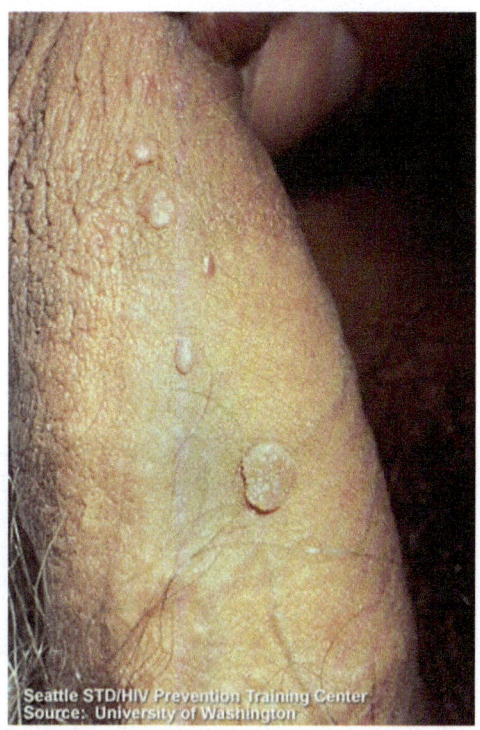

Role of STIs in HIV Transmission

Studies and meta-analyses have confirmed an association between a recent STI and the acquisition and transmission of HIV. This conclusion is based on ecological, cross sectional, case control, and cohort studies.

A cohort study using data from a male circumcision trial in South Africa examined the association between HPV and HIV incidence. Although there was no association between low-risk HPV and HIV, there was a fourfold increased risk in men with high-risk HPV. The incidence increased with the number of high-risk HPV genotypes detected.

Another cohort study on two African countries followed 4,439 women every 3 months for up to 2 years. Reproductive tract infections were associated with HIV in at least one statistical model. The strongest risk was from gonorrhea but HSV-2 and bacterial vaginosis also confirmed risk for HIV acquisition.

In a large systematic review and meta-analysis, data from 25 study populations were summarized to estimate the risk of HIV transmission per act in heterosexuals. The study authors found that current or past genital ulcers in the HIV susceptible partner increased per-act infectivity fivefold compared with no STI.

The risk factors for STI and HIV and mode of transmission are very similar. This association underscores the importance of STI prevention and treatment as part of HIV prevention.

Syndromic Management

Most STIs can be effectively treated if detected early. However, diagnosis is based on collection of samples, transportation to laboratories and sophisticated testing. In many developing countries, evaluation and treatment of these infections are limited by the following factors:

- Lack of knowledge of STIs and their consequences.
- Lack of confidential adolescent friendly services.
- Lack of medical providers that have the expertise to diagnose accurately the infection.
- Limited availability of transportation and laboratory facilities that could process sample accurately.

To overcome these barriers the WHO has recommended a syndromic rather than an etiologic approach to management of STIs (Table 12.4). This allows trained healthcare workers to identify STIs earlier based on clinical signs and symptoms, and supplemented by a "risk assessment" approach in case of vaginitis (Table 12.5). The "syndromic modules" then guide the healthcare worker in treating patients based on embedded algorithms.

Each syndromic management module consists of:

(a) *Problem box*: Defines the symptoms and signs.
(b) *Decision box*: Helps worker decide what the possible diagnoses are.
(c) *Action box*: Determines the course of Treatment and/or referral.

Table 12.4 Syndromic versus etiologic management of STIs

Etiologic	Syndromic
Treatment does not begin until the organism is identified	Treatment is problem-oriented
Requires lab facilities which may not be available and will delay treatment	Highly sensitive but less specific
More specific as treatment targets etiologic agent	Provider may treat the wrong infection and miss mixed infections
Delays treatment. Requires a second visit before treatment is started	Treats the patient at the *first* visit and so makes STI care more accessible
Patient will continue to transmit disease until treatment started	Uses flowcharts that guide the health worker through logical steps
More accurate and needed in case of syphilis	Provides opportunity and time for education and counseling

Table 12.5 Risk assessment approach

Risk factor	Score
Partner has urethral discharge	2
New partner in last 3 months	1
More than one partner in last 3 months	1
Not living with steady partner	1
Age less than 21 years	1
If risk score 2 and over treat for cervicitis	

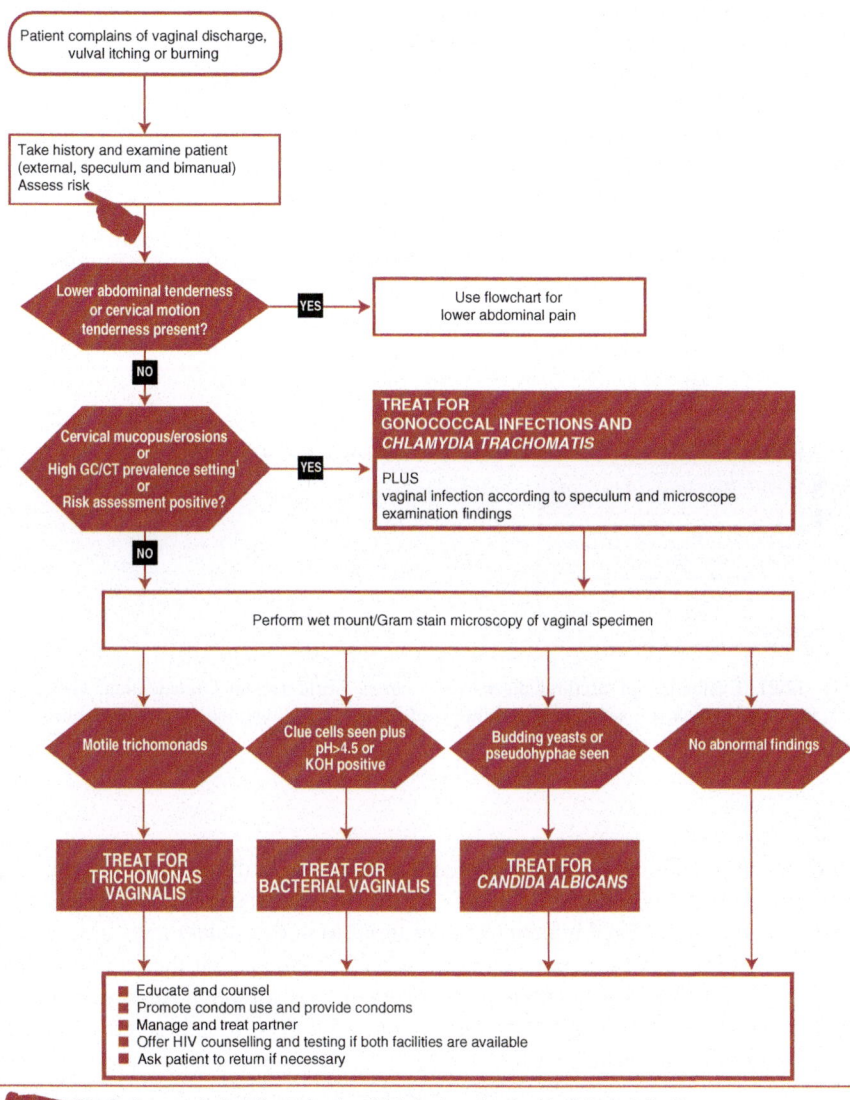

Fig. 12.20 Evaluation of vaginal discharge: bimanual, speculum with or without microscope. *Source*: World Health Organization. Guidelines for the management of sexually transmitted infections. http://whqlibdoc.who.int/publications/2003/9241546263.pdf

Examples of syndromic management modules include those for vaginal discharge, urethral discharge, genital ulcers, and for females with abdominal pain (Figs. 12.20, 12.21, 12.22, and 12.23).

In case of symptoms of vaginal discharge the WHO recommends caution while using the syndromic modules as this could be indicative of a vaginal or cervical

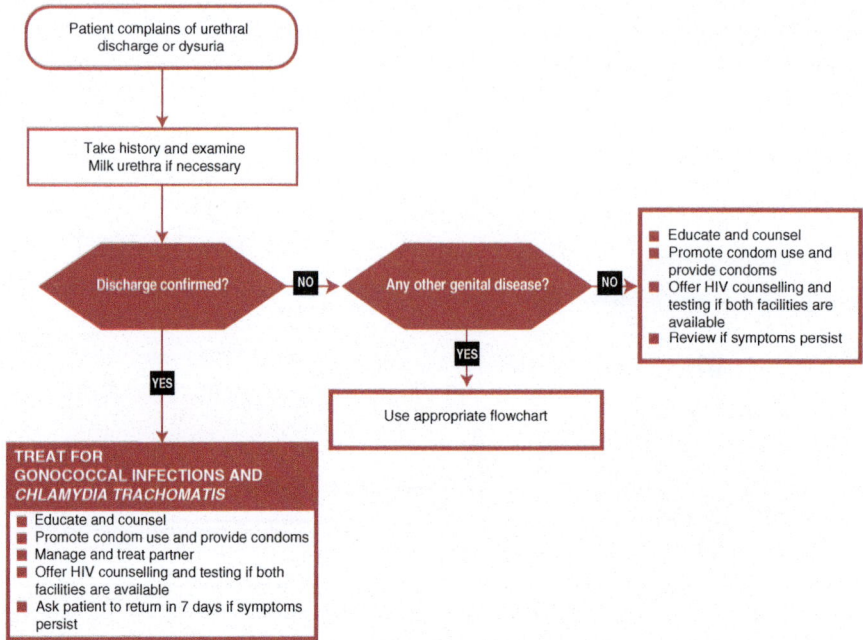

Fig. 12.21 Evaluation of urethral discharge. *Source*: World Health Organization. Guidelines for the management of sexually transmitted infections. http://whqlibdoc.who.int/publications/2003/9241546263.pdf

infection. The algorithms are considered sensitive in identifying causes of vaginitis but less specific for cervical infection. Thus it is recommended that treatment be instituted for trichomonal infection and bacterial vaginosis unless there are signs of cervical infection. If examination is not allowed by the patient then a risk assessment approach has been recommended (Table 12.5). Although this increases the specificity of the algorithm it still tends to have a low positive predictive value in areas where the prevalence of STIs is low.

Public Health Package for STI Prevention and Control

Young people are more likely to have STIs and to not seek treatment for the same.

They are also more likely to be reinfected after having being treated and more than 40 % of adolescents subsequently develop another STI other than the one they initially presented with. Thus it is important to provide a public health intervention that provides primary, secondary, and tertiary services.

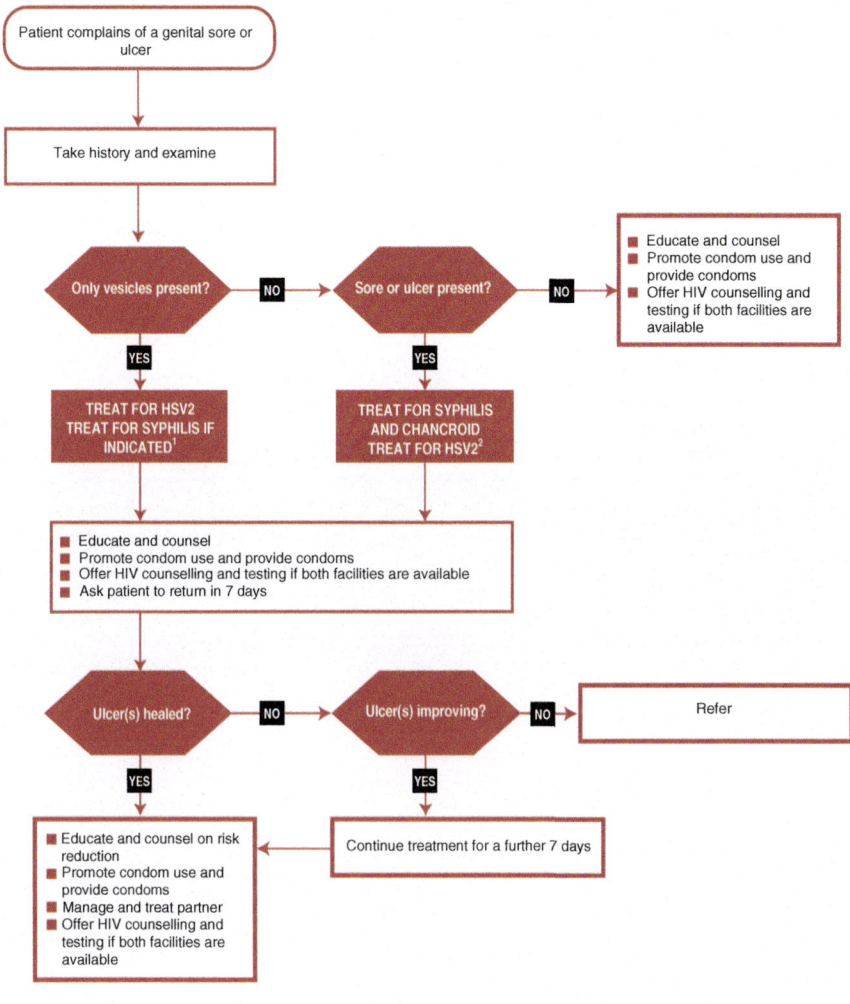

1 Indications for syphilis treatment:
   - RPR positive; and
   - Patient has not been treated for syphilis recently.
2 Treat for HSV2 where prevalence is 30% or higher, of adapt to local conditions.

Fig. 12.22 Evaluation of genital ulcers. *Source*: World Health Organization. Guidelines for the management of sexually transmitted infections. http://whqlibdoc.who.int/publications/2003/9241546263.pdf

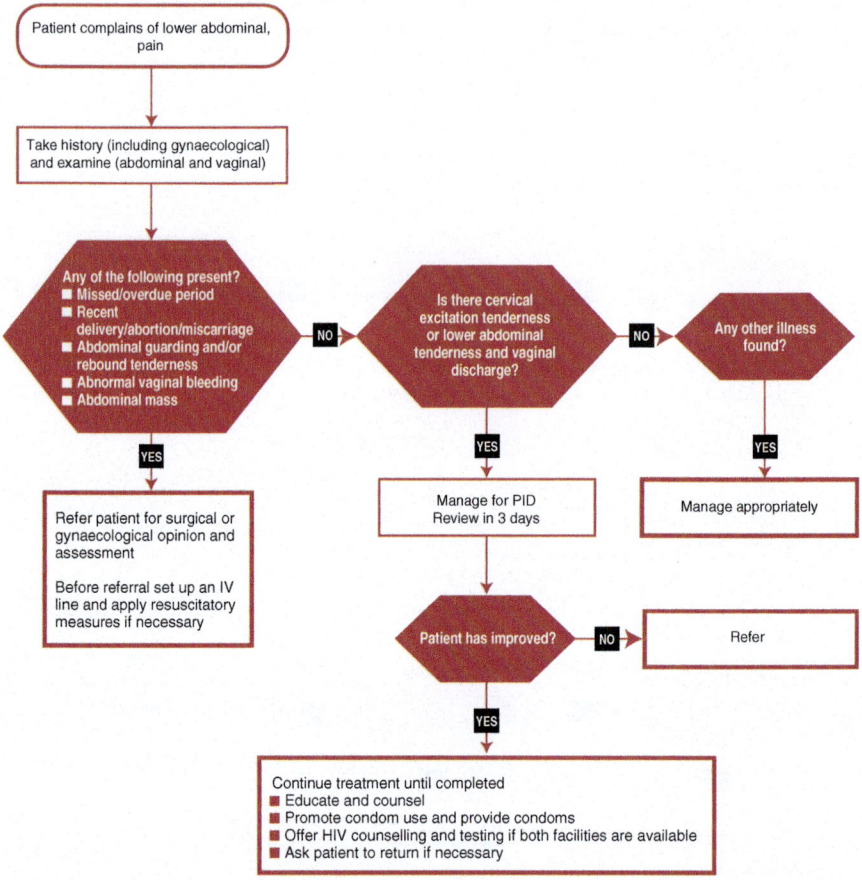

Fig. 12.23 Evaluation of adolescent female with abdominal pain. *Source*: World Health Organization. Guidelines for the management of sexually transmitted infections. http://whqlibdoc.who.int/publications/2003/9241546263.pdf

Primary Measures

1. Educate and counsel patients at risk about STIs, including modes of transmission, signs and symptoms of STIs, and correct use of condoms.
2. Educate and counsel adolescents about postponing sexual activity and limiting sexual partners.
3. Diagnose and treat patients and partners of patients with an STI.
4. Identify and immunize patients at risk for vaccine preventable STI.
5. Research and development of vaccines against STIs.

Secondary Measures

1. Early detection and treatment of asymptomatic cases which would involve routine screening of all adolescents.
2. Partner notification and treatment.

Tertiary Measures

1. Management of sequelae of untreated STIs.

Special Adolescent Populations

Adolescent sex workers and street youth: Little data are available on these adolescents in general, but they constitute an important but often neglected population and are at high risk for STIs.

Females: Higher reported rates of STI may suffer more complications including ectopic pregnancy, PID, infertility, and pelvic pain. Untreated STIs in pregnant adolescents can have severe consequences for her offspring.

Race and Ethnicity: African Americans and Hispanics have higher STI prevalence rates in comparison to non-Hispanic whites.

Males who have sex with males: Some are at higher risk for HIV and other STI.

Women who have sex with women (WSW): Few data are available on the risks associated with sex between women. Most WSW report one or more lifetime male sexual partners and thus can acquire and transmit STIs to their female partners as well.

Recommended Reading

1. Centers for Disease Control and Prevention. Sexually transmitted diseases treatment guidelines, 2010. MMWR 2010;59 (No. RR12).
2. Goldstein MA. Sexually transmitted infections in adolescents. In: Goldstein MA, ed. *The MassGeneral Hospital for Children adolescent medicine handbook*. New York, NY: Springer; 2011.
3. Ward H, Ronn M. The contribution of STIs to the sexual transmission of HIV. Curr Opin HIV AIDS. 2010;5:305–10.
4. World Health Organization. Guidelines for management of sexually transmitted infections. Geneva: WHO; 2003.
5. Karl L Dehne, Gabriele Riedner. Sexually transmitted infections amongst adolescents. The need for adequate health services. World Health Organization and Deutsche Gesellschaft fuer Technische Zusammenarbeit (GTZ) GmbH 2005.

Chapter 13
Contraceptive Options for Adolescents

Nupur Gupta

Keywords Adolescents • Pregnancy prevention • Hormonal contraception • Natural family planning

Overview

- The oral contraceptive pill (OCP) remains the most common form of contraception for adolescents and reproductive-age women in the US.
- Resource-limited settings require contraceptive methods that are more effective, less user dependent, and confidential. Several newer hormonal methods that fulfill these criteria have been developed but may or may not be available around the world.
- This chapter discusses different hormonal and nonhormonal methods that are available, their mechanism of action, side effects, and efficacy.
- Emergency contraception using progestin-only pills (POPs), the "Yuzpe Regimen," and the copper intrauterine device (IUD) are also reviewed.

History

1. *Gynecological history*:
    a) Menstrual history including age of menarche, regularity of menses, date of last menstrual period, cycle length, and history of dysmenorrhea.
    b) Ask about pregnancies, previous deliveries, and abortions.

N. Gupta, M.D., M.P.H. (✉)
MassGeneral Hospital for Children, Harvard Medical School, 55 Fruit Street, Boston, MA 02114, USA
e-mail: ngupta3@partners.org

c) Possibility of female circumcision should be considered and carefully questioned for, taking into consideration cultural issues, depending on which country the provider is practicing in; this may contribute towards severe dysmenorrhea, and may be life threatening at the time of delivery.

2. *Personal history*: History of thrombosis or migraine with aura or focal neurological deficits should be taken as this could affect their choice of contraception.
3. *Family history*: History suggestive of thromboembolism, e.g., strokes, myocardial infarction, pulmonary embolism, or deaths at an early age. If positive patient should have basic workup to rule out prothrombotic disorders. This is not often available in developing countries and using the WHO/CDC guidelines for contraindications to hormonal contraception might be useful in guiding the provider (http://www.cdc.gov/mmwr/pdf/rr/rr59e0528.pdf).

Absolute contraindications to combined hormonal contraception

1. Patients with personal history of venous thromboembolism
2. Patients with known Factor V Leiden mutation (risk of clot increased 30-fold) or other thrombophilia condition (e.g., prothrombin gene mutation, protein C or S deficiency)
3. Smokers 35 years of age or older
4. Personal history of breast cancer
5. Uncontrolled hypertension
6. History of stroke
7. History of migraine with neurologic symptoms (there is some controversy to this recommendation; this is a relative contraindication)
8. Undiagnosed uterine bleeding
9. Liver disease

Types of Contraception

1. Hormonal
2. Nonhormonal IUD
3. Traditional family planning methods
4. Surgical methods

1. Hormonal
    a) Combined, with estrogen and progestin, including the OCP, the contraceptive patch, the vaginal ring, and monthly injectables.
    b) Progestin-only methods include injectable three-monthly depot medroxyprogesterone acetate (DMPA), the subcutaneous progestin-containing rod (Implanon®), and the progestin-containing IUD (Mirena®).
    c) Emergency contraception

a) Combined Hormonal Contraception

1) The oral contraceptive pill (OCP)

Description and method of use: Contains a synthetic estrogen, usually ethinyl estradiol, and different types of progestins. Adolescents should preferably start on a low-dose formulation containing 20 or 30 μg of estrogen if available.

Mechanism of action:

a. Prevents ovulation by inhibiting the gonadotropin-releasing hormone (GnRH) axis
b. Thickens cervical mucus to prevent sperm penetration
c. Inhibits capacitation of the sperm
d. Creates endometrial atrophy

If side effects occur the pill could be switched to a different formulation, but a trial of 3 months is recommended prior to changing.

Counseling:

a. Patient should start pill on either day 1 of the menstrual cycle or on the Sunday after menstruation begins. OR use the "quick start method" which entails starting on the day of the visit as long as they have a negative pregnancy test.
b. The pill should be taken at about the same time every day. Taking at night might reduce initial nausea associated with hormonal contraception.
c. If a pill is missed, then the patient may double up for up to 2 days. If more than two pills missed it would be better to stop, get a withdrawal bleed, and then start a new pack.
d. Teens do not need a pelvic exam to initiate birth control.
e. Counsel about condom use and STI and HIV acquisition.
f. Discuss risks and side effects particularly signs of thromboembolic phenomenon. Counsel patients to seek care immediately for severe chest pain, shortness of breath, severe headaches, vision changes, and severe leg or abdominal pain.

Efficacy: Perfect use: Failure rate is 0.3 %. Typical use: Failure rate is 8 %.

Side effects:

Minor: Irregular menstrual bleeding, nausea, increased appetite, weight gain, breast tenderness, fluid retention, bloating, headache, mood changes. Rare: Acne, hirsutism, and male-pattern hair loss
Major: Hypertension, thromboembolic phenomenon

Newer oral contraceptives

Extended cycle regimes can be prescribed for those in whom extended cycles are indicated due to medical conditions like premenstrual dysphoric disorder (PMDD) or endometriosis. This may also be beneficial in those with anemia where continued blood loss could worsen the anemia. These can include OCPs that have 84 days of active hormone tablets followed by 7 inactive ones providing an extended cycle of 91 days; this could also be done using regular monophasic OCPs by missing the inert pills at the end of the pack. These would give the user only four "menstrual" periods a year potentially reducing other side effects that occur because of hormone withdrawal like premenstrual symptoms, headaches and migraines, mood changes, and heavy or painful monthly bleeding.

2) Transdermal Contraception

Description: Transdermal contraception that is currently available in some areas around the world is a 20 cm two plastic patch that contains a combination of the progestin, norelgestromin (NGMN) and ethinyl estradiol. The patch has three layers, the translucent, flexible polyester backing layer film, a middle drug containing adhesive layer, and a clear, polyester film that protects the adhesive layer during storage and is removed just before application. The hormones are released from the adhesive layer and absorbed across the skin, and allow for a fairly constant level to be maintained.

Mechanism of action: Similar to the OCP.

Method of use: A new patch is placed on the skin once a week for 3 weeks. The fourth week is patch-free which allows for a withdrawal bleed to occur.

Efficacy: Perfect use: 0.3 % failure rate. Typical use: 8 % failure rate. The patch may be less efficacious in heavier women, >90 kg.

Counseling:

a. The patch may be applied anywhere on the body where it is likely to stay adherent as on the skin of the buttocks, upper outer arm, lower abdomen, or back. It should NOT be applied on the skin of the breasts. All sites are equally effective.
b. The site should preferably be changed every time a new patch is applied and should be free of creams, oils, and cosmetics.
c. Regular activities including exercise, bathing, and swimming do not usually cause patch detachment.
d. If patch becomes detached it may be reapplied or a new patch must be applied immediately to maintain hormone levels and efficacy. The patch is then changed on the regular patch change day. However if unclear when detachment occurred then a new cycle should be started and efficacy then cannot be guaranteed. Detachment rate: 3–5 %, but in adolescents may be as high as 35 %.

Side effects: Similar to the OCP, plus skin irritation or rash at the site of application, greater likelihood of breast discomfort, engorgement or pain, and dysmenorrhea compared with the pill user. Women are exposed to 60 % more total estrogen in their blood as compared to someone taking a 35 µg OCP, and this increased estrogen may increase the risk of adverse events.

3) Vaginal Ring

Description: The vaginal ring (Nuva Ring®) is a silicone ring about 2 in. in diameter, containing a combination of a progestin, etonogestrel, and ethinyl estradiol implanted in the core of the ring.

Mechanism of action: Similar to the OCP. The hormones are released slowly and constantly into the vagina from the ring, and subsequently absorbed through the vaginal mucosa into the general circulation.

Method of use: The ring is flexible and is inserted intravaginally by the user by pressing the two sides together, usually on the last day of her menstrual period. A tampon applicator may also be used for this purpose. It is removed 3 weeks later and the user then experiences a withdrawal bleed within a few days after removal resulting in a menstrual period. A new ring is then reinserted 1 week later.

Efficacy: Perfect use: 0.3 % failure rate. Typical use: 8 % failure rate.

Counseling:

a. The ring may be removed for up to 3 h during coitus if the user so desires, without the use of a backup method, but must then be reinserted by the user after intercourse.
b. The ring should be refrigerated at 4–8 °C when not dispensed. However after dispensing it can be kept in its packet at room temperature (less than 30 °C) for up to 4 months.
c. If the ring falls out, it should be washed with lukewarm water and reinserted.

Side effects: Similar to the OCP, plus nonspecific vaginitis, leucorrhea, and occasionally vaginal discomfort. Some patients may discontinue the ring because of repeated device-related events like expulsion, foreign body sensation, or coital discomfort.

4) Combined Injectable Contraception

Description: Combined injectable contraceptives contain both progestin and estrogen and are injected intramuscularly once a month to achieve contraception. They cause fewer side effects than the progestin-only contraceptives that are administered once every 2–3 months. These are not currently available, or approved for use in the US. Injectables like Cyclofem®, Cyclo-Provera®, and Feminena® are however available in different parts of the world and in resource-limited settings. The Program for Approved Technology in Health (PATH) has also created a single-use, prefilled, nonreusable syringe, Uniject®, which allows community workers or women themselves to administer the injection. A study in Brazil showed that of the women who agreed to self-administer after receiving training, 93 % were able to correctly administer and 57 % preferred self-injection at home to clinic visits.

Method of use: Deep intramuscular injection in the gluteal or deltoid muscle

Efficacy: 0.1–0.4 pregnancies per 100 women per year of typical use.

Counseling: Return to fertility is more rapid and may be as soon as 6 weeks after the last injection compared to DMPA, where the time to conception after stopping DMPA may be as long as 10 months.

Side effects: Similar to OCPs, plus menstrual irregularity, which may include amenorrhea.

b) Progestin-Only Contraception

Progestin-only contraception is indicated particularly in women who cannot use estrogen (see contraindications above). The WHO and the CDC have some CI to the progestin-only methods as well including personal history of breast cancer, severe decompensated cirrhosis of the liver, liver tumors, acute or recurrent deep vein thrombosis or pulmonary embolism, and stroke.

I. Progestin-only pills (POPs):

Description: These pills contain only a progestin and are indicated in those patients in whom estrogens are contraindicated. These can also be used by breastfeeding teenage mothers. Those available in the US contain norethindrone, but desogestrel- and LNG-containing POPs are also available internationally.

Mechanism of action:

a. Inhibit ovulation (less than with implants and injectables)
b. Thicken cervical mucus
c. Cause endometrial atrophy

Method of use: These must be taken every day at almost the same time. There is no pill-free or hormone-free week as in the combined OCPS.

Efficacy: Perfect use: 0.3 % failure rate. Typical use: 8–9 % failure rate.

Side effects: Irregular menses.

Counseling: Women must be reminded to take the POP pills at the same time every day. Also if they are very late or miss a day they must use emergency contraceptive methods to prevent pregnancy.

II. Injectable depot medroxyprogesterone acetate (DMPA):

Description: DMPA provides 3 months of contraception. As it does not contain estrogen, it can be used by women in whom estrogen is contraindicated.

Mechanism of action:

a. Inhibits ovulation
b. Thickens cervical mucus
c. Causes endometrial atrophy

Method of use: Deep intramuscular injection in the gluteal or deltoid muscle every 3 months in a dose of 150 mg.
Efficacy: Perfect use: 0.3 % failure rate. Typical use: 3 % failure rate.

Side effects: Menstrual irregularities (irregular bleeding or amenorrhea) and weight gain (54 %). It may also cause reduction in bone mineral density and delay in return to fertility (usually about 10 months). Discontinuation rates for Depo-Provera are exceedingly high with 33 % of adolescents not choosing to get a second injection at 3 months and 75 % discontinuing use by 12 months. Weight gain is one of the most important reasons for discontinuation of DMPA.

III. Subcutaneous DMPA Formulation:

Subcutaneous depot-medroxyprogesterone acetate (DMPA-SC) contains 104 mg of MPA and is administered every 3 months by the subcutaneous route. It provides slower and more sustained absorption of the DMPA and is just as efficacious in preventing ovulation. It is less painful and is available only in a prefilled Uniject syringe. Self-administration is possible and this may increase compliance.

IV. Subdermal Contraceptive Implant:

Description: This implant is an ethylene vinyl acetate rod, 4 cm in length and 2 mm in diameter containing 68 mg of etonogestrel. The hormone is released into the circulation from its subdermal location through the thin membrane covering the matrix. It provides 3 years of contraception. It is available as Implanon® in the US.

Mechanism of action:

a. Suppresses ovulation (especially in the first few years). This does not suppress follicular activity and so estrogen levels are maintained.
b. Increases viscosity of cervical mucus.

Method of use: The implant is inserted subdermally using a preloaded disposable applicator and takes less than 1 minute to insert. Providers do need some basic training to administer this device. Removal requires a 2 mm skin incision and some finger pressure. Newer implants, like Jadelle®, take less than 5 minutes to insert.

Efficacy: Failure rate: 0.38 %.

Side effects:

Due to medication: Acne, emotional lability, headache, weight gain, dysmenorrhea, and depression. Weight gain is much less than what occurs with injectable DMPA and no significant changes in bone mineral density have been reported.

Implant site symptoms: Mild pain of short duration: <5 %.

V. Levonorgestrel-releasing intrauterine contraceptive system (LNG-IUS):

Description: The device has a 32 mm T-shaped polyethylene frame with a cylinder wrapped around its stem. The cylinder contains 52 mg of LNG mixed with polydimethyl siloxane. This allows for the slow and sustained release of the hormone providing contraception for 5 years. The amount of LNG released decreases over the years but contraceptive efficacy is maintained. Impregnation of the device with barium sulfate allows easy visualization on X-ray or ultrasound.

The WHO states that women who are at high risk for pelvic inflammatory disease (PID) are not good candidates, but those women who have had PID and have demonstrated their fertility may use the LNG IUS if they are now at a low risk for sexually transmitted infections (STIs). Contraindications are similar to those for other IUDs including a specific contraindication for women who have a past history of and/or are at continuing risk for ectopic pregnancy.

Mechanism of action:

a. Thickens cervical mucus
b. Inhibits sperm motility and function
c. Causes endometrial atrophy
d. Suppresses ovulation (25–50 % of users)
e. Foreign body reaction

Method of use: Inserted intrauterine. It is usually recommended for use by parous women with no history of PID. However it can be used for adolescents who have never been pregnant as well especially if estrogens are contraindicated. Basic training is required for insertion. The size of uterus should be assessed before insertion and should be at least 6–9 cm in length and unobstructed. The device is usually administered with applicator using one-hand technique ideally within 7 days of menses or 4 or more weeks postpartum. WHO also recommends that it could be inserted immediately post abortion.

Efficacy: It has a first-year failure rate of 0.14 pregnancies per 100 women and gross cumulative rate at 5 years of 0.71 pregnancies per 100 women.

Side effects: Irregular menstrual bleeding is common in the first 1–4 months after insertion, but as the topical effect of the hormone results in atrophy of the endometrium this usually resolves with amenorrhea occurring by 1 year in 20–50 % of users. This method actually causes less bleeding as compared to a copper-bearing IUD. Other side effects include acne, dizziness, headaches, breast tenderness, nausea, vomiting, weight gain, and ovarian cysts. The chances of ectopic pregnancy are less than 1 per 1,000 women years of use (slightly less than a copper-containing IUD).

c) Emergency Contraception (EC)

In the developing world about 50 % of female adolescents have an unmet need for contraception and thus the chances of unwanted pregnancies are high. In 2012, the developing world witnessed about 80 million unintended pregnancies, 30 million unplanned births, 40 million abortions, and 10 million miscarriages. Nearly half of all abortions are unsafe and 98 % of these take place in developing countries. Even in the US although the use of contraceptives by adolescents is increasing and pregnancy rates are falling, eight out of ten adolescent pregnancies are still unintended. Appropriate use of emergency contraception could reduce the risk of pregnancy by 89–99 % and more than a million pregnancies per year could be prevented. Although not an ideal form of contraception it should be easily available to all adolescents.

Indications: It is indicated in any woman who has a risk of pregnancy by virtue of having unprotected intercourse; in cases of potential failure of contraceptive methods such as broken condoms, delayed withdrawal, displaced diaphragms, incorrect usage of the contraceptive patch, ring or OCP; when DMPA is more than 4 weeks and combined monthly injectable more than 7 days late; or in cases of expulsion of an IUD or hormonal contraceptive implant. It also indicated in case of failure of natural family planning methods such as failed withdrawal or incorrect calculation of safe or fertile periods and in all cases of sexual assault.

Description: Available hormonal methods including POPs, combined OCPs and mifepristone. The copper-releasing IUD may also be used as a non-hormonal method for the purpose of emergency contraception.

I. *POPs*: The WHO recommends one dose of a progestin-only pill that contain 1.5 mg of levonorgestrel (LNG). This should be taken as soon after unprotected intercourse as possible but has been shown to be efficacious if taken within 5 days (120 hours) of the event. This is available in the US as Plan B One-step® now Two step regimens that contain two tablets of LNG (0.75 mg) taken 12 hours apart are also available but are now phasing out.

   Mechanism of Action: LNG emergency contraception acts by preventing ovulation; It may also prevent fertilization of the egg by thickening cervical mucus and preventing the ability of the sperm to bind to the ovum. It has no effect after implantation has begun and does not cause abortion.

II. *The "Yuzpe regime"*: This involves the use of combined oral contraceptives (COCs) for the purpose of emergency contraception. This may be particularly useful in developing countries where emergency contraception formulations may not be available. This involves taking two doses of OCP that contain at least 100 µg of ethinyl estradiol and a minimum of 0.5 mg of LNG. As LNG is the active isomer of norgestrel, doubling the dose of this may be needed to achieve the same effect. This may involve taking a large number of pills and the patient is likely to get nauseous and administering an antiemetic 30–60 min before the first COC dose is advisable.

III. *Ulipristal acetate*: This is administered as a single 30 mg pill, up to 120 h after unprotected intercourse. In this case pregnancy must be excluded because of the risk of fetal loss if this medication is given in the first trimester. Thus, patients who have a delayed period for more than 7 days after taking the medication must be advised to come in for a pregnancy test.

   Mechanism of Action: This acts by preventing the binding of progesterone to its receptors.

IV. *Copper IUD*: The WHO recommends that this should be inserted within 5 days of unprotected intercourse. It is really effective and can continue to be used as a form of long-term contraception.

   Mechanism of action: The Copper IUD acts by causing a chemical change that prevents fertilization by damaging the sperm and the egg before they can meet.

Efficacy: LNG: Chance of pregnancy was 1.1 %; Yuzpe: 3.2 % (both taken within 72 h of unprotected sex). Most studies show increased efficacy of LNG emergency contraception the sooner it is administered after unprotected intercourse. In a large study conducted by Glasier et al., ulipristal (30 mg) was found to be as efficacious as 1.5 mg of LNG (1.8 % versus 2.6 %) if taken within 72 h but was found to be more effective than in preventing pregnancy if taken between 72 and 120 h.

The copper IUD is the most effective, preventing 99 % of pregnancies if inserted within 120 h of unprotected intercourse.

Side Effects:

Side effects are more commonly seen after taking emergency contraception with the "Yuzpe regime" especially if using COCPs; they are less when using POPs for EC; with the POPs the most common side effects are headache, fatigue, nausea, and dizziness reported in the first week after taking the EC. While with the COCPs the estrogen-related symptoms are more common including nausea, vomiting, breast tenderness, and headache. Vaginal spotting occurs with both.

Contraindications to the use of POPs are allergy, pregnancy, and undiagnosed genital bleeding, while those to COCPs also include the contraindications to estrogen. *Although a personal history of deep vein thrombosis and pulmonary embolism is an absolute contraindication to ongoing contraception with the combined OC it is not to emergency contraception, although it would be prudent to use a POP in such circumstances.* If a pregnant woman does inadvertently take LNG as a form of emergency contraception there is no evidence to show that this will harm the mother or the fetus.

Ulipristal can cause headache, nausea, and abdominal pain. There is a risk of fetal loss if given in first trimester and a risk of ectopic if pregnancy continues with the patient presenting with severe abdominal pain at 3–5 weeks.

The copper IUD is contraindicated only if the woman is already pregnant.

2. Nonhormonal IUD: Copper IUD

Description: This is a plastic device that contains copper sleeves or wire. It has threads at the end that extend into the vagina so that women can make sure that the device has not been expelled. This gives contraceptive protection for 10 years.

Mechanism of action: Copper component of the device damages the sperm and prevents fertilization of the egg. It also induces a foreign body reaction that prevents the sperms from reaching the fallopian tubes.

Method of use: It is inserted intrauterine usually within 12 days of the start of the woman's last menstrual cycle, within 48 h of giving birth, or after 4 weeks of child birth. If she is switching from another method it can be inserted on any day as long as the patient is not pregnant. Basic provider training is needed for insertion. Further information about precautions with inserting an IUD can be found in the WHO handbook (http://whqlibdoc.who.int/publications/2011/9780978856373_eng.pdf).

Side effects:

Severe menstrual cramping.

Increased risk of PID but only for the first 20 days after insertion. Risk of expulsion and perforation are very low.

Efficacy: 99 %.

Counseling: Ask patient if she has had any STIs and whether she has been treated for the same; screen for tuberculosis and HIV. If the patient has had STIs but has been treated she can still have the Cu IUD inserted. If she has HIV, is under treatment and is well she can still have the IUD inserted.

3. Traditional Methods

a) Withdrawal or Coitus Interruptus:

Description: In this the male partner withdraws at the time of ejaculation so that the semen is kept away from the external genitalia.

Mechanism of action: The sperm is prevented from coming in contact with the egg preventing fertilization.

Efficacy: 96 % with correct and consistent use of this method (ideal); 76 % is what is typically observed as timing of withdrawal is hard to determine.

b) Fertility Awareness Methods:

Description: The adolescent female is educated about the fertile days in her menstrual cycle and uses either the menstrual calendar or a symptom-based approach, i.e., by assessing cervical mucus or basal body temperature to assess when she has a higher chance of pregnancy. This awareness allows her to either abstain or have protected intercourse during those days to achieve contraception. The WHO also endorses the Standard Days Method® (SDM) which is an inexpensive and easy way for women to keep track of their fertile days. For women whose cycles range from 26–32 days, days 8 through 19 (from the first day of the menstrual cycle) are considered potentially fertile days and intercourse should be avoided during those days. CycleBeads® are color coded beads that can help women identify these days. http://www.cyclebeads.com/cyclebeads

Mechanism of action: By avoiding unprotected intercourse during the female partner's fertile period, couples are able to prevent pregnancy.

Efficacy: 95–97 % with correct use of this method (ideal); 75 % is what is typically observed.

c) Lactational Amenorrhea (LAM):

Description: This is a temporary method of contraception that is available to new teenage mothers who are lactating; the women should be amenorrheic and solely breast-feeding day and night to use this successfully as a method of contraception.

Mechanism of action: Exclusive breastfeeding will physiologically prevent ovulation and, thus, prevent pregnancy.

Efficacy: 99 % with correct and consistent use (ideal); 98 % is what is typically observed.

4. Surgical Methods

Female sterilization (tubal ligation) and male sterilization (vasectomy) may be offered to adolescents and young adults who are married or have completed families and also in those cases where future pregnancies may serve as a risk to the physical or emotional well-being of the mother. Surgical or gynecological referral should be sought.

Suggested Reading

Department of Health and Human Services, Centers for Disease Control and Prevention. Morbidity and Mortality Weekly Report, U.S. Medical Eligibility, Criteria for Contraceptive Use, 2010. 28 May 2010/Vol. 59. http://www.cdc.gov/mmwr/pdf/rr/rr59e0528.pdf. Accessed 26 Dec 2012.

Emergency Contraception. Committee on adolescence. Pediatrics. 2012. doi:10.1542/peds.2012-2962. originally published online November 26.

Glasier AF, Cameron ST, Fine PM, et al. Ulipristal acetate versus levonorgestrel for emergency contraception: a randomised non-inferiority trial and meta-analysis. Lancet. 2010; 375(9714):555–62.

Gupta N, Corrado S, Goldstein M, Gupta N, Corrado S, Goldstein M. Hormonal contraception for the adolescent. Pediatr Rev. 2008;29(11):386–96.

Guttmacher Institute. Contraception. http://www.guttmacher.org/sections/contraception.php

World Health Organization. Family planning: a global handbook for providers, 2011 Update. http://whqlibdoc.who.int/publications/2011/9780978856373_eng.pdf. Accessed 26 Dec 2012.

World Health Organization. Medical Eligibility Criteria for Contraceptive Use, 2008 update. http://whqlibdoc.who.int/hq/2008/WHO_RHR_08.19_eng.pdf. Accessed 26 Dec 2012.

Part IV
Communicable Diseases

Chapter 14
Acute Respiratory Infections

David A. Lyczkowski, Peter P. Moschovis, and Shamim Qazi

Keywords Acute respiratory infection • Children • Pneumonia • Assessment • Treatment

Overview

- Acute respiratory infection is the leading cause of death worldwide in children <5 years of age, with over 1.2 million deaths annually.
- Risk factors include malnutrition, prematurity, medical comorbidities including HIV/AIDS, and environmental exposures.
- The primary focus of assessment is determining the severity of illness (based on exam findings and pulse oximetry); identification of the culprit organism is rare and usually unnecessary.
- Other causes of respiratory distress should be considered including upper respiratory infections, noninfectious causes of respiratory illness, and cardiac or other systemic diseases.

D.A. Lyczkowski, M.D. (✉)
Harvard MGH Medicine-Pediatrics Residency Program Massachusetts
General Hospital, Boston, MA, USA
e-mail: lyczkows@post.harvard.edu

P.P. Moschovis, M.D., M.P.H.
Division of Pulmonary and Critical Care, Department of Medicine,
Massachusetts General Hospital, Boston, MA, USA

Department of Pediatrics, Division of Global Health, Massachusetts General Hospital,
Boston, MA, USA

S. Qazi, M.B.B.S., M.Sc., M.D.
Department of Maternal, Newborn, Child and Adolescent Health, World Health Organization,
Geneva, Switzerland

- Mild or moderate disease can generally be managed in the outpatient setting, while children with severe pneumonia or hypoxemia require inpatient admission.
- Treatment may include antibiotics, bronchodilators, oxygen, and supportive care. Management differs for children with stridor, wheeze, HIV/AIDS, malnutrition, and complicated pneumonia.

Epidemiology

Acute respiratory infection, which includes pneumonia, bronchitis, and bronchiolitis, is the leading cause of death worldwide in children under 5 years of age. An estimated 156 million cases occur each year globally, of which 97 % are in low- and middle-income countries, resulting in over 1.2 million deaths annually. To address this burden of disease, the WHO and UNICEF launched a Global Action Plan for the Prevention and Control of Pneumonia (GAPP) in 2009 with a focus on case management, vaccination, and elimination of risk factors.

Risk Factors

Several well-established factors increase both the risk of developing infection and the severity of disease once a child is infected.

- Nutritional:
  - Protein–energy malnutrition.
  - Micronutrient deficiency (especially vitamin D and zinc).
  - Lack of breastfeeding.
- Environmental:
  - House air pollution, parental smoking, crowding.
  - Lack of sunshine, time indoors.
  - High altitude.
- Comorbidities: Prematurity, low birth weight, HIV, chronic lung disease, heart disease, asthma.

Assessment

Case management of children with acute respiratory infection in resource-limited settings poses unique challenges. The primary goals of the initial assessment are to determine (1) the severity of illness, (2) the most likely responsible pathogen(s), and (3) relevant comorbidities.

Table 14.1 WHO classification of a child with cough or difficult breathing

WHO classification of a child with cough or difficult breathing	Signs and symptoms
Severe pneumonia	Central cyanosis, severe respiratory distress (e.g., head nodding), convulsions, lethargy, unconsciousness, inability to drink, or vomiting all oral intake or grunting
Pneumonia	Lower chest indrawing or fast breathing (≥ 60 breaths/min in a child <2 months; ≥ 50 breaths/min in a child 2–11 months; ≥ 40 breaths/min in a child 1–5 years)

Source: World Health Organization. Pocket book of hospital care for children: guidelines of the management of common illnesses with limited resources. Second edition. *Geneva: WHO Press, 2013*

Severity of Illness

WHO guidelines define pneumonia simply as cough or difficult breathing associated with rapid breathing or lower chest indrawing. Additional criteria are used to distinguish pneumonia from severe pneumonia (Table 14.1). Of note, the most recent revision of WHO guidelines, published in 2013, eliminated a third category of "very severe pneumonia" and simplified the treatment algorithm. Recommendations below are based on the 2013 WHO guidelines.

Although these definitions allow rapid classification without the need for a stethoscope, pulse oximeter, radiograph, or other diagnostic tools, the WHO classification system does cause some confusion because it uses the term "pneumonia" to describe all acute respiratory illnesses with tachypnea and chest indrawing, which may include such common illnesses as croup, asthma, or bronchiolitis in addition to the clinicopathologic entity usually understood by the term "pneumonia." As a result, the WHO definition lacks specificity and is 80 % sensitive for children with true bacterial pneumonia. Nevertheless, assessment of disease severity is an essential first step in the management of acute respiratory illness regardless of cause, and the WHO classification system remains a useful tool for triaging and guiding treatment for children with acute respiratory illness.

Physical Examination and Chest Radiography

The clinician should assess for other signs of pneumonia on chest auscultation, including decreased or bronchial breath sounds, crackles, increased vocal resonance, and pleural rub. However, under the WHO classification, these signs are not necessary for the diagnosis of pneumonia, and absence of these signs does not exclude the diagnosis of pneumonia. For children with severe pneumonia, acute decompensation, or clinical deterioration despite treatment, chest X-ray should be obtained to identify patients with complications such as pleural effusion, empyema,

Table 14.2 Differential diagnosis of acute respiratory illness

	Etiology	Clinical diagnosis or diagnostic testing
Upper respiratory	Viral upper respiratory infection (e.g., adenovirus, human metapneumovirus, parainfluenza)	Nasal congestion, rhinorrhea, other upper respiratory tract symptoms
	Acute otitis media	Otoscopy showing dull or bulging tympanic membranes
	Viral or bacterial rhinosinusitis	Mucopurulent nasal discharge, sinus tenderness
	Croup (laryngotracheobronchitis)	Barking cough
	Complications of pharyngitis (peritonsillar or retropharyngeal abscess)	Deviated uvula, oropharyngeal swelling, meningismus
	Laryngomalacia, tracheomalacia, or bronchomalacia	Laryngoscopy, bronchoscopy where available
	Bacterial tracheitis or epiglottitis	Lateral neck radiograph
Lower respiratory	Viral pneumonia or bronchiolitis (e.g., RSV, influenza)	
	Bacterial pneumonia (e.g., S. pneumoniae, H. influenzae, S. aureus)	Sputum gram stain/culture, blood culture
	Atypical bacterial pneumonia (e.g., C. pneumoniae, pertussis)	
	Tuberculosis	Chest radiograph, induced sputum for acid-fast bacilli (AFB) smear and culture
Asthma		
	Foreign body aspiration	Chest radiograph
	Pleural effusion/empyema	Chest radiograph, chest ultrasound
	Interstitial lung disease	Chest radiograph
	Pneumothorax	Chest radiograph
Cardiac	Congestive heart failure	Chest radiograph, echocardiography
	Congenital heart diseases (cyanotic and noncyanotic)	Chest radiograph, echocardiography
	Acquired valvular diseases	Chest radiograph, echocardiography, ECG
	Myocarditis	ECG
	Pericardial tamponade	Pulsus paradoxus, ECG, echocardiography
HIV-associated illnesses	P. jirovecii pneumonia	Chest radiograph, sputum silver stain or PAS stain
	CMV pneumonia	Fundoscopy for retinitis, PCR where available
	Atypical mycobacterial infection (e.g., M. avium intracellulare)	Chest radiograph, induced sputum AFB smear and culture
	Lymphoid interstitial pneumonitis	Chest radiograph with bilateral reticulo-nodular interstitial pattern and hilar adenopathy
Other	Severe anemia	Blood count
	Malaria	Thick and thin smear, rapid diagnostic testing
	Severe dehydration	
	Other causes of metabolic acidosis	Chemistry panel, blood gas
	Organophosphate poisoning	Fundoscopy, neurologic examination
	Illness complicated by malnutrition	
	Elevated intracranial pressure	

pneumothorax, pneumatocele, interstitial pneumonia, or pericardial effusion. For children without severe pneumonia, chest radiography is not routinely recommended because it does not often change the management.

Pulse Oximetry

Hypoxemia is associated with a two- to fivefold increased risk of death. Pulse oximetry is an important tool for identifying which children with pneumonia need oxygen therapy, and is recommended by the WHO for assessment of children with respiratory distress. When pulse oximetry is not available, cyanosis and head nodding have good specificity but poor sensitivity for hypoxemia; other signs including a respiratory rate >70, chest indrawing, inability to feed due to respiratory distress, and altered mental status may be suggestive but have poor sensitivity and specificity.

Etiology and Differential Diagnosis

The most common bacterial pathogens causing pneumonia among children in developing countries are *S. pneumoniae* (30–50 %), *H. influenzae*, *S. aureus*, and *K. pneumoniae*. RSV has been isolated in 15–40 % of children hospitalized with pneumonia or bronchiolitis; adenovirus, parainfluenza, influenza A and B, human rhinovirus, and human metapneumovirus are also widely prevalent. Viral and bacterial respiratory illnesses may coexist.

Particular attention should be paid to differentiating illnesses that may require a different course of treatment. Croup, asthma, other wheezing syndromes, pulmonary tuberculosis, and viral bronchiolitis are common and require different treatment than does pneumonia. Non-respiratory causes of rapid breathing should also be considered. Children with HIV frequently have typical etiologies of respiratory illness (e.g., pneumococcal pneumonia, tuberculosis) but are also at risk for a range of other respiratory pathogens, Table 14.2.

Management

The management of acute respiratory infection includes diagnostic evaluation, triage to an appropriate venue (i.e., inpatient versus outpatient care), and treatment (including antibiotic therapy, oxygen, bronchodilators, antipyretics, and/or hydration).

Table 14.3 Management of pneumonia in children 2 months to 5 years

	Pneumonia	Severe pneumonia
Location of treatment	Outpatient (unless supplemental O_2 is required)	Inpatient
Diagnostic testing	If no improvement in 72 h, obtain chest radiograph	Consider chest radiograph. If no improvement in 48 h, obtain chest radiograph
Antibiotics	Amoxicillin 40 mg/kg PO twice daily × 5 days (or ×3 days in HIV-negative child with no chest indrawing)	Ampicillin 50 mg/kg IM/IV (or benzylpenicillin 50,000 U/kg IM/IV) every 6 h and gentamicin 7.5 mg/kg IM daily × 5 days or more. Alternate: Ceftriaxone 80 mg/kg IM/IV daily × 5 days or more
		If not improved within 48 h of first treatment regimen, switch to gentamicin 7.5 mg/kg IM/IV daily and cloxacillin 50 mg/kg IM/IV every 6 h followed by cloxacillin or dicloxacillin 50 mg/kg PO four times daily to complete 21 days
Antibiotics in HIV-infected or HIV-exposed children	Amoxicillin 40 mg/kg PO twice daily × 5 days if no chest indrawing. If chest indrawing, treat as for severe pneumonia	Ampicillin 50 mg/kg IM/IV (or benzylpenicillin 50,000 mg/kg IM/IV) every 6 h and gentamicin 7.5 mg/kg IM/IV daily × 5 days. Alternate: Ceftriaxone 80 mg/kg IM/IV daily × 5 days
		If not improved within 48 h on ampicillin/gentamicin, switch to ceftriaxone 80 mg/kg if available or to gentamicin and cloxacillin as for very severe pneumonia
		After 5 days of parenteral treatment, if improving, switch to amoxicillin 40 mg/kg PO twice daily for an additional 5 days
		For children with clinical signs of PCP (e.g., interstitial pneumonia on chest radiograph) and for all children 2–11 months, also give high-dose cotrimoxazole 8 + 40 mg/kg IV or PO every 8 h × 21 days
Oxygen	If SpO_2<90 % (<87 % at altitudes >2500 m), give supplemental O_2 via nasal prongs (nasal or nasopharyngeal catheters are acceptable alternatives). If pulse oximetry not available, give supplemental O_2 to children with signs of hypoxia (see "Pulse oximetry," above). Discontinue supplemental O_2 after SpO_2 stably >90 % while breathing room air	
Other interventions	Return for follow-up in 3 days or sooner if danger signs develop. For children >1 year, offer a safe remedy for sore throat and cough (e.g., hot tea with honey and lemon)	Treat complications if identified. Paracetamol if fever >39°C that causes distress. Bronchodilator if wheeze (see "Asthma and other wheezing illnesses," below). Suction secretions as needed. Encourage breastfeeding and oral fluids or place nasogastric tube if necessary for daily maintenance fluids. Reassessment by nurse every 3 h and by doctor twice daily

Sources: World Health Organization. Evidence for technical update of pocket book recommendations. Recommendations for management of common childhood conditions. Geneva: WHO Press, 2012; *World Health Organization*. Integrated Management of Childhood Illness (IMCI) pneumonia case management guidelines. Geneva: WHO Press, 2013; *World Health Organization*. Pocket book of hospital care for children: guidelines of the management of common illnesses with limited resources. Second edition. Geneva: WHO Press, 2013

Pneumonia

Unless another etiology for the acute respiratory illness can be clearly and rapidly identified, it is generally prudent to initiate treatment for bacterial pneumonia, Table 14.3.

Reevaluation is an important part of the management of acute respiratory infection. After 3 days of treatment, improvement is defined (by WHO guidelines) as slower breathing, less fever, eating better, and disappearance of chest indrawing. Lack of improvement after 3 days of treatment should prompt the clinician to consider switching therapies; worsening after 3 days of treatment should prompt the clinician to switch therapies and reevaluate for other diagnoses.

Complicated Pneumonia

Necrotizing pneumonia (commonly due to *S. pneumoniae, S. aureus, or Group A streptococci*), lung abscess (commonly due to *S. aureus*), parapneumonic effusion, and empyema may complicate pneumonia. If such complications are suspected, chest radiograph should be obtained. For Gram-negative coverage, ceftriaxone or amoxicillin/clavulanic acid may be used. When *S. aureus* infection is suspected or proven, Gram-positive coverage should include an agent active against methicillin-sensitive *S. aureus* (MSSA) (e.g., cloxacillin) or, if the local prevalence of methicillin-resistant *S. aureus* (MRSA) is high, an agent active against MRSA (e.g., vancomycin or clindamycin). In complicated pneumonia, a prolonged course of antibiotic therapy is indicated; in general, following defervescence, a good general rule is 5 days of IV antibiotics followed by 2 weeks of oral antibiotics.

If parapneumonic effusion or empyema is present, thoracentesis (consider ultrasound guidance) should be performed to evaluate fluid pH, cell count, LDH, total protein, glucose, Gram stain, and cultures. AFB smear/culture and cytology may be indicated as well. A chest tube is recommended for large effusions occupying greater than half the hemithorax, effusions causing hypoxia or hypercapnia, complicated effusions (positive Gram stain or culture, pH < 7.2, or glucose < 60 mg/dL [3.3 mmol/L]), empyemas (frank pus), or failure to improve with 48–72 h of antibiotic therapy. If the effusion is multiloculated and in cases that present late (>1 week of symptoms), surgical debridement or decortication may be necessary.

Pneumonia in Children with HIV/AIDS

Children with HIV and community-acquired pneumonia have sixfold higher case-fatality rates than do HIV-uninfected children with community-acquired pneumonia; the effect is greatest in infants under 12 months. Antibiotic selection for such children is described in Table 14.3 above.

Although *P. jirovecii* pneumonia is common among children with HIV, empiric therapy with cotrimoxazole is only recommended for children aged 2–11 months, for those with high clinical suspicion of *P. jirovecii* pneumonia (e.g., bilateral interstitial pattern on chest radiograph, mild fever, and/or severe respiratory distress), or for those with positive sputum silver stain or PAS. Peak incidence is in children aged 4–6 months. For children with confirmed or suspected *P. jirovecii* pneumonia, treatment consists of cotrimoxazole 8+40 mg/kg/dose, three times daily for 3 weeks (or for sulfa-allergic children, pentamidine 4 mg/kg daily for 3 weeks). The IV route is preferred over PO. After treatment is completed, routine cotrimoxazole prophylaxis should follow. Although the WHO makes no recommendation concerning corticosteroids, a joint statement by the CDC, NIH, IDSA, AAP, and others makes a grade AI recommendation partly based on extrapolation from adult studies. Thus, corticosteroids may be considered for children with *P. jirovecii* pneumonia and $PaO_2 < 70$ mmHg on room air or alveolar-arterial O_2 gradient >35 mmHg. Prednisone is dosed 1 mg/kg/dose (maximum 40 mg/dose) twice daily for 5 days, then 0.5 mg/kg/dose (maximum 20 mg/dose) twice daily for 5 days, and then 0.5 mg/kg/dose (maximum 20 mg/dose) daily for 5 days.

Tuberculosis is prevalent in approximately 8–8.5 % of children with HIV and acute respiratory infection and in 20.7 % of such children who fail therapy for community-acquired pneumonia. Coinfection with typical bacterial pathogens and mycobacteria is also common. The WHO does not make any recommendation on the basis of available data regarding empiric therapy for tuberculosis in children presenting with acute respiratory infection, but a high level of suspicion and low threshold for testing or empiric therapy must be maintained. See Chaps. 18 and 19 for further discussion of HIV and TB coinfection.

The role of empiric antiviral therapy for CMV pneumonitis in children with HIV and acute respiratory infection remains uncertain. For confirmed disseminated CMV disease, the preferred agent is ganciclovir 5 mg/kg IV every 12 h for 14–21 days followed by chronic suppressive therapy with 5 mg/kg daily for 5–7 days per week.

Pneumonia Complicated by Malnutrition

Severely malnourished children, like other immunosuppressed children, are susceptible to a wide range of infections including typical causes of pneumonia and also many opportunistic infections. Compared with pneumonia in a well-nourished child, pneumonia in a malnourished child is more likely to be caused by Gram-negative bacteria (*Klebsiella pneumoniae, Escherichia coli, Haemophilus influenzae*) or *Staphylococcus aureus*. In view of the nutritional consequences and immunological impairment associated with HIV, any malnourished child with pneumonia should be tested for HIV. Tuberculosis and *P. jirovecii* pneumonia should be considered; if suspected, evaluation should include chest radiograph, induced sputum for acid-fast bacilli (smear and culture), and sputum for silver or PAS staining. Nutritional supplementation should be provided during and after antibiotic therapy for all children with malnutrition and pneumonia. Children with severe acute malnutrition and pneumonia should also receive care and interventions to prevent and treat hypoglycemia, hypothermia, and other specific complications. See chapter 22 for management of acute malnutrition.

Asthma and Other Wheezing Illnesses

Diffuse wheeze suggests bronchospasm, and is most commonly caused by viral illness (upper respiratory infection with reactive airways, viral pneumonia, or, in children under 2 years of age, bronchiolitis) or asthma. Obstructive lung disease such as asthma or reactive airways disease may be associated with prolonged expiratory phase, hyperresonance on percussion, and hyperinflated chest. Focal wheeze, asymmetric chest excursion, and dullness on percussion may be caused by a foreign body lodged in the airway. It is important to distinguish wheeze from stridor (see "Croup and Other Conditions That Cause Stridor," below).

To distinguish among possible causes of respiratory illness associated with wheeze, a trial of a short-acting bronchodilator such as salbutamol (or albuterol) can be useful. Administer salbutamol (or albuterol) by metered-dose inhaler with spacer (2 puffs or 200 mcg), or by nebulizer (2.5 mg salbutamol with 4–6 mL sterile water), up to three times in rapid succession. If inhaled salbutamol is not available, subcutaneous epinephrine (0.01 mL/kg of 1:1,000 solution, maximum 0.3 mL) may be used instead.

1. If there is a good response to bronchodilator (decreased respiratory distress, decreased wheeze, and increased air movement), the most likely diagnosis is asthma or reactive airways disease.

    (a) If respiratory distress (tachypnea, retractions, nasal flaring, or grunting) is absent or resolves after administration of a fast-acting bronchodilator, manage at home with inhaled salbutamol via metered-dose inhaler with spacer, via nebulizer, or if inhaled formulations are not available, oral salbutamol (2 mg every 6–8 h for children 1–5 years of age).

    (b) If respiratory distress persists despite bronchodilator, admit to a hospital. In the hospital, give three doses of a rapid-acting bronchodilator as above, followed by repeated administrations up to every hour as needed; a corticosteroid such as oral prednisolone 1 mg/kg daily × 3 days or until improved; and oxygen therapy if the child is hypoxemic.

    (c) If a hospitalized child has not responded to the interventions above, add aminophylline IV (5 mg/kg loading dose, maximum 300 mg, if the child has not received aminophylline in the prior 24 h, followed by 5 mg/kg every 6 h). Each dose of aminophylline should be run over at least 20 min (preferably 1 h). Aminophylline should be stopped immediately if the child develops vomiting, headache, seizure, or heart rate >180/min.

2. If there is minimal or no response to an adequate trial of a short-acting bronchodilator, suspect bronchiolitis or foreign body. Although bronchiolitis is most commonly viral in etiology, it can be difficult to distinguish from bacterial pneumonia and, therefore, is treated as pneumonia (Table 14.3).

Croup and Other Conditions That Cause Stridor

Stridor is a noise heard on inspiration, and in severe cases also on exhalation, caused by narrowing and increased air turbulence in the upper airways (larynx, pharynx, or trachea). It can be distinguished from wheezing (of lower airways origin) by using a stethoscope to listen in front of the mouth, over the throat, and on the chest. The most common cause of acute stridor in young children is croup (viral laryngotracheobronchitis), which can be due to parainfluenza, influenza, measles, or other viruses. Other common causes of stridor in children include:

- Foreign body lodged in the large airways.
- Bacterial tracheitis or epiglottitis.
- Peritonsillar or retropharyngeal abscess.
- Diphtheria.
- Subglottic stenosis or airway edema.
- Laryngomalacia or tracheomalacia.
- Tumor or extrinsic mass causing airway compression.
- Vocal cord dysfunction.

It is necessary to identify rapidly patients with foreign body, tracheitis, epiglottitis, and abscesses based on history and exam because urgent treatment with antibiotics and/or operative intervention may be needed to address the underlying cause of airway obstruction. Regardless of cause, the severity of stridor must be assessed. In mild cases, stridor is present only when the child is agitated or crying. In severe cases, stridor is present at rest; other signs of respiratory distress including chest wall retractions, tachypnea, or nasal flaring may be present as well.

Patients with mild stridor may be managed expectantly at home, unless another condition requiring treatment (e.g., retropharyngeal abscess) is also present. Patients with stridor at rest or with other signs of respiratory distress should receive the following:

- Systemic steroids (dexamethasone 0.6 mg/kg [maximum 9 mg] PO or IV once, or an equivalent dose of prednisone or prednisolone).
- Nebulized epinephrine 1:1,000 solution. If effective in improving symptoms, repeat hourly and monitor heart rate.

Children with persistent signs of severe respiratory distress may be at risk of airway collapse. In these cases, children may require:

- Endotracheal intubation and/or emergency tracheostomy (to be performed only by an experienced provider).
- Oxygen therapy (which should be provided by nasal cannula, and only if the need for intubation/tracheostomy is imminent).

Recommended Reading

Bari A, Sadruddin S, Khan A, et al. Community case management of severe pneumonia with oral amoxicillin in children aged 2-59 months in Haripur district, Pakistan: a cluster randomised trial. Lancet. 2011;378:1796–803.

Rudan I, Boschi-Pinto C, Biloglav Z, et al. Epidemiology and etiology of childhood pneumonia. Bull World Health Organ. 2008;86:408–16.

Singh V, Aneja S. Pneumonia—management in the developing world. Paediatr Respir Rev. 2011;12:52–9.

World Health Organization. Pocket book of hospital care for children: guidelines of the management of common illnesses with limited resources. 2nd ed. Geneva: WHO Press; 2013.

World Health Organization. Recommendations for management of common childhood conditions: evidence for technical update of pocket book recommendations: newborn conditions, dysentery, pneumonia, oxygen use and delivery, common causes of fever, severe acute malnutrition and supportive care. Geneva: WHO Press; 2012.

World Health Orgnization. WHO recommendations on the management of diarrhoea and pneumonia in HIV-infected infants and children: integrated management of childhood illness (IMCI). Geneva: WHO Press; 2010.

Chapter 15
Diarrheal Illnesses

A. Kaytee Welsh and Archana Patel

Keywords Diarrhea • Dehydration • Gastroenteritis • Oral rehydration therapy • Malnutrition • Zinc

Overview

- Diarrheal illness is a leading cause of morbidity and mortality in the pediatric population worldwide.
- Diarrheal illness is both largely preventable and treatable.
- Rehydration is the mainstay of treatment.
- Early refeeding during diarrheal illnesses is important in prevention and treatment of malnutrition.
- Improved water, hand, and sanitation hygiene is key to prevention of diarrheal illnesses.

Introduction

There are more than two billion cases of diarrheal illness every year in the pediatric population worldwide. Diarrheal illness is the third leading cause of death in children under five according to the WHO, accounting for 1.5–2 million deaths per year,

---

A.K. Welsh, M.D. (✉)
Massachusetts General Hospital, Boston, MA, USA
e-mail: awelsh@partners.org

A. Patel, M.D., Ph.D., D.N.B.
Clinical Epidemiology Unit, Department of Pediatrics,
Indira Gandhi Government Medical College, Nagpur, India

and is the leading cause of malnutrition in children under 5. Eighty percent of deaths related to diarrheal illnesses occur in toddlers less than 2 years of age. On average, infants have six episodes of diarrheal illness per year, with children experiencing an average of three episodes per year. Due to worsening sanitation, food and water hygiene, and malnutrition, diarrhea is one of the leading causes of death during periods of major conflict, natural disasters, and population displacements. The mainstay of treatment is oral rehydration therapy (ORT) with oral rehydration salts (ORS), early refeeding, and zinc supplementation.

Definitions

Diarrhea is defined by the WHO as the passage of at least three loose or watery stools in a 24-h period. Diarrhea has four syndromic presentations: acute watery, acute invasive (bloody), or persistent ($\geq$2 weeks duration), and diarrhea with malnutrition.

1) Acute watery diarrhea is most commonly viral, specifically due to rotavirus, although cases of norovirus are likely underestimated. In older children, *Enterotoxigenic Escherichia coli* (ETEC) is a common pathogen causing acute watery diarrhea.
2) Invasive diarrhea is defined by frank blood in the stool, often associated with fever, and is caused by exudative inflammation in the colon. Most common cause is shigellosis.
3) Persistent diarrhea is defined by diarrheal illness that lasts greater than 2 weeks. Persistent diarrhea is both a common cause as well as a common complication of malnutrition.
4) Diarrhea with malnutrition is more likely to cause significant electrolyte abnormalities, specifically hypernatremia and hypokalemia, has a higher risk of systemic infection, and has a higher risk of complications, such as heart failure, during rehydration therapy.

History/Clinical Assessment

1) Characterization of diarrhea.
    a) Length of illness: acute versus chronic.
    b) Onset: acute versus gradual.
    c) Presenting symptoms.
    d) Amount of diarrhea (estimation of the amount of fluid loss).
    e) Blood or mucus in the stool.

2) Review of systems: Important to elicit symptoms such as fever, cough, vomiting, abdominal pain, urinary symptoms, rash, bilious vomiting, jaundice, and muscle and joint aches that could suggest etiologies other than infectious gastroenteritis. These include but are not limited to non-GI infections, surgical (appendicitis, intussusception), systemic illnesses (pneumonia, UTI, HIV, hepatitis, measles), Hirschsprung's disease, and necrotizing enterocolitis.
3) Hydration status: WHO dehydration classification: Severe dehydration, some dehydration, no dehydration.
   a) *Severe dehydration*: Two or more of the following signs—lethargy/unconsciousness, sunken eyes, unable to drink or drinks poorly, skin pinch goes back very slowly (>2 s), >10 % body weight deficit, >100 ml/kg fluid deficit.
   b) *Some dehydration*: Two or more of the following signs—restlessness, irritability, sunken eyes, drinks eagerly, thirsty, skin pinch goes back slowly, 5–10 % body weight deficit, 50–100 ml/kg fluid deficit.
   c) *No dehydration*: Not enough signs to classify as some or severe dehydration. <5 % body deficit, <50 ml/kg fluid deficit.
4) Types of dehydration:
   a) Hypertonic dehydration (plasma sodium >150 mmol/l): Excess loss of water compared to salt. Occurs when the body starts to retain salt to help preserve intravascular volume. Can also occur when fluids high in salt (chicken soup) are used to rehydrate without another source of water.
   b) Isotonic dehydration (plasma sodium 130–150 mmol/l): Equal net loss of water and salt. Most common.
   c) Hypotonic dehydration (plasma sodium <130 mmol/l): Excess net sodium loss compared to water. Most commonly occurs when water is exclusively used for rehydration.
5) Clinical signs of malnutrition: Visible signs of wasting (marasmus), presence of bilateral hand and feet edema (kwashiorkor).
   a) Definitions of malnutrition: Severe: weight for height > −3 SD; moderate: weight for height between >−2 SD, but <−3 SD; mild: >−1 SD, but <−2 SD.
   b) Moderate dehydration with signs of malnutrition is classified by the WHO as seriously ill and should be treated in the hospital.
6) Warning signs: Rigid abdomen (suggestive of appendicitis, bowel perforation, and need for surgical intervention), abdominal mass (intussusception), petechiae (sepsis, hemolytic uremic syndrome (HUS), meningococcal infection), jaundice (hepatitis), attacks of crying (intussusception), undue sleepiness (severe dehydration, sepsis), fever.
7) Assessment of comorbid conditions: Immunocompromised patients, pregnancy, diabetes, renal or liver disease.

Syndromic Presentations of Diarrheal Illness

Acute Watery Diarrhea

In children ≤5 years of age, viral infections account for approximately 60 % of all acute diarrheal illnesses. Most causes are indistinguishable, and treatment is supportive (Table 15.1).

Invasive (Bloody) Diarrhea

This is also often referred to as dysentery. The most common cause of invasive diarrhea or diarrhea with fever is shigellosis (Table 15.2).

Treatment

a) *Largely supportive care*, with primary focus on rehydration (see Fig. 15.1) due to diarrhea causing increased loss of fluid and electrolytes.
b) *ORT* has been shown to be as effective as IV fluids in mild-to-moderate dehydration.
   - ORS—Utilize Na/glucose transporter in the intestinal lumen, move glucose and sodium into the cell, creating an osmotic gradient that allows water to be absorbed into the body. The sodium–glucose transporter is one of the few mucosal transporters not disrupted during intestinal infections.
   - Originally created to treat dehydration associated with cholera infections.
   - Equimolar concentration of glucose and sodium is key.
   - Too much glucose (fruit juice) or sodium (chicken soup) can worsen diarrhea by increasing the osmotic gradient inside the intestinal lumen.
   - *Vibrio cholera* toxin causes active transport of sodium into the intestinal lumen, which causes the high-volume stool. The first popular ORS had high osmolality of glucose and sodium to compensate. More commonly, ORS has been used for diarrhea caused by rotavirus. Concern that treatment with high-osmolality ORS would cause hypernatremia in patients with diarrhea not caused by vibrio led to the creation of lower osmolality ORS and it is becoming the new standard.
   - Avoid using ORS in patients with impaired mental status, abdominal ileus, or inability to absorb fluid from intestinal tract.
   - Oral rehydration with water alone can cause hyponatremia, which can lead to lethargy and seizures.
   - *ORS recipe*:
     a. WHO recommends using the following: Sucrose 27 g, sodium bicarbonate 2.5 g; dissolve sugar and salts in 1 liter of clean water (boiled, chlorinated",

Table 15.1 Acute watery diarrhea, common etiologies, transmission, symptoms, complications, and management considerations

Infectious etiology	Transmission	Symptoms	Complications	Management
Viral: Rotavirus, noro-viruses, astrovirus, enteric adenovirus (most common cause of diarrhea)	Fecal oral route, contaminated water and food	Vomiting (usually most severe in norovirus infection), fever, watery diarrhea, usually large volume, colicky abdominal pain, exaggerated bowel sounds	Significant dehydration	Rehydration Continue breastfeeding Early refeeding to prevent malnutrition
Cholera: *Vibrio cholerae*	Contaminated food or water, can survive in seawater, copepods and zooplankton, often outbreaks occur during times of upheaval	Vomiting, mild to severe, watery "rice-water" diarrhea, significant volume loss, muscle and abdominal cramping, local outbreaks	Severe and life-threatening dehydration, electrolyte imbalances, metabolic acidosis, hypoglycemia, shock, renal failure, ileus, cardiac arrhythmias	Aggressive rehydration with ORS, sucrose or rice-water-based solutions, IV fluid hydration for severe cases when available, antibiotics in severe cases: azithromycin, erythromycin, furazolidone, cotrimoxazole, all for 3 days
E. coli: ETEC, Enteropathogenic *Escherichia coli* (EPEC) (second most common cause of diarrhea, most common cause of travelers' diarrhea)	Contaminated food, fecal-oral route; EPEC is often a hospital-acquired infection	Watery diarrhea, often large volume, vomiting, abdominal pain	Dehydration, electrolyte abnormalities	Rehydration, antibiotics can be given for suspected EPEC in young infants: cotrimoxazole 15 mg/kg daily for 5 days for infants >1 month old depending on local resistance patterns
Giardiasis	Contaminated water with cysts, not killed by chlorination, direct person-to-person contact	Watery diarrhea which often turns steatorrheic, with nausea, abdominal bloating	Fat malabsorption, weight loss, vitamin deficiencies, chronic giardiasis, lactose intolerance	Rehydration, antibiotics if symptoms persist: metronidazole for 3-day course or single-dose tinidazole
Cryptosporidiosis	Contaminated water	Diarrhea, abdominal cramping	Severe infection mimicking cholera can occur in patients with AIDS, can cause chronic diarrhea	Rehydration, HAART in patients with AIDS

Table 15.2 Invasive diarrhea—common etiologies, transmission, symptoms, complications, and management considerations

Infectious etiology	Transmission	Symptoms	Complications	Management
Shigellosis: *Shigella dysenteriae*, *S. flexneri*, *S. boydii*, *S. sonneii*	Humans only natural host, person-to-person contact, contaminated water or food	Tenesmus, fever, passage of frequent bloody stools	Dehydration, hypoglycemia, hyponatremia, hemolytic-uremic syndrome (HUS), thrombotic thrombocytopenic purpura (TTP), convulsions, "rose spot" rash, Reiter's syndrome	Rehydration, antibiotics for persistent bloody diarrhea, or systemic symptoms/infection: ampicillin, cotrimoxazole (resistance is increasing), quinolones
EHEC: *E. coli* 0157	Contaminated food: beef, milk, fruit, and vegetables	2–3-day watery diarrhea followed by bloody diarrhea, vomiting, abdominal pain	Dehydration, HUS, severe hemorrhagic colitis	Rehydration, antibiotics are not indicated, antibiotics have been associated with increased risk of HUS
Campylobacter enterocolitis	Contact with infected animals, commonly birds, ubiquitous zoonosis, contaminated food or water, infected individuals can continue to excrete bacteria in feces for up to 3 weeks after illness	Fever, abdominal pain, may be followed by bloody diarrhea	In the presence of other systemic illnesses—malnutrition, liver disease, malignancy, diabetes, renal failure, and immunodeficiency can cause severe disseminated infection (meningitis, abscesses, Reiter's syndrome, reactive arthritis), Guillain–Barré syndrome	Rehydration, supportive care, in severe case antibiotics: erythromycin, cotrimoxazole, ciprofloxacin, azithromycin

Salmonella enterocolitis: *S. typhi*, *S. enteritidis*	Contact with infected animals, person-to-person contact, infected individuals can continue to excrete bacteria in feces for up to 8 weeks after illness, chronic carrier state occurs in 2–5 % of patients infected	Nausea, vomiting, headache, fever, watery diarrhea, which turns bloody, cramping abdominal pain which can be severe and mimic appendicitis	Toxic megacolon; bacteremia; infection of meninges, bones, joints, lungs, heart valves, liver, spleen, ovaries, kidneys	Rehydration, supportive care, in severe cases or risk of developing severe disease, treat with antibiotics: ciprofloxacin for systemic illness: chloramphenicol, amoxicillin, cotrimoxazole, azithromycin, cefotaxime, ceftriaxone
Amoebic dysentery: *Entamoeba histolytica*	Contaminated food and drink (human feces), sexual transmission	Abdominal pain, diarrhea, as infection progresses diarrhea becomes bloody with mucous and tenesmus	Toxic megacolon, bowel perforation, systemic infection (parasite can infect almost any tissue in the body causing abscesses) Risk factors for severe infections: pregnancy, malnourishment, immunosupression, young children	Rehydration metronidazole for 5-day course, followed by diloxanide furoate for 10 days (for treatment of cysts); if signs of peritonitis, add a broad-spectrum antibiotic

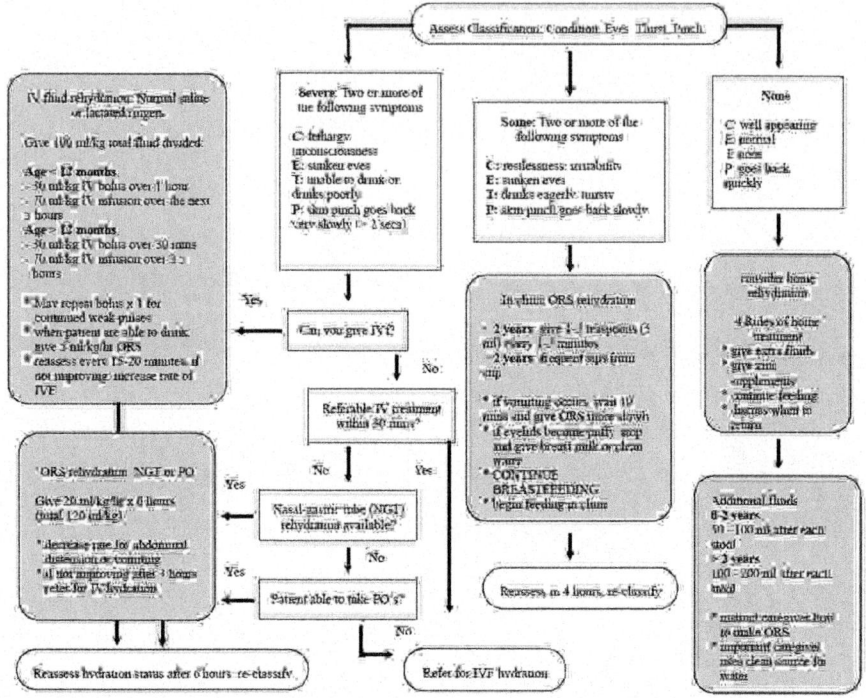

Fig. 15.1 WHO Pocket Book of Hospital care for children classification of severity of dehydration in children with diarrhea and recommended treatment plan

or filtered); alternatively, add six-level small spoons (i.e., teaspoons) of sugar and a half small spoon of salt to 1 of clean water.
  b. Rice-based ORS: Boil 50 g of rice powder in 1 liter. of water, and add sugar and salts as above (use within 12 h of preparation).
  c. In children with severe malnutrition full-strength ORS solution should not be used. Instead, ReSoMal, which is an ORS solution that is higher in potassium and lower in sodium, should be used. However a simple solution can also be prepared by adding 1 liter plain water to the oral rehydration solution and adding 45 ml of potassium chloride (from a stock solution containing 100 g KCl/l). Children receiving the solution should also receive 2 ml intramuscularly of 50 % magnesium sulfate solution once and 1 ml/kg/day of zinc chloride (10 g/l) orally daily until diarrhea stops.

c) *Antibiotics*: Not routinely used, but could be considered in the following:

- Suspicion of cholera: Endemic areas, recent local outbreaks, large-volume "rice-water" diarrhea—important to treat early with antibiotics as well as aggressive rehydration.
- Concern for systemic illness—fever, sepsis, especially related to invasive systemic shigellosis or Salmonella Typhi (*S. Typhi*).

- Comorbid illness increasing the risk for severe illness—immunocompromised patients, severe malnutrition, infants with invasive disease, pregnancy, diabetes, renal or liver disease.
- Chronic infection, which can occur with giardia, cryptosporidiosis, and *S. typhi*.

d) *Zinc supplementation*:
  - Zinc is an important micronutrient for health and development.
  - Increased losses of zinc occur during episodes of diarrhea.
  - Zinc supplementation has been shown to reduce severity and duration of diarrheal illness and protect against future episodes for 2–3 months following illness.
  - WHO recommends zinc supplementation during diarrheal illnesses as follows:

    <6 months of age: 10 mg once a day, by mouth, for 10–14 days.
    6 months—5 years: 20 mg once a day, by mouth, for 10–14 days.

e) *Early refeeding*: Early refeeding during acute illness has been shown to be safe and effective and not doing so may prolong the course and worsen the severity of illness. It is also important for treatment and prevention of malnutrition, which is often caused by recurrent episodes of diarrhea.
  WHO recommends the following:
  – Continue breastfeeding throughout diarrheal illness and rehydration therapy; infants not exclusively breastfeed and children should be fed every 3–4 h (six meals a day). Suggested foods include starches, cereal, rice, vegetables, meat, fish, fresh fruit juice, or banana to add potassium.
  – 1–2 teaspoons of vegetable oil with each serving of food to provide extra calories to diet.
  – Offer an extra meal a day for 2 weeks following illness to replenish and maintain nutrition.

f) *Antidiarrheal agents* These are not recommended, do not prevent dehydration or malnutrition, and can cause dangerous side effects.

g) *Follow-up recommendations*: Recommend that parents return to the clinic if the patient is unable to drink or breastfeed, becomes more sick, diarrhea worsens, or with the development of fever and/ or bloody stools. If the patient does not worsen, but diarrhea persists, the patient should return to clinic in 5 days.

Persistent Diarrheal Illness

- Etiology of persistent diarrhea is multi-factorial including acute infection and malnutrition with delayed mucosal healing, diminished digestion, decreased absorptive capacity and repeated infections. The subsequent reduction in nutrient absorption with increased requirements often worsens nutritional status and creates a vicious cycle. It is important to always consider HIV in high-risk areas.

Treatment

a) Evaluate for dehydration, systemic infection, and other non-intestinal infections (pneumonia, UTI, sepsis, HIV, measles, otitis media) and treat as needed.
b) Refer for inpatient treatment patients with moderate to severe malnutrition, dehydration, systemic infections, age <4 months (Table 15.3).
c) Treat dehydration according to dehydration flow sheet.
d) Bloody stool—Treat with antibiotics for shigella infection. If the patient continues to have bloody diarrhea repeat treatment with second antibiotic depending on local sensitivities. WHO recommends treating for *Entamoeba histolytica* if bloody stools continue after treatment for Shigella, or microscopic examination of stool shows *Entamoeba histolytica* trophozoites within RBCs.
e) *Giardia lamblia*: WHO recommends only treating for Giardia if microscopic examination of stool is positive for Giardia cysts or trophozoites.
f) Maintain nutrition: Minimum of 110 cal per kilogram daily.
g) Transient lactose intolerance can occur following an intestinal infection, consider decreasing or eliminating dairy from the diet. Do not decrease breastfeeding.
h) Vitamin supplementation: WHO recommends giving double the recommended daily allowances (RDA) of selective vitamins and minerals for 2 weeks in children with persistent diarrhea. RDA for child >1 year: folate 50 micrograms, zinc 10 mg, vitamin A 400 micrograms, iron 10 mg, copper 1 mg, magnesium 80 mg.

Diarrhea with Malnutrition

For treatment considerations for the severely malnourished, see Chap. 22.

Table 15.3 Indications for hospitalization

Absolute	Relative
Severe dehydration	Neonatal age
Neurological involvement	Febrile infant <6 months with bloody diarrhea
Severe systemic illness (e.g., pneumonia, sepsis, shock)	Immune deficiency
Life-threatening causes of diarrhea	Malnutrition
Severe vomiting	Parents unable to manage the problem
Bloody diarrhea with malnutrition, dehydration, age, <1 year, or measles in past 6 months	
Severe malnutrition (weight for height >−3 SD)	
Persistent diarrhea in age <4 months or with moderate malnutrition (weight for height <−3 SD but >−2 SD)	

Prevention

Exclusive breastfeeding for the first 6 months, improved access to clean drinking water by chlorination, filtration or boiling water when clear water is not available; hand hygiene (washing hands with soap); food hygiene; improved community sanitation; vitamin A supplementation, rotavirus and measles vaccination.

Recommended Reading

1. American Academy of Pediatrics. Red book: 2009 report of the committee on infectious diseases. 28th ed. Elk Grove Village, IL: American Academy of Pediatrics; 2009.
2. Eddleston M, Davidson R, Brent A, Wilkinson R. Oxford handbook of tropical medicine. 3rd ed. New York: Oxford University Press Inc.; 2008.
3. Stanton B, Evans J. Oral rehydration therapy. UpToDate. 2012.
4. The United Nations Children's Fund (UNICEF)/World Health Organization (WHO). Diarrhea: why children are still dying and what can be done. The United Nations Children's Fund/World Health Organization. 2009.
5. World Health Organization. Pocket book of hospital care for children: guidelines for the management of common illnesses with limited resources. Geneva: World Health Organization; 2005.

Chapter 16
Malaria

Paul J. Krezanoski and Davidson H. Hamer

Keywords Malaria • *Plasmodium falciparum* • *Plasmodium vivax* • *Plasmodium malariae* • *Plasmodium ovale* • Artemisinin-based combination therapy • Rapid diagnostic test • Anemia • Cerebral malaria

Overview

- Malaria is responsible for substantial morbidity and mortality worldwide (in 2010, ~216,000,000 episodes and 655,000 or more deaths).
- Four species of *Plasmodium* responsible for most human cases (*P. falciparum, P. vivax, P. ovale*, and *P. malariae*).
- Clinically, malaria ranges from asymptomatic parasitemia to uncomplicated malaria to severe malaria (manifested typically to be cerebral malaria, severe anemia, hypoglycemia, and potentially multisystem organ failure).

P.J. Krezanoski, M.D.
Department of Pediatrics, Massachusetts General Hospital, Boston, MA, USA

Department of Internal Medicine, Massachusetts General Hospital, Boston, MA, USA

D.H. Hamer, M.D (✉)
Center for Global Health and Development, Boston University, Crosstown 3rd Floor, 801 Massachusetts Ave., Boston, MA 02118, USA

Department of International Health, Boston University School of Public Health, Boston, MA, USA

Section of Infectious Diseases, Department of Medicine, Boston University School of Medicine, Boston, MA, USA

Zambia Centre for Applied Health Research and Development, Lusaka, Zambia
e-mail: dhamer@bu.edu

- While thick and thin blood smears have been the mainstay of diagnosis for decades, recent years have seen the widespread use of rapid diagnostic, antigen-based tests (RDTs) with high sensitivity and specificity.
- Artemisinin-based combination therapy is the preferred treatment modality for uncomplicated and severe disease due to *P. falciparum*, while chloroquine remains the treatment of choice for the other three species in most regions of the world.

Malaria Epidemiology

- Substantial progress has been made in the last decade in reducing malaria-associated morbidity and mortality worldwide.
- In some endemic countries, aggressive malaria control has reduced the malaria burden to a point where malaria elimination is becoming a feasible reality either nationally or sub-nationally.
- In 2010 there were an estimated 216 million episodes of malaria with more than 80 % occurring in sub-Saharan Africa.
- Worldwide malaria mortality estimates for 2010 ranged from approximately 655,000 deaths to as high as 1,238,000, with most of these deaths occurring in children under 5 in sub-Saharan Africa.
- Between 2000 and 2010, malaria transmission decreased by >50 % in 43 of 99 countries reporting active transmission.
- Despite the substantial improvements in the global burden of malaria, the disease continues to cause substantial household-level economic burden in many endemic areas.

Malaria Parasites

- Four major species of *Plasmodium* cause disease in humans.
- *P. falciparum* occurs in nearly all areas of the world where there is malaria transmission. Intensity of transmission is greatest in sub-Saharan Africa.
- *P. vivax* transmission occurs throughout the malarious areas of the Americas, Asia, the Middle East, North Africa, and parts of East Africa but does not occur in West or Central Africa.
- *P. ovale* is found mainly in sub-Saharan Africa.
- In recent years, a species that predominantly infects Old World monkeys (macaques), *Plasmodium knowlesi*, has been increasingly recognized as a cause of malaria in humans in parts of South East Asia (especially in Peninsular Malaysia and Malaysian Borneo).
- *P. malariae* occurs in a patchy distribution in low levels in all areas where malaria occurs.

Life Cycle

Members of the genus *Plasmodium* undergo:

- Sexual multiplication termed sporogony in the mosquito host
- Two types of asexual division termed schizogony in the vertebrate host (Fig. 16.1).
- Mosquitoes of the *Anopheles* genus are the main vectors for transmission of malaria to humans.
- While feeding on an infected human, female *Anopheles* mosquitoes ingest gametocytes.
- Gamete formation occurs in the stomach of the mosquito with eventual release of microgametes, which fertilize macrogametes to form oocysts.
- The oocyst progressively enlarges and then ruptures, releasing thousands of sporozoites.
- The sporozoites migrate to the salivary glands of the female mosquito and then are injected into humans when she takes a blood meal.
- In humans, a cycle of asexual division takes place in the liver.
- During this phase, sporozoites divide asexually with the eventual release of thousands of merozoites.
- Upon rupture of the tissue schizont, the merozoites enter the circulation where they invade red blood cells.
- During the erythrocytic phase, another cycle of asexual division takes place during which trophozoites (early—ring forms; later—mature trophozoites) grow.
- Subsequently merozoites are formed which eventually cause rupture of the red blood cell while subpopulations of merozoites differentiate into gametocytes.
- In people who become infected with *P. vivax* or *P. ovale*, a latent form of infection may develop in liver cells (known as hypnozoites). They may reawaken weeks to months after the initial infection and lead to a relapse of malaria.

Modes of Acquisition of Malaria

- Bite of female anopheline mosquitoes (most common mode)
- Transplacental (vertical)
- Direct inoculation of infected red blood cells via transfusion or from contaminated needles

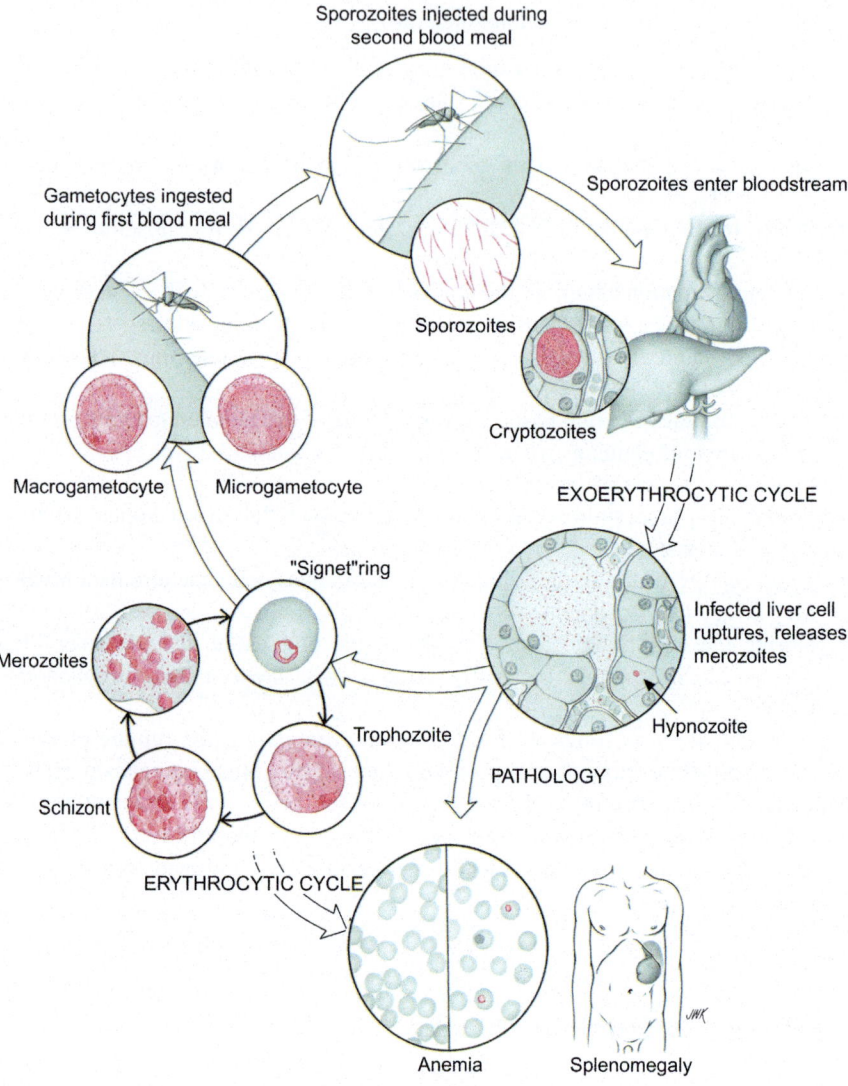

Fig. 16.1 Life cycle of *Plasmodium vivax* in humans (schizogony). From Parasitic Diseases, 5th edition, Eds. Despommier, Gwadz, Hotez, Knirsch. 2005, Apple Tree Productions, New York, NY. Reprinted with permission from Dickson Despommier

Description of Vector and Host Characteristics Influencing Malaria Transmission

Intensity of transmission is influenced by the following:

- Seasonal incidence and prevalence of infection in humans
- Presence of a susceptible human population
- Vector characteristics including their feeding patterns, relative abundance, resting behavior, susceptibility to infection, and effectiveness as a vector. Some anopheline species such as *An. gambiae*, found in many parts of Africa, are highly effective vectors.
- Local climatic and environmental features that affect vector breeding and the rate of sporogony. Seasonal variation of humidity, temperature, and rainfall greatly influence patterns of transmission in many areas of the world.

Host factors that influence the incidence and severity of malaria infections include:

- Underlying immunity, which may be present in populations continuously exposed to malaria in endemic areas
- Occupation, social behavior, and migration (which all affect vector–human interactions)
- Genetic factors. Examples include the following:
  - Suppression of *P. falciparum* development in the presence of fetal hemoglobin or hemoglobin S. Consequently, heterozygotic persons with sickle cell trait have less severe falciparum malaria infections.
  - People whose red blood cells lack the Duffy a and b blood group determinants are resistant to infection with *P. vivax*. As many Africans are Duffy negative, there is a very low incidence of *P. vivax* malaria in sub-Saharan Africa.

Vulnerable Groups

- Children under 5 years: Young children in areas with moderate to intense malaria transmission are at highest risk due to their lack of immunity. Consequently, they are at increased risk of severe malaria including cerebral malaria, severe anemia, and other complications. With repeated infections, partial immunity develops which helps reduce the frequency and severity of clinical episodes of malaria.
- Pregnant women: Malaria in pregnancy poses substantial risk to the mother, fetus, and neonate.
  - In areas of stable malaria transmission, clinically symptomatic infections are rare and the main consequence is an increased risk of:
    - Maternal anemia
    - Low birth weight
    - Neonatal and infant deaths

- In areas with low or unstable malaria transmission, pregnant women have little acquired immunity to malaria and are, therefore, at increased risk of:
  - Symptomatic malaria
  - Severe malaria with central nervous system complications
  - Anemia
  - Adverse birth outcomes including abortion, preterm labor, and stillbirths.
- Primigravidae at the highest risk due to their lack of immunity at the level of the placenta.

Clinical Manifestations

Categorized as uncomplicated versus severe (complicated) malaria.

- **Uncomplicated malaria**
  - Classic attacks (infrequently observed) last 6–10 h separated into three stages:
    - Cold stage of chills and rigors
    - Hot stage of fever, headaches, vomiting, seizures in children <5 years
    - Sweating with fatigue
  - Signs:
    - Fever is the classic sign of malaria infection.
      - Initially, fevers occur at irregular intervals and can be very high, >40 °C, especially in children and nonimmune adults.
      - Seizures in the setting of malaria are concerning for cerebral malaria—be careful attributing seizures to simple febrile seizures.
      - Later fevers may have periodicity. *P. falciparum* typically is described as aperiodic, but classic description of *P. vivax* and *P. ovale* with periodic fevers q48hrs and *P. malariae* every 72 h.
      - Note that young children may also present with hypothermia.
    - Hepatomegaly/splenomegaly
    - Jaundice
    - Tachypnea
    - Diaphoresis
    - Lab values: Mild anemia, mild thrombocytopenia, elevation of bilirubin, and LFTs
  - Symptoms: Nonspecific symptoms commonly occur
    - Chills
    - Rigors

- Headaches
- Abdominal pain
- Vomiting
- Lethargy/malaise

- **Severe malaria**
  Definition: Patient is unable to take anything by mouth and/or obtunded at presentation. With delayed or ineffective treatment, may progress from uncomplicated to severe malaria within hours.
  - Most frequently due to *P. falciparum*, but occasionally *P. vivax* or *P. knowlesi*.
  - RBCs adhere to blood vessels ("cytoadherence") and cause microvascular sludging, infarcts, capillary leak, and end-organ damage.
  - In areas of stable transmission, where the population typically has frequent exposure and thus has developed protective immunity, severe malaria is typically confined to young children, who have not yet developed immunity, and pregnant women whose immune systems are altered due to pregnancy and lack of placental immunity.
  - Organ systems:
    - Severe anemia
    - Hypoglycemia
    - Seizures
    - Respiratory collapse
    - Metabolic acidosis
    - Renal failure (less frequently in children)
    - Coagulopathy ± DIC
    - Hypotension
  - Physical findings include pallor, petechiae, decreased peripheral perfusion, altered mental status, severe hepatomegaly, and splenomegaly.
  - Cerebral malaria: Encephalopathic presentation, seizures, delirium. CSF findings typically with elevated opening pressure (mean 16 cm H_2O) and low glucose concentration. Retinal hemorrhages in 30–40 % of cases.
  - Severe malaria is a predisposing factor to other infections, e.g., *Salmonella* and other gram-negative bacilli bacteremia concurrent with *P. falciparum* and aspiration pneumonias after seizures.

Diagnosis

Diagnosis of malaria is often challenging because symptoms are typically nonspecific (see clinical manifestations). In addition, even when parasites are seen on blood smears, there is the possibility that the parasitemia is unrelated to a serious non-malarial illness (e.g., bacteremia).

- Clinical diagnosis
  - Often over-diagnosed given non-specificity of symptoms.
  - Clinical signs and symptoms have low sensitivity and specificity except in areas with high transmission (e.g., fever, thrombocytopenia, and splenomegaly only had sensitivity of 71 % and specificity of 88 % in African children).
- Light microscopy
  - Microscopic examination of blood smears remains the gold standard for diagnosis of malaria, determination of the malarial species, quantification of parasitemia, and monitoring of treatment efficacy.
  - Given fever periodicity, smears are typically required every 6–12 h for 48 h to rule out malaria. However, in smear-positive patients, the first smear is positive ~95 % of the time.
  - Examining blood smears, gathered by finger stick or venipuncture:
    - Thin smear: Identification of species, stage, and parasite density
    - Thick smear: Parasite density, allowing for screening of larger quantity of blood than thin smear (increasing diagnostic sensitivity)
    - Parasite density determination. Scan 200–500 fields with oil immersion lens (~100×), ~20 min per slide.
      - Thin smear: % of infected RBCs, counting a minimum of 500 RBCs
    - (# of infected RBCs/# of RBCs counted) ×100 = % of infected RBCs
      - Thick smear: # of parasites/µL of blood in relation to standardized 8,000 WBCs/µL.
    - # of parasites × (8,000/# of WBCs counted) = # of parasites/µL
  - Common reasons for false negatives:
    - Smears are typically not useful at very low parasite density (e.g., 5–10 parasites/µL).
    - Inadequate materials (lancets for blood collection, chemicals for Giemsa staining, slides, microscope, and power source).
    - Insufficient expertise in preparing and examining smears.
  - See Fig. 16.2 for parasite ring forms for microscopic identification.
- Rapid diagnostic tests (RDTs)
  - Description: To put testing and clinical decisions in the hands of the prescriber or provide diagnostic services in settings where microscopy is not available or cannot be effectively supported. The use and availability of RDTs have greatly increased in the last decade. These come in a range of formats (e.g., dipsticks, immunochromatographic cards, and cassettes). Some only detect *P. falciparum*, while others are designed to detect both *P. falciparum* and non-falciparum

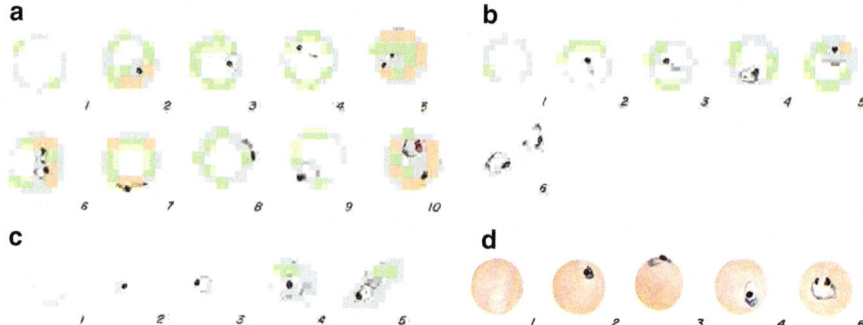

Fig. 16.2 Malaria parasite ring forms of (**a**) *P. falciparum*, (**b**) *P. vivax*, (**c**) *P. ovale*, and (**d**) *P. malariae*. From Coatney, Collins, Warren, Contacos. The Primate Malarias. Bethesda: U.S. Department of Health, Education and Welfare; 1971. (*Source*: CDC. Available at http://www.dpd.cdc.gov/dpdx/HTML/Frames/M-R/Malaria/body_Malariadiagfind2.htm)

species of *Plasmodia*. Histidine-rich protein 2 (HRP-2) and *P. falciparum*-specific parasite LDH are the two antigens used to identify *P. falciparum*, and aldolase or non-*P. falciparum* parasite LDH are used to identify *P. vivax*, *P. ovale*, and *P. malariae*.

- Specificity/sensitivity: Varies with different RDTs. Higher quality tests generally have a sensitivity ≥95 % for detection of *P. falciparum* when there are ≥100 asexual forms per μL of blood and specificity >95 %. Sensitivity declines rapidly when parasite density is low (<100 asexual forms per μL of blood).
- Role in diagnosis: In order to reduce the overuse of the newer, costly antimalarial drugs—artemisinin-based combination therapy (ACT)—there has been a push to scale up the availability and use of diagnostics including RDTs.
- In 2010, the WHO recommended that all children under the age of 5 years suspected to have malaria should have a malaria diagnostic test (rather than empiric therapy for fever).
- Since RDTs are easy to use and do not require electricity or expertise in blood smear interpretation, they are now widely available at the primary health level in many parts of the world. They also are being widely used by community health workers as part of integrated community case management of common childhood diseases (malaria, pneumonia, and diarrhea).

Treatment

Initial decisions about malaria treatment need to take into account where the malaria was acquired, species of *Plasmodium* responsible for the infection, severity of the infection, and host characteristics such as age, weight, and pregnancy status.

- Antimalarial resistance and regional variation
  - In much of the world, *P. falciparum* is resistant to many formerly commonly used antimalarial drugs including chloroquine and sulfadoxine-pyrimethamine (SP, Fansidar).
  - Chloroquine remains effective in Mexico, Central America, Haiti, Dominican Republic, and parts of the Middle East and China. Recent reports from Haiti suggest that chloroquine resistance may be present.
  - Mefloquine resistance is well described in Thailand and Cambodia, and has sporadically occurred in parts of Africa and South America.
  - Artemisinin resistance has recently been identified in Cambodia and, to a lesser extent, in Thailand.
  - Chloroquine-resistant *P. vivax* occurs in Indonesia, Oceania, and Peru.
- ABCs first
  - Adjunctive and supportive treatment

Although antimalarials play a central role in therapy of malaria, it is also important to consider adjunctive measures:

  - Antipyretics (or non-pharmacologic measures) for fever
  - Oral rehydration therapy for mild-to-moderate dehydration or IV rehydration for severe dehydration
  - Antiemetics for nausea and vomiting

- Uncomplicated malaria
  - ACTs are the treatment of choice for uncomplicated falciparum malaria, with major combinations available worldwide including artemether–lumefantrine, amodiaquine–artesunate, artesunate–mefloquine, and dihydroartemisinin–piperaquine. Monotherapy with artemisinin derivatives should be avoided.
  - As treatment regimens vary by region, consult local recommendations for treatment guidelines.
  - Choice of treatment medication based on the risk of resistance in malaria-endemic regions and dosing guidelines for the United States are provided in Table 16.1.
  - A detailed algorithm for the diagnosis and treatment of malaria in returning travelers, immigrants, and refugees has been developed by the CDC and is available at http://www.cdc.gov/immigrantrefugeehealth/pdf/malaria-domestic.pdf.
- Severe malaria
  - ABCs and adjunctive therapy: Severe malaria is a medical emergency! Supportive treatment of complications is critically important. These measures include the following (adapted from WHO 2010 Malaria Treatment Guidelines):
    - Coma: Maintain airway, intubate if necessary, and place patient on his/her side (note: heparin, adrenaline, and corticosteroids have not been shown to improve outcomes and may be harmful).

Table 16.1 Choice of treatment medication based on the risk of resistance in malaria-endemic regions and dosing guidelines for the United States

Guidelines for Treatment of Malaria in the United States

(Based on drugs currently available for use in the United States—updated September 23, 2011)

CDC Malaria Hotline: (770) 488-7788 or (855) 856-4713 toll-free Monday-Friday 9 am to 5 pm EST—(770) 488-7100 after hours, weekends and holidays

Clinical diagnosis/*Plasmodium* species	Region infection acquired	Recommended drug and adult dose[a]	Recommended drug and pediatric dose[a] *Pediatric dose should NEVER exceed adult dose*
Uncomplicated malaria/ P. falciparum or Species not identified If "species not identified" is subsequently diagnosed as *P. vivax* or *P. ovale*: see *P. vivax* and *P ovale* (below) re. treatment with primaquine	Chloroquine-resistant or unknown resistance[b] (All malarious regions except those specified as chloroquine-sensitive listed in the box below)	A. *Atovaquone-proguanil (Malarone™)*[c] Adult tab = 250 mg atovaquone/100 mg proguanil 4 adult tabs po qd × 3 days B. *Artemether-lumefantrine (Coartem™)*[c] 1 tablet = 20 mg artemether and 120 mg lumefantrine A 3-day treatment schedule with a total of 6 oral doses is recommended for both adult and pediatric patients based on weight. The patient should receive the initial dose, followed by the second dose 8 h later, then 1 dose po bid for the following 2 days 5 to <15 kg: 1 tablet per dose 15 to <25 kg: 2 tablets per dose 25 to <35 kg: 3 tablets per dose ≥35 kg: 4 tablets per dose	A. *Atovaquone-proguanil (Malarone™)*[c] Adult tab = 250 mg atovaquone/100 mg proguanil Peds tab = 62.5 mg atovaquone/25 mg proguanil 5–8 kg: 2 peds tabs po qd × 3 days 9–10 kg: 3 peds tabs po qd × 3 days 11–20 kg: 1 adult tab po qd × 3 days 21–30 kg: 2 adult tabs po qd × 3 days 31–40 kg: 3 adult tabs po qd × 3 days >40 kg: 4 adult tabs po qd × 3 days

(continued)

Table 16.1 (continued)

Guidelines for Treatment of Malaria in the United States

(Based on drugs currently available for use in the United States—updated September 23, 2011)

CDC Malaria Hotline: (770) 488-7788 or (855) 856-4713 toll-free Monday-Friday 9 am to 5 pm EST—(770) 488-7100 after hours, weekends and holidays

Clinical diagnosis/*Plasmodium* species	Region infection acquired	Recommended drug and adult dose[a]	Recommended drug and pediatric dose[a] *Pediatric dose should NEVER exceed adult dose*
		C. *Quinine sulfate plus one of the following: Doxycycline, Tetracycline, or Clindamycin*	C. *Quinine sulfate[d] plus one of the following: Doxycycline[f], Tetracycline[f] or Clindamycin*
		Quinine sulfate: 542 mg base (=650 mg salt)[d] po tid×3 or 7 days[e]	Quinine sulfate: 8.3 mg base/kg (=10 mg salt/kg) po tid×3 or 7 days[e]
		Doxycycline: 100 mg po bid×7 days	Doxycycline: 2.2 mg/kg po every 12 h×7 days
		Tetracycline: 250 mg po qid×7 days	Tetracycline: 25 mg/kg/day po divided qid×7 days
		Clindamycin: 20 mg base/kg/day po divided tid×7 days	Clindamycin: 20 mg base/kg/day po divided tid×7 days
		D. *Mefloquine (Lariam™ and generics)[g]*	D. *Mefloquine (Lariam™ and generics)[g]*
		684 mg base (=750 mg salt) po as initial dose, followed by 456 mg base (=500 mg salt) po given 6–12 h after initial dose Total dose=1,250 mg salt	13.7 mg base/kg (=15 mg salt/kg) po as initial dose, followed by 9.1 mg base/kg (=10 mg salt/kg) po given 6–12 h after initial dose. Total dose=25 mg salt/kg

Uncomplicated malaria/ P. falciparum or Species not identified	*Chloroquine-sensitive* (Central America west of Panama Canal; Haiti; the Dominican Republic;; and most of the Middle East)	*Chloroquine phosphate (Aralen™ and generics)*[h] 600 mg base (=1,000 mg salt) po immediately, followed by 300 mg base (=500 mg salt) po at 6, 24, and 48 h Total dose: 1,500 mg base (=2,500 mg salt) OR *Hydroxychloroquine (Plaquenil™ and generics)* 620 mg base (=800 mg salt) po immediately, followed by 310 mg base (=400 mg salt) po at 6, 24, and 48 h Total dose: 1,550 mg base (=2,000 mg salt)	*Chloroquine phosphate (Aralen™ and generics)*[h] 10 mg base/kg po immediately, followed by 5 mg base/kg po at 6, 24, and 48 h Total dose: 25 mg base/kg OR *Hydroxychloroquine (Plaquenil™ and generics)* 10 mg base/kg po immediately, followed by 5 mg base/kg po at 6, 24, and 48 h Total dose: 25 mg base/kg
Uncomplicated malaria/ P. malariae or P. knowlesi	All regions	*Chloroquine phosphate*[h]: Treatment as above OR *Hydroxychloroquine*: Treatment as above	*Chloroquine phosphate*[h]: Treatment as above OR *Hydroxychloroquine*: Treatment as above
Uncomplicated malaria/ P.vivax or P. ovale	All regions Note: for suspected chloroquine-resistant *P. vivax*, see row below	*Chloroquine phosphate*[h] plus *Primaquine phosphate*[i] *Chloroquine phosphate*: Treatment as above *Primaquine phosphate*: 30 mg base po qd×14 days OR *Hydroxychloroquine plus Primaquine phosphate*[i] *Hydroxychloroquine*: Treatment as above *Primaquine phosphate*: 30 mg base po qd×14 days	*Chloroquine phosphate*[h] plus *Primaquine phosphate*[i] *Chloroquine phosphate*: Treatment as above *Primaquine phosphate*: 0.5 mg base/kg po qd×14 days OR *Hydroxychloroquine plus Primaquine phosphate*[i] *Hydroxychloroquine*: Treatment as above *Primaquine phosphate*: 0.5 mg base/kg po qd×14 days

(continued)

Table 16.1 (continued)

Guidelines for Treatment of Malaria in the United States

(Based on drugs currently available for use in the United States—updated September 23, 2011)

CDC Malaria Hotline: (770) 488-7788 or (855) 856-4713 toll-free Monday-Friday 9 am to 5 pm EST—(770) 488-7100 after hours, weekends and holidays

Clinical diagnosis/*Plasmodium* species	Region infection acquired	Recommended drug and adult dose[a]	Recommended drug and pediatric dose[a] Pediatric dose should NEVER exceed adult dose
Uncomplicated malaria/ P. vivax	*Chloroquine-resistant*[j] (Papua New Guinea and Indonesia)	A. Quinine sulfate plus either Doxycycline or Tetracycline plus Primaquine phosphate[i] Quinine sulfate: Treatment as above Doxycycline or Tetracycline: Treatment as above Primaquine phosphate: Treatment as above B. Atovaquone-proguanil plus Primaquine phosphate[i] Atovaquone-proguanil: Treatment as above Primaquine phosphate: Treatment as above C. Mefloquine plus Primaquine phosphate[i] Mefloquine: Treatment as above Primaquine phosphate: Treatment as above	A. Quinine sulfate plus either Doxycycline[f] or Tetracycline[f] plus Primaquine phosphate[i] Quinine sulfate: Treatment as above Doxycycline or Tetracycline: Treatment as above Primaquine phosphate: Treatment as above B. Atovaquone-proguanil plus Primaquine phosphate[i] Atovaquone-proguanil: Treatment as above Primaquine phosphate: Treatment as above C. Mefloquine plus Primaquine phosphate[i] Mefloquine: Treatment as above Primaquine phosphate: Treatment as above
Uncomplicated malaria: alternatives for pregnant women[k,l,m]	*Chloroquine-sensitive* (see uncomplicated malaria sections above for chloroquine-sensitive species by region)	Chloroquine phosphate: Treatment as above *OR* Hydroxychloroquine: Treatment as above	Not applicable

Chloroquine-resistant (see sections above for regions with chloroquine resistant *P. falciparum* and *P. vivax*)		*Quinine sulfate plus Clindamycin* Quinine sulfate: Treatment as above Clindamycin: Treatment as above OR Mefloquine: Treatment as above	Not applicable
Severe malaria[a,o,p,q]	All regions	*Quinidine gluconate*[a] *plus one of the following: Doxycycline, Tetracycline, or Clindamycin* Quinidine gluconate: 6.25 mg base/kg (=10 mg salt/kg) loading dose IV over 1–2 h, then 0.0125 mg base/kg/min (=0.02 mg salt/kg/min) continuous infusion for at least 24 h. An alternative regimen is 15 mg base/kg (=24 mg salt/kg) loading dose IV infused over 4 h, followed by 7.5 mg base/kg (=12 mg salt/kg) infused over 4 h every 8 h, starting 8 h after the loading dose (see package insert). Once parasite density <1% and patient can take oral medication, complete treatment with oral quinine, dose as above. Quinidine/quinine course = 7 days in Southeast Asia; =3 days in Africa or South America	*Quinidine gluconate*[a] *plus one of the following: Doxycycline*[d], *Tetracycline*[d], *or Clindamycin* Quinidine gluconate: Same mg/kg dosing and recommendations as for adults Doxycycline: Treatment as above. If patient not able to take oral medication, may give IV. For children <45 kg, give 2.2 mg/kg IV every 12 h and then switch to oral doxycycline (dose as above) as soon as patient can take oral medication. For children >45 kg, use same dosing as for adults. For IV use, avoid rapid administration. Treatment course = 7 days Tetracycline: Treatment as above Clindamycin: Treatment as above. If patient not able to take oral medication, give 10 mg base/kg loading dose IV followed by 5 mg base/kg IV every 8 h. Switch to oral clindamycin (oral dose as above) as soon as patient can take oral medication. For IV use, avoid rapid administration. Treatment course = 7 days *Investigational new drug (contact CDC for information):* Artesunate followed by one of the following: Atovaquone-proguanil (Malarone™), Clindamycin, or Mefloquine

(continued)

Table 16.1 (continued)

Guidelines for Treatment of Malaria in the United States

(Based on drugs currently available for use in the United States—updated September 23, 2011)

CDC Malaria Hotline: (770) 488-7788 or (855) 856-4713 toll-free Monday-Friday 9 am to 5 pm EST—(770) 488-7100 after hours, weekends and holidays

Clinical diagnosis/*Plasmodium* species	Region infection acquired	Recommended drug and adult dose[a]	Recommended drug and pediatric dose[a] *Pediatric dose should NEVER exceed adult dose*
		Doxycycline: Treatment as above. If patient not able to take oral medication, give 100 mg IV every 12 h and then switch to oral doxycycline (as above) as soon as patient can take oral medication. For IV use, avoid rapid administration. Treatment course = 7 days	
		Tetracycline: Treatment as above	
		Clindamycin: Treatment as above. If patient not able to take oral medication, give 10 mg base/kg loading dose IV followed by 5 mg base/kg IV every 8 h. Switch to oral clindamycin (oral dose as above) as soon as patient can take oral medication. For IV use, avoid rapid administration. Treatment course = 7 days	
		Investigational new drug (contact CDC for information): Artesunate followed by one of the following: Atovaquone-proguanil (Malarone™), Doxycycline (Clindamycin in pregnant women), or Mefloquine	

Source: CDC. Available at http://www.cdc.gov/malaria/resources/pdf/treatmenttable.pdf

[a] If a person develops malaria despite taking chemoprophylaxis, that particular medicine should not be used as a part of their treatment regimen. Use one of the other options instead

[b] There are four options (A, B, C, or D) available for treatment of uncomplicated malaria caused by chloroquine-resistant *P. falciparum*. Options A, B, and C are equally recommended. Because of a higher rate of severe neuropsychiatric reactions seen at treatment doses, we do not recommend option D (mefloquine) unless the other options cannot be used. For option C, because there is more data on the efficacy of quinine in combination with doxycycline or tetracycline, these treatment combinations are generally preferred to quinine in combination with clindamycin

[c] Take with with food or whole milk. If patient vomits within 30 min of taking a dose, then they should repeat the dose

[d] US manufactured quinine sulfate capsule is in a 324 mg dosage; therefore two capsules should be sufficient for adult dosing. Pediatric dosing may be difficult due to unavailability of non-capsule forms of quinine

[e] For infections acquired in Southeast Asia, quinine treatment should continue for 7 days. For infections acquired elsewhere, quinine treatment should continue for 3 days

[f] Doxycycline and tetracycline are not indicated for use in children less than 8 years old. For children less than 8 years old with chloroquine-resistant *P. falciparum*, atovaquone-proguanil and artemether-lumefantrine are recommended treatment options; mefloquine can be considered if no other options are available. For children less than 8 years old with chloroquine-resistant *P. vivax*, mefloquine is the recommended treatment. If it is not available or is not being tolerated and if the treatment benefits outweigh the risks, atovaquone-proguanil or artemether-lumefantrine should be used instead

[g] Treatment with mefloquine is not recommended in persons who have acquired infections from Southeast Asia due to drug resistance

[h] When treating chloroquine-sensitive infections, chloroquine and hydroxychloroquine are recommended options. However, regimens used to treat chloroquine-resistant infections may also be used if available, more convenient, or preferred

[i] Primaquine is used to eradicate any hypnozoites that may remain dormant in the liver, and thus prevent relapses, in *P. vivax* and *P. ovale* infections. Because primaquine can cause hemolytic anemia in G6PD-deficient persons, G6PD screening must occur prior to starting treatment with primaquine. For persons with borderline G6PD deficiency or as an alternate to the above regimen, primaquine may be given 45 mg orally one time per week for 8 weeks; consultation with an expert in infectious disease and/or tropical medicine is advised if this alternative regimen is considered in G6PD-deficient persons. Primaquine must not be used during pregnancy

[j] There are three options (A, B, or C) available for treatment of uncomplicated malaria caused by chloroquine-resistant *P. vivax*. High treatment failure rates due to chloroquine-resistant *P. vivax* have been well documented in Papua New Guinea and Indonesia. Rare case reports of chloroquine-resistant *P. vivax* have also been documented in Burma (Myanmar), India, and Central and South America. Persons acquiring *P. vivax* infections outside of Papua New Guinea or Indonesia should be started on chloroquine. If the patient does not respond, the treatment should be changed to a chloroquine-resistant *P. vivax* regimen and CDC should be notified (Malaria Hotline number listed above). For treatment of chloroquine-resistant *P. vivax* infections, options A, B, and C are equally recommended

[k] For pregnant women diagnosed with uncomplicated malaria caused by chloroquine-resistant *P. falciparum* or chloroquine-resistant *P. vivax* infection, treatment with doxycycline or tetracycline is generally not indicated. However, doxycycline or tetracycline may be used in combination with quinine (as recommended for non-pregnant adults) if other treatment options are not available or are not being tolerated, and the benefit is judged to outweigh the risks

(continued)

Table 16.1 (continued)

[l]Atovaquone-proguanil and artemether-lumefantrine are generally not recommended for use in pregnant women, particularly in the first trimester due to lack of sufficient safety data. For pregnant women diagnosed with uncomplicated malaria caused by chloroquine-resistant *P. falciparum* infection, atovaquone-proguanil or artemether-lumefantrine may be used if other treatment options are not available or are not being tolerated, and if the potential benefit is judged to outweigh the potential risks

[m]For *P. vivax* and *P. ovale* infections, primaquine phosphate for radical treatment of hypnozoites should not be given during pregnancy. Pregnant patients with *P. vivax* and *P. ovale* infections should be maintained on chloroquine prophylaxis for the duration of their pregnancy. The chemoprophylactic dose of chloroquine phosphate is 300 mg base (=500 mg salt) orally once per week. After delivery, pregnant patients who do not have G6PD deficiency should be treated with primaquine

[n]Persons with a positive blood smear OR history of recent possible exposure and no other recognized pathology who have one or more of the following clinical criteria (impaired consciousness/coma, severe normocytic anemia, renal failure, pulmonary edema, acute respiratory distress syndrome, circulatory shock, disseminated intravascular coagulation, spontaneous bleeding, acidosis, hemoglobinuria, jaundice, repeated generalized convulsions, and/or parasitemia of >5%) are considered to have manifestations of more severe disease. Severe malaria is most often caused by *P. falciparum*

[o]Patients diagnosed with severe malaria should be treated aggressively with parenteral antimalarial therapy. Treatment with IV quinidine should be initiated as soon as possible after the diagnosis has been made. Patients with severe malaria should be given an intravenous loading dose of quinidine unless they have received more than 40 mg/kg of quinine in the preceding 48 h or if they have received mefloquine within the preceding 12 h. Consultation with a cardiologist and a physician with experience treating malaria is advised when treating malaria patients with quinidine. During administration of quinidine, blood pressure monitoring (for hypotension) and cardiac monitoring (for widening of the QRS complex and/or lengthening of the QTc interval) should be monitored continuously and blood glucose (for hypoglycemia) should be monitored periodically. Cardiac complications, if severe, may warrant temporary discontinuation of the drug or slowing of the intravenous infusion

[p]Consider exchange transfusion if the parasite density (i.e. parasitemia) is >10% OR if the patient has altered mental status, non-volume overload pulmonary edema, or renal complications. The parasite density can be estimated by examining a monolayer of red blood cells (RBCs) on the thin smear under oil immersion magnification. The slide should be examined where the RBCs are more or less touching (approximately 400 RBCs per field). The parasite density can then be estimated from the percentage of infected RBCs and should be monitored every 12 h. Exchange transfusion should be continued until the parasite density is <1 % (usually requires 8–10 units). IV quinidine administration should not be delayed for an exchange transfusion and can be given concurrently throughout the exchange transfusion

[q]Pregnant women diagnosed with severe malaria should be treated aggressively with parenteral antimalarial therapy

- Hyperpyrexia: Acetaminophen (paracetamol) plus mechanical measures to lower body temperature (e.g., fanning, tepid sponging, cooling blanket).
- Convulsions: Maintain airway, check blood glucose, and treat with IV or rectal diazepam or IM paraldehyde.
- Severe anemia: Transfuse with screened whole blood or packed RBCs.
- Hypoglycemia: Check blood glucose, correct hypoglycemia, and maintain with glucose-containing infusion.
- Acute pulmonary edema: Prop patient at an angle of 45°, administer oxygen, give diuretic, hold IV fluids, and consider intubation with addition of PEEP.
- Acute renal failure: Exclude pre-renal causes, and monitor fluid balance and urinary sodium, hemofiltration, or hemodialysis if full renal failure occurs.
- Spontaneous bleeding and coagulopathy: Transfuse with fresh whole blood or PRBCs plus cryoprecipitate, FFP, and platelets, if available; administer vitamin K injection.
- Metabolic acidosis: Exclude or treat hypoglycemia, hypovolemia, and bacteremia.
- Shock: Obtain blood cultures and administer parenteral broad-spectrum antibiotics; correct hemodynamic disturbances.
- Choice of antimalarial drug in severe malaria.
  - In 2011, the WHO recommended the use of parenteral artesunate for the treatment of severe malaria rather than IV quinine. In countries, such as the United States, where IV artesunate is not yet commercially available (but is available from the CDC for compassionate use), IV quinidine or quinine remain the first-line agents.
  - Detailed descriptions of drug doses are provided in Table 16.1.
- High-grade parasitemia
  - Consider exchange transfusion if parasitemia ≥ 10 %, and patient has altered mental status, ARDS, or acute renal failure.

Prevention

Prevention of malaria in poor countries is approached on multiple levels:

- Personal protection:
  - Avoid outside activities from dusk to dawn.
  - Cover exposed area with long sleeves and pants.
  - Use insect repellants (DEET or picaridin) on exposed skin.

- Household protection:
  - Burning mosquito coils and other space repellants
  - Insecticide-treated bednets (ITNs)
    - Most important and most effective form of malaria prevention:
    - Long-lasting nets with embedded insecticide (LLIN) protect the individual under the net, but also provide vector control by killing off mosquitoes before they can transmit malaria.
    - Unfurl around bed, and tuck under mattress.
- Vector control:
  - Indoor residual spraying (IRS): Insecticide treatments for the inside of homes, on walls and roofs. Lasts for months. Kills mosquitoes after they have taken a blood meal, so need large coverage to be effective in reducing community levels of malaria.
    - Environmental approaches: Mosquito breeding grounds can be reduced by permanently removing water-gathering areas, i.e., puddles, open barrels, and standing water.
    - Chemical treatment of water sources can limit malaria breeding as well.
  - Treatment as protection:
    - Within ecological niches (villages and neighborhoods), unchecked malaria leads to more malaria through propagation in human hosts.
    - Effective and early treatment of affected individuals leads to decreased potential for transmission of parasites to the community as a whole.
    - Thus, effective treatment for symptomatic patients is critical for individual and community protection (see IPT below).
- Intermittent preventive treatment (IPT) in pregnant women and children
  - IPT in pregnancy (IPTp)
    - WHO currently recommends a package of interventions for controlling malaria during pregnancy in areas with stable *P. falciparum* transmission, including the use of ITNs, administration during pregnancy of monthly sulfadoxine–pyrimethamine (SP) after quickening, and effective case management of malaria.
    - New guidelines have recently been released by the WHO recommend monthly dosing of SP-IPTp after the first trimester as a result of the waning efficacy of SP in many areas of Africa.
    - IPTp, especially when used with ITNs, helps reduce maternal anemia, placental malaria, and the risk of low birth weight and neonatal mortality.

- IPT in infants (IPTi) and children (IPTc)
    - SP-IPTi involves the administration of a full therapeutic course of SP delivered through the Expanded Program on Immunization (EPI) at defined intervals corresponding to routine vaccination schedules—usually at 10 weeks, 14 weeks, and ~9 months of age—to infants at risk of malaria.
    - In 2010, the WHO recommended the use of IPTi in areas with moderate-to-high malaria transmission (annual entomological inoculation rate ≥ 10 infective bites per year) and where SP resistance is low (defined as a prevalence of the pf dhps 540 mutation of <50 %).
    - IPTi has been shown to provide protection against clinical malaria, anemia, malaria-related hospitalizations, and all-cause hospitalizations of infants.
    - SP-IPTi should be avoided in infants taking cotrimoxazole due to increased potential for allergic reactions.
- Malaria prevention for travelers (IDSA Travel Medicine Guidelines)
    - Importance
        - Most common febrile illness in returning travelers, with around 1,300 cases and several deaths reported to the CDC annually, most secondary to *P. falciparum*
        - Very dangerous in travelers because of their lack of protective immunity
    - Risk assessment
        - Evaluated with a detailed itinerary and comparison to published maps of known malaria risk zones and parasite resistance patterns
        - Other factors include length of stay, rainy vs. dry season, types of accommodations, elevation, and ability to adhere to chemoprophylaxis and other prevention measures
    - Guidelines (Table 16.2)
- All travelers in affected areas should use personal protection, including avoiding insect exposure through insect repellent and rigorous ITN use.
- Chemoprophylaxis is recommended to travelers to much of sub-Saharan Africa, Latin and South America, and Southeast Asia.
- Individual risk depends on specific activities; see maps at www.cdc.gov/travel.
- Most common chemoprophylaxis medications are daily atovaquone–proguanil (Malarone), doxycycline, or chloroquine (in selected areas of efficacy), or once-weekly mefloquine (Larium).
- See Table 16.2 for dosing and side effect profiles for chemoprophylaxis options.

Table 16.2 Antimalarial drugs for prophylaxis and self-treatment

Generic name	Trade name	Tablet size	Adult dosage	Pediatric dosage	Adverse effects
Prophylaxis					
Chloroquine phosphate	Aralen[a]	500 mg salt (300 mg base)	One tablet orally once per week; begin 1 week before travel and continue for 4 weeks after travel	8.3 mg/kg of body weight salt (5 mg/kg of body weight base) orally once per week	May exacerbate psoriasis; common adverse effects include bitter taste, headache, pruritus in persons of African descent; occasional adverse effects include skin eruptions, reversible corneal opacity, transient visual blurring, and partial alopecia; rare adverse events include retinopathy (>100 g base total dose), blood dyscrasias, nail and mucous membrane discoloration, nerve deafness, myopathy, and photophobia
Hydroxychloroquine	—	200 mg salt (155 mg base)	Two tablets orally once per week, as for chloroquine	6.5 mg/kg of body weight salt (5 mg/kg of body weight base) orally once per week (maximum 310 mg base)	As for chloroquine
Atovaquone-proguanil	Malarone[b]	250 mg atovaquone and 100 mg proguanil (adult tablet); 62.5 mg atovaquone and 25 mg proguanil (pediatric tablet)	One tablet orally once daily; begin 1–2 days before travel and continue for 7 days after travel	Body weight 11–20 kg, one pediatric tablet daily; body weight 21–30 kg, two pediatric tablets daily; body weight 31–40 kg, three pediatric tablets daily; body weight ≥41 kg, one adult tablet daily	Take with food; do not use in persons with creatinine clearance <30 mL/min; common adverse events include nausea, abdominal pain, and headache; occasional adverse events include transient increase in transaminase levels with treatment doses; rare adverse events include rash

Doxycycline	—	100 mg	One tablet orally once daily; begin 1–2 days before travel and continue for 4 weeks after travel	≥8 years old, 2 mg/kg of body weight orally once daily (maximum dosage, 100 mg/day)	Stains teeth in children <8 years old and fetuses; should be taken in upright position to avoid esophageal irritation; common adverse events include GI upset, photosensitivity, and *Candida* vaginitis; rare adverse events include allergic reactions, blood dyscrasias, azotemia in renal disease, and esophageal ulceration
Mefloquine	Lariam[c]	250 mg salt (228 mg base)	One tablet orally once per week; begin 1 week before travel and continue for 4 weeks after travel	Body weight ≤9 kg, 5 mg salt per kg weekly; body weight 10–19 kg, one-quarter tablet; body weight 20–30 kg, one-half tablet; body weight 31–45 kg, three-quarters tablet; body weight ≥46 kg, one tablet	Contraindicated in patients with active depression, history of psychosis, seizure disorder, or cardiac conduction abnormality; common adverse events include dizziness, nausea, diarrhea, headache, nightmares, insomnia, and mood alteration; rare adverse events include seizures and psychosis
Primaquine	—	26.3 mg salt (15 mg base)			Hemolysis with G6PD deficiency; take with food; common adverse events include GI upset
For presumptive antirelapse therapy (terminal prophylaxis)			Two tablets orally once daily for 14 days	0.8 mg/kg of body weight salt (0.5 mg/kg of body weight base) orally once daily for 14 days	
For primary prophylaxis			Two tablets orally once daily; begin 1–2 days before travel and continue for 7 days after travel	0.8 mg/kg of body weight salt (0.5 mg/kg of body weight base) orally; begin 1–2 days before travel and continue for 7 days after travel	

(continued)

Table 16.2 (continued)

Generic name	Trade name	Tablet size	Adult dosage	Pediatric dosage	Adverse effects
Self-treatment					
Atovaquone-proguanil	Malarone[b]	250 mg atovaquone and 100 mg proguanil (adult dose)	Four tablets orally once daily (can be divided into two doses) for 3 days	body weight 5–8 kg, two pediatric tablets for 3 days; body weight 9–10 kg, three pediatric tablets for 3 days; body weight 11–20 kg, one adult tablet for 3 days; body weight 21–30 kg, two adult tablets for 3 days; body weight 31–40 kg, three adult tablets for 3 days; body weight ≥41 kg, four adult tablets for 3 days	Take with food; do not use in persons with creatinine clearance <30 mL/min; common adverse events include nausea, abdominal pain, and headache; occasional adverse events include transient increase in transaminase levels; rare adverse events include rash

From Hill et al. The practice of travel medicine: Guidelines by the Infectious Diseases society of America. Clin Infect Dis. 2006;43:1499–1539. Reprinted with permission from Oxford University Press

G6PD glucose-6-phosphate dehydrogenase, *GI* gastrointestinal

[a]Abbott Laboratories
[b]GlaxoSmithKline
[c]Roche

Recommended Reading

1. World Health Organisation. World Malaria Report. 2011. Available from: http://www.who.int/malaria/world_malaria_report_2010/en/index.html
2. World Health Organization. Severe and complicated malaria. Trans R Soc Trop Med Hyg. 2000;94 suppl 1:1–90.
3. World Health Organisation. Guidelines for the treatment of malaria. 2010. Available from: http://whqlibdoc.who.int/publications/2010/9789241547925_eng.pdf
4. Hill DR, Ericsson CD, Pearson RD, Keystone JS, Freedman DO, Kozarsky PE, DuPont HL, Bia FJ, Fischer PR, Ryan ET. The practice of travel medicine: guidelines by the Infectious Diseases Society of America. Clin Infect Dis. 2006;43:1499–539.
5. Centers for Disease Control. Malaria. Available from: http://www.cdc.gov/malaria/malaria_worldwide/reduction/mda_mft.html

Chapter 17
Measles

Elizabeth R. Wolf and Elisa Margolis

Keywords Measles • Vitamin A • Koplik • Bitot • Pneumonia • Encephalitis • Rash • Fever • Conjunctivitis • Coryza

Overview

- Measles (also known as rubeola) is a highly contagious viral illness.
- Measles is characterized by fever, an erythematous maculopapular rash, cough, conjunctivitis, and coryza.
- Severe complications include pneumonia, blindness, and encephalitis.
- The recommended treatment is vitamin A.
- Widespread vaccination campaigns over the past several decades have dramatically decreased the incidence of this disease, but it is still a significant public health problem worldwide due to suboptimal vaccination rates.

E.R. Wolf, M.D., D.T.M.&H. (✉)
Pediatrics Department, Center for Child Health, Behavior and Development,
University of Washington, Mailstop CW8-6, PO Box 5371, Seattle, WA 98145, USA
e-mail: ewolf@uw.edu

E. Margolis, M.D., Ph.D.
Infectious Disease Division, Pediatrics Department, Seattle Childrens Hospital,
4800 Sand Point Way NE, Room A-5950, Seattle, WA 98105, USA
e-mail: emarg2@uw.edu

Epidemiology

Global Burden of Disease

The measles vaccine has dramatically altered the global distribution of this disease. Measles now occurs primarily in areas of low vaccination coverage, namely, Africa and Southeast Asia. Even with increasing vaccination coverage rates, parts of the world with high HIV prevalence have continued to have measles outbreaks because of inadequate immunity in this population. Smaller outbreaks of measles also occur in the developed world, where anti-vaccination movements have recently gained popularity.

Transmission

Measles is one of the most contagious viral illnesses. In a susceptible population, a single measles case can result in 12 or more new cases. Outbreaks can occur even when less than 10 % of the population is unvaccinated. In crowded conditions, such as refugee camps, measles can spread rapidly.

Transmission occurs via the respiratory tract through infectious droplets. Droplets from an infectious patient can remain airborne for several hours and can persist in the environment even after an infectious patient has left. Patients are contagious between 4 days before the rash to 4 days after the rash onset.

Age of Presentation

In populations with low vaccination coverage, measles typically affects infants and young children. Neonates are initially protected by maternal antibodies (this protection is stronger for mothers with previous measles infection than mothers who have been immunized). In HIV-unexposed infants, the loss of maternal antibodies occurs by 6 months of age. In HIV-exposed infants, the nadir of maternal measles immunity occurs earlier due to passing of fewer maternal antibodies. As measles vaccine coverage increases, the affected age distribution shifts towards older children and adolescents.

Clinical Presentation

The incubation period for measles lasts about 8–12 days from exposure to onset of symptoms. The first stage of measles is prodromal, characterized by fever, conjunctivitis, runny nose (coryza), cough, and fussiness. Pathognomonic spots on buccal

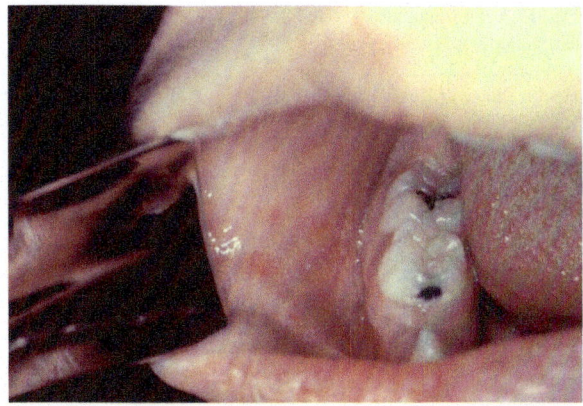

Fig. 17.1 Koplik spots (courtesy of CDC Public Health Images Library)

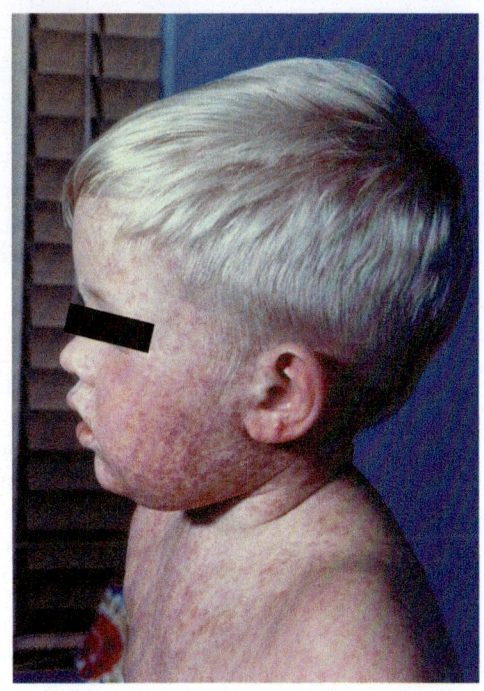

Fig. 17.2 Classic measles exanthem (courtesy of CDC Public Health Images Library)

mucosa (Koplik spots), characterized by an erythematous base with central raised white hue (Fig. 17.1), usually appear 48 h before the rash. The measles rash, which is maculopapular and erythematous in light-skinned individuals (Fig. 17.2), then appears around day 4 of the illness and lasts for 3–5 days. The rash begins on the face (sometimes behind the ears) and then spreads caudally to the trunk and the rest of the body. In malnourished children, the rash can appear deeply pigmented or hemorrhagic. As the rash fades, it may desquamate (Fig. 17.3).

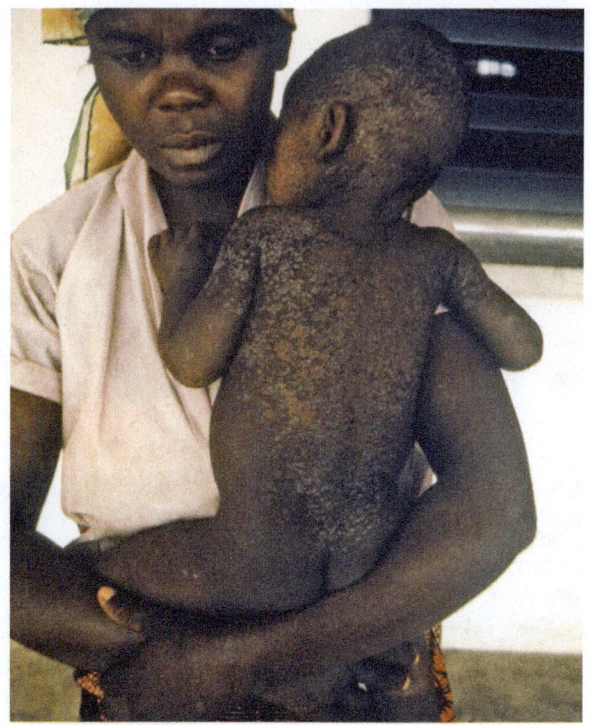

Fig. 17.3 Desquamation associated with measles rash (courtesy of CDC Public Health Images Library and Dr. Lyle Conrad)

The differential for the measles rash includes Scarlet fever, Kawasaki disease, rubella, parvovirus, coxsackie virus, HHV6, and erythema multiforme or other drug reactions.

A milder form of measles may occur in children with preexisting partial immunity (from passive maternal antibodies, IVIG, partial vaccination response, or previous measles disease). It is characterized by mild respiratory symptoms, with or without a rash or fever. Immunocompromised children may not display the characteristic rash.

Diagnosis

Measles in the developing world is most often diagnosed clinically during epidemics. The WHO clinical case definition is the following: any person in whom a clinician suspects measles infection, or any person with fever and maculopapular (i.e., nonvesicular) rash with cough, coryza (i.e., runny nose), or conjunctivitis (i.e., red eyes). Laboratory confirmation with measles IgM assay is not required for diagnosis but may be used early in epidemics for disease verification or in cases where the clinical presentation is unclear. The sensitivity of IgM varies with the type of assay used and may be diminished during the first 72 h after rash onset. Measles IgM may not be available in low-resource settings. Other laboratory means of measles diagnosis (such as paired acute and convalescent IgG, and PCR) are also unlikely to be available in the developing world.

Complications

The rate of complications with measles is quite variable and ranges from 10 to 40 % depending on the population studied. Groups at higher risk of complications include the immunocompromised, pregnant, malnourished, infants, and the elderly. In developing countries, the case fatality rate can be as high as 4–6 %, with highest rates in children under 5 years. The most common complications in children are otitis media, pneumonia, diarrhea, and croup. Pneumonia is the most common fatal complication and can result from measles itself or a bacterial superinfection.

Ophthalmologic complications of measles can be particularly devastating and overlap those caused by vitamin A deficiency. The spectrum of ophthalmologic complications includes xerophthalmia (dry eyes), Bitot's spots (gray, triangular spots of keratinized epithelium on the conjunctivae) (Fig. 17.4), corneal ulceration, night blindness, and total blindness.

Central nervous system complications of measles are rare but quite serious. Approximately 1 in 1,000 children with measles suffers from acute encephalitis within two weeks of their measles infection. Acute disseminated encephalomyelitis (ADEM) can also follow measles. In both cases, the cerebrospinal fluid typically shows a lymphocytic pleocytosis, increased protein and normal glucose. Both measles-related acute encephalitis and ADEM have a 10–20 % risk of mortality. Subacute sclerosing panencephalitis (SSPE) is an extremely rare complication (4–11 cases per 100,000 cases) that typically occurs 7–10 years after measles illness. It progresses from personality changes to myoclonic jerks to a vegetative state and finally, death. SSPE can be treated symptomatically with anti-spasmodics and anti-convulsants but is incurable. The gravity of these neurologic complications underscores the importance of measles prevention.

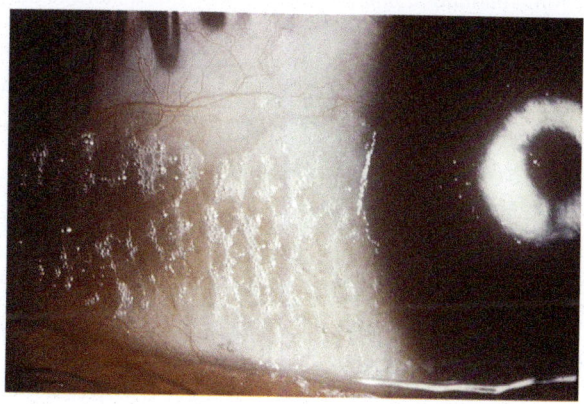

Fig. 17.4 Bitot's spots (courtesy of CDC Public Health Images Library)

Management

Besides supportive care, the only recommended treatment for uncomplicated measles is vitamin A. Vitamin A (Table 17.1) has been shown to reduce mortality, complications, and time to recovery in children with measles. In the developed world, ribavirin and/or IVIG can also be used as adjuvant therapies in severely immunocompromised individuals.

Acetaminophen can be used for symptomatic reduction of fever. Patients with measles should be isolated either at home or in isolation wards of hospitals for the duration of their contagious period. Hospitalization is indicated for the severely malnourished, those with respiratory, neurologic, or ophthamologic complications, and those who require IV antibiotics, fluid resuscitation, or oxygen therapy.

Conjunctivitis

Measles conjunctivitis may be associated with a watery discharge. Ophthalmologic antibiotic ointments are not necessary unless an ophthamologic complication or bacterial superinfection is suspected (e.g., draining pus). In these cases, the WHO recommends tetracycline eye ointment three times a day for 7 days. A protective pad can be placed to prevent additional infections. Steroid eye ointments and traditional local remedies should be *avoided* as these may worsen ophthalmologic complications.

Pneumonia

The use of prophylactic antibiotics to prevent measles-related bacterial pneumonia is controversial. Antibiotics are indicated, however, once a bacterial pneumonia is suspected. Pathogens that have been implicated in measles-related bacterial pneumonia include *S. pneumoniae*, *H. influenzae*, and *S. aureus*.

Table 17.1 Dosing of vitamin A in pediatric measles

Vitamin A on days 1 and 2
200,000 IU orally for children ≥12 months of age
100,000 IU orally for infants 6–11 months of age
50,000 IU orally for infants <6 months of age
An additional (i.e., a third) age-specific dose should be given 2–4 weeks later to children with clinical signs and symptoms of vitamin A deficiency. (Signs of vitamin A deficiency include night blindness, Bitot's spots, xerosis (dryness) of conjunctivae and cornea, pruritus, and growth retardation (see Chap. 22)
Data taken from the 2004 WHO paper "Treating Measles in Children" Slide 34. Can be accessed from http://www.who.int/immunization_delivery/interventions/TreatingMeaslesENG300.pdf

Measles Croup

Measles croup should be treated as other types of viral croup with regard to supportive care and, in severe cases, nebulized epinephrine. Although corticosteroids are regularly used in the treatment of non-measles-related croup, the WHO recommends against corticosteroids for measles-related croup.

Mouth Ulcers

The WHO recommends saltwater rinses (pinch of salt in a cup of clean water) four times a day if the child is able to eat and drink. Then, gentian violet 0.25 % solution is applied. If the ulcers are foul-smelling or severe, IM/IV benzylpenicillin (50,000 U/kg every 6 h) plus PO metronidazole (7.5 mg/kg three times a day) for 5 days should be administered. Nasogastric feedings may be required for ulcers that prevent adequate oral intake.

Prevention

Vaccination

In 2010, the WHO estimated that about 85 % of the world's children received one dose of measles vaccine by age 1. In most countries in the developing world, measles vaccine is given as a single live-attenuated vaccine rather than in combination with rubella, mumps, and/or varicella. The Measles Rubella Initiative and the Global Alliance for Vaccines and Immunization (GAVI) are working to expand global coverage of the combination measles–rubella vaccine.

The measles vaccine is recommended for all HIV-positive individuals except those who are severely immunocompromised. Many clinicians exclude those with absolute CD4 counts ≤200 (children over 5) or CD4 % ≤15 % (children under 5).

In areas where measles is endemic, the first dose of the measles vaccine is typically given at 9 months of age. In non-endemic areas, the first dose is given at 12–15 months of age for a higher likelihood of seroconversion (95 % compared to 85 %). In 2008, the WHO recommended a second dose of the vaccine for countries with adequate healthcare delivery systems and high coverage of the single dose. The second dose of the measles vaccine is recommended no less than 28 days from the first dose.

During a measles outbreak, supplementary immunization activities (SIAs) are used to augment standard vaccination regimens. These are widespread vaccination campaigns in which children who have never been vaccinated or have received only one dose of measles vaccine are immunized.

Measles infection confers lifelong immunity. Vaccination, particularly with the two-dose series, is felt to confer long-term immunity for several decades. HIV-positive individuals (particularly those not on HAART) have high rates of primary and secondary vaccine failure.

Recommended Reading

American Academy of Pediatrics. Red Book: 2012 Report of the Committee on Infectious Diseases. 29th edition. In: Pickering LK, editor. Elk Grove Village, IL: American Academy of Pediatrics; 2012.

Duke T, Mgone CS. Measles: not just another viral exanthem. Lancet. 2003;361:763–73.

Hussey GD, Klein M. A randomized, controlled trial of vitamin A in children with severe measles. N Engl J Med. 1990;323(3):160–4.

WHO. Measles Vaccines: WHO position paper. 2009;35:349–60.

Moss WJ, Griffin DE. Global measles elimination. Nat Rev Microbiol. 2006;4:900–8.

Chapter 18
HIV/AIDS

Kathleen M. Powis and Aura M. Obando

Keywords Pediatric HIV treatment • Infant HIV prophylaxis • Pediatric opportunistic infections

Overview

- 33 million people worldwide have HIV/AIDS as of the end of 2009. Global estimated HIV incidence was 2.6 million individuals in 2009 across all ages; 370,000 (12 %) were children under age 15.
- Four million children have died from HIV/AIDS and half of HIV-infected infants will die in the first 2 years of life without ARV treatment.
- Over 90 % of HIV infection in pediatrics occurs through vertical transmission.
- Yet in 2009, only 53 % of HIV+pregnant women in low- and middle-income countries received ARVs for prevention of mother-to-child HIV transmission (PMTCT). Without ARV therapy, the rate of mother-to-child transmission (MTCT) is estimated to range from 20 to 30 %.
- Elimination of MTCT is possible with comprehensive care delivery/education programs.

K.M. Powis, M.D., M.P.H., M.B.A.
Internal Medicine and Pediatrics, Pediatric Global Health, Massachusetts General Hospital, Boston, MA, USA

Department of Immunology and Infectious Diseases, Harvard School of Public Health, Boston, MA, USA

A.M. Obando, M.D. (✉)
Internal Medicine/Pediatrics, Massachusetts General Hospital,
175 Cambridge St, 5th Floor, Boston MA 02114, USA
e-mail: AOBANDO@partners.org

Global Burden of Disease

- 33 million people worldwide have HIV/AIDS as of the end of 2009; two-thirds are in sub-Saharan Africa.
- Global estimated HIV incidence was 2.6 million individuals in 2009 across all ages; 370,000 (12 %) were children under age 15.
- 2.5 Million children estimated to be living with HIV at the end of 2009.
- Approximately 450,000 or 23 % of children qualifying for treatment received antiretrovirals (ARV) in 2010.
- Four million children have died from HIV/AIDS.
- Half of HIV-infected infants will die in the first 2 years of life without ARV treatment.
- Over 90 % of HIV-infected children reside in sub-Saharan Africa.
- In many developed countries, vertical HIV transmission has been virtually eliminated.

Modes of Transmission

- Over 90 % of HIV infection in pediatrics occurs through vertical transmission. Yet in 2009, only 53 % of HIV+pregnant women in low- and middle-income countries received ARVs for PMTCT. Without ARV therapy, the rate of MTCT is estimated to range from 20 to 30 %.
- Rates of MTCT are doubled in populations of HIV+women that breastfeed. Expanding ARV treatment through the breastfeeding period can reduce risk of transmission to 5 % or less.

Preventing Mother-to-Child Transmission of HIV

Elimination of MTCT is possible with comprehensive care delivery/education programs. Program success requires the following:

- Diagnosis of HIV prior to conception or early in pregnancy.
- Maternal access/adherence to ARV treatment.
- ARV prophylactic treatment of HIV-exposed infants within hours of delivery through the first 4–6 weeks of life.
- Selection of infant feeding choice that optimizes HIV-free survival.
- Access/adherence to ARVs for either the mother or the infant throughout breastfeeding, if breastfeeding presents the safest feeding option.

Prevention Strategies

a) *Early maternal diagnosis and diagnostic studies*:
- Antenatal clinics (ANC) should offer HIV testing and counseling (HTC) to all pregnant women.
- Rapid HIV testing detects HIV antibodies within 6–12 weeks after infection. A negative rapid HIV test early in pregnancy warrants retesting prior to or at delivery.
- ARV regimens have a variety of toxicity profiles including anemia, neutropenia, hepatotoxicity, and decreased renal function. Drawing safety labs at diagnosis minimizes treatment initiation delay.

b) *Early initiation of maternal antiretroviral treatment*:
The World Health Organization (WHO) recommendations for treatment of HIV during pregnancy are presented in Table 18.1. For WHO-recommended specific ARVs regimens in pregnancy, refer to http://whqlibdoc.who.int/publications/2010/9789241599818_eng.pdf.

c) *Infant prophylaxis*:
- All HIV-exposed uninfected infants require ARV prophylaxis (Table 18.2). Treatment is only effective if started within 72 h of delivery, but should be initiated as soon after delivery as possible. Acceptable regimens are listed in Table 18.2.
- Trimethoprim/Sulfamethoxazole (TMP/SMZ) (Cotrimoxazole, Septrim®, Bactrim®) prevents morbidity/mortality in HIV-infected infants. TMP/SMZ should be initiated at 6 weeks of life and continued until transmission risk is eliminated and testing confirms HIV-negative status.
- Breastfed infants will require TMP/SMZ prophylaxis until testing negative for HIV 6 weeks after breastfeeding cessation.
- Exclusively formula fed infants may not require TMP/SMZ prophylaxis, if HIV testing at 6 weeks of life is negative.
- Refer to Table 18.9 for dosing guidelines.

d) *Infant feeding options*:
WHO policy recommends that national/regional authorities decide which infant feeding practice, will be primarily promoted. A country's approach should be based upon:

- Socioeconomic/cultural contexts of populations served by maternal–child health services
- Availability and quality of health services
- Local epidemiology including HIV prevalence among pregnant women
- Main causes of maternal/child undernutrition and infant/child mortality

The feeding policy should promote HIV-infant survival and maternal health. The policy must balance risk of MTCT inherent with breastfeeding with meeting infant nutritional needs and protecting against non-HIV morbidity/mortality (e.g., diarrheal disease).

Table 18.1 WHO PMTCT mother–infant treatment guidelines

	Woman receives		Infant receives
	Treatment (for CD4 count ≤350 cells/mm^3)	Prophylaxis (for CD4 count >350 cells/mm^3)	
Option A	Triple ARVs starting as soon as diagnosed, continued for life	*Antepartum*: AZT twice daily starting as early as 14 weeks gestation *Intrapartum*: at onset of labor, sdNVP if treated with AZT less than 4 weeks prior to delivery *Postpartum*: daily AZT/3TC twice daily through 7 days postpartum, if sdNVP required at labor onset	For breastfed infant, daily NVP from birth through 1 week beyond complete cessation of breastfeeding, if mother is not on triple ARVs If not breastfeeding or breastfeeding and mother is taking triple ARVs, either daily NVP or twice daily AZT through age 4–6 weeks
Option B	*Same initial ARVs for both* Triple ARVs starting as soon as diagnosed, continued for life	Triple ARVs starting as early as 14 weeks gestation and continued intrapartum and through childbirth if not breastfeeding or until 1 week after cessation of all breastfeeding	
Option B+	*Same for treatment and prophylaxis* Regardless of CD4 count, triple ARVs starting as soon as diagnosed, continued for life		

Source: World Health Organization HIV/AIDS Programmatic Update: Use of Antiretroviral Drugs for Treating Pregnant Women and Preventing HIV Infection in Infants; Executive Summary April 2012, p. 2. http://www.who.int/hiv/PMTCT_update.pdf Reprinted with permission
3TC lamivudine, *ARV* antiretroviral, *AZT* zidovudine, *sdNVP* single-dose Nevirapine

Table 18.2 NVP or AZT prophylactic dosing for HIV-exposed uninfected infants

	Newborn ≥2.5 kg	Newborn preterm (<35 weeks) or with low birth weight (<2.5 kg)	Treatment duration
NVP syrup	6 mg orally once daily	2 mg/kg once daily	Option for formula fed infants or breastfed infants born to women on a triple ARV regimen <6 weeks prior to delivery: Treat for 4–6 weeks from date of delivery
			Option for breastfed infants born to women not taking triple ARV regimen during breastfeeding. Treat from delivery throughout breastfeeding to be stopped 1 week after breastfeeding cessation.
AZT syrup	4 mg/kg orally every 12 h	2 mg/kg orally every 12 h for the first 2 weeks of life, increasing to 2 mg/kg orally every 8 h (three times/day)	Regimen can be used in formula fed infants or in breastfeed infants born to women who will remain on triple ARV regimens throughout breastfeeding and should be initiated at delivery and continued for 4–6 weeks

Infant feeding options include the following:

- For infants known to be HIV infected from birth, breastfeeding should be continued at least through the first year of life.
- For HIV-exposed infants, exclusive breastfeeding for the first 6 months of life is an option, so long as:
    - Infant has received 4–6 weeks of NVP prophylaxis after delivery.
    - Mother remains on HAART throughout breastfeeding or the infant continues on NVP until 1 week after last breast milk exposure if the mother not on HAART.
- Among breastfed infants of mothers who are HAART non-adherent or lack viral suppression, daily infant NVP can reduce MTCT risk.
- Another option for HIV-exposed infants is exclusive formula feeding with education on formula preparation and adequate storage.

Age appropriate complementary foods should be introduced by 6 months of life for all infants.

HIV-infected pregnant women should be informed of the nationally promoted infant feeding practice, apprised of the risks/benefits of alternatives, and be supported once an appropriate feeding choice is elected.

e) *Infant testing*:
Over 30 % of untreated HIV-infected infants will die within the first year of life. Survival can be improved to 95 % if HAART is started as early as 6 weeks of life. Provider-initiated HTC, and timely access to HIV care/services are imperative for:

- Infants presenting to health facilities with signs/symptoms of HIV infection
- Infants born to HIV-infected women as routine follow-up care
- Infants with an HIV-infected sibling or parent

Through the first 18 months of life, HIV DNA or RNA testing is necessary, since maternal antibodies transferred passively during pregnancy to infants cloud interpretation of rapid HIV antibody testing. Infant HIV testing should be incorporated into routine well-child and immunizations visits. Testing should occur as follows:

- Between 4 and 6 weeks of life or sooner if presenting to a health facility with acute illness concerning for HIV (e.g., pneumonia, diarrhea, malnutrition). Infants tested prior to 4 weeks due to acute illness with an initial negative test should be retested at 6 weeks of life.
- Breastfed asymptomatic infants should be tested 6 weeks after breastfeeding cessation. If the previously breast fed child is ≥ 18 months, a rapid HIV antibody test can be performed.

Signs/Symptoms of HIV in the Pediatric Population

The WHO Clinical Staging Tables (Tables 18.3 and 18.4) are used for patients diagnosed with HIV. Yet clinical presentations in these tables should prompt providers to consider HIV in the differential diagnosis, particularly if an infant/child was exposed to HIV in utero or resides in a region of high HIV prevalence.

Staging and Treatment of HIV

a) The WHO Clinical Stages (Table 18.3 and 18.4) are associated with HIV disease progression in the absence of ARV treatment. Staging should guide treatment initiation and use of TMP/SMZ prophylaxis. In the first 24 weeks after triple ARV treatment initiation, clinical events noted in the staging tables may reflect immune reconstitution events. After 24 weeks, events likely reflect immune deterioration and should be monitored closely, particularly if access to CD4 count/viral load is not available.
b) *Rationale and Criteria for Treatment Initiation*
   50% of HIV-infected infants will die before age 2, if untreated. Initiation of and daily compliance with combination ARVs significantly reduces HIV morbidity/mortality (Table 18.5).
c) *WHO Recommendations Antiretroviral Treatment Regimens* (Table 18.6)
d) *Selected Antiretroviral Formulations, Dosing, Adverse Reactions, and Side Effect Profiles* (Table 18.7)

   For an incremented, weight range dosing table of commonly used ARVs, refer to http://www.columbia-icap.org/resources/peds/files/dosingguide/pedsdosingguideltrSEC.pdf

e) *Schedule of health visits*
   Recommended clinical care timing of HIV-infected patients on treatment:

   - Infants: 2, 4, 8 weeks, then every 4 weeks in first year of life
   - Children: 2, 4, 8, 12 weeks, then every 2–3 months once stabilized on therapy
   - Adolescents: 2, 4, 12 weeks, then every 3–6 months once stabilized on therapy

- In the event of illness, medication adverse reaction, virological/immunologic failure, patients should be seen more frequently.

f) *Immunization of HIV-infected infants/children*
   WHO recommends the following immunizations for HIV-infected children (Table 18.8):
g) *Prophylactic Medications*
   Trimethoprim/Sulfamethoxazole (TMP/SMZ): Decreases morbidity/mortality among HIV-infected infant/children (Table 18.9). Prophylactic eligibility:

   - Infants in the first year of life
   - Children age 12–60 months with a CD4 cell % <25 %

Table 18.3 WHO clinical staging of HIV/AIDS for infants and children

Clinical Stage 1
Asymptomatic
Persistent generalized lymphadenopathy

Clinical Stage 2
Hepatosplenomegaly
Papular pruritic eruptions
Seborrhoeic dermatitis
Extensive human papilloma virus infection
Extensive molluscum contagiosum
Fungal nail infections
Recurrent oral ulcers
Linear gingival erythema
Angular cheilitis
Parotid enlargement
Herpes zoster
Recurrent or chronic respiratory infections (sinusitis, tonsillitis, otitis media, and pharyngitis)

Clinical Stage 3
Moderated unexplained malnutrition not adequately responding to standard therapy
Unexplained persistent diarrhea (14 days or more)
Unexplained persistent fever (above 37.5 °C intermittent or constant, for longer than 1 month)
Oral candidiasis (after the first 6–8 weeks of life)
Oral hairy leukoplakia
Acute necrotizing ulcerative gingivitis/periodontitis
Lymph node tuberculosis
Pulmonary tuberculosis
Severe recurrent bacterial pneumonia
Symptomatic lymphoid interstitial pneumonitis
Chronic HIV-associated lung disease including bronchiectasis
Unexplained anemia (<8 g/dl), neutropenia (<0.5 × 10^9/L), and/or chronic thrombocytopenia (<50 × 10^9/L)

Clinical Stage 4
Unexplained severe wasting, stunting, or severe malnutrition not responding to standard therapy
Pneumocystis pneumonia
Recurrent severe bacterial infections (e.g., empyema, pyomyositis, osteomyelitis, meningitis, excluding PNA)
Chronic herpes simplex infection (orolabial or cutaneous >1 month's duration or visceral at any site)
Esophageal candidiasis (or candidiasis of the trachea, bronchi or lungs)
Extrapulmonary tuberculosis
Kaposi sarcoma
Cytomegalovirus (CMV) infection: retinitis or CMV infection affecting another organ after 1 month of age
Central nervous system toxoplasmosis (after 1 month of life)
Extrapulmonary cryptococcosis (including meningitis)
HIV encephalopathy
Disseminated endemic mycosis (coccidiomycosis or histoplasmosis)

(continued)

Table 18.3 (continued)

Chronic cryptosporidiosis (with diarrhea)
Chronic isosporiasis
Cerebral or B-cell non-Hodgkin lymphoma
Progressive multifocal leukoencephalopathy
Symptomatic HIV-associated nephropathy or HIV-associated cardiomyopathy

Source: WHO Case Definitions of HIV for Surveillance and Revised Clinical Staging and Immunological Classification of HIV-Related Disease in Adults and Children 2007, pages 17–18, http://www.who.int/hiv/pub/guidelines/HIVstaging150307.pdf<http://www.who.int/hiv/pub/guidelines/HIVstaging150307.pdf
Reprinted with permission

- Children and adolescents over 60 months of age with CD4 cell % <15 % or an absolute CD4 cell count <200
- Children or adolescents who are no longer virally suppressed on a triple ARV regimen.
- Children or adolescents who discontinue a triple ARV regimen

Management of Selected Opportunistic Infections (OIs)

a) *Introduction*

- In pre-HAART era, OIs were primary cause of death
- OIs continue to be the presenting symptoms in untreated HIV + children
- OI treatment/prophylaxis may lead to drug–drug interactions with ARVs, resulting in adverse effects or subtherapeutic ARV levels, limiting HAART and OI options
- Immune reconstitution inflammatory syndrome (IRIS) can complicate OI treatment

    – May occur after initiating HAART, as CD4 counts recover, evoking immune response to active/latent/occult OIs
    – OIs more likely to occur in children starting ARVs at lower CD4 counts; can be seen up to 4 months after initiating HAART
  – There may be significant mortality with simultaneous treatment of OIs and HAART initiation, particularly with CNS IRIS; risks must be balanced against potential mortality associated with delayed ARV initiation.
  – For TB, *P. jiroveci*, Cryptococcus, OI treatment may be warranted prior to ARV initiation.
  – Treatment to mitigate inflammatory response is variable: can include observation, NSAIDs, corticosteroids, depending on severity of response.

b) *Selected Opportunistic Infections* (Table 18.10)
c) *Lymphoid Interstitial Pneumonitis*:

Table 18.4 World Health Organization Clinical Staging of HIV/AIDS for adolescents and adults

Clinical Stage 1
  Asymptomatic
  Persistent generalized lymphadenopathy

Clinical Stage 2
  Moderate unexplained weight loss (<10 % of presumed or measured body weight)
  Recurrent respiratory infections (sinusitis, tonsillitis, otitis media, and pharyngitis)
  Herpes zoster
  Angular cheilitis
  Recurrent oral ulcerations
  Papular pruritic eruptions
  Seborrheic dermatitis
  Fungal nail infections

Clinical Stage 3
  Unexplained severe weight loss (>10 % of presumed or measured body weight)
  Unexplained chronic diarrhea for >1 month
  Unexplained persistent fever for >1 month (>37.6 °C, intermittent or constant)
  Persistent oral candidiasis (thrush)
  Oral hairy leukoplakia
  Pulmonary tuberculosis (current)
  Severe presumed bacterial infections (e.g., pneumonia, empyema, osteomyelitis, meningitis, bacteremia)
  Acute necrotizing ulcerative stomatitis, gingivitis, or periodontitis
  Unexplained anemia (hemoglobin <8 g/dL), neutropenia (<0.5×10^9/L), or chronic thrombocytopenia (<50×10^9/L)

Clinical Stage 4
  HIV wasting syndrome
  Pneumocystis pneumonia
  Recurrent severe bacterial pneumonia
  Chronic herpes simplex infection (orolabial, genital, anorectal >1 month or visceral at any site)
  Esophageal candidiasis (or candidiasis of trachea, bronchi or lungs)
  Extrapulmonary tuberculosis
  Kaposi Sarcoma
  Cytomegalovirus infection (retinitis or infection of other organs)
  Central nervous system toxoplasmosis
  HIV encephalopathy
  Extrapulmonary cryptococcosis including meningitis
  Disseminated non-tuberculous mycobacterium infection
  Progressive multifocal leukoencephalopathy
  Chronic cryptosporidiosis (with diarrhea)
  Chronic isoporiasis
  Disseminated mycosis (coccidiodomycosis or histoplasmosis)
  Recurrent non-typhyoidal Salmonella bacteremia
  Lymphoma (cerebral or B-cell non-Hodgkin) or other solid HIV-associated tumors
  Invasive cervical carcinoma
  Atypical disseminated leishmaniasis
  Symptomatic HIV-associated nephropathy or symptomatic HIV-associated cardiomyopathy
  Symptomatic HIV-associated cardiomyopathy
  Reactivation of American trypanosomiasis (meningoencephalitis or myocarditis)

Source: WHO Case Definitions of HIV for Surveillance and Revised Clinical Staging and Immunological Classification of HIV-Related Disease in Adults and Children 2007, pages 15–16, http://www.who.int/hiv/pub/guidelines/HIVstaging150307.pdf<http://www.who.int/hiv/pub/guidelines/HIVstaging150307.pdf
Reprinted with permission

Table 18.5 Criteria for initiating treatment in infants, children, and adolescents with confirmed or suspected HIV

WHO antiretroviral treatment initiation criteria for infants, children, and adolescents
Infants
• Initiate combination ARVs for all HIV-infected infants diagnosed in the first year of life, irrespective of CD4 cell count or WHO clinical stage
Children/adolescents
• Initiate combination ARVs for all HIV-infected children between 12 and 24 months of age, irrespective of CD4 cell count or WHO clinical stage
• Initiate combination ARVs for all HIV-infected children between 24 and 59 months of age with CD4 cell percentage $\leq 25\%$ or with absolute CD4 cell count ≤ 750 cells/mm^3, irrespective of WHO clinical stage
• Initiate combination ARVs for all HIV-infected children ≥ 5 years old with CD4 cell count ≤ 350 cells/mm^3, irrespective of WHO clinical stage
• Initiate combination ARVs for all HIV-infected children or adolescents with WHO clinical stages 3 or 4, irrespective of CD4 cell count
• Initiate combination ARVs for any child less than 18 months of age given a presumptive clinical diagnosis of HIV infection

Lymphoid interstitial pneumonitis (LIP) is not an opportunistic infection, rather a complication of pediatric HIV disease, occurring in 25–40 % of children with perinatally acquired HIV. It is a pediatric AIDS-defining illness, presenting in the 3rd–4th year of life. Characterized by diffuse infiltrate of lymphocytes, plasma cells, and histiocytes in the pulmonary interstitium, the pathogenesis is not well understood, but may result from an exaggerated immune response to inhaled antigens or EBV infection.

Onset tends to be insidious, characterized by cough, tachypnea, and digital clubbing. Lymphadenopathy, hepatosplenomegaly, and salivary gland enlargement may exist. Clinical course can range from spontaneous remission, to viral respiratory infection induced exacerbations, or progression to respiratory failure. CXR has classic findings of diffuse, symmetric micronodular infiltrates with mediastinal or hilar adenopathy. Pulmonary function tests demonstrated restrictive pattern.

Treatment requires a fully suppressive ARV regimen. IV gammaglobulin administered periodically may slow/halt disease progression. Pulmonary toilet is important, as LIP patients experience bronchiectasis.

Health Challenges of the HIV-Exposed Uninfected Infant/Children

HIV-exposed uninfected infants/children experience higher morbidity/mortality in the first 2 years of life compared with infants born to HIV-uninfected women. Frequent health visits with close monitoring of growth failure and illnesses can optimize survival.

Table 18.6 WHO pediatric HIV treatment guidelines for infants and children

WHO general guidelines for ARV class selection and first-line treatment regimens

Infants
- For infants with no prior exposure to ARVs either in utero or prophylactically, start nevirapine (NVP)+2 nucleoside reverse transcriptase inhibitors (NRTIs)
- For infants exposed to maternal or infant NVP or other maternal non-nucleoside reverse transcriptase inhibitors (NNRTIs), start lopinavir/ritonavir (LPV/r)+2 NRTIs
- For infants whose exposure to ARVs is unknown, start NVP+2 NRTIs

Children
- For children between 12 and 24 months of age exposed to maternal or infant NVP or other NNRTIs used for maternal treatment or PMTCT, start LPV/r+2 NRTIs
- For children between 12 and 24 months of age not exposed to NNRTIs, start NVP+2 NRTIs
- For children >24 months but <36 months of age, start NVP+2 NRTIs
- For children ≥3 years of age, start NVP or efavirenz (EFV)+2 NRTIs

For infants and children, the NRTI backbone should be one of the following regimens in preferential order
1. Lamivudine (3TC)+zidovudine (AZT)
2. 3TC+Abacavir (ABC)
3. 3TC+Stavudine (d4T)

Note: AZT and d4T should never be use in the same regimen, due to antagonistic effect of concurrent use

Concurrent treatment of Tuberculosis and HIV
- For infants and children <2 years of age, with exposure to NVP who are taking a rifampicin-containing tuberculosis (TB) regimen, triple NRTI regimen is the preferred first line (e.g., 3TC-ZDV-ABC)
- Make adjustments to ARV regimens, as needed, to decrease potential for toxicities and drug–drug interactions
  - If on a regimen of NVP+2 NRTIs, substitute EFV for NVP is child is ≥3 years of age
  - If on a regimen of NVP+2 NRTIs, and EFV substitution is not possible, ensure that NVP dosing is at maximum dose of 200 mg/m^2 (max 200 mg) twice daily
  - If on any regimen containing LPV/r, consider doubling the dose or adding RTV at a 1:1 ratio of LPV:RTV to achieve the full therapeutic dose of LPV with concurrent use of rifampicin-containing regimens

WHO guidelines for second-line treatment regimens
- After virological failure on a first-line NNRTI-based regimen, a protease inhibitor (PI) boosted with ritonavir (r)+2 NRTIs are recommended with modification of two of the three drugs in the triple regimen, so long as nonadherence has been excluded as the cause of virological failure
  - LPV/r is the preferred boosted PI for second-line ARV regimen after failure on a first-line NNRTI-based regimen
  - After failure on a first-line regimen of 3TC+AZT or d4T, ABC+3TC is the preferred NRTI backbone for second-line regimen
  - After failure on a first-line regimen of 3TC+ABC, 3TC+AZT is the preferred NRTI back-bone option for second-line regimen

Table 18.7 Selected antiretroviral formulations, dosing, adverse reactions, and side effect profiles

Drug name	Formulations	Dosing	Side effect profile	Comments
Nucleoside reverse transcriptase inhibitors				
Abacavir (ABC)	Tablet: 300 mg Liquid: 20 mg/ml	Target dose: 8 mg/kg/dose twice daily to maximum of 300 mg twice daily	Potential for hypersensitivity reaction Hepatotoxicity Lipodystrophy Increased risk of coronary heart disease in adults	May be used from 3 months of age or older, but not prior to 3 months ABC should be stopped immediately and never used again if hypersensitivity reaction is noted No food restrictions Tablet can be crushed and mixed with a small amount of water or food if taken immediately Dose adjustment required for hepatic impairment
Didanosine (DDI)	Chewable tablets: 25, 50, 100, 150, 200 mg Enteric-coated tablets: 125, 200, 250, 400 mg (designed for once daily dosing) Powder for oral solution: 10 mg/ml when reconstituted with water and may requiring buffering	Target dose: <3 months: 50 mg/m² /dose twice daily ≥3 months to <13 years: 90–120 mg/m²/dose twice daily Maximum dosing: 200 mg/dose twice daily or 400 mg once daily, applicable at 13 years of age or older and at >60 kg	Peripheral neuropathy (although rare in infants/children) Diarrhea Pancreatitis Lactic acidosis	This regimen is being phased out of many national regimens in resource-limited settings due to its side effect profile and need for buffering DDI is degraded rapidly unless given as an enteric-coated formulation or combined with buffering agents or antacids. It is recommended to administer DDI 30 min before or 2 h after meals Requires dose adjust with renal impairment
Emtricitabine (FTC)	Tablet: 200 mg Liquid: 10 mg/ml	Target dose: <3 months: 3 mg/kg once daily ≥3 months and up: 6 mg/kg once daily to maximum dose of 200 mg per day	GI upset including nausea, vomiting, and/or diarrhea	Co-formulated option with Tenofovir and with Tenofovir and Efavirenz Requires dose adjust with renal impairment

Lamivudine (3TC)	Tablet: 150 mg Liquid: 10 mg/ml	Target dose: 4 mg/kg/dose twice daily to maximum of 150 mg/dose twice daily <30 days: 2 mg/kg/dose twice daily	Nausea/vomiting	Well tolerated without food restrictions Tablet can be crushed and mixed with a small amount of water or food if taken immediately Active against Hepatitis B Requires dose adjust with renal impairment
Stavudine (d4T)	Capsules: 15, 20, 30 mg Liquid: 1 mg/ml	Target dose: 1 mg/kg/dose twice daily Dose at <30 kg: 1 mg/kg/dose twice daily Dose at 30–60 kg: 30 mg twice daily Dose at >60 kg: 40 mg twice daily	Lactic acidosis Hepatotoxicity Pancreatitis Peripheral Neuropathy Lipodystrophy Metabolic Syndrome	Do not use with AZT due to antagonistic effect Tablet can be opened and mixed with small amount of food or water and remains stable in solution up to 24 h if refrigerated Requires dose adjust with renal impairment
Tenofovir (TDF)	Tablet: 150, 250, 300 mg Powder: 40 mg/g	Target dose: ≥ 2 years of age: 8 mg/kg once daily to a maximum of 300 mg	Decreased bone mineral density Renal toxicity Lactic acidosis Hepatotoxicity	Co-formulated with FTC and EFV Powder should be mixed with 2–4 oz of soft food and taken immediately Concerning for use in children given potential for loss of bone mineral density. Use of calcium and vitamin D supplementation may be appropriate in adolescents Should not be used concurrently with DDI given increased risk of pancreatitis and virologic failure when co-administered Active against Hepatitis B

(continued)

Table 18.7 (continued)

Drug name	Formulations	Dosing	Side effect profile	Comments
Zidovudine (AZT)	Tablet: 300 mg Capsule: 100; 250 mg Liquid: 10 mg/ml	Target dose: 180–240 mg/m^2 per dose given twice daily with maximum dose of 300 mg/dose twice daily	Anemia Neutropenia Lactic acidosis Hepatotoxicity Nausea/vomiting Diarrhea	Co-formulated with 3TC Do not use with d4T due to antagonistic effect Liquid is light sensitive and should be stored in a glass jar Capsules may be opened and tablets may be crushed, mixing with small amounts of water or food, if taken immediately Requires dose adjustment for Cr Cl <15 or on hemo-/peritoneal dialysis
Non-nucleoside reverse transcriptase inhibitors				
Efavirenz (EFV)	Tablet: 600 mg Capsule: 50, 100, 200 mg Liquid: 30 mg/ml	*Only approved for use in ages 3 years or older* Target dose: 15 mg/kg/day for capsule or tablet and 19.5 mg/kg/day in the liquid formulation	Headaches Vivid dreams (resolves on treatment) Worsening of baseline psychiatric disorders Persistent and severe CNS toxicity Lipodystrophy Rash Use with caution in patients with seizure disorder Possibly teratogenic, with question of association with neural tube defects	Liquid has lower bioavailability and ration of 1.3 liquid to solid formulation is recommended for dosing equivalency Can be dosed with food, but if taken with food, especially fatty meals, absorption is increased by an average of 50 % Dosing more common at bedtime to reduce CNS side effects Capsules can be opened and mixed with a small amount of food or water but may require mixing with sweet foods, as the medication has a peppery taste

| Nevirapine (NVP) | Tablet: 200 mg
Liquid: 10 mg/ml | Target dose: Induction: 160–200 mg/m²/dose once daily with maximum dose 200 mg × 14 days
Maintenance dose: 160–200 mg/m²/dose twice daily to maximum dose of 200 mg | Steven Johnson Syndrome
Hepatotoxicity | Symptomatic hepatotoxicity is rare in children prior to adolescence
If mild rash occurs during the first 14 days of induction dosing, continue once daily dosing and only escalate dose once the rash has subsided and the dose is well tolerated
If severe rash occurs, especially accompanied by fever, blistering, oral lesions, and/or conjunctival injection, permanently discontinue drug
For children 14–24.9 kg the suggested dose is 1 tablet in the a.m. and 0.5 tablets in the p.m.
Tablets can be crushed and combined with a small amount of water or food if taken immediately
Contraindicated with moderate to severe liver impairment
Increased risk of hepatotoxicity in females with CD4 > 250 and males with CD4 > 350 who are ARV treatment naïve |

(continued)

Table 18.7 (continued)

Drug name	Formulations	Dosing	Side effect profile	Comments
Protease inhibitors				
Atazanvir/ritonovir (ATV/r)	Tablet: 100, 150, 200, 300 mg Ritonavir: 100 mg	Treatment-Naïve Children only: 15 to <25 kg: ATV 150 mg + r 80 mg once daily Both treatment naïve and experienced children: 15 to <32 kg: ATV 200 mg + r 100 mg once daily 32 to <39 kg: ATV 250 mg + r 100 mg once daily ≥39 kg: ATV 300 mg + r 100 mg once daily	Hyperbilirubinemia Stevens Johnson Syndrome DRESS syndrome Nephrolithiasis Prolonged PR interval Insulin Intolerance Hepatotoxicity	Must be administered with food, as it enhances absorption ATV can prolong PR interval and should be used with caution in pediatric patients with cardiac conduction disease Do not use in less than 3 months of age due to risk of kernicterus Data are insufficient to recommend dosing of ATV in children younger or in treatment—experienced children weighing less than 25 kg
Kaletra (LPV/r)	Tablet: 200 mg lopinavir/50 mg ritonavir Capsule: 133.3 mg lopinavir/33.3 mg ritonavir Liquid: 80 mg/ml lopinavir and 20 mg/ml ritonavir	Lopinavir target dose: 5–7.9 kg: 16 mg/kg/dose twice daily 8–9.9 kg: 14 mg/kg/dose twice daily 10–13.9 kg: 12 mg/kg/dose twice daily 14–39.9 kg 10 mg/kg/dose twice daily Ritonavir target dose: 7–14.9 kg: 3 mg/kg/dose twice daily 15–40 kg: 2.5 mg/kg/dose twice daily Max dose: 400 mg Lopinavir and 100 mg Ritonavir twice daily	Severe diarrhea Nausea/vomiting Dyslipidemia Metabolic Syndrome	Should be taken with food Liquid formulation requires refrigeration Ritonavir component inhibits the cytochrome P450 system, resulting in drug–drug interactions, particularly when dosed with rifampicin in a TB–HIV coinfected patient With moderate to severe liver impairment Lopinavir levels may be increased by 30 %

Table 18.8 WHO Immunization Recommendations for HIV-infected infants/children/adolescents

Immunization	Recommendation
BCG	HIV-infected infants or infants of HIV-unknown status with symptoms consistent with HIV should not be vaccinated
Hepatitis B	Recommended
Polio	Recommended and choice of OPV or IPV dictated by absence/presence of polio in the community OPV recommended in polio endemic areas and areas at high risk of polio importation and spread. However, the OPV vaccine is a live attenuated vaccine and should not be given to infants/children with severe HIV infection (WHO stage III or IV or CD4 % <15 % or absolute CD4 count <200)
Diphtheria–Tetanus–Pertussis	Recommended
Haemophilus influenzae—Type B	Recommended
Pneumococcal (conjugated) [PCV]	HIV-infected infants who have received their three primary PCV vaccinations before 12 months of age may benefit from a booster vaccination in the second year of life
Rotavirus	Recommended
Measles	Contraindicated in infants with severe HIV infection (WHO stage III or IV, or CD4 % <15 % or absolute CD4 cell count <200), but recommended for all other HIV-infected infants/children
	In areas with high incidence of both HIV infection and measles, the measles immunization may be offered as early as 6 months of life to asymptomatic or mildly symptomatic HIV-infected infants. Infants receiving early administration of measles vaccine should receive two additional doses in accordance with the national immunization schedule
Mumps	Contraindicated in infants with severe HIV infection (WHO stage III or IV, or CD4 % <15 % or < absolute CD4 count 200), but recommended for all other HIV-infected infants/children
Rubella	Contraindicated in infants with severe HIV infection (WHO stage III or IV, or CD4 % <15 % or absolute CD4 count <200), but recommended for all other HIV-infected infants/children
Varicella	Recommended only in asymptomatic, non-immunosuppressed, HIV-infected children
	MMRV vaccine has not been studied in HIV-infected children and should not be used in place of MMR vaccinations
	Should be given 28 days or greater after MMR vaccination to optimize the immunogenicity
Yellow Fever	Recommended in areas with endemic Yellow Fever
Human Papilloma Virus	Recommended for females; not yet recommended by WHO for males

Table 18.9 TMP/SMZ dosing recommendations for infant, children, and adolescents

Age range	Suspension 40 mg TMP/200 mg SMZ per 5 ml	Single Strength Tablet 80 mg TMP/400 mg SMZ
≥ 6 weeks to <6 months	2.5 ml once daily	¼ tablet once daily
6 months to 60 months	5 ml once daily	½ tablet once daily
5 years to 14 years	10 ml once daily	1 tablet daily
>14 years		Two single strength tablets or one double strength tablet once daily

Where an allergy to TMP/SMZ or sulfa containing medication is noted, Dapsone 2 mg/kg dosed once daily to a maximum of 100 mg can be substituted

Adolescents and HIV

a) *Introduction*

- In regions with generalized HIV epidemics females age 15–24 experience highest incidence of new infections.
- Adolescents may engage in risky sexual behaviors
- HIV medication adherence challenges are common in adolescents
- Adolescents with perinatally acquired HIV may experience physical/developmental delays leading to stigmatization
- WHO recommends selection of adolescent treatment regimens based upon sexual maturity rating with Tanner stage ≤3 receiving pediatric dosing/regimens, adolescent ≥ stage 4 receiving adult dosing/regimens.

b) *Prevention Programs*

Prevention programs targeted to adolescents include:

- HIV education
- Social messaging promoting delayed sexual debut and discouraging multiple concurrent partners
- Promotion and availability of condoms
- Promotion of HTC services
- Promotion of safe male circumcision programs

- No single adolescent prevention program has successfully reduced HIV incidence in high prevalence settings. The selected combination of programs must be contextually acceptable/applicable to the community. Understanding culture, nature of the HIV epidemic in a particular community and creating a peer driven program, condoned by community leaders, parents and educators is likely to have the greatest traction in preventing incident HIV infections among adolescents.

Table 18.10 Risk factors, prevention, clinical presentation, and treatment of selected opportunistic infections

Tuberculosis	Risk factors and prevention	Increased risk of TB coinfection in any patient with HIV, regardless of CD4 count, although there is a stronger association of TB disease with degree of immunodeficiency. Congenital TB is a rare occurrence, in children born to women with active infection, and has a high mortality rate. More commonly, children are infected by an adult with active TB residing within the household
		Risk of progressing from latent TB infection to active TB when coinfected with HIV is 10 % per year (compared to incidence of 1 in 10 over a lifespan in non-HIV-infected hosts). HIV also increases risk of rapid TB progression, with more severe manifestations
		WHO prevention guidelines advocate initiation of ARVs, in that restoring the immune system and reducing the viral load significantly reduces HIV and TB coinfection. ARV should be started per standard WHO recommendations (see above) and in all patients infected with TB regardless of CD4 count. The WHO also recommends implementation of the "Three I's for HIV/TB," a program that emphasizes *I*ntensified TB case finding, *I*soniazid preventative therapy, and TB *I*nfection control. All patients with TB should have HIV testing particularly in areas of high prevalence. WHO recommends 6 months of isoniazid preventative therapy in HIV-infected TB-exposed infants
		Given evidence of BCG-associated complications in HIV-infected infants, the WHO deems HIV infection in infants a contraindication to administering BCG vaccine. For HIV-exposed infants, however, who may have difficulties obtaining a delayed BCG vaccine, consensus recommendations are to continue administering BCG vaccine at birth in countries where TB and HIV are endemic
	Clinical notes	Rates of TB incidence in HIV-infected children is 1595/100,000 in ages 0–12 months, and 5930/100,000 in ages 15 months–15 years, compared to rates in HIV-uninfected children: 659/100,000 ages 0–12 months and 3588/100,000 ages 0–5 years
		Manifestations of TB: extrathoracic TB more common in HIV-uninfected children and they often have positive tuberculin skin test (TSTs) and normal CXRs. In HIV-infected may see: prolonged cough and fever, more severe weight loss or failure to thrive, generalized lymphadenopathy, splenomegaly, finger clubbing, and diarrhea. TSTs are often false-negative in this population and they often have abnormal CXRs with lung cavities, infiltrations/opacifications
	Diagnosis	WHO diagnostic criteria includes the presence of 3 or more of the following: (1) chronic symptoms suggestive of TB, (2) physical signs suggestive of TB, (3) positive TST (among persons with HIV infection, >5 mm of induration is considered a positive reaction), (4) CXR findings suggestive of TB. HIV-infected children should be screened annually with a TST

(continued)

Table 18.10 (continued)

	Challenges in diagnosing TB in HIV-infected children include high rates of false-negative TSTs. Newer interferon-γ assays have significantly higher sensitivity but have limited availability and are more prone to indeterminate results in younger children. Young children unable to expectorate can be tested by obtaining three morning gastric aspirates on 3 separate days. Furthermore, CXR interpretation is limited in detection of pulmonary TB in HIV+ children due to similarities to other HIV-related lung diseases
	Other potential modes of diagnosis include: fine needle aspiration of lymph nodes in TB lymphadenitis, nasopharyngeal aspiration, sputum induction, and string test (well tolerated in children as young as 4 years). Sputum induction thought to yield superior culture results to gastric aspirates but in several studies HIV infection has been linked to less culture positive sputa or gastric aspirates when compared to that of children who are noninfected with HIV
Treatment	Please see Chap. 19 for recommended treatment regimens. Please see Table 18.6 for adjustments to ARV regimens when on TB treatment
	Below are notes specific to TB/HIV coinfection
	WHO recommends a 6–9 months standard quadruple therapy for pulmonary TB as in HIV-uninfected children, and 12 months for extrapulmonary TB involving the bones or joints, CNS, or miliary disease
	Coadministration of rifamycins and ARVs results in increased metabolism of NNRTIs and PIs due to CP450 induction by rifamycins
	Triple NRTI treatments (treatment of choice in age <2 years exposed to sdNVP when also treating TB with rifamycins) may be associated with more rapid acquisition of viral resistance and inferior antiviral activity
	Optimal timing of initiating HAART in HIV–TB coinfected children unknown
	For children already on HAART, treatment for TB should be initiated as soon as possible
	For ARV-naïve children, some experts recommend deferral of ARV until completion of TB therapy given the important effects of rifamycins and potential for toxicity and nonadherence given complicated multiple drug regimens. Others recommend initiating anti-TB treatment in ART-naïve children 2–8 weeks prior to initiating ARVs to improve adherence and differentiate side effects. Patient factors (immune status, likelihood of adherence, etc.) must be considered. For the most immunocompromised children, benefits of earlier ARV initiation (2 weeks after anti-TB therapy) may outweigh the potential risks of IRIS

		IRIS associated with TB in children characterized by fevers and lymphadenopathy. The TST may revert to positive and CXR may show lymphadenopathy and new infiltrates. Studies in children have found rate of IRIS to be about 20 % when on ARVs. Approximately half of those cases are attributed to unmasking TB infection. Time of onset varied from 4 to 6 weeks after initiation of ARVs. TB-IRIS needs to be distinguished from other infections, tumors, side effects of ARVs, and failure of TB treatment due to resistance of poor adherence
Pneumocystis jiroveci		*Pneumocystis* spp. are one of the most common causes of infection in humans, symptomatic disease (Pneumocystis pneumonia, PCP) is seen almost exclusively in immunocompromised hosts. PCP cases peak in children at age 3–6 months and is a major cause of death of HIV-infected children and infants in resource-limited settings. However, there has been a sharp decline in PCP cases in children with implementation of PMTCT programs and PCP prophylaxis
	Risk factors and prevention	*Prevention* The primary risk factor for acquisition of infection is degree of immunocompromise as measured by CD4 count. Prophylaxis is recommended for all HIV-infected children 1. Aged >6 years with CD4 <200 c/mm^3 or CD4 <15 % 2. Aged 1–5 years with CD4 <500 c/mm^3 or CD4 <15 % 3. All HIV-infected infants <12 months regardless of CD4 count or percentage 4. HIV-exposed infants should initiate prophylaxis at 4–6 weeks of age until they are determined to be uninfected with HIV Prophylaxis regimens 1. First-line prophylaxis is with TMP–SMX. Please see Table 18.9 for dosing recommendations for prophylaxis with TMP–SMX 2. Atovaquone is second-line prophylaxis, is tolerated well but expensive, and is dosed at 30 mg/kg/day for patients 1–3 months and >24 months of age, and 45 mg/kg/day for infants aged 4–24 months. Azithromycin can be used to supplement atovaquone for broader bacterial prophylaxis 3. Dapsone is effective and inexpensive but associated with more adverse effects than atovaquone. Dapsone is dosed on a daily or weekly schedule as 2 mg/kg/day (max total dose of 100 mg/day) or 4 mg/kg/week (maximum total dosage of 200 mg/week) orally 4. Aerosolized pentamidine is recommended for children who are unable to tolerate TMP–SMX, atovaquone, or Dapsone. The dosage for all ages is 300 mg once a month

(continued)

Table 18.10 (continued)

	Primary prophylaxis may be discontinued in children who have achieved immune reconstitution and are over 1 year of age if they have received ARVs for >6 months, CD4 percentage >15 % or CD4 count >200 cells/mm^3 for patients aged >6 years, and CD4 percentage >15 % or CD4 count >500 cells/mm^3 for patients aged 1–5 years for >3 consecutive months
Clinical notes	Clinical presentation is typically with fever, tachypnea, dyspnea, and cough. Onset can be insidious or abrupt. On exam, children may have basilar rales and substantial hypoxia. Four variables associated with Pneumocystis pneumonia in HIV-infected children who present with pneumonia: age <6 months, respiratory rate >59 bpm, arterial percentage Hgb saturation <92 %, and absence of vomiting. CD4 count is often <200 cells/mm^3 and the CD4 percentage <15 % in children aged >5 years. Lactic dehydrogenase may be elevated but is not specific to PCP. CXR commonly demonstrate diffuse parenchymal infiltrates with a ground-glass appearance, although they can also be normal or with only mild infiltrates. Early infiltrates are perihilar and progress toward the periphery and apically
Diagnosis	Definitive diagnosis of PCP is through demonstration of organism in pulmonary tissue along with evidence of pneumonitis. Induced sputum may not be tolerated in young children. If induced sputum analysis is negative a bronchoalveolar lavage (BAL) may be necessary. Nasogastric aspirates may also help with diagnosis and can be obtained on three consecutive mornings to maximize yield of organism. However, bronchoscopy and BAL remains diagnostic procedure of choice for most children/infants. Results may remain positive for 72 h after initiation of PCP treatment and thus results should not delay initiation of treatment. Transbronchial biopsy may be necessary if BAL is negative with a clinical picture of PCP, with a sensitivity of 87–95 %; cysts may still be seen on biopsy up to 10 days after initiating treatment. Open-lung biopsy is the most sensitive and specific modality for diagnosis but as it requires thoracotomy and is not recommended routinely. Definite diagnosis may not be possible in resource-limited settings and absence of ability to definitively diagnosis should not delay timely treatment initiation if a clinical suspicion of PCP exists
Treatment	*Treatment options in order of recommendation* 1. TMP–SMX is the first-line treatment for PCP. For HIV-infected children aged >2 months dosing is 15–20 mg/kg/day of the TMP component and 75–100 mg/kg/day of the SMX component administered intravenously in 3 or 4 divided doses, with the dose infused over 1 h for 21 days. In mild to moderate disease, oral TMP–SMX may be substituted after the acute pneumonitis improves to complete 21 days of treatment 2. IV pentamidine isethionate once daily is used in patients who are unable to tolerate TMP–SMX or who do not demonstrate clinical improvement after 5–7 days of therapy. This course may be completed in patients demonstrating clinical improvement after 7–10 days of IV treatment with an oral regimen such as atovaquone or TMP/Dapsone to complete 21 days of treatment

3. Atovaquone is an alternative for treatment in adults with limited data in children. The dosage is 30–40 mg/kg/day in two divided doses administered orally is established for children <3 and >24 months of age. Children aged 3–24 months require a higher dosage of 45 mg/kg/day. In adolescents and adults atovaquone is dosed 750 mg twice daily

4. Dapsone/TMP can be effective in treating mild/moderate PCP in adults with limited data in children. In adolescents and adults the dose is 100 mg (total dose) orally once daily and TMP 15 mg/kg/day divided into three daily doses administered for 21 days. Among children aged <13 years, a Dapsone dosage of 2 mg/kg/day is required to achieve therapeutic levels. The pediatric dose of TMP is 15 mg/kg/day divided into three daily doses. Dapsone is less effective than when combined with TMP

In moderate to severe PCP, a short course of corticosteroids can help reduce acute respiratory failure, need for ventilation, and mortality with early implementation (within 72 h of diagnosis). Suggested regimen: prednisone on days 1–5, 1 mg/kg/dose twice daily; days 6–10, 0.5 mg/kg/dose twice daily; and days 11–21, 0.5 mg/kg once daily

Oral/esophageal candidiasis	Risk factors and prevention	Candida species, particularly *c. albicans*, account for the most common fungal OIs in HIV-infected infants/children, with oral thrush and diaper dermatitis occurring in 50–85 % of these patients. Invasive candidiasis occurs when mucosal surface is penetrated and hematogenous spread takes place. Oropharyngeal candidiasis (OPC) is seen in as many as 28 % of children on ARVs. Candida esophagitis is seen more in children who are not responding to ARVs. These patients may not have the typical symptoms of odynophagia or concomitant OPC, whereas 94 % of HIV-infected children not on ARVs with esophageal candidiasis will also have OPC. Having CD4 <100 cells/mm^3, high viral loads and neutropenia, are risk factors for candida esophagitis
		Disseminated candidiasis is not common in HIV+ children. Risk factors for disseminated candidiasis in HIV-infected children include coinfection with HSV or CMV esophagitis, resulting in dissemination of candidal esophagitis. Other risk factors include having a chronically indwelling central venous catheter and parenteral nutrition
		There is no way to prevent exposure, as candida species are commensals on human mucosal surfaces. Routine prophylaxis of candidiasis in HIV-infected children is not indicated given the general benign nature of infection and the availability of treatment

(continued)

Table 18.10 (continued)

Clinical notes	OPC manifests most commonly as pseudomembranous patches (thrush) that are creamy white and can be scraped off, with underlying erythematous mucosa, and can be found throughout the oropharynx. Erythematous OPC (atrophic) can appear as flat erythematous lesions on mucosal surfaces. Hyperplastic candidiasis: raised white plaques that cannot be removed and are found on lower surface of tongue, palate, and buccal mucosa. Angular cheilitis appears as red fissures in the corners of the mouth
	Esophageal candidiasis manifests commonly with odynophagia, dysphagia, chest pain, and in children, with nausea and vomiting (and consequently weight loss or dehydration)
	Candidemia presents most commonly as new onset fever, particularly in children with indwelling central venous catheters. Candidemia can lead to endophthalmitis and requires an eye exam by an ophthalmologist
Diagnosis	OPC can be diagnosed clinically and confirmed by KOH wet mounts demonstrating budding yeast
	Esophageal candidiasis has a classic cobblestoning appearance on barium swallow. Endoscopy can also be performed to explore other causes of esophagitis (e.g., CMV) in cases that are refractory. On endoscopy, small white plaques and confluent plaques will be seen on a hyperemic surface with extensive ulceration
	Candidemia is diagnosed via blood cultures
Treatment	*Oropharyngeal*
	1. Uncomplicated infection: topical therapy with clotrimazole troches or nystatin or amphotericin B suspension
	2. Fluconazole 3–6 mg/kg (max 400 mg) daily × 7–14 days or itraconazole 2.5 mg/kg (max 200–400 mg) twice daily × 7–14 days (can also use ketoconazole but may have lower efficacy) more effective than nystatin, particularly in infants, and is recommended if systemic therapy being used
	Esophageal: Requires systemic therapy
	1. PO or IV fluconazole or oral itraconazole are first line dosed as above, with a course of 14–21 days
	2. Voriconazole or caspofungin also effective but have limited availability and have not been used extensively in children
	Invasive
	1. Amphotericin B is drug of choice, dosed at 0.5–1.5 mg/kg IV daily. Duration depends on the extent of infection and clinical response. Generally, children should be treated until 2–3 weeks after the last positive blood culture and there are signs of resolution of infection
	2. Flucytosine + Amphotericin B used in some children with invasive disease but flucytosine has narrow therapeutic index
	3. Fluconazole (high dose at 5–6 mg/kg twice daily max of 800/day) can be used as alternative to amphotericin B in children who have not recently received azole therapy. Alternatively, initial course can be with amphotericin B and completed with fluconazole

18 HIV/AIDS

	Monitoring	Azoles can inhibit CYP450 and can interact with other drugs, resulting in lower plasma concentrations of the azole. There is potential for drug–drug interactions particularly with PIs All drugs associated with increase in transaminases and potentially hepatitis Amphotericin B requires monitoring for nephrotoxicity and hypokalemia IRIS due to candida infection has yet to be described in children Secondary prophylaxis of recurrent OPC is not recommended If recurrences severe, could consider suppressive therapy with a systemic azole
Cryptococcal meningitis	Risk factors and prevention	Early initiation of ARVs is the most cost-effective preventative measure
	Clinical notes	Routine antifungal prophylaxis is not recommended prior to ARV initiation in children or adolescents Early diagnosis and treatment reduces morbidity/mortality. Mortality rates of HIV-related cryptococcal disease (in adults) as high as 35–65 % in sub-Saharan Africa (compared to 10–20 % in developed world). Reasons for high fatality rates include: (1) presentation late in course of disease when treatment is less effective, (2) delays in diagnosis due to limited access to LP and rapid assays, (3) poor access to and high cost of IV amphotericin B (first-line induction treatment), (4) inability to monitor for toxicity of amphotericin B (hypokalemia and nephrotoxicity) Immediate initiation of ARVs is not recommended in patients with cryptococcal meningitis due to risk of IRIS. ARVs should be initiated once response to antifungal therapy is noted 2–4 weeks after initiation of amphotericin B or 4–6 weeks after initiation of high-dose fluconazole
	Diagnosis	Obtain CSF opening pressure at initial LP (lumbar puncture) In order of level of preference 1. LP + rapid CSF CrAg assay (rapid cryptococcal antigen assay) (when results are assured <24 h) 2. LP + CSF India Ink test (when CrAg assay results not available in <24 h) 3. When LP contraindicated (e.g., focal neurological signs, seizures) obtain rapid serum or plasma CrAg (if positive initiate treatment) 4. If CrAg not available, rapid referral for further investigation *n.b.* Fungal culture is gold standard for confirmation of diagnosis

(continued)

Table 18.10 (continued)

Treatment	Amphotericin B use requires at least minimal monitoring for toxicity (baseline and twice weekly for electrolyte abnormalities and nephrotoxicity) as well as adequate pre-hydration
	Induction Phase: (in order of preference for 2 weeks of induction)
	1. Amphotericin B 0.7–1 mg/kg/day + flucytosine 100 mg/kg/day
	2. Amphotericin B 0.7–1 mg/kg/day + fluconazole 12 mg/kg/day up to 800 mg/day
	3. Amphotericin B 0.7–1 mg/kg/day short course (5–7 days) + high-dose fluconazole 12 mg/kg/day up to 800 mg/day to complete 2 weeks when hydration, electrolyte monitoring, and toxicity monitoring cannot be provided for 2 week period
	d. Fluconazole 12 mg/kg/day up to 1200 mg/kg/day ± flucytosine 100 mg/kg/day, when amphotericin B is not available
	e. Fluconazole high dose alone 12 mg/kg/day up to 1200 mg/day, when amphotericin B is not available
	Consolidation Phase (8 weeks of treatment)
	1. Fluconazole 400–800 mg/day after a 2-week induction with amphotericin B (6–12 mg/kg/day up to 400–800 mg/day if below 19 years)
	2. Fluconazole 800 mg/day after induction treatment with short-course amphotericin B or a fluconazole-based induction regimen (fluconazole 12 mg/kg/day up to 800 mg/day if below 19 years)
	Maintenance treatment (and secondary prophylaxis)
	Oral fluconazole 200 mg daily (6 mg/kg/day up to 200 mg/day if below 19 years). In children <2 years old, this antifungal maintenance should NOT be discontinued. In HIV + adolescents, and children >2 years old who have been successfully treated, discontinuation of maintenance is recommended when the patient has been adherent to ARV and antifungal maintenance for at least 1 year and have demonstrated immune reconstitution (CD4 count ≥200 c/mm^3, or ≥100 c/mm^3 with suppressed viral load, or a CD4 cell count percentage greater than 25 % or absolute count greater than 750 cells/mm^3 in children aged 2–5 years old). Maintenance should be restarted if CD4 count drops ≤100 cells/mm^3 or ≤25 % or 750 cells/mm^3 in children aged 2–5 years old

Centers for Disease Control and Prevention. Guidelines for the Prevention and Treatment of Opportunistic Infections Among HIV-Exposed and HIV-Infected Children. MMWR 2009;58(No. RR-11): 1–176

Rapid advice: diagnosis, prevention, and management of cryptococcal disease in HIV-infected adults, adolescents. WHO. December 2011

Human immunodeficiency virus and tuberculosis coinfection in children: challenges in diagnosis and treatment. Pediatr Infect Dis J. 2010 Oct;29(10):e63–70. http://www.who.int/hiv/topics/tb/hiv_tb_factsheet_june_2011.pdf.

c) *Adherence for HIV-positive Adolescents on Treatment*
   Adherence to long-term daily therapy can be a challenge for anyone, but is particularly challenging for some adolescents. In order to optimize adherence, adolescents require care that addresses:

   - Perception of being immortal
   - Desire for independence
   - Parental disclosure of HIV status for adolescents with newly acquired infection
   - Parental disclosure of HIV status to adolescents infected via MTCT

(d) *Support for HIV-Positive Adolescents*
   As HIV-infected adolescents become sexually active, or consider marriage and reproductive health issues, additional support, counseling, and education are required. Establishing supportive services to address evolving needs of HIV-infected adolescents and assisting in transferring to an adult provider are essential.

Recommended Reading

1. World Health Organization. Antiretroviral drugs for treating pregnant women and preventing HIV infection in infants: recommendations for a public health approach. 2010. http://whqlibdoc.who.int/publications/2010/9789241599818_eng.pdf.
2. World Health Organization. Guidelines on HIV and infant feeding: Principles and recommendations for infant feeding in the context of HIV and a summary of evidence. 2010. http://whqlibdoc.who.int/publications/2010/9789241599535_eng.pdf.
3. International Center for AIDS Care and Treatment Programs. Pediatric antiretroviral dosing in resource-limited settings. 2006. http://www.columbia-icap.org/resources/peds/files/dosing-guide/pedsdosingguideltrSEC.pdf.
4. World Health Organization. WHO case definitions of HIV for surveillance and revised clinical staging and immunological classification of HIV-related disease in adults and children. 2007 http://www.who.int/hiv/pub/guidelines/HIVstaging150307.pdf.
5. World Health Organization HIV/AIDS Programmatic Update: Use of antiretroviral drugs for treating pregnant women and preventing HIV infection in infants; executive summary. April 2012. http://www.who.int/hiv/PMTCT_update.pdf.

Chapter 19
Tuberculosis

Rinn Song and Kristian R. Olson

Keywords Tuberculosis • Children • Clinical presentation • Diagnosis • Treatment • HIV • MDR-TB • Prevention

Overview

- TB is one of the leading global infectious causes of morbidity and mortality.
- Younger children and children with HIV are at highest risk of severe forms of TB and TB-associated death.
- A high index of suspicion is required as clinical presentation is nonspecific and diagnosis is challenging.
- TB treatment requires multiple antibiotics for 6 months or longer.
- Prevention is based on BCG vaccination and isoniazid preventive therapy for children with HIV.

R. Song, M.D., Dr.Med., M.P.H. (✉)
Division of Infectious Diseases, Children's Hospital Boston,
300 Longwood Avenue, Boston, MA 02115, USA
e-mail: rinn.song@childrens.harvard.edu

K.R. Olson, M.D., M.P.H., D.T.M.&H.
Department of Pediatrics, Mass General Center for Global Health,
Massachusetts General Hospital, Boston, MA, USA

Internal Medicine, Inpatient Clinician Educator Service,
Massachusetts General Hospital, Boston, MA, USA

Introduction/Epidemiology

Tuberculosis (TB) is caused by infection with mycobacteria of the *Mycobacterium tuberculosis complex* group (*M. tuberculosis, M. bovis,* and *M. africanum*). By far the most prevalent of these causing disease among children is *M. tuberculosis* (Mtb). TB can be found worldwide and is among the leading, often unrecognized infectious causes of morbidity and mortality among children in resource-limited settings in the world. Due to diagnostic challenges and poor reporting, the global disease burden is difficult to ascertain. However, it is estimated that children younger than 15 years of age account for approximately 11 % of the total global TB case burden per year (at least 0.9–1.0 million pediatric TB cases annually). The majority of pediatric TB cases, approximately 75–80 % or more, occur among children living in 22 high-burden countries (primarily countries in sub-Saharan Africa, South-East Asia, the former Soviet Union, India, and China). Limited pediatric TB surveillance data hampers reliable estimates of TB-related deaths among children, but the WHO estimates that up to 400,000–500,000 children die worldwide annually due to TB.

Transmission of TB is airborne following inhalation of droplet nuclei containing mycobacteria produced usually by an adult or occasionally an adolescent with active TB. Children younger than 10 years of age with pulmonary TB very rarely infect other children due to their low number of mycobacteria in their respiratory secretions. Following infection, children have a higher risk of progression to active TB disease and also a higher risk of disseminated TB and death due to TB compared to adults. This applies particularly to children younger than 2 years of age and children with conditions that impair immune competence (specifically HIV infection, but also moderate to severe malnutrition).

Clinical Presentation

TB infection is not synonymous with disease. Following inhalation of droplet nuclei from an infectious patient with TB, infected children can remain asymptomatic and without evidence of active disease if the infection is being controlled by their host immune response.

Children unable to contain their primary infection progress to develop active TB disease. Most childhood TB disease (>90 %) occurs within the first year following infection. Thus, reactivation of latent TB infection is relatively rare but can occur among older children and adolescents. Clinical manifestations of TB include pulmonary and extrapulmonary TB. The latter is more common among children than adults (up to 20–25 % of all pediatric TB cases). During the first few months of disease progression, pulmonary TB manifests initially with uncomplicated intrathoracic lymph-node disease, primarily affecting the hilar or mediastinal lymph nodes. Subsequently, children can develop intraparenchymal pulmonary disease (also called a Ghon focus), which can later progress to present as complicated lymph node disease with further intraparenchymal abnormalities on chest radiography. Enlargement of the intrathoracic lymph nodes can lead to partial or complete bronchial obstruction. Children present most commonly with chronic cough (>3 weeks) that has often not responded to standard antibiotic therapy for community-acquired bacterial pneumonia. In addition, prolonged fever or night sweats (>2 weeks) despite empiric antimalarial therapy in settings with high malaria prevalence and weight loss or failure to thrive are common symptoms of TB. During later stages of pulmonary TB, associated with worsening parenchymal involvement, children can also present with respiratory distress and tachypnea, as well as localized wheezing and hypoxia.

If early stages of TB disease are not recognized and treated, hematogenous spread may occur, leading to extrapulmonary TB and disseminated TB. Children can rapidly develop disseminated TB, with miliary TB with multi-organ involvement (>2 organ systems) and TB meningitis being the most clinically significant manifestations as both are associated with high mortality rates. Both miliary TB and TB meningitis are most common among infants, younger children, and children with HIV. Miliary TB presents with high unremitting fevers, generalized lymphadenopathy, and hepatosplenomegaly in approximately 50 % of affected children. TB meningitis presents in the early stage with irritability, fever, headaches, and decreased activity level. In the later stage, children present with vomiting, lethargy, neck stiffness, and abnormal focal neurological findings.

Among other manifestations of extra-pulmonary TB, TB of peripheral lymph nodes is the most common form, accounting for approximately 65 % of all pediatric extrapulmonary TB cases. TB lymphadenitis (also known as "scrofula") affects primarily the supraclavicular, submandibular, and cervical lymph nodes of the neck. It is more commonly unilateral, but it can be bilateral and present with or without fistulae. Pleural TB, most often presenting with a unilateral pleural effusion, is one of the other more common manifestations of extrapulmonary TB, accounting for approximately 6–7 % of all TB cases. Other forms of extrapulmonary TB include abdominal TB, where the ileum, jejunum, and appendix represent the most commonly affected sites, often with concomitant intra-abdominal lymphadenopathy, chronic diarrhea, and ascites on clinical examination. TB can also affect bones and joints, particularly weight-bearing sites, such as the lower thoracic and upper lumbar vertebrae of the spine (also called "Pott disease"), which presents with gibbus (an anterior angular deformity of the spine), back pain, or refusal to walk. Other common osteoarticular sites for TB include the hip, knees, ankles, and elbows. TB can also affect the pericardium, while TB involving the kidneys, skin, or eyes is relatively rare.

Untreated TB disease mortality can be as high as 30–50 % among children, but with adequate therapy, cure rates of higher than 95 % can be achieved. Notable exceptions include miliary TB and TB meningitis in which mortality estimates range widely from 17 to 69 %.

Differential Diagnosis

Due to the non-specificity of the common symptoms associated with TB, the differential diagnosis for TB is broad among children without HIV and even broader among children with HIV. For pulmonary TB, the differential includes primarily bacterial pneumonia, but also viral respiratory diseases during the earlier stages of TB, as well as fungal infections such as histoplasmosis, coccidioidomycosis, blastomycosis, or cryptococcosis. Among children with HIV, lymphocytic interstitial pneumonia or pneumonia due to *Pneumocystis jiroveci* should be considered. The differential diagnosis for extrapulmonary TB depends on the location of the disease, but it also very broad and requires a high index of suspicion, particularly if the child has been exposed to an adult with TB.

Diagnosis

The diagnosis of TB among children is difficult. Sputum-smear microscopy, the most readily available and applied diagnostic method for TB diagnosis among adults in resource-limited settings, has very low sensitivity in children due to the paucibacillary nature of TB among children and their inability to produce adequate sputum specimens. Among children younger than 5 years of age, early morning gastric aspirates are the most commonly used specimens for TB diagnosis, but these require hospitalization. Induced sputum specimens can be collected from children of all ages but require a fairly sophisticated clinical setting. Among children with clinical-compatible TB, at best, only 30–40 % will have positive TB cultures.

If TB is suspected, the diagnostic evaluation should include the following:

(a) Clinical examination including assessment of growth parameters.
(b) Thorough medical history, including careful assessment of any TB contact history (members of the household and frequent contacts of the child outside of the household).
(c) Chest radiography (if available).
(d) Tuberculin skin test (TST) (if available).
(e) Collection of specimens for laboratory diagnosis of TB. If facilities and resources are available, at least two gastric aspirates should be obtained from younger children and at least two induced sputum or sputum specimens from older children. If extrapulmonary TB is suspected, specimen collection from the suspected sites should be attempted (e.g., CSF for TB meningitis, lymph node aspirate for TB lymphadenitis, ascitic fluid for abdominal TB, pleural fluid for pleural TB).
(f) In countries with high HIV prevalence, HIV testing should also be considered for a child suspected of having TB.

Mycobacteriologic Modalities

All obtained specimens should be examined for presence of acid-fast bacilli (AFB) using light microscopy. Based on the low sensitivity of smear microscopy among children, specimens should ideally also be sent for detection of *Mtb* using culture methods. However, in many resource-limited settings, TB culture capacities are highly limited and often only available at district or national reference laboratories. Despite the limited availability and its low sensitivity for pediatric TB diagnosis, identification of *Mtb* using culture remains the preferred method for definite laboratory confirmation of TB. *Mtb* are slowly replicating bacteria and culture results can take up to 2–6 weeks. Therefore, if there is a strong clinical suspicion for TB, empiric TB treatment should be initiated while awaiting TB culture results. In 2010, the WHO endorsed an automated real-time PCR platform for TB diagnosis among both adults and children, the Xpert MTB/RIF. Though less sensitive than liquid culture, it provides results within less than 2 h, detects rifampin resistance, has excellent specificity, and is currently being widely implemented in many high-burden TB countries. Pediatric studies of the Xpert MTB/RIF have shown a sensitivity of 60–70 % using induced sputum, sputum, or nasopharyngeal aspirates compared to TB culture.

Imaging Modalities

Chest X-rays (CXRs) play an important role in the diagnosis of pulmonary TB. Both anterior-posterior (AP) and lateral views should be obtained. Lateral views are useful to evaluate the hilar and mediastinal thoracic areas for lymphadenopathy. CXR abnormalities vary based on the disease stage, but hilar or mediastinal lymph node enlargement with intraparenchymal lesions are suggestive of pulmonary TB. Hilar lymphadenopathy can lead to segmental or lobar atelectasis or hyperinflation due to airway compression. Cavitary disease is rare before the age of 10 years. CXRs are also important for diagnosis of miliary TB with presence of numerous bilateral lung nodules as well for the assessment for pleural or pericardial effusions. Ultrasound can be useful to detect ascites or intraabdominal lymphadenopathy, but these findings are also nonspecific.

Immunologic Diagnostic Modalities

The TST is the standard method for diagnosis of TB infection. It is based on the detection of a delayed-type hypersensitivity response to purified protein derivative (PPD), a combination of several antigens present in *Mycobacterium tuberculosis complex*, *Mycobacterium bovis Bacille Calmette-Guerin* (BCG), and several non-tuberculous mycobacteria (NTM). Following intradermal injection with PPD, the induration is measured 48–72 h later. A positive TST is defined as an induration of ≥ 10 mm. In children with HIV or severe malnutrition, an induration of ≥ 5 mm is considered positive. False-positive results can be due to prior BCG vaccination (especially among infants and younger children) and NTMs. False-negative results can be seen among children with HIV, severe malnutrition, or infants younger than 6 months, but also among children with active TB. The WHO recommends not taking prior BCG vaccination into account when interpreting TST results.

The interferon-gamma release assays (IGRAs) are whole-blood ELISA assays that detect interferon-gamma production by lymphocytes following in vitro stimulation with fairly Mtb-specific antigens. Two IGRAs are commercially available: the Quantiferon Assay and the T.Spot-TB. Their main advantage is higher specificity compared to the TST, but their sensitivity is not higher than the TST and may be lower in active disease. In addition, the IGRAs require a sophisticated laboratory setup, a blood draw, and are expensive. Therefore, the WHO released a policy in 2011 discouraging usage of IGRA in resource-limited settings.

Clinical Diagnosis

In the absence of laboratory confirmation of TB and, therefore, in the majority of settings with high-TB burden in resource-limited countries, the diagnosis of TB is usually made on clinical grounds. The WHO advises to strongly consider a diagnosis of TB if three or more of the four following parameters are fulfilled:

(a) Chronic symptoms suggestive of TB (chronic cough >3 weeks, fever >2 weeks, malnutrition, or failure to thrive).
(b) Physical signs highly suggestive of TB (e.g., signs of meningitis, gibbus, lymphadenitis).
(c) A positive TST or close contact to an infectious TB case.
(d) CXR findings suggestive of TB.

Multiple clinical scoring algorithms for pediatric TB diagnosis are used in high-burden countries, but they are poorly validated and none of them were developed in the era of the HIV epidemic.

Treatment

Treatment for TB disease is divided into an intensive phase of 2 months with more than two antibiotics, followed by a continuation phase of two antibiotics. Children with pulmonary TB or TB lymphadenitis who live in settings with low HIV prevalence and settings with low drug-resistance to isoniazid should be treated with

Table 19.1 Recommended doses of first-line anti-TB medications for children

Isoniazid (H)	10 mg/kg (range 10–15 mg/kg) PO once daily; maximum dose 300 mg/day PO once daily
Rifampicin (R)	15 mg/kg (range 10–20 mg/kg) PO once daily ; maximum dose 600 mg/day PO once daily
Pyrazinamide (Z)	35 mg/kg (30–40 mg/kg) PO once daily
Ethambutol (E)	20 mg/kg (15–25 mg/kg) PO once daily

Streptomycin should not be used as part of first-line treatment regimens for children with pulmonary tuberculosis or tuberculous peripheral lymphadenitis. (Source: WHO. Rapid Advice: Treatment of tuberculosis in children. Geneva. 2010)

isoniazid, rifampin, and pyrazinamide for 2 months, followed by isoniazid and rifampin for 4 months (Table 19.1). By contrast, children with pulmonary TB or TB lymphadenitis who live in settings with high HIV prevalence or settings with high levels of isoniazid resistance should receive ethambutol in addition to isoniazid, rifampin, and pyrazinamide for the first 2 months, followed by 4 months of isoniazid and rifampin. This regimen also applies for children with extensive pulmonary disease, regardless of HIV or drug-resistance country data.

Children with extrapulmonary TB, specifically TB meningitis, should receive a 12-month total treatment course (2 months of isoniazid, rifampin, pyrazinamide, and ethambutol, followed by 10 months of isoniazid and rifampin). Adjunctive steroid treatment has been shown to reduce mortality and morbidity among children with TB meningitis.

During TB treatment, children should be monitored for drug toxicities. The most common is hepatotoxicity due to isoniazid or rifampin. However, in general, the standard antibiotic therapy is well-tolerated. Adherence facilitation and caregiver training is required to avoid treatment failure and the development of resistance.

Among children with HIV who are diagnosed with TB, antiretroviral therapy (ART) should be initiated for all children regardless of CD4 count or WHO clinical stage. Ideally, ART should be started as soon as possible after TB treatment has been initiated (within 2–8 weeks). (In adults, concurrent ART and TB treatment is recommended. However, there are not clear data for optimal timing of ART and TB treatment for children with HIV-TB co-infection.) TB therapy guidelines follow the above outlined recommendations with the exception that children should be carefully evaluated at the end of the routine TB therapy treatment to assess whether the continuation phase may have to be prolonged.

Immune reconstitution inflammatory syndrome (IRIS) represents a clinical manifestation when the child's clinical status worsens after ART has been introduced. Paradoxical IRIS applies to children with TB who had previously responded well to TB therapy. It tends to occur within the first 3 months of ART initiation and is more common among children with advanced AIDS. Mild to moderate IRIS is relatively common (up to one-third of children in some studies) but usually self-resolves and does not require further interventions. Severe IRIS may require steroid treatment.

Children with latent TB infection (LTBI) (i.e., TB infection without disease) should receive 9 months of isoniazid.

Treatment of drug-resistant TB requires a longer treatment duration (up to 18–24 months) and second-line antibiotics including injectables, with often unfavorable toxicity profiles. The selection of a regimen for drug-resistant TB for children is fairly complex and input from local or international experts may be necessary.

Prevention

Vaccination with Bacille Calmette-Guérin (BCG) at birth, a live attenuated vaccine, is universally recommended by the WHO in moderate- to high-burden TB countries. BCG vaccination has shown to have moderate efficacy against disseminated TB and TB meningitis. Protection by the vaccine wanes over time, leading to inconsistent or low protection against adult-type TB. Among children with immunodeficiencies including HIV, BCG vaccination is contraindicated due to the risk of disseminated BCG disease. Moreover, it offers no documented protection against TB among HIV-infected children.

For post-exposure prophylaxis, the WHO recommends isoniazid preventive therapy (IPT)—consisting of isoniazid for 6 months—for children younger than 5 years of age and for all children with HIV who have had documented close contact to adults with TB and in whom active TB has been ruled out.

Even in the absence of a documented TB exposure history, HIV-infected children older than 12 months of age should be offered IPT if a symptom-based screening tool (fever, weight loss, cough, or a TB contact history in the past month) is negative for active TB. This is referred to as pre-exposure prophylaxis.

Recommended Reading

1. Newton SM, Brent AJ, Anderson S, Whittaker E, Kampmann B. Paediatric tuberculosis. Lancet Infect Dis. 2008;8:498–510.
2. Perez-Velez CM, Marais BJ. Tuberculosis in children. N Engl J Med. 2012;367(4):348–61.
3. World Health Organization. Guidance for national tuberculosis programmes on the management of tuberculosis in children. Geneva: World Health Organization; 2006.
4. World Health Organization. Guidelines for intensified tuberculosis case-finding and isoniazid preventive therapy for people living with HIV in resource-constrained settings. Geneva: World Health Organization; 2010.
5. World Health Organization. Rapid advice: treatment of tuberculosis in children. Geneva: World Health Organization; 2010.

Chapter 20
Parasitic Diseases

Amanda P. Garcia and LeAnne M. Fox

Keywords Neglected tropical diseases • Lymphatic filariasis • Elephantiasis • Onchocerciasis • River blindness • Schistosomiasis • Bilharzia • American trypanosomiasis • Chagas disease • Visceral leishmaniasis • *Kala-azar* • Acute dermatolymphangioadenitis • Immunochromatographic card test • Diethylcarbamazine • Ivermectin • Praziquantel • Benznidazole

Overview

- Neglected tropical diseases (NTDs) are a group of infectious diseases that cause substantial illness for more than a billion people globally.
- Lymphatic filariasis affects 120 million people in 72 countries and causes lymphedema and hydrocele.
- Onchocerciasis affects 37 million people worldwide—of these, 270,000 have become blind due to the disease.
- Schistosomiasis affects more than 200 million people worldwide and causes gastrointestinal, liver, and urinary pathology.
- It is estimated that 8–11 million people in Mexico, Central America, and South America have Chagas disease, most of whom are asymptomatic, but some of whom have severe cardiac or gastrointestinal manifestations.
- Visceral leishmaniasis causes a severe, systemic disease that is usually fatal without treatment—90 % of cases occur in India, Bangladesh, Nepal, Sudan, Ethiopia, and Brazil.

A.P. Garcia, M.P.H. (✉) • L.M. Fox, M.D., M.P.H., D.T.M.&H.
Division of Parasitic Diseases and Malaria, Center for Global Health,
Centers for Disease Control and Prevention, Atlanta, GA, USA
e-mail: aburke@cdc.gov

Global Burden of Parasitic Diseases

The burden of parasitic diseases is great in developing countries. Many parasitic diseases of importance are often neglected from a global community viewpoint. This chapter highlights five neglected parasitic diseases of global significance: lymphatic filariasis, onchocerciasis, schistosomiasis, American trypanosomiasis (Chagas disease), and visceral leishmaniasis. These parasitic diseases are among the NTDs, a group of infectious diseases that have been eradicated in more developed parts of the world and persist only in the poorest, most marginalized communities and conflict areas (Fig. 20.1). NTDs cause substantial illness for more than 1 billion people globally and are a source of tremendous suffering because of their disfiguring, debilitating, and sometimes deadly impact. It is estimated that every year, NTDs kill 534,000 people worldwide. NTDs affect the world's poorest people, impairing physical and cognitive development and ultimately trapping the poor in a cycle of poverty and disease.

Lymphatic Filariasis

Lymphatic filariasis (LF) is caused by the filarial nematodes, *Wuchereria bancrofti*, *Brugia malayi*, and *Brugia timori*. The nematodes are transmitted by the bite of infected *Aedes, Culex, Anopheles,* and *Mansonia* mosquito species. The adult filarial worms live in the human lymph system. 120 million people are infected

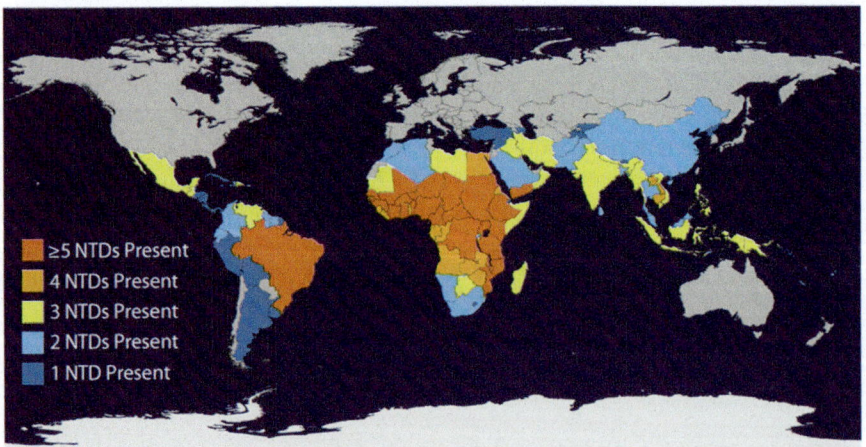

Fig. 20.1 Global overlap of six of the common NTDs. Specifically guinea worm disease, lymphatic filariasis, onchocerciasis, schistosomiasis, soil-transmitted helminths, and trachoma (Credit: CDC)

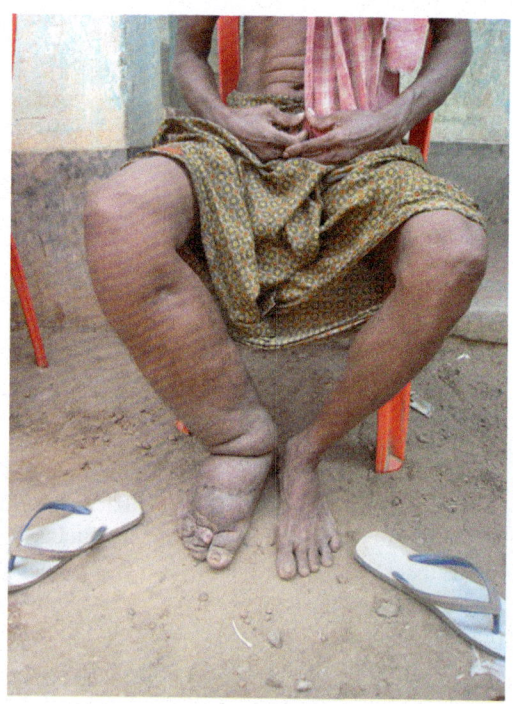

Fig. 20.2 Young adult in India with unilateral lymphedema. (Photo Credit: Mr. Jonathan Rout, Church's Auxiliary for Social Action, India)

throughout the subtropics of Asia, Africa, the Western Pacific, and parts of the Caribbean and South America. Forty million persons have clinical disease that manifests as lymphedema (Fig. 20.2) and/or elephantiasis or hydrocele in men.

Clinical Presentation

Most filarial infections are asymptomatic, but living worms can cause progressive lymphatic vessel dilation and dysfunction, leading to lymphedema of the leg, scrotum, penis, arm, or breast, as well as hydrocele in men. Filarial lymphadenopathy is commonly seen in infected children. Prior to a child reaching puberty, adult filarial worms can be detected by ultrasonography of the inguinal, crural, and axillary lymph nodes and vessels. Death of the adult worm triggers an acute inflammatory response, which progresses distally (retrograde) along the affected lymphatic vessel, usually in the limbs, and is termed acute filarial lymphangitis (AFL). If present, systemic symptoms, such as headache or fever, are generally mild. Death of the adult worm can cause inflammation and may present as funiculitis, epididymitis, or orchitis, particularly in adolescent or adult men. A tender granulomatous nodule may be palpable at the site of the dead worm. Infected persons may exhibit acute

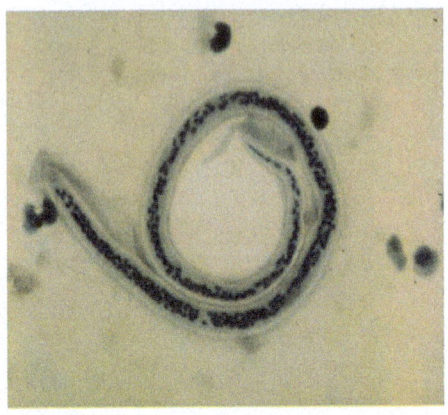

Fig. 20.3 Microfilaria of *Wuchereria bancrofti* on a thick blood film stained with hematoxylin. (Credit: Mark L. Eberhard, Ph.D., Division of Parasitic Diseases and Malaria, Centers for Disease Control and Prevention, Atlanta, GA)

manifestations, particularly acute dermatolymphangioadenitis (ADLA), a clinically distinct syndrome that is caused by bacterial infection of the small collecting lymphatic vessels in areas of lymphatic dysfunction. This syndrome develops in a reticular rather than a linear pattern and is associated with severe pain, fever, and chills. There is often a history of injury to the skin, such as trauma, insect bites, or interdigital fungal infections. ADLA is often diagnosed as cellulitis, and symptoms can last 3–15 days.

Differential Diagnosis

The differential diagnosis varies based on the clinical presentation. Bacterial infection, thrombophlebitis, or trauma can be mistaken for acute filarial adenolymphangitis. Tuberculosis, leprosy, sarcoidosis, and other systemic granulomatous diseases may be confused with filarial disease. Chronic lymphedema can be caused by malignancy, postoperative changes, congenital malformations, or a hereditary form of lymphostasis (Milroy's disease), as well as renal or cardiac failure. A foreign body reaction to silica dust introduced into traumatized legs, termed podoconiosis, accounts for some of the burden of elephantiasis in some parts of the world.

Diagnosis

The standard method for diagnosing an active lymphatic filarial infection is the identification of microfilariae in a thick blood smear by microscopic examination (Fig. 20.3). A rapid-format immunochromatographic card test (ICT) is available for identifying circulating filarial antigen in most LF-endemic countries and has a high sensitivity and specificity. Determination of serum antifilarial IgG is also a diagnostically useful test.

Treatment

The antiparasitic treatment of choice for LF is diethylcarbamazine (DEC). Physicians can either give DEC in a 1-day or 12-day treatment (6 mg/kg/day); 1-day treatment is generally as effective as the 12-day regimen (Table 20.1). DEC is typically well-tolerated. Side effects are, in general, limited and depend on the number of microfilariae in the blood, but include dizziness, nausea, fever, headache, or pain in muscles or joints. For the chronic manifestations of lymphedema, treatment recommendations include proper hygiene, skin care, physiotherapy, and in some cases antibiotics. For hydrocele, surgical repair is curative.

Prevention

No vaccine is available for lymphatic filariasis. Yearly administration of (DEC) or ivermectin to populations at risk will treat infection and can assist with elimination of lymphatic filariasis in disease-endemic countries. Protective measures include avoidance of mosquito bites through mosquito nets and repellants and wearing long sleeves and trousers between dusk and dawn.

Onchocerciasis

Onchocerciasis, also known as River Blindness, is caused by the filarial nematode, *Onchocerca volvulus*. It is transmitted by the bite of female *Simulium* blackflies, which bite during the day and are found near flowing rivers and streams in tropical climates. The greatest burden of onchocerciasis is in sub-Saharan Africa, though the parasite is found in limited areas in the Americas and in Yemen in the Middle East. The World Health Organization (WHO) estimates that 37 million people are infected with *O. volvulus* worldwide; of these people, 270,000 are blind and 500,000 have some sort of visual impairment. Some 90 million people are at risk for becoming infected with the parasite, and in hyperendemic areas, up to 90 % of children younger than 15 years have microfilariae detected in the skin.

Clinical Presentation

The *O. volvulus* adult worms develop 6–12 months after initial infection and can involve the skin, subcutaneous tissues, and lymphatic system. In patients in Africa, the disease presents as nodules found on the lower torso, pelvis, and lower

Table 20.1 Drug treatment table

Disease	Drug	Adult dosage	Pediatric dosage
Lymphatic filariasis	Diethylcarbamazine citrate (DEC)	1 day or 12 day course 6 mg/kg per day	1 day or 12 day course 6 mg/kg per day
Onchocerciasis microfilariae	Ivermectin	150 mcg/kg orally in one dose every 6 months	150 mcg/kg orally in one dose every 6 months[a]
Schistosomiasis			
S. mansoni	Praziquantel	40 mg/kg per day orally in two divided doses for 1 day	40 mg/kg per day orally in two divided doses for 1 day[b]
S. haematobium	Praziquantel	40 mg/kg per day orally in two divided doses for 1 day	40 mg/kg per day orally in two divided doses for 1 day[b]
S. japonicum	Praziquantel	60 mg/kg per day orally in three divided doses for 1 day	60 mg/kg per day orally in three divided doses for 1 day[b]
American trypanosomiasis (Chagas disease)	Benznidazole	≥12 years: 5–7 mg/kg per day orally in two divided doses for 60 days	10 mg/kg per day orally in two divided doses for 60 days
	Nifurtimox	≥17 years: 8–10 mg/kg per day orally in 3 or 4 divided doses for 90 days	≤10 years: 15–20 mg/kg per day orally in 3 or 4 divided doses for 90 days 11–16 years: 12.5–15 mg/kg/day orally in 3 or 4 divided doses for 90 days
Visceral leishmaniasis	Liposomal amphotericin B[c]	3 mg/kg IV daily on days 1–5, 14 and 21 (total dose 21 mg/kg)	3 mg/kg IV daily on days 1–5, 14 and 21 (total dose 21 mg/kg)
	Conventional amphotericin B deoxycholate[d]	0.75–1.0 mg/kg per day for 15–20 days	0.75–1.0 mg/kg per day for 15–20 days
		0.75–1.0 mg/kg every other day for 30–40 days	0.75–1.0 mg/kg every other day for 30–40 days

[a]The safety of ivermectin in children who weigh less than 15 kg has not been demonstrated. Doxycycline is contraindicated in children less than 9 years old and has not been studied in the treatment of onchocerciasis in children less than 12 years old

[b]There is a lack of safety trial data for the use of praziquantel in children less than 4 years of age or pregnant women. However, this drug has been distributed widely in mass drug administration programs and WHO now recommends that pregnant women should be treated as part of those campaigns based on extensive experience with the drug and review of the veterinary and human evidence

[c]Drug with highest therapeutic efficacy and most favorable safety profile for visceral leishmaniasis

[d]Has a high antileishmanial efficacy but is associated with high risk of renal toxicity and other side effects. Alternate day dosing and pretreatment saline loading may decrease risk of renal toxicity and other adverse effects

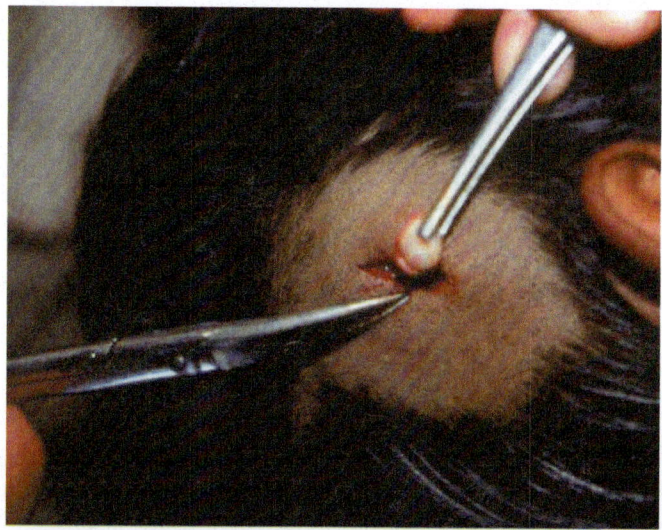

Fig. 20.4 Onchocercal nodule being removed from the head of a Guatemalan child (Credit: Frank O. Richards M.D., The Carter Center, Atlanta, GA)

extremities. In patients in Central and South America, the disease often presents as nodules found on the upper body, but they may also occur in extremities. Clinical manifestations also include highly pruritic, papular dermatitis, lymphadenitis, and ocular lesions, which can lead to visual loss and blindness. Spotted depigmentation of the skin can also occur, termed "leopard skin." Children who have not been residents in endemic areas for long periods have a very low chance of infection. Infected children generally present with acute manifestations such as acute papular dermatitis or punctate keratitis or may present with a palpable subcutaneous nodule (Fig. 20.4).

Differential Diagnosis

Early onchodermatitis must be distinguished from atopic dermatitis, food allergies, contact dermatitis, insect bites, and scabies. The chronic skin lesions may be mistaken for severe chronic eczema or malnutrition. "Leopard skin" must be distinguished from other causes of hypopigmentation including vitiligo and leprosy.

Diagnosis

Diagnosis of onchocerciasis is made through finding microfilariae in skin shavings or punch biopsy, finding adult worms in histologic lesions of excised nodules, or by characteristic eye lesions. Serologic testing is also available.

Treatment

Ivermectin is the treatment of choice for onchocerciasis, typically given at 150 mcg/kg orally in one dose every 6 months, the same dosage for children as adults. Repeated annual or semiannual doses may be required because the drug kills the microfilariae but not the adult worms, which can live for many years and continue to produce microfilariae.

Prevention

No vaccine is available for onchocerciasis. Yearly administration of ivermectin to populations at risk will treat infection and can assist with control/elimination of onchocerciasis in disease-endemic countries. Protective measures include avoiding blackfly habitats and the use of personal protection measures against biting insects.

Schistosomiasis

Schistosomiasis, also known as bilharzia, is primarily caused by helminth infection with *Schistosoma mansoni*, *Schistosoma haematobium*, or *Schistosoma japonicum*. More than 200 million people are infected worldwide. Water transmission occurs via penetration of larval cercariae through human skin in contaminated bodies of freshwater.

Clinical Presentation

The incubation period for schistosomiasis is usually 14–84 days. Many people are asymptomatic and have subclinical disease during both the acute and chronic stages of infection. During an acute infection, patients may present with rash, fever, headache, myalgia, and respiratory symptoms. Often, eosinophilia is present with hepatomegaly and/or splenomegaly. Clinical manifestations of chronic disease result from host immune responses to schistosome eggs. *S. mansoni* and *S. japonicum* eggs most commonly lodge in the blood vessels of the liver or intestine and can cause diarrhea, constipation, and blood in the stool. Chronic inflammation can lead to bowel wall ulceration, hyperplasia, and polyposis and, with heavy infections, to liver fibrosis and periportal hypertension. *S. haematobium* eggs tend to lodge in the urinary tract, causing bladder damage, dysuria, and hematuria. Chronic infections may increase the risk of bladder cancer.

Fig. 20.5 *S. mansoni* egg in unstained wet mounts showing the characteristic lateral spine. Image courtesy of the CDC-DPDx and the Wisconsin State Laboratory of Hygiene

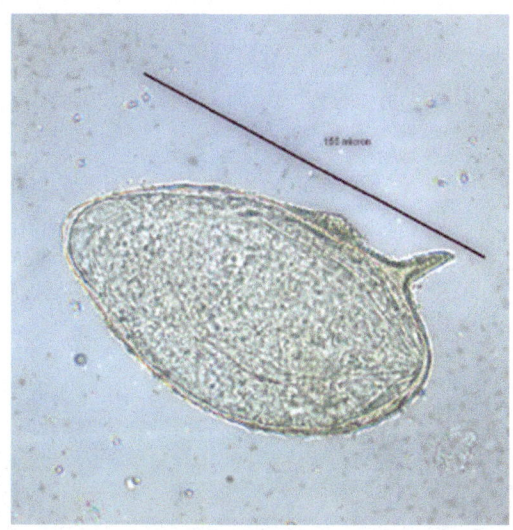

Differential Diagnosis

Fever and rash with eosinophilia can be due to other helminth infections or drug reactions. Hepatic and intestinal symptoms may be confused with inflammatory bowel disease, cirrhosis from other causes, visceral leishmaniasis, tropical splenomegaly, appendicitis, pancreatitis, and *Salmonella* infection. Renal symptoms, including hematuria, may indicate other disorders including urinary tract infection, renal tuberculosis, acute nephritis, or urogenital cancer.

Diagnosis

Diagnosis of schistosomiasis is made by microscopic identification of parasite eggs in stool (*S. mansoni* or *S. japonicum*, Figs. 20.5 and 20.6) or urine (*S. haematobium*, Fig. 20.7). Serologic tests are useful to diagnose mild infections where egg shedding may not be consistent. It is also important to screen asymptomatic people who may have been exposed during travel.

Treatment

Praziquantel is most effective against the adult forms of the *Schistosoma* parasites. For *S. mansoni* and *S. haematobium*, praziquantel at 40 mg/kg per day orally in two divided doses for 1 day is recommended. For *S. japonicum*, praziquantel at 60 mg/kg per day orally in three divided doses for 1 day is recommended.

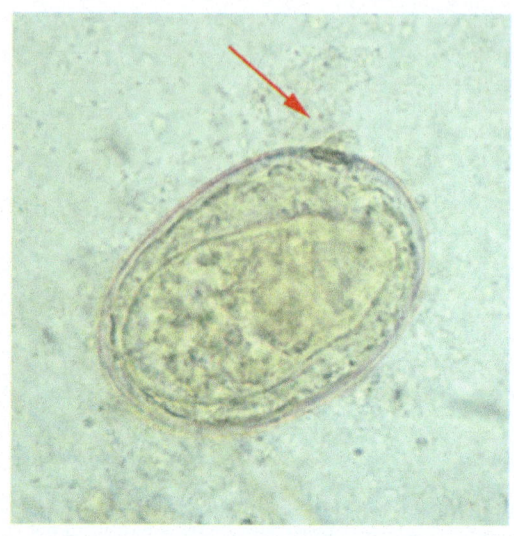

Fig. 20.6 *S. japonicum* egg in unstained wet mount. Note the small, inconspicuous spines (*arrow*). Image courtesy of the CDC-DPDx and the Wisconsin State Laboratory of Hygiene

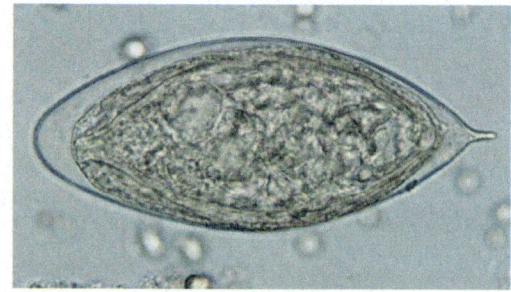

Fig. 20.7 *S. haematobium egg* in wet mount of urine concentrate, showing the characteristic terminal spine. Image courtesy of the CDC-DPDx and the Wisconsin State Laboratory of Hygiene

Prevention

No vaccine is available for schistosomiasis. Yearly administration of praziquantel to populations at risk will treat infection and can assist with control or elimination of schistosomiasis in disease-endemic countries. Preventive measures include avoiding wading, swimming, or other contact with freshwater. Filtering water with fine-mesh filters, heating bathing water to 50 °C for 5 min, or allowing water to stand for over 24 h before exposure can eliminate risk of infection.

American Trypanosomiasis (Chagas Disease)

Chagas disease, also known as American trypanosomiasis, is caused by the protozoan, *Trypanosoma cruzi*. Infection occurs through vector-borne transmission in endemic countries via feces of triatomine insects, where the feces are inadvertently inoculated into the skin or the mucosa of the eye, nose, or mouth when the insect's bite is scratched and rubbed. An estimated 8–11 million people in Mexico, Central America, and South America have Chagas disease.

Clinical Presentation

Acute Chagas disease occurs immediately after infection and may last up to a few weeks or months, and parasites may be found in the circulating blood. Infection may be mild or asymptomatic. There may be fever or swelling around the site of inoculation where the parasite entered into the skin or mucous membrane. When this occurs around the eye, it is called "Romaña's sign." Rarely, acute infection may result in myocarditis, encephalitis, or meningitis. Following the acute phase, most infected people enter into a prolonged asymptomatic form of disease (called "chronic indeterminate") during which few or no parasites are found in the blood. During this time, most people are unaware of their infection. Many people may remain asymptomatic for life and never develop Chagas-related symptoms. However, an estimated 20–30 % of infected people will develop debilitating and sometimes life-threatening medical problems over the course of their lives. Some complications of chronic Chagas disease include conduction abnormalities such as right bundle branch block and/or left anterior fascicular block, which may be followed years later by dilated cardiomyopathy. Later cardiac disease is sometimes accompanied by apical aneurysm and thrombus formation. Less frequently, patients with Chagas disease experience gastrointestinal disease (megasyndromes). Once the characteristic pathology is established (e.g., dilated cardiomyopathy, megaesophagus), antiparasitic treatment will not reverse it.

Differential Diagnosis

The differential diagnoses for acute Chagas disease include typhoid fever, visceral leishmaniasis, schistosomiasis, malaria, brucellosis, infectious mononucleosis, and toxoplasmosis among others. Romaña's sign must be differentiated from a local allergic reaction with edema, such as an insect bite, which resolves more rapidly, or severe conjunctivitis or trauma. Cardiomyopathy due to Chagas disease must be differentiated from myocarditis or pericarditis due to other causes such as rheumatic fever or viral myocarditis.

Diagnosis

Parasitologic methods, including identification of trypomastigotes in blood by microscopy, are most effective during acute infections. Circulating parasite levels decrease rapidly within a few months and are undetectable by most methods during the chronic phase. Diagnosis of chronic infection is made by serologic tests for antibody to the parasite. A single test is not sufficiently sensitive or specific to make the diagnosis. For this reason, the standard approach is to apply two or more tests that use different techniques and/or that detect antibodies to different antigens. Two commonly used techniques are enzyme-linked immunosorbent assay (ELISA) and immunofluorescent antibody test (IFA). To increase accuracy of diagnosis, careful consideration of the patient's history to identify possible risks for infection can be helpful.

Treatment

Antiparasitic treatment is indicated for all cases of acute or reactivated Chagas disease and for chronic *T. cruzi* infection in children up through age 18. Congenital infections are considered acute disease. Treatment is strongly recommended for adults up to 50 years old with chronic infection who do not already have advanced Chagas cardiomyopathy. Physicians should consider factors such as the patient's age, clinical status, preference for treatment, and overall health. The two drugs used to treat infection with *T. cruzi* are nifurtimox and benznidazole. For benznidazole, the treatment recommendation for children under 12 years is 10 mg/kg per day orally in two divided doses for 60 days and for children 12 years or older, 5–7 mg/kg per day orally in two divided doses for 60 days. For nifurtimox, the treatment recommendation for children less than 10 years is 15–20 mg/kg per day orally in three or four divided doses for 90 days and for children 11–16 years, 12.5–15 mg/kg per day orally in three or four divided doses for 90 days.

Prevention

In endemic areas, improved housing and spraying insecticide inside housing to eliminate triatomine bugs has significantly decreased the spread of Chagas disease. Further, screening for Chagas disease in blood donations is another important public health tool in helping to prevent transfusion-acquired disease. Early detection and treatment of new cases, including mother-to-child (congenital) cases, also helps to reduce the burden of disease.

Visceral Leishmaniasis

Visceral leishmaniasis (VL), also known as *kala-azar*, is caused by obligate intracellular protozoans, particularly of the species *Leishmania donovani* and *Leishmania infantum*. 90 % of VL cases occur in India, Bangladesh, Nepal, Sudan, Ethiopia, and Brazil. VL can also be found in southern Europe. VL is predominantly transmitted through the bite of infected female phlebotomine sandflies. Congenital and blood-borne transmission of VL has also been reported. Cutaneous leishmaniasis is another form of the disease that is caused by the same protozoan and is also transmitted by the bite of the sandfly.

Clinical Presentation

The time from an infective sandfly bite to the onset of VL is typically 2–6 months, but onset can range from 2 weeks to more than 2 years. The onset is usually insidious, with worsening symptoms over a period of weeks to months. The typical patient presents with fever lasting at least 2 weeks, malaise, and weight loss, and may complain of abdominal fullness related to organomegaly. Common clinical features include fever, wasting, splenomegaly, hepatomegaly, hypergammaglobulinemia, and pancytopenia. Hepatomegaly is usually less prominent than splenomegaly.

Differential Diagnosis

The differential diagnosis of VL is broad and can include hepatosplenic schistosomiasis, myeloproliferative diseases, and tropical splenomegaly due to chronic malaria. Other possibilities include miliary tuberculosis, histoplasmosis, brucellosis, subacute bacterial endocarditis, infectious mononucleosis, *Salmonella* bacteremia, lymphoma, or leukemia.

Diagnosis

Definitive diagnosis of VL requires the demonstration of the parasite by smear or culture in tissue, usually bone marrow or spleen, and thus entails an invasive procedure (Fig. 20.8).

Treatment

The main constraints on the choice of antileishmanial drug are cost and availability. Drug resistance must also be considered, especially for VL originating in the Indian

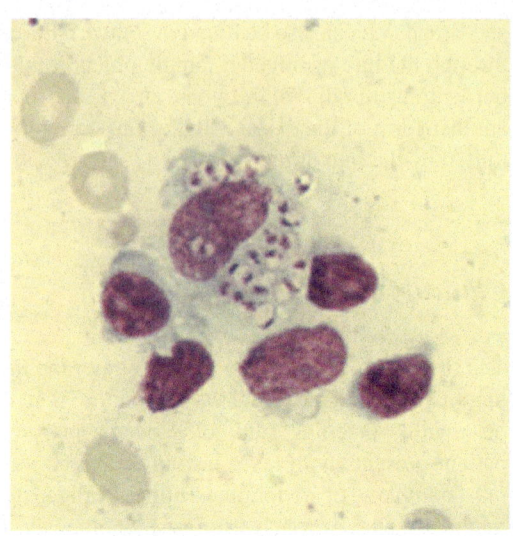

Fig. 20.8 *Leishmania* spp. amastigotes in a Giemsa-stained tissue scraping. Image courtesy of CDC-DPDx

subcontinent. The drugs of choice are liposomal amphotericin B and conventional amphotericin B deoxycholate. Liposomal amphotericin B is the drug with the highest therapeutic efficacy and the most favorable safety profile. The FDA-approved regimen consists of 3 mg/kg IV daily on days 1–5, 14, and 21 (total dose 21 mg/kg); other shorter regimens with similar total dose also have high efficacy. Conventional amphotericin B deoxycholate has high antileishmanial efficacy but is associated with high risk of renal toxicity and other side effects. Effective regimens include 0.75–1.0 mg/kg IV daily for 15–20 days or 0.75–1.0 mg/kg IV every other day for 30–40 days. Alternate day dosing and pretreatment saline loading may decrease risk of renal toxicity and other adverse effects.

Prevention

No vaccine or drugs to prevent *Leishmania* infection are available. Prevention is based on two major modalities: measures to decrease human exposure to sandfly bites and interventions to decrease the infection reservoir. Preventive measures also include wearing protective clothing, applying insect repellent to exposed skin, using bed nets treated with a pyrethroid-containing insecticide, and spraying dwellings with residual-action insecticides.

Recommended Reading

1. Centers for Disease Control and Prevention. Parasites. http://www.cdc.gov/parasites/. Accessed 26 Jul 2012.
2. CDC Health Information for International Travel: the Yellow Book 2012. New York: Oxford University Press; 2012.
3. Fox LM, King C. Filarial infections. In: Magill A, Hill D, Ryan E, Solomon T, editors. Hunter's tropical medicine and emerging infectious diseases. 9th ed. London: Saunders; 2012.
4. Onchocerciasis. In: Pickering LK, Baker CJ, Kimberlin DW, Long SS, editors. The American Academy of Pediatrics. Red Book: 2012 Report of the Committee on Infectious Diseases. Elk Grove Village, IL: American Academy of Pediatrics; 2012. p. 522.
5. Control of the Leishmaniases, Report of a meeting of the WHO Expert Committee on the Control of Leishmaniases, Geneva, 22–26 Mar 2010, WHO Technical Report Series, no 949; 2010.

Chapter 21
Vaccine-Preventable Diseases

Michele S. Duke and Vandana L. Madhavan

Keywords Vaccine-preventable diseases/illnesses • Immunization/vaccine schedule • Immunization/vaccine contraindications • Immunization/vaccine administration • Global burden of disease/illness • Anthrax • Cholera • Diphtheria • Hepatitis A (HAV) • Hepatitis B (HBV) • Haemophilus influenzae B (Hib) • Japanese encephalitis (JE) • Meningococcal/meningitis/Neisseria meningitides • Mumps • Bordatella pertussis • Pneumococcal/Streptococcus pneumoniae • Polio • Rabies • Rubella • Tetanus/Clostridium tetani • Typhoid/enteric fever/Salmonella typhi/Salmonella paratyphi • Varicella/Chickenpox • Yellow fever

Overview

- A substantial proportion of deaths in children worldwide are from vaccine-preventable illnesses, with the largest disease burden occurring in select countries in Africa and Asia.
- Millions of deaths are averted each year as a result of immunization.
- We review the specific vaccine-preventable diseases, summarizing the microbiology, epidemiology, and clinical presentations as well as treatment, infection control, and post-exposure recommendations.
- Additionally, we review the World Health Organization immunization recommendations, contraindications, precautions, and the data regarding coverage rates.

M.S. Duke, M.D. (✉)
Division of Global Health, MassGeneral Hospital for Children,
100 Cambridge Street, 15th Floor, Boston, MA 02114, USA
e-mail: msduke@partners.org

V.L. Madhavan, M.D., M.P.H.
Pediatric Infectious Disease, MassGeneral Hospital for Children, Boston, MA, USA

Global Burden of Vaccine-Preventable Diseases

- In 2011, the estimated number of all deaths in children under 5 was 6.9 million, with nearly 4.4 million of these deaths from preventable infectious diseases. In 2008, the WHO estimated that 1.5 million deaths in children under 5 were from the following vaccine-preventable diseases: pneumococcal disease (476,000), rotavirus (453,000), Hib (199,000), pertussis (195,000), measles (118,000), and tetanus (61,000).
- Annually, 2–3 million deaths are averted due to immunization against diphtheria, tetanus, pertussis, and measles.
- In 2010, there was greater than 90 % immunization coverage for DTP3 in 130 countries, the majority of which occurred in the Americas, Europe, and Western Pacific.
- Overall vaccine coverage trends are positive, with increased uptake of both DTP3 and new/underused vaccines (e.g., Hep B, Hib, PCV, and rotavirus).
- Nearly 70 % of children without DTP3 live in ten countries: Afghanistan, Democratic Republic of Congo, Ethiopia, India, Indonesia, Iraq, Nigeria, Pakistan, South Africa, and Uganda.

List of Specific Diseases

Due to varying prevalence rates worldwide, diseases are listed alphabetically. As these diseases may be reportable to local and global authorities, check local and regional reporting requirements following diagnosis.

Anthrax

- Intro—Caused by *Bacillus anthracis*, a spore-forming Gram-positive bacilli. Anthrax is a zoonotic infection that results from exposure to infected livestock/animal products; anthrax can infect skin, lungs, GI tract, and meninges. The vaccine is typically only for military personnel in some countries, and is not WHO-recommended.
- Clinical presentation (1) Cutaneous: pruritic papule/vesicle → ulceration → black painless eschar. (2) GI: oropharyngeal (ulcers/unilateral neck swelling) or intestinal (hematemesis, bloody diarrhea, ascites). (3) Inhalational: nonspecific prodrome → fulminant phase with hypoxia and shock 2–5 days later; a widened mediastinum is often seen on CXR. All three presentations can cause CNS disease with hematogenous seeding of meninges.

- Differential diagnosis—Cutaneous: spider bite, leishmaniasis, diphtheria. GI: bacterial gastroenteritis (if bloody diarrhea present), tularemia (if oropharyngeal lesions), scrofula (neck swelling). Inhalational: TB (similar prodrome but shorter), pulmonary plague (*Yersinia pestis*).
- Diagnostic studies—Gram stain and culture of affected area(s), CXR.
- Management—Cutaneous: penicillin or tetracyclines PO 7–10 days. Systemic disease: ciprofloxacin or doxycycline IV ≥60 days.
- Post-exposure prophylaxis—Ciprofloxacin or doxycycline PO.

Cholera (also see Chap. 15 for more information).

- Intro—Caused by *Vibrio cholerae*, a Gram-negative bacilli. Infection results from ingestion of contaminated water (epidemic) or food. Cholera is now endemic in many countries, especially in Africa, Asia, and recently Haiti. Two oral vaccines (one killed whole-cell, one live attenuated) are available outside the U.S. Oral vaccine is WHO-recommended only for children in high-risk populations.
- Clinical presentation—Most patients are asymptomatic or have mild disease. Fewer than 5 % develop cholera gravis: no fever, frequent, voluminous, painless, watery stools with flecks of mucus ("rice water stools"), which can progress to hypovolemic shock within hours.
- Differential diagnosis—If symptoms are mild, consider typical causes of gastroenteritis (viral, bacterial, parasitic).
- Diagnosis—Clinical. Gram stain and culture of stool/vomitus (culture requires thiosulfate citrate bile salts sucrose agar, which needs to be specially requested).
- Management—ORT is preferred for mild-to-moderate dehydration (see Chap. 15 for recipes) or IV rehydration for severe dehydration. Doxycycline or tetracycline is indicated in severe cases. Prevent additional cases by treating the water supplies.
- Post-exposure prophylaxis—Not routinely recommended (secondary transmission is rare).

Diphtheria

- Intro—Caused by *Corynebacterium diphtheriae*, a Gram-positive pleomorphic bacillus. Diphtheria remains endemic in Africa, Asia, Latin America, Middle East, as well as former Soviet republics. Disease is spread by droplets or contact with active skin lesions. Routine WHO-recommended vaccine.
- Clinical presentation (1) Respiratory: low-grade fever, mild prodrome over 1–2 days → membranous nasopharyngitis or obstructive laryngotracheitis with classic gray membrane. (2) Cutaneous: chronic ulcer with dirty gray membrane. Can also have vaginal, conjunctival, or otic disease. Complications include severe neck swelling (bull neck), airway obstruction, myocarditis, peripheral neuropathy.

- Differential diagnosis—Cutaneous: anthrax, leishmaniasis, spider bite. Respiratory: anthrax, tularemia, viral diseases (oral ulcers), Lemierre's syndrome (bull neck).
- Diagnosis—Culture of affected area(s) (needs cystine-tellurite blood agar or modified Tinsdale agar); isolates should be tested for toxin production.
- Management—Equine antitoxin IV (when diphtheria suspected) plus erythromycin or penicillin (PO or IV). Perform a scratch test for sensitivity to toxin, as 5–20 % of people will have allergic reactions.
- Post-exposure prophylaxis—Indicated for all close contacts: penicillin IM or erythromycin PO, throat culture, close surveillance for 7 days PLUS vaccine, if unimmunized.

Hepatitis A

- Intro—Caused by a Picornavirus (RNA), which can be found worldwide. Infection is spread via fecal-oral transmission; the average incubation period is 28 days, and the highest risk of transmission occurs 1–2 weeks prior to the onset of jaundice. It is a self-limited illness (<2–6 months) without chronic state. Vaccine is WHO-recommended for high-risk populations, including residents of and travelers to endemic countries.
- Clinical presentation—Acute illness with fever, nausea/anorexia → jaundice (in 30 % of children <6 years old; in 70 % of older children and adults).
- Differential diagnosis—Broad: consider all causes of acute jaundice (including malaria, fulminant HBV/HCV).
- Diagnosis—Clinical and serology (IgM and IgG).
- Management—Supportive care, no evidence for antiviral therapy.
- Post-exposure prophylaxis—Vaccine (preferred). Immune globulin IM (when administered within 2 weeks of exposure).

Hepatitis B

- Intro—Caused by a DNA virus, which can be found worldwide (highest rates are found in Africa, Southeast Asia, and Pacific Islands). Transmission may be vertical or through bodily fluids (blood, semen, saliva, etc.); incubation period is 45–160 days. Infection can be an acute self-limited illness or result in chronic infection (up to 90 % of children, 5–10 % of adults). Routine WHO-recommended vaccine, including all neonates, even in low-endemicity countries, and all high-risk adolescents and adults. Standard precautions.
- Clinical presentation—Variable: asymptomatic, nonspecific symptoms (malaise, nausea, anorexia), jaundice, or fulminant hepatitis; may also produce arthralgias, arthritis, thrombocytopenia, or rashes (e.g., Gianotti-Crosti). If infection is not

Table 21.1 Serologic markers of Hepatitis B infection

HBsAg (Hepatitis B surface antigen)	Positive in acute and chronic HBV (false negative may occur in "window" phase)
Anti-HBs (antibody to HBsAg)	Positive in resolved HBV and immunization
HBeAg (Hepatitis B e antigen)	Positive in HBV cases with increased infectivity
Anti-HBe (antibody to HBeAg)	Positive in HBV cases with decreased infectivity
IgG anti-HBc (IgG antibody to HBcAg)	Positive in acute, resolved, and chronic HBV (not present after immunization)
IgM anti-HBc (IgM antibody to HBcAg)	Positive in acute and recent HBV (including HBsAg-negative "window" phase)

Adapted from: American Academy of Pediatrics. *2012 Red Book*; Mandell GL, Bennett JE, Dolin R. *Principles and Practice of Infectious Diseases*. 6th ed. Philadelphia: Elsevier Churchill Livingstone; 2005

Table 21.2 Interpretation of serologic markers of Heptatits B infection

	HBsAg	Anti-HBs	HBeAg	Anti-HBe	IgG anti-HBc	IgM anti-HBc
Immunized	−	+	−	−	−	−
Acute	+	−	+	−	+	+
Resolved	−	+	−	+/−	+	−
Chronic	+	−	+/−	+/−	+	−

Adapted from: Mandell GL, Bennett JE, Dolin R. *Principles and Practice of Infectious Diseases*. 6th ed. Philadelphia: Elsevier Churchill Livingstone; 2005

cleared, it will progress to chronic infection (can be asymptomatic, with an increased risk of cirrhosis or hepatocellular carcinoma).
- Differential diagnosis—Broad: consider all causes of acute jaundice (including malaria, HAV, fulminant HCV, etc.) as well as chronic liver disease.
- Diagnosis—Clinical and serology, see Tables 21.1 and 21.2.
- Management—Acute infection is managed supportively. Chronic infection: Regular monitoring is recommended. Treat with lamivudine plus interferon for significant laboratory or pathologic abnormalities; additional antiviral agents may be considered in adults.
- Post-exposure prophylaxis—Initiate or continue vaccine series if incomplete; in addition, give HBIG if source case is known to be HBsAg-positive. For neonates, if a mother is HBsAg positive, give vaccine and HBIG 0.5 ml (in different sites) to newborn within 12 h of birth. If maternal status is unknown, give vaccine within 12 h, obtain Ag testing, and give HBIG if positive, or if testing is unable to be obtained. Complete immunization 3-dose series as scheduled; birth dose of vaccine does not count if newborn is pre-term/<2 kg. All of these infants should be tested for HBsAb and HBsAg at 9–18 months of age (after completion of 3-dose series) to identify chronically infected children requiring further management.

Haemophilus Influenzae B (Hib)

- Intro—Caused by *Haemophilus influenzae* serotype B, a gram-negative coccobacillus, which can be part of normal respiratory flora. Infection is spread by respiratory tract droplets or contact with secretions. Routine WHO-recommended vaccine. Droplet precautions for first 24 h of antibacterial treatment.
- Clinical presentation—Many manifestations of infection: (1) Systemic (occult bacteremia, septicemia). (2) CNS (meningitis, subdural effusions, endophthalmitis). (3) Respiratory/ENT (epiglottitis, pneumonia, otitis media). (4) Cardiac (purulent pericarditis, endocarditis). (5) Skin/musculoskeletal (cellulitis, septic arthritis, osteomyelitis). (6) Other (peritonitis, chorioamnionitis).
- Differential diagnosis—Dependent on clinical presentation.
- Diagnosis—Gram stain and culture; latex agglutination of CSF (false negatives possible).
- Management—Third-generation cephalosporin (first choice), carbapenem, ampicillin/chloramphenicol for invasive disease. Add dexamethasone in meningitis to prevent hearing loss. For empiric coverage of presumed meningitis, for neonates use ampicillin and gentamicin (plus acyclovir if concerned about HSV); for infants use ampicillin and ceftriaxone (if *Listeria* is a concern); for older infants and children use ceftriaxone/cefotaxime (plus vancomycin if concerned about resistant pneumococci).
- Post-exposure prophylaxis—Rifampin for contacts in selected cases (including households with underimmunized children <4 years old, immunocompromised, index case treated with non-cephalosporin, or two or more cases within community).

Influenza—see Chap. 14.

Japanese Encephalitis

- Intro—Caused by a Flavivirus (single-stranded RNA virus), which is found in most of Asia and parts of Western Pacific. Virus is transmitted by mosquitoes (mostly *Culex* species). Incubation period is 5–15 days. WHO-recommended vaccine for children residing in certain regions and for travelers staying for >1 month or in highly rural area during transmission season; the current available vaccine is a 2-dose series for patients ≥17 years. It is important to weigh vaccine benefits vs. risks of hypersensitivity (immediate through 2 weeks post-vaccination.) Standard precautions.
- Clinical presentation—Systemic febrile illness, aseptic meningitis, acute encephalitis (headache, vomiting, mental status changes, focal neurologic deficits, weakness/flaccid paralysis, parkinsonian syndrome, seizures). Mortality rate is 20–30 %, with up to 50 % of survivors developing significant neurologic sequelae.

- Differential diagnosis—Other viral etiologies of encephalitis.
- Diagnosis—Clinical. Leukocytosis, anemia, hyponatremia may be noted. CSF shows lymphocytic pleocytosis. IgM ELISA acute and convalescent titers may be obtained from serum and/or CSF.
- Management—Supportive.

Measles—see Chap. 17.

Meningococcal

- Intro—Caused by *Neisseria meningitidis,* a gram-negative diplococcus, with multiple serogroups (including A, B, C, Y, W-135). Infection spreads from asymptomatic colonization of upper respiratory tract. Found worldwide, with epidemics in sub-Saharan Africa (A) and in Hajj pilgrims (W-135). Quadrivalent (ACYW) polysaccharide and conjugate vaccines are available; the vaccine is WHO-recommended for children in high-risk populations. Droplet precautions.
- Clinical presentation (1) Meningococcemia (fever, prostration, gun-metal gray petechial rash, adrenal hemorrhage, DIC, death). (2) Acute meningitis. (3) Pneumonia. (4) Conjunctivitis. Complications include arthritis, myocarditis, and endophthalmitis; long-term sequelae include hearing loss and neurologic disability.
- Differential diagnosis—Other etiologies of sepsis and/or acute meningitis.
- Diagnosis—Gram stain and culture of blood and/or CSF; petechial lesions are suggestive but not diagnostic.
- Management—Penicillin G, ampicillin, or third-generation cephalosporin IV×5–7 days (if allergic, chloramphenicol is an alternative). Check culture and sensitivities and tailor antibiotics accordingly; moderate penicillin-resistance is more common in parts of Europe and Africa, but can be overcome with high-dose penicillin or cephalosporin (ceftriaxone, cefotaxime). For empiric coverage of presumed meningitis, for neonates use ampicillin and gentamicin (plus acyclovir if concerned about HSV); for infants use ampicillin and ceftriaxone (if *Listeria* is a concern); for older infants and children use ceftriaxone/cefotaxime (plus vancomycin if concerned about resistant pneumococci).
- Post-exposure prophylaxis—Ceftriaxone or rifampin for pediatric patients; ciprofloxacin for adults. Indicated for close contacts (e.g., household members, school classmates, direct exposure to oral secretions).

Mumps

- Intro—Caused by a Paramyxovirus (RNA virus), which is found worldwide; humans are the only host. Spreads through respiratory secretions. Incubation period is 12–25 days. WHO-recommended vaccine only in countries with high-performing

immunization programs, as part of MMR vaccine. Droplet precautions for 9 days from parotid swelling.
- Clinical presentation—Systemic illness with parotitis and in males, orchitis. CNS symptoms may occur in 10 %, but 50 % will have pleiocytosis. Other rare significant manifestations include myocardidis, cerebellar ataxia, pancreatitis, and in females, oophoritis. One-third may only have respiratory infection. Sterility or other long-term sequelae rarely occur.
- Differential diagnosis—Bacterial (*S. aureus,* other gram negatives), viral (HIV, LCMV, CMV, paraflu/flu, enterovirus), non-TB mycobacteria, salivary duct calculi, metabolic (diabetes mellitus, cirrhosis, malnutrition).
- Diagnosis—Serology (IgM), PCR.
- Management—Supportive.
- Post-exposure prophylaxis—None. However, after exposure unvaccinated persons need quarantine for 3 weeks.

Pertussis

- Intro—Caused by *Bordetella pertussis*, a gram-negative bacillus, which is found worldwide; humans are the only host. Infection spreads through respiratory secretions. Incubation period is 5–21 days. Routine WHO-recommended vaccine; an adult booster to combat waning immunity is less standardized. Neither vaccination nor disease confers lifelong immunity. Droplet precautions.
- Clinical presentation—Catarrhal stage (URI symptoms) → Paroxysmal stage (6–10 weeks, coughing paroxysms with inspiratory whoop, vomiting; in infants gagging and apnea) → Convalescent stage. Complications include pneumonia, seizures, encephalopathy, and sudden death.
- Differential diagnosis—*Bordetella parapertussis/bronchiseptica*, *Mycoplasma pneumoniae, Chlamydia trachomatis/pneumoniae*, adenovirus, RSV.
- Diagnosis—Serology, PCR, culture.
- Management—Macrolide antibiotics (azithromycin preferred) or TMP-SMX; may shorten duration of illness if given during catarrhal stage, otherwise decreases contagion only.
- Post-exposure prophylaxis—For household or close health care contacts; PEP is same as treatment.

Pneumococcal

- Intro—Caused by *Streptococcus pneumoniae,* a lancet-shaped gram-positive coccus, with numerous serotypes. Organism is found worldwide; up to 90 % of

humans have nasopharyngeal carriage. Infection spreads via respiratory droplets. Very young, very old, immunocompromised, patients with cochlear implants are at greater risk. Conjugate (7- and 13-valent) and polysaccharide (23-valent) vaccines are available. Routine WHO-recommended vaccine. Standard precautions.
- Clinical presentation—Wide range of manifestations include: otitis media, conjunctivitis, sinusitis, skin/soft tissue infections, pneumonia/empyema, bacteremia, peritonitis, meningitis, and sepsis.
- Differential diagnosis—Extremely broad, treat empirically until diagnosis is made.
- Diagnosis—Gram stain and culture; latex agglutination (CSF); PCR is investigational.
- Management—Tailored according to susceptibility testing and site of infection. Third-generation cephalosporins are usually first-line for invasive disease but consider adding a second agent if there is local increased resistance and/or CNS infection; consider dexamethasone for meningitis in children >6 weeks (give with first dose of antibiotics). For empiric coverage of presumed meningitis, for neonates use ampicillin and gentamicin (plus acyclovir if concerned about HSV); for infants use ampicillin and ceftriaxone (if *Listeria* is a concern); for older infants and children use ceftriaxone/cefotaxime (plus vancomycin if concerned about resistant pneumococci).
- Post-exposure prophylaxis—None, but check vaccination status.

Polio

- Intro—Caused by poliovirus (Enterovirus family, serotypes 1, 2, 3). Disease is largely eradicated through vaccines, but remains endemic in Nigeria, Pakistan, and Afghanistan, with sporadic importation cases in other countries. India is on track to be polio-free as of 2012. Humans are the only host. Infection is spread by fecal-oral and respiratory secretions; can also be vaccine-acquired. Incubation period 3–6 days, for paralysis 7–21 days. Routine WHO-recommended vaccine; injectable/killed (IPV) and oral/live-attenuated (OPV) formulations are available. Contact precautions for infants/young children.
- Clinical presentation—~70 % are asymptomatic, ~25 % mild illness only (fever, sore throat). 1–5 % develop aseptic meningitis, of which a small subset (<1 %) have acute flaccid paralysis (rapid onset, asymmetric, can involve cranial nerves and/or respiratory tract musculature), and two-thirds of these patients have permanent paralysis. Postpolio syndrome may occur in adult survivors (decades later, irreversible/progressive muscle weakness).
- Differential diagnosis—ARI (initial symptoms); Guillain-Barre syndrome, botulism (paralysis).

- Diagnosis—Clinical. Cell culture or PCR from stool, pharynx, urine, or CSF; stool of highest yield.
- Management—Supportive.
- Post-exposure prophylaxis—None.

Rabies

- Intro—Caused by Rabiesvirus, an RNA lyssavirus. Virus is found worldwide but 95 % of human cases occur in Asia/Africa. 99 % of infections are transmitted from rabid dogs, but bat rabies is increasing. Infection can occur from any carnivorous mammal, but there is less risk from rodents and lagomorphs; transmission can also be transplant- or laboratory-acquired. The average incubation period is 1–3 months, but can be days to over 1 year. WHO-recommended vaccine for children in high-risk populations; a 4-vaccine series is recommended for high-risk travelers and workers (five doses for immunocompromised patients). Standard precautions.
- Clinical presentation—Rapid progression of neuropsychiatric symptoms (including anxiety, hydrophobia, radicular pain, dysautonomia, and dysesthesia; paralysis is also possible). Inexorable progression toward death in almost all cases.
- Differential diagnosis—Acute encephalitis, Guillain-Barrè syndrome.
- Diagnosis—Culture (saliva); antibody titer (serum if unimmunized, CSF); PCR (affected tissues); fluorescent microscopy (skin biopsy).
- Management—Supportive; Wisconsin protocol can be attempted (three survivors).
- Post-exposure prophylaxis—Local wound care (15-min wash with soap). Passive immunization: rabies immune globulin (20 IU/kg) on Day 0 (administer as much as possible at wound site, give remainder IM) and Active immunization: Rabies vaccine (1 ml in deltoid or thigh) on Days 0, 3, 7, 14 (or as soon as available).

Rubella

- Intro—Caused by Rubivirus, RNA virus in Togaviridae family. Infection spreads through nasopharyngeal secretions. The incubation period is 2–3 weeks; patients are most infective 7 days before to 14 days after the rash, although neonates may shed virus for more than 1 year. Routine WHO-recommended vaccine. Droplet precautions for 7 days after rash; contact precautions for congenital rubella syndrome (CRS) patients for 1 year.
- Clinical presentation (1) Postnatal rubella—often subclinical (25–50 % of cases) or mild disease: erythematous maculopapular rash (starts on face then generalizes), lymphadenopathy, low-grade fever, conjunctivitis, polyarthralgias/arthritis (more common in teens). (2) CRS—ocular (cataracts, glaucoma, microphthalmos),

cardiac (PDA, PPS), auditory (sensorineural loss), neurologic (microcephaly, meningoencephalitis, mental retardation), IUGR, interstitial pneumonitis, hepatosplenomegaly, thrombocytopenia, "blueberry muffin" rash (dermal erythropoiesis).
- Differential diagnosis—Neonatal leukemia, CMV, galactosemia (CRS); mild rubeola (postnatal).
- Diagnosis—Rubella-specific IgM suggests congenital infection or recent postnatal infection; a fourfold increase in IgG between acute and convalescent phases suggests postnatal disease. Cell culture or PCR from nasopharynx/urine is diagnostic.
- Management—Supportive.
- Post-exposure prophylaxis—If pregnant, test IgG and IgM; +IgG indicates immunity, repeat test in 3 and 6 weeks to assess for seroconversion. If not pregnant, may consider vaccination within 3 days of exposure, although not shown to prevent illness.

Tetanus

- Intro—Caused by a neuromuscular toxin from *Clostridium tetani* (a spore-forming soil/intestinal anaerobic bacillus), which is found worldwide although is more prevalent in the tropics. Infection results from contaminated wounds or umbilical stumps. Incubation period is up to 21 days (average 8 days), less for neonatal tetanus. Routine WHO-recommended vaccine; periodic boosters are required. Not transmissible by humans; standard precautions.
- Clinical presentation (1) Generalized tetanus: most common presentation; progressive trismus and muscular spasms. (2) Neonatal tetanus—generalized illness in infants who lack maternal antibody, typically from suboptimal umbilical care. (3) Cephalic tetanus—involvement of cranial nerves due to contaminated head/neck wound, can progress to generalized illness. (4) Localized tetanus—focal spasms near wound, also usually evolves into generalized tetanus.
- Differential diagnosis—Hypocalcemia, poisoning/overdose (e.g., strychnine, phenothiazine), conversion disorder.
- Diagnosis—Clinical. (Positive anti-tetanus titer cannot rule out tetanus illness.)
- Management—Pharmacologic: Tetanus immune globulin (TIG) IM 500–6,000 U (debated) and metronidazole 30 mg/kg/day PO or IV × 10–14 days. Equine tetanus antitoxin or IVIG (200–400 mg/kg) are alternatives if TIG is not available. Penicillin 100,000 U/kg/day is an alternative antibiotic. Non-pharmacologic: Appropriate wound cleaning/debridement. Adequate pain control and sedation as needed. Low-light and low-stimuli environment. Ventilatory support may be required.
- Post-exposure prophylaxis—Wound care; TIG for high-risk wounds, undervaccination, or immunocompromised; Td(aP) if undervaccinated.

Tuberculosis—see Chap. 19.

Typhoid/Enteric Fever

- Intro—Also known as enteric fever. Life-threatening, acute, generalized infection caused by *Salmonella typhi* and *S. paratyphi*. Fecal-oral transmission. Prevalent in settings with limited hygiene. Asymptomatic carriers most important reservoirs (e.g., "Typhoid Mary"). Bacteria ingested in contaminated water/food, attach and penetrate GI, spread through body via macrophages. Two vaccines: inactivated/killed IM vaccine (requires booster after 2 years) and live oral Ty21a vaccine (requires 3–4 doses over 5 days and booster after 5 years). Not among WHO routine vaccinations, although commonly given to travelers to typhoid-endemic regions.
- Clinical presentation—Fever (usually increasing over first week, then high and sustained), quite unwell, malaise, abdominal pain, diarrhea, rose spots (in fairer-skinned individuals); complications: intestinal perforation/hemorrhage, shock, organ failures.
- Differential diagnosis—Any abdominal/gastrointestinal infection (e.g., dysentery, appendicitis), dengue, influenza, malaria, visceral leishmaniasis, rickettsial diseases, etc.
- Diagnosis—Blood culture (best). Other: string capsule; aspirate of rose spots, CSF, abscess, marrow; Widal test (low sensitivity and specificity).
- Management—Historically, first-line treatment was chloramphenicol (or amoxicillin, cotrimoxazole). Due to increasing resistance, flouroquinolones (e.g., ciprofloxacin), ceftriaxone, azithromycin now recommended. Steroids if severe disease (delirium, coma, shock). Surgical resection (not just suturing) of GI perforations.
- Post-exposure prophylaxis—None.

Varicella

- Intro—Caused by a herpesvirus (DNA virus); humans are the only reservoir and incidence varies with season in temperate zones. Infection is spread via airborne secretions. Incubation period is 10–21 days (longer in immunocompromised patients). Vaccine is not WHO-recommended, but there is increasing worldwide availability of the vaccine. Patients contagious until all lesions have crusted. Airborne precautions for varicella; contact precautions for shingles.
- Clinical presentation—Initial viremia → low-grade fever, malaise, coryza → pruritic rash (rapid development of clear vesicles on erythematous base, typically 200–500 in wild-type disease, lesions initially on trunk and move outward, can be in multiple stages). Disease course may be modified if vaccinated or after IG products. Complications include bacterial superinfection, pneumonia, ataxia/encephalitis, Reye's syndrome (from concurrent salicylate use), glomerulonephritis, arthritis, and hepatitis. After varicella infection, virus lies latent in dorsal root ganglia; reactivation yields herpes zoster/shingles. Clinical course is most severe in infants, adolescents/adults, and immunocompromised patients.

- Differential diagnosis—Nonspecific viral illness prior to onset of rash.
- Diagnosis—Clinical; PCR (or DFA, culture) from lesion; acute/convalescent IgG titers.
- Management—Supportive; acyclovir/valacyclovir PO or IV if at risk for severe disease (underlying or iatrogenic immunodeficiency, comorbidities).
- Post-exposure prophylaxis—Vaccination given <3–5 days post-exposure. ZIG up to 10 days post-exposure (can use IVIG). Consider oral acyclovir, especially in higher-risk patients.

Yellow Fever

- Intro—Caused by an arbovirus (RNA Flavivirus) that is endemic in tropical areas of South America and Africa. Transmission occurs from bites of *Aedes aegypti* or *Haemagogus* spp mosquitoes; rare cases of in utero and breastfeeding transmission have been documented. Incubation period is 2–15 days. WHO-recommended vaccine for children residing in certain regions. Live-attenuated single-dose vaccine confers immunity for 10 years, and is recommended for all persons ≥9 months traveling to endemic areas, and required for travel to/from certain countries by international regulations. Contraindicated in egg-allergic or immunocompromised persons including symptomatic HIV; take precaution if pregnant/breastfeeding (only give if significant risk of infection outweighs risks of immunization). Standard precautions.
- Clinical presentations (1) Systemic febrile illness: fever, headache, arthralgia/myalgia, jaundice; most patients recover in 3–4 days. (2) Hemorrhagic fever: after several days of nonspecific symptoms, 15 % of patients develop hemorrhage and septic shock with 50 % mortality; the remainder recover after ~14 days.
- Differential diagnosis—In early stages consider all causes of jaundice; once hemorrhagic, consider Lassa, Ebola, Marburg viruses and other hemorrhagic viruses.
- Diagnosis—Serologic testing for virus-specific IgM; if negative within 10 days of illness, repeat test.
- Management—Supportive. Preventative through vector reduction.
- Post-exposure prophylaxis—None.

Immunizations (see Appendix 13, 14, 15)

I. WHO vaccine schedule (Table 21.3)
- WHO routine immunization recommendations are intended to assist program managers in developing country-specific immunization schedules. Health care workers should refer to national immunization schedules.

Table 21.3 WHO-recommended vaccines for all children (contraindications apply)

Vaccine	Birth	6 Weeks	10 Weeks	14 Weeks	9 Months	Booster
BCG	X					
Hep B	X	X	(+/− extra dose)	X		
OPV	X[a]	X	X	X		
DTP		X	X	X		(Booster age 1–6 years)
Hib		X	X	X		
Pneumococcal		X	X	X		
Rotavirus		X	X	X[b]		
Measles					X[c]	Booster ≥15 months
Rubella					X	
HPV	2–3 doses, starting at 9–10 years, depending on vaccine formulation					

Adapted from: World Health Organization. http://www.who.int/en/; World Health Organization. *Pocket Book of Hospital Care for Children.* 2005
[a]Birth dose of OPV given if endemic country, or risk of importation and risk of transmission is high
[b]Third dose needed if RotaTeq formulation is used
[c]May administer first dose as early as 6 months, but does not count towards 2-dose series

- Ten vaccines are currently WHO-recommended for all children (contraindications are discussed below): BCG, Hepatitis B, polio, DTP, Hib, pneumococcal, rotavirus, measles, rubella, and HPV.
- For children residing in certain regions, the following vaccines are WHO-recommended: Japanese encephalitis, yellow fever, tick-borne encephalitis.
- For high-risk populations, the following vaccines are WHO-recommended: typhoid, cholera, meningococcal, rabies, Hepatitis A.
- In countries with program capacity, the following vaccines are WHO-recommended: mumps, influenza.

II. Contraindications and considerations for *routinely* recommended vaccines

- General contraindications—History of anaphylaxis to vaccine or vaccine component.
- BCG—Contraindicated in symptomatic HIV infection (okay in asymptomatic HIV.)
- Hep B—Doses given to infants <2,000 g do not count towards series.
- OPV—Doses given during diarrheal illness do not count towards series.
- DTP—Contraindicated in patients with a history of seizures or shock within 3 days of prior DTP, and in any child with poorly controlled seizures or active CNS disease (give DT instead, to avoid possible encephalopathy to pertussis component.)
- Measles—Pregnancy, immunocompromised state.
- Rubella—Pregnancy.

III. Administration
- IM—Sites include outer thigh midway between hip and knee, deltoid muscle, or (for children >2 years) upper- outer quadrant of buttock. Insert needle at a 90° angle into muscle.
- SQ—Sites as above. Insert needle at a 45° angle into subcutaneous fatty tissue, taking care not to go deep into underlying muscle.
- Intradermal—Any undamaged, uninfected site is acceptable, such as anterior forearm. Insert needle bevel upwards at an angle almost parallel to surface of the skin, about 2 mm deep. Drug administration produces a blanched, raised bleb.

Recommended Reading

1. World Health Organization. http://www.who.int/en/ (including http://www.who.int/immunization_monitoring/diseases/en/, http://www.who.int/topics/cholera/en/, http://www.who.int/rabies/en/, http://www.who.int/immunization/policy/immunization_tables/en/)
2. American Academy of Pediatrics. 2012 Red Book. http://aapredbook.aappublications.org/
3. Centers for Disease Control and Prevention. http://www.cdc.gov
4. Mandell GL, Bennett JE, Dolin R. Principles and practice of infectious diseases. 6th ed. Philadelphia: Elsevier Churchill Livingstone; 2005.
5. World Health Organization. Pocket Book of Hospital Care for Children. 2005. http://www.who.int/maternal_child_adolescent/documents/9241546700/en/index.html
6. UNICEF. http://www.unicef.org/videoaudio/PDFs/UNICEF_2012_child_mortality_for_web_0904.pdf

Part V
Non-Communicable Diseases

Chapter 22
Malnutrition

Pornthep Tanpowpong, Sarah Messmer, Jennifer Kasper, and Ronald E. Kleinman

Keywords Malnutrition • Growth • Anthropometrics • Marasmus • Kwashiorkor • Ready to use therapeutic formula

Overview

- Malnutrition is a major public health problem worldwide and is related to increased risk of infectious disease and death.
- Assessment of nutrition status should be done using standardized growth charts (e.g., WHO, CDC). Wasting is a sign of acute malnutrition, whereas stunting is a sign of chronic malnutrition.

P. Tanpowpong, M.D., M.P.H.
Pediatric Gastroenterology, Hepatology and Nutrition, Department of Pediatrics, Harvard Medical School, MassGeneral Hospital for Children, Boston, MA, USA

S. Messmer, M.S4
Harvard Medical School, Boston, MA, USA

J. Kasper, M.D., M.P.H.
Division of Global Health, MassGeneral Hospital for Children, 100 Cambridge St., 15th Floor, Boston, MA 02114, USA
e-mail: jkasper1@partners.org

R.E. Kleinman, M.D. (✉)
Division of Pediatric Gastroenterology and Nutrition, Department of Paediatrics, MassGeneral Hospital for Children, 175 Cambridge Street, CPZS 578, Boston, MA 02114, USA
e-mail: rkleinman@partners.org

- Marasmus is a result of severe calorie deprivation; it is characterized by muscle wasting and severe growth retardation. Kwashiorkor is a condition that occurs when protein in the diet is insufficient to meet needs for maintenance and growth; it is characterized by edema, muscle wasting, and lightening of hair color.
- Inpatient or outpatient management depends on the severity of the malnutrition, the presence or absence of anorexia, and signs of infection.

Background on Malnutrition

Malnutrition is a major public health problem worldwide. According to the United Nations Food and Agriculture Organization, 12 % of the world's population is undernourished, and approximately 20 % of the global disease burden is a result of protein-energy and micronutrient deficiency; over the last two decades, the number of undernourished people in every region of the world, except sub-Saharan Africa, has decreased (Fig. 22.1). Malnutrition can vary in degree and be due to insufficient intake of food, increased nutrient requirements, inadequate utilization, excessive loss of nutrients, or a combination of these. Generally, underweight children are at increased risk of morbidity and mortality from common infectious illnesses. The WHO estimated that in 2010 approximately 20 % of children younger than 5 years were at least moderately underweight (defined as a weight-for-age z-score <2 SD). Weight-for-height demonstrates a direct relationship with childhood mortality from malnutrition. In several countries the mortality rate of children with severe acute malnutrition (weight-for-height <−3 SD) was found to be approximately 20 %. Furthermore, systemic translocation of bacteria from the bowel during a malnourished state contributes to deaths from pneumonia, diarrhea, bacteremia, and sepsis. Severe enteropathy (pathology of the intestine, often due to infectious processes) is also well known to be associated with more severe degrees of malnutrition; and children with more severe enteropathy have a much worse long-term prognosis for clinical recovery. In the following discussion we will provide a very broad overview of the assessment of growth and nutritional status, the classification of those with clinically apparent malnutrition, and interventions to rehabilitate the patient with protein-energy malnutrition.

Assessment of Growth and Nutritional Status

The assessment of growth and nutritional status is an essential part of the evaluation and management of all children, including those with acute and chronic diseases, and is the first step in evaluating all children whose growth differs from the norm. A thorough dietary history, physical examination, and measurement of trend in changes in height, weight, and body mass index are sufficient to assess the nutritional status for most children. Each method of nutritional assessment has its own strengths and weaknesses, and no single approach is perfectly sensitive or specific in detecting malnutrition. Therefore, applying various clinical, anthropometric, and laboratory measurements to help assess growth and nutritional status is crucial in children with or at risk for malnutrition.

22 Malnutrition

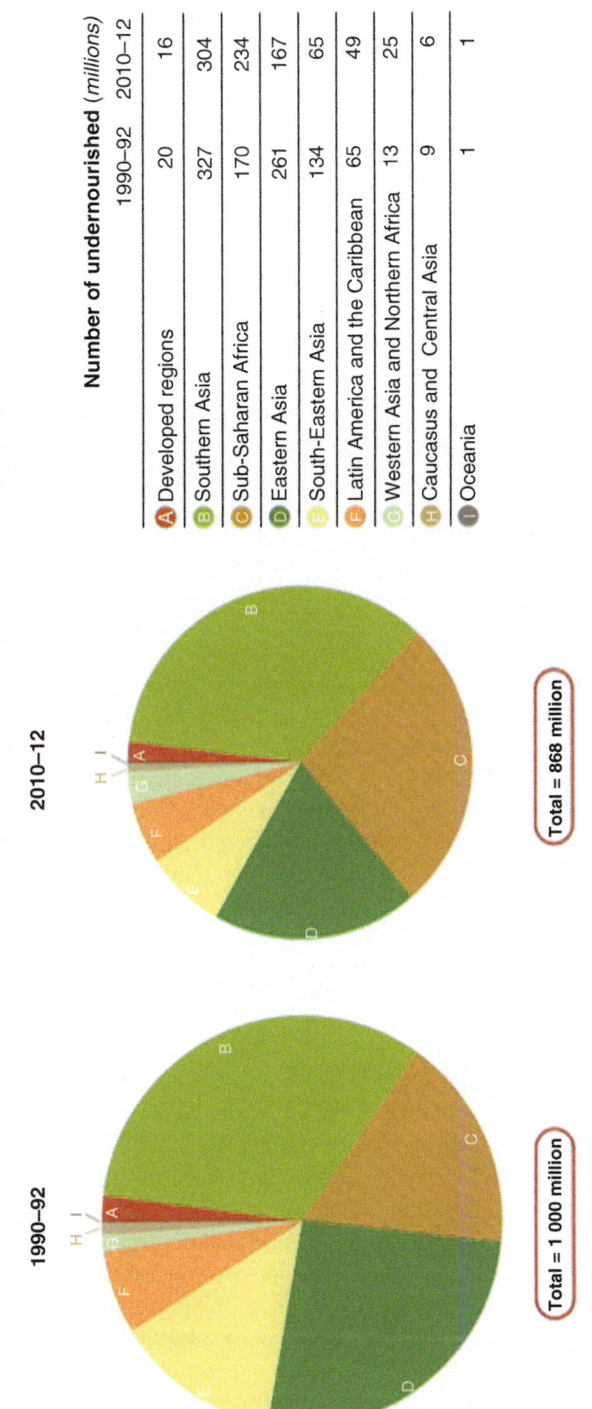

Fig. 22.1 Prevalence of undernourishment by region. (Source: Food and Agriculture Organization, www.fao.org/hunger. Accessed at: http://www.fao.org/docrep/016/i3027e/i3027e02.pdf)

Assessment by History

Whenever resources allow, experienced health care providers should carefully obtain details regarding the quality and quantity of macronutrients and micronutrients consumed. Information regarding meal plans and time spent for each meal and snack should be directly gathered from the patient and/or primary caregivers. A history of the development of feeding skills and dietary patterns should also be obtained. Dietary patterns include family eating patterns and the degree of control exerted by caregivers over the child's feeding. The current ideal method of dietary intake assessment is a 3- to 5-day diet diary to account for the daily variation in diet. A registered dietitian would ideally also perform a complete nutrient analysis, but this may be unavailable in resource-poor settings. The socioeconomic conditions and degree of food security should also be evaluated, inquiring about parental employment, salary, type of housing, number of people in the household, number of children <5 years of age, and number and types of animals as proxies of wealth.

Clinical Assessment

In conjunction with a detailed dietary history, a thorough physical examination for the signs associated with nutritional deficiencies (both macronutrients and micronutrients) should be performed. Clinical signs associated with nutritional inadequacy (both macronutrients and micronutrients) are shown in Table 22.1. Generally, distinguishing wasting from stunting in young children is difficult, and wasting is sometimes not easily determined by the general appearance alone. Therefore, the use of clinical and anthropometric measures is required for the early detection of nutritional inadequacy, particularly in the screening of children who are at high risk for malnutrition.

Anthropometric Evaluation

The measurement of growth in children can be performed both in a cross-sectional and a longitudinal fashion. Anthropometric measurements should always be compared to the reference standard for age, gender, race/ethnicity, and specific health conditions/diseases, if applicable. Various anthropometric reference data are publicly available (e.g., WHO [http://www.cdc.gov/growthcharts/who_charts.htm], CDC [http://www.cdc.gov/growthcharts/]). Special attention should be given to the use of age-appropriate techniques and equipment for measuring these parameters. Single measurements can be useful in screening children who may be at risk for nutritional deficiency and determining the need for a further, more comprehensive medical evaluation. The proper use of longitudinal measures, rather than the use of single time point measurements, is more valuable in determining nutritional status and making a decision to implement nutritional interventions. Different scales of

Table 22.1 Clinical signs associated with nutritional deficiencies

Organ	Clinical sign(s)	Nutritional deficiency
Hair	Thin, sparse, easily fragile	Protein, energy, zinc
Face	Diffuse pigmentation	Protein, energy
	Moon face	Protein (kwashiorkor)
	Nasolabial seborrhea	Riboflavin, niacin, or pyridoxine
Eyes	Pale conjunctivae (anemia)	Iron, folate, or vitamin B12
	Bitot spots, conjunctival xerosis	Vitamin A
Lips	Angular stomatitis or cheilosis	Riboflavin, niacin, or pyridoxine
Mouth	Ageusia or dysgeusia	Zinc
Tongue	Magenta tongue	Riboflavin
	Atrophic filiform papillae	Riboflavin, niacin, folate, iron, or vitamin B12
	Glossitis	Riboflavin, niacin, folate, iron, or vitamin B12
Teeth	Caries	Fluoride, vitamin D
Gums	Swollen, bleeding, gingivitis	Vitamin C
Glands	Parotid enlargement	Protein, energy
	Thyroid enlargement	Iodine
Skin	Xerosis, follicular keratosis	Vitamin A, biotin, essential fatty acids
	Perifolliculosis with blood, petechiae, poor wound healing	Vitamin C
	Dry, depigmented, easily pluckable hair	Protein
	Scrotal or vulvar dermatosis	Riboflavin
Nails	Koilonychia	Iron
Subcutaneous tissues	Edema	Protein, thiamine
	Decreased subcutaneous fat	Protein, energy
Bone	Epiphyseal enlargement	Vitamin C, vitamin D
	Joint tenderness	Vitamin C
	Craniotabes, frontal blossing, rachitic rosary, bowed legs, rickets	Vitamin D
Heart	Cardiomegaly, tachycardia	Thiamine
Liver	Hepatomegaly	Protein, energy
Nervous system	Psychomotor changes, confusion, irritability	Protein
	Sensory loss, motor weakness, calf tenderness	Thiamine
	Loss of vibratory sense, decreased deep tendon reflexes	Thiamine, vitamin B12, or vitamin E

comparison, such as percentiles, z score (i.e., the number of standard deviations above or below the reference median value) or percent of the median, have been used to standardize anthropometric measurements. The primary aim of the comparison is to determine a degree of deviation from normal values. Abnormal growth over time may predict subsequent health problems, especially morbidity, mortality, intellectual development, work capacity, reproductive performance, and risk of chronic diseases.

Weight should be recorded as nude weight, particularly in infants. *Length or height* is currently the most useful indicator of growth status, although it is difficult to obtain accurately and maintain validity and reproducibility, especially in younger children. Infants and children less than 24 months of age should have their lengths measured while lying down/supine; children greater than 24 months of age should be measured while standing erect and ideally one should take the average of three readings. For simplicity, however, infants and children less than 87 cm should be measured supine and those greater than 87 cm should be measured while standing, These measurements should always be referenced by age and gender. *Weight-for-height (or length)* is used to differentiate wasting from stunting and is independent of age and gender. Wasting is a consequence of short-term inadequate nutrition that results in a decreased weight-for-height ratio, while stunting is a longer-term consequence of malnutrition leading to growth failure, but often a proportionate weight-for-height ratio.

Mid-upper arm circumference (MUAC) is an anthropometric measurement used frequently in resource-poor settings to evaluate malnutrition in children aged 6–60 months. The MUAC is measured at the mid-point between the elbow and shoulder while the arm is relaxed. Easy-to-use four-color MUAC tapes are available to allow for triage of patients into risk groups: properly nourished, at risk, moderately malnourished, and severely malnourished (Figs. 22.2 and 22.3). Studies have shown that in a well-nourished population, very few children in this age group have a MUAC <115 mm, and that those children who do have a MUAC <115 mm have a significantly elevated risk of death compared to those who do not. As the MUAC is quick, accurate, and easy to measure, it is a reliable way to triage children who require prompt nutritional interventions.

Anthropometric Classification of Malnutrition

The degree of malnutrition is determined based on the aforementioned anthropometric measurements (Table 22.2).

Stunting is a deficit in height-for-age and signifies slowing of skeletal growth. It usually reflects a chronic process. If a normal 12-month-old child stops growing completely, then he/she will take 6 months to fall below the -2 z-score for height-for-age (i.e., become stunted), whereas a 36-month-old child will take 13 months to do the same. Furthermore, because stunting results from a chronic insult, the older and the more stunted a child is, the longer he will have to grow at an accelerated rate before full catch-up growth is achieved.

Wasting is defined by weight-for-height, as it is a better index of acute risk than weight-for-age, which is often decreased in the setting of stunting. The World

22 Malnutrition

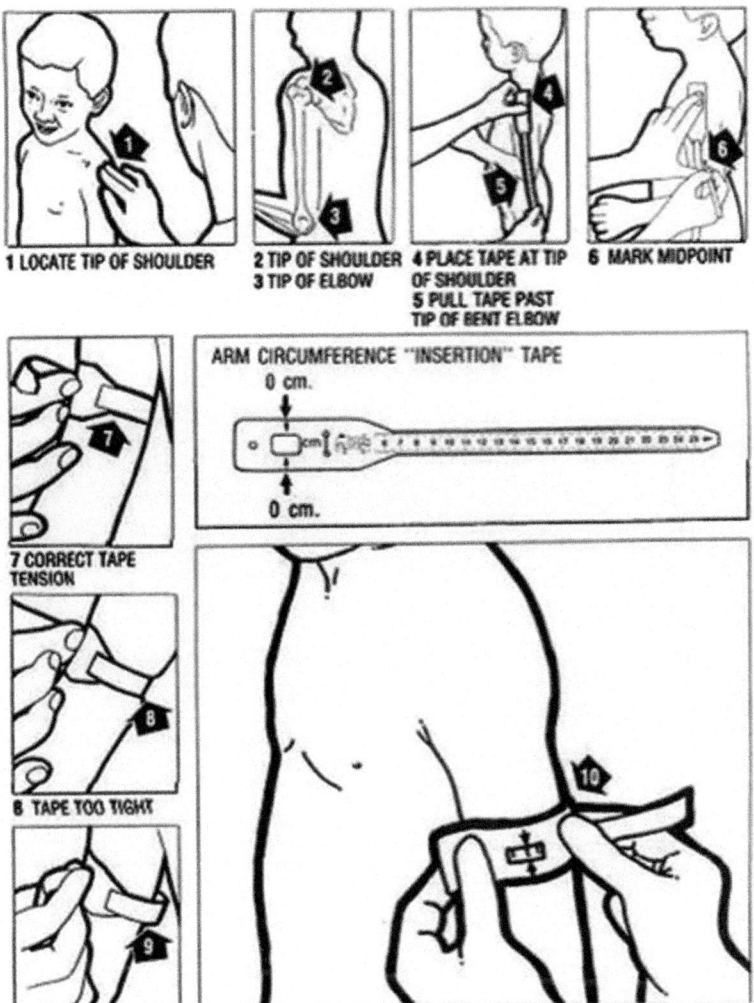

Fig. 22.2 How to measure mid-upper arm circumference (MUAC). (Source: UNICEF. http://motherchildnutrition.org/early-malnutrition-detection/detection-referral-children-with-acute-malnutrition/screening-for-acute-malnutrition.html)

Health Organization defines severe acute malnutrition (SAM) by the degree of wasting. SAM can be diagnosed using any of the following criteria:

1. Weight-for-height <-3 z-score.
2. MUAC <115 mm.
3. Bilateral pedal edema.

The definition of SAM is critical in clinical settings, as it is an indicator for the need for prompt medical attention.

Fig. 22.3 How to measure mid-upper arm circumference. (Source: WHO Joint Committee http://whqlibdoc.who.int/hq/1999/a57361.pdf)

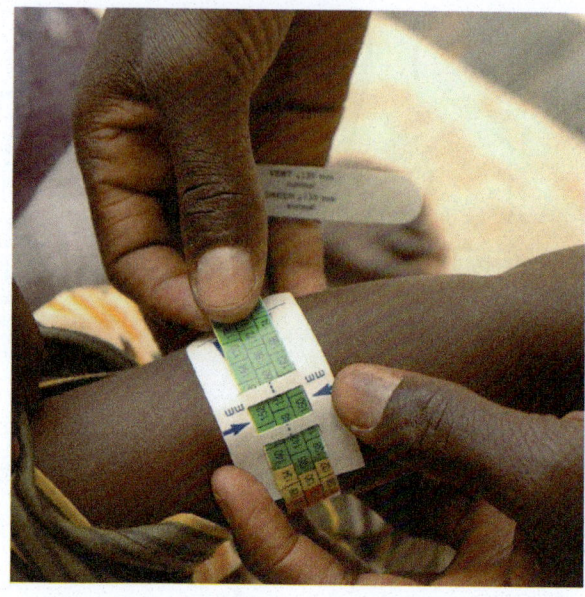

Table 22.2 WHO classification of protein energy malnutrition

Characteristic	Mild	Moderate	Severe
Edema	No	No	Yes
WT/HT deficit (standard deviation from and % of the median of the reference population)	1–2 (80–89)	2–3 (70–79)	>3 (<70)
HT/age deficit (standard deviation from and % of the median of the reference population) (%)	1–2 (80–89)	2–3 (85–89)	>3 (<85)

Clinical Classification of Malnourished States

Marasmus is a result of severe calorie deprivation; it is characterized by muscle wasting and severe growth retardation (Fig. 22.4).

Kwashiorkor is a condition that occurs when protein in the diet is insufficient to meet needs for maintenance and growth. Edema due to low plasma oncotic pressure in conjunction with muscle wasting is a classic clinical sign of kwashiorkor. In childhood, kwashiorkor is often precipitated by conditions that increase protein needs, such as trauma, diarrhea, or systemic infection. In reality, kwashiorkor is most often a result of both energy (calorie) and protein insufficiency, and the term has largely been replaced by "protein-energy malnutrition" (Fig. 22.5).

Marasmic kwashiorkor is a third classification, in which the edema of kwashiorkor occurs in the setting of underlying muscle wasting consistent with marasmus.

Children with severe malnutrition of any form can present with apathy, fatigue, mood changes, and learning disabilities. Furthermore, anorexia and irritability can make nutrition support even more difficult. As malnutrition progresses, the risks of

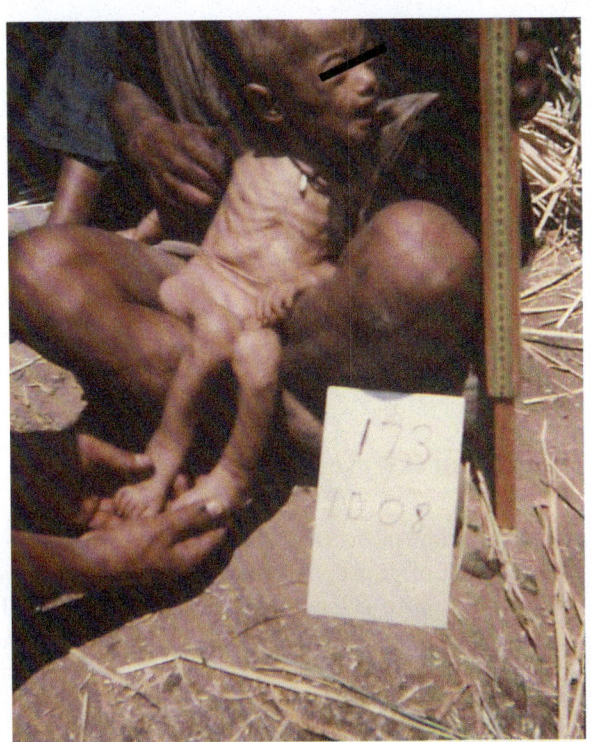

Fig. 22.4 Marasmus. Source: Public Health Image Library. Image #3994. http://phil.cdc.gov/phil/home.asp

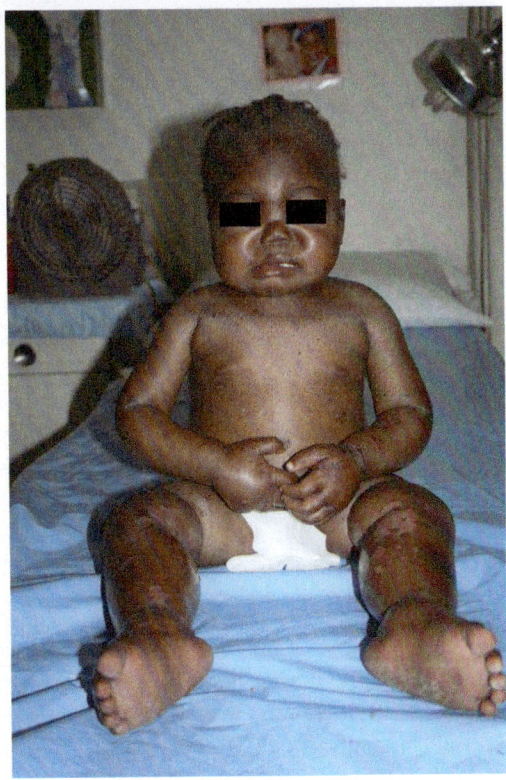

Fig. 22.5 Kwashiorkor. Source: http://artistsforhope.blogspot.com/2010/10/what-is-kwashiorkor.html

significant morbidity and mortality increase. Severely malnourished children have eightfold greater risk of death overall and eight, nine and ten times the risk of dying from pneumonia, malaria and diarrhea than their better-nourished peers respectively. Marasmic kwashiorkor and kwashiorkor are associated with significantly higher morbidity and mortality than marasmus and require immediate medical attention. Severe malnutrition can cause permanent developmental insults such as lower IQ, worse cognitive ability, poorer school performance, and behavioral problems. Therefore, it is crucial to identify children at high risk for malnutrition and provide nutritional support to prevent these conditions.

Nutritional Interventions

After completing the nutritional assessment of the child with malnutrition, including an evaluation of growth, degree of malnutrition, and any factors that may affect dietary intake, such as socioeconomic and psychological factors, it is also important to understand the child's and family's cultural background. Food choices and/or preferences and eating habits are one of the most important parts of individual culture, and these need to be considered in the longer-term plans for successful nutritional support. Using staple foods familiar to the family have the highest chance of long-term acceptance. Primary caregivers' (usually mothers) decisions regarding feeding practices may be influenced by several factors, including food availability, time allocation, the presence of alternative caregivers, religious or cultural beliefs and values. Effective nutritional interventions require multidisciplinary approaches to deal with several interrelated socioeconomic, community health, and condition-specific factors.

For mild to moderate malnutrition, encouraging oral feedings remains essential, and caregivers should be counseled on ways to provide an appropriate daily protein intake and increase the caloric density of the food along with appropriate supplementation of vitamins and minerals.

For children meeting the WHO criteria for SAM (Fig. 22.6 and Table 22.3), more intensive management is necessary. Treatment may be community-based or inpatient-based, depending on the presence or absence of medical complications and whether or not the child has an appetite. There is a growing emphasis on community-based treatment, as it is generally more acceptable to families and cost-effective in resource-poor settings, and there is less risk of morbidity and mortality due to nosocomial infections during hospitalization.

Community-Based Intervention

For patients who meet criteria for community-based intervention, children remain at home with the family, with a focus on intensive nutrition with the use of ready-to-use therapeutic foods (RUTF), which are equivalent to F-100 and fulfill the daily

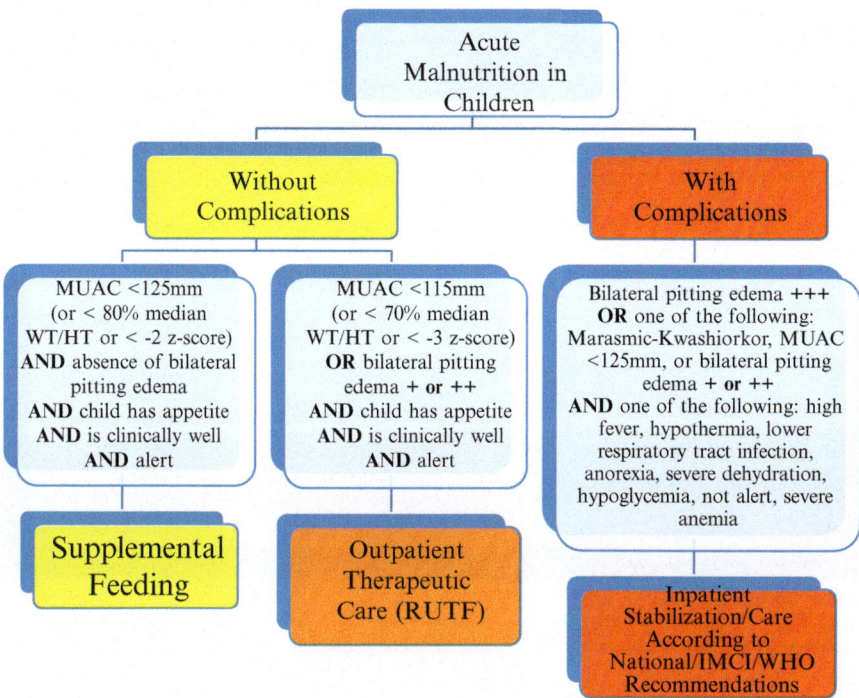

Fig. 22.6 Classification of Acute Malnutrition. Adapted from Valid International. CTC Field Manual. 2006

Table 22.3 Classification of edema

Grade of edema	Definition
Grade 1	Mild: both feet and ankles
Grade 2	Moderate: both feet, and legs, lower arms, and hands
Grade 3	Severe: generalized edema, including both feet, legs, arms, hands, and face

requirements for many critical nutrients. Initially these formulas were milk-based, but soy-based, corn-based, and peanut-based formulas have since been developed. Recently, more peanut-based products such as Plumpy'nut© are being used, as these formulas can be eaten directly from the packet and are safe for consumption for up to 2 years after production date. They do not require mixing with water; thus children are not at increased risk of waterborne illnesses. Figure 22.7 is weight-based approach to Plumpy'nut© supplementation. Finding a food that is culturally acceptable as well as locally produced are primary concerns while choosing a therapeutic food.

Plumpy'nut©
Each packet contains 500kcal
Goal is to provide a child 200kcals/kg/day

Weight of Child (kg)	Packets of Plumpy'nut per Day	Packets of Plumpy'nut per Week
3.5-3.9	1.5	11
4.0-5.4	2	14
5.5-6.9	2.5	18
7.0-8.4	3	21
8.5-9.4	3.5	25
9.5-10.4	4	28
10.5-11.9	4.5	32
>12	5	35

Fig. 22.7 Weight-based approach to PlumpyNut supplementation for malnourished child. Adapted from Valid International. CTC Field Manual. 2006

Inpatient Treatment

For patients who require inpatient treatment, algorithms exist to guide therapy (Table 22.4), with a focus on dividing treatment into phases: initial treatment (treating life-threatening problems such as metabolic abnormalities and deficiencies), rehabilitation (intensive feeding to recover lost weight), and follow-up (after discharge to prevent relapse).

Two different formulas were developed for the treatment of severe malnutrition, F-75 and F-100, and provide 75 kcals/100 ml and 100 kcals/100 ml respectively, with F-75 used for initial treatment and F-100 for the rehabilitation phase. During the initial phase, the goal is 80–100 kcals/kg per day, gradually transitioning to an equivalent amount of F-100 during the first 2 days of the rehabilitation phase, and then increasing feed size gradually until the child no longer finishes the feed, aiming for 150–220 kcals/kg per day. For children over 24 months, solid foods may also be introduced during the rehabilitation phase. Per the WHO algorithm, patients may be transferred from inpatient to community-based programs or begin with community-based therapy as long as they are able to tolerate feeding at home.

Tolerance of foods with higher caloric density and of increased overall intake should be closely monitored for the development of refeeding syndrome, especially in children with severe malnutrition. Refeeding syndrome is a constellation of fluid,

22 Malnutrition

Table 22.4 Management of a child with severe malnutrition

Initial treatment days 1–2	Initial treatment days 3–7	Rehabilitation days 14–42	Follow-up days 43–182
Treat or prevent hypoglycemia, hypothermia, dehydration	Correct electrolyte imbalances	Correct electrolyte imbalances	Increase feeding to recover lost weight ("catch-up growth") using ready to use therapeutic food (e.g., Plumpy'nut©)
Correct electrolyte imbalances	Treat infections	Correct micronutrient deficiencies with iron	Stimulate emotional and sensory development
Treat infections	Correct micronutrient deficiencies without iron	Increase feeding to recover lost weight ("catch-up growth") using F100	
Correct micronutrient deficiencies without iron	Continue feeding with F75	Stimulate emotional and sensory development	
Begin feeding with F75	Stimulate emotional and sensory development	Prepare for discharge	
Stimulate emotional and sensory development			

(Adapted from: WHO Joint Committee http://whqlibdoc.who.int/hq/1999/a57361.pdf)

electrolyte, and metabolic derangements that arise from an overly aggressive attempt at nutritional rehabilitation in the severely malnourished child. Upon rapid refeeding of calories and protein, hypophosphatemia, hemolytic anemia, muscle weakness (including the diaphragm), decreased cardiac output, hypokalemia, hypomagnesemia, cardiac-respiratory failure, and volume overload can develop, and if unaddressed, can lead to death. The symptoms of refeeding syndrome are variable and can occur early or late in the course of refeeding; symptoms can be nonspecific (e.g., nausea, vomiting, lethargy) or progress to hypotension, arrhythmias, respiratory depression, seizures, coma, and death. Practitioners need to maintain a high level of suspicion. Children at high risk of refeeding syndrome include those with significant weight loss or severe malnutrition. Progressively increasing the calorie and protein intake over several days along with serial monitoring of serum electrolytes in the early phase of nutritional rehabilitation is indicated, along with appropriate supplementation of vitamins, potassium, and magnesium. Digestion and absorption are usually adequate to allow oral feeding in most children. In those with severe enteropathy and persistent diarrhea, a combination of intravenous and oral feedings may be required.

Conclusion

Malnutrition is a major threat to the growth and well-being of children in the resource-poor world, particularly among infant and preschool children. Significant long-term morbidities follow prolonged subtle and clinically apparent states of malnutrition. Social and environmental factors that limit access to food or decrease the availability of food for families are often the cause of malnutrition in childhood. New preparations of single food that are culturally acceptable have been used in those parts of the world where nutritional deprivation is highly prevalent and shows great promise to lessen the risk of severe malnutrition and its long-term consequences. Prompt nutritional rehabilitation is essential when severe malnutrition has been identified.

Recommended Reading

1. Kleinman RE. Pediatric nutrition handbook. 7th ed. Elk Grove Village, IL: American Academy of Pediatrics; 2013.
2. Walker WA. Pediatric gastrointestinal disease: pathophysiology, diagnosis, management. 5th ed. Hamilton, ON: BC Decker; 2008.
3. World Health Organization. Management of severe malnutrition: a manual for physicians and other senior health workers. Geneva; 1999. http://whqlibdoc.who.int/hq/1999/a57361.pdf

4. Community-based management of severe acute malnutrition. A joint statement by the World Health Organization, the World Food Programme, the United Nations System Standing Committee on Nutrition and the United Nations Children's Fund. May 2007. http://www.who.int/nutrition/publications/severemalnutrition/978-92-806-4147-9_eng.pdf
5. WHO child growth standards and the identification of severe acute malnutrition in infants and children. A joint statement by the World Health Organization and the United Nations Children's Fund. 2009. http://www.who.int/nutrition/publications/severemalnutrition/9789241598163_eng.pdf
6. Valid International and Concern Worldwide. Community-based therapeutic care (CTC): a field manual. Oxford, UK: Valid International; 2006.

Chapter 23
Micronutrient Deficiencies

Jyoti Ramakrishna and Jay Thiagarajah

Keywords Micronutrient • Iron • Iodine • Vitamin A • Zinc • Supplementation • Folic acid • B vitamins

Overview

- Micronutrients are vitamins and minerals needed in small amounts for normal growth, development, and immune system function.
- Globally, the most important deficiencies are iron, iodine, vitamin A, and zinc.
- Vitamin and mineral supplementation in disease-prone areas is an effective strategy in reducing mortality and morbidity.

Introduction

Micronutrients are important trace elements required for growth, metabolism, and the normal functioning of the immune system. Micronutrient deficiencies either manifest as specific deficiency diseases with clinical signs (Vitamins A–E, iron, iodine) or deficiencies that affect growth, development, and immune function

---

J. Ramakrishna, M.B.B.S., M.D. (✉)
Division of Global Health, MassGeneral Hospital for Children,
Harvard University, Boston, MA 02114, USA
e-mail: jramakrishna@partners.org

J. Thiagarajah, M.B.B.S., Ph.D.
Department of Pediatrics, MassGeneral Hospital for Children, Boston, MA, USA

throughout the body initially without overt signs (zinc, phosphorus, magnesium). In resource-limited settings, micronutrient deficiencies contribute significantly to increased child and maternal mortality and morbidity, and they are a major focus of international public health interventions.

Global Burden of Micronutrient Disease

- *Prevalence*: More than two billion people worldwide are affected by micronutrient deficiencies and many have multiple deficiencies (Fig. 23.1); the majority of those impacted live in developing countries. Micronutrient deficiencies disproportionately affect the most vulnerable populations, such as infants and pregnant women.
- *Etiology and causes*
    - Food insecurity—poor and inconsistent access to nutrient-rich foods, such as fresh fruits and vegetables, meats, and dairy products. Fortification of foods is not available in many developing countries.
    - Inadequate care—poverty, leading to fractured and inconsistent presence of caregivers and consequent lack of appropriate food provision for children and mothers.
    - Lack of health services/unhealthy environment—Chronic micronutrient deficiencies are not screened for, diagnosed, or treated early enough, leading to long-term morbidities. A lack of education in the importance of a varied diet inclusive of micronutrient-rich foods in caregivers may lead to deficiencies.

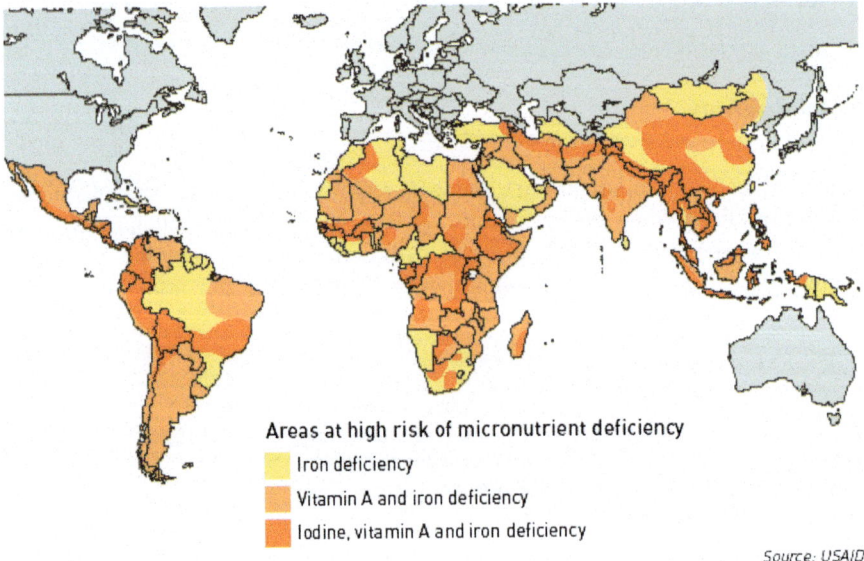

Fig. 23.1 Geographic prevalence of micronutrient deficiency. Source: United States Agency for International Development (USAID)

- *Consequences*
  - Short-term:
    - Iron deficiency is the most prevalent micronutrient deficiency, affecting half of all pregnant women and 40 % of preschool children in developing countries. It is implicated in the death of an estimated 800,000 people annually.
    - 250 million preschool children are vitamin A deficient worldwide; 250–500,000 children become blind every year; half of them die within 12 months of related illnesses such as diarrhea and other infections.
    - Iodine deficiency is the most prevalent cause of preventable cognitive impairment in the world; 18 million babies are born mentally impaired because of maternal iodine deficiency. The WHO estimates 54 countries are still at risk with the median urinary concentration below 100 µg/l, or endemic goiter affecting >5 % of children 6–12 years of age.
    - 150,000 babies are born each year with neural tube defects due to inadequate maternal folate intake.
    - The extent of zinc deficiency worldwide is unknown since it does not occur in isolation. Deficiency specifically affects rapidly dividing and differentiating cells such as the immune system and the gastrointestinal tract. It is thought to be more prevalent in infants and young children, playing a role in susceptibility to infections and diarrheal illness.
- Long-term: An estimated 1.6 billion people globally suffer from compromised intellectual ability and reduced productive capacity as a result of micronutrient deficiencies. For instance, congenital hypothyroidism leads to mental impairment; iodine deficiency can lead to diminished IQ by as much as 10–15 points in affected children less than 6 years of age; and adults with iron and iodine deficiency are fatigued and unable to work. Vitamin A and zinc deficiencies lead to days lost at work and school due to illness. This contributes to a vicious cycle of poverty, malnutrition, specific deficiencies, and infections. Adult height and weight are also affected, both by the deficiencies themselves such as iodine and zinc, but also due to the burden of chronic illness and malnutrition caused by them. Life expectancy is shortened both due to specific deficiency states and increased infection risks. Maternal malnutrition further affects the nutrition of infants, having a ripple effect from one generation to the next.

Iron Deficiency

- Clinical signs and symptoms: Symptoms of anemia (skin pallor, conjunctival pallor, tachycardia, tachypnea, edema).
- Etiology/pathogenesis: Poor intake of iron rich foods such as red meats, dark green leafy vegetables and fortified grains, which are expensive and unavailable. Compounded by losses in women of childbearing age, and infections such as malaria and hookworms.

Table 23.1 Diagnostic testing in resource poor and rich settings

	Resource poor	Resource rich
Iron	Clinical: anemia. WHO hemoglobin color scale (commercially available)	Hemoglobin, RBC morphology including MCV/MCH/MCHC, Ferritin, TIBC
Vitamin A	Clinical: Visual impairment, corneal ulceration, Bitot's spots on conjunctiva, xerophthalmia	Serum retinol levels Full ophthalmolgical evaluation
Iodine	Clinical: Goiter, signs of hypothyroidism	24 h urine iodine, thyroid function testing, ultrasound
Zinc	Clinical: reduced immune function, poor wound healing, dermatitis, diarrhea	Plasma zinc levels
Folic acid	Clinical: anemia. WHO hemoglobin color scale	Hemoglobin, RBC morphology including MCV/MCH/MCHC. Plasma folate and cobalamin levels
Vitamin D	Clinical: bone abnormalities	Serum vitamin D levels
Vitamin C	Tourniquet test—appearance of petechiae on arm when occluding venous return with blood pressure cuff	Urinary vitamin C: decreased after high dose ascorbic acid
Vitamin B1 (thiamine)	Clinical: right heart failure/neuropathy	EKG, CXR, plasma pyruvate, lactate
Vitamin B2 (riboflavin)	Clinical: stomatitis, dermatitis	Plasma B2 levels
Vitamin B12 (cobalamin)	Clinical: peripheral sensory/motor neuropathy	CBC, RBC morphology—megaloblastic anemia. Plasma B12 level, Schilling test
Niacin	Clinical: triad of GI, CNS, skin findings	Plasma niacin levels

- Diagnosis and testing: Primarily a clinical diagnosis. Supportive laboratory tests include CBC, although hemoglobin alone is sufficient; RBC morphology including MCV/MCH/MCHC. Iron studies are expensive and mostly unnecessary (Table 23.1).
- Management:
  - Individual field management: Anemia is classified by blood hemoglobin concentration as mild (10–10.9 g/dl), moderate (7–9.9 g/dl) and severe (<7 g/dl) based on age and gender. Mild anemia can be addressed with iron supplementation for 6–12 weeks. (1–2 mg/kg/day elemental iron), prevention of ongoing losses, and treating underlying infections. Moderate to severe anemia may require hospitalization and cautious transfusion if in heart failure. If available, check hemoglobin electrophoresis.
  - Prevention: Dietary counselling is useful but iron rich diets (see above) are often not affordable. Spacing of pregnancies and prenatal supplementation are helpful (Table 23.2). Sanitation helps to reduce infections.
- Prognosis: Excellent if treated.

Table 23.2 International public health programs for micronutrient deficiency

Maternal	Iron and folate supplementation in pregnancy
	Calcium supplementation
	Iodization of salt
Neonate	Promotion of breastfeeding
Children	Zinc supplementation/fortification
	Vitamin A supplementation/fortification
	Iodization of salt

Vitamin A

- Clinical signs and symptoms: Night blindness: stumbling after dark, poor vision in dim light. Bitot's spots: foamy grey opacities on cornea; keratomalacia: dry cornea; and xerophthalmia: dry eyes, no tears. Also dry skin, dry hair, broken nails, increased number of respiratory and diarrheal illnesses.
- Etiology/pathogenesis: Beta carotene is the provitamin in plant sources—fruits and vegetables; retinol is found in meats, eggs, and dairy. Fat-soluble, stored in the liver. Dietary insufficiency causes deficiency. Dry cornea becomes opaque, breaks down, becomes infected, and ulcerates, causing blindness.
- Diagnosis and testing: Primarily clinical diagnosis, based on above signs and symptoms. Serum retinol <0.7 µM/l.
- Management:
  - Individual field management: Recognition of early stage with night blindness and Bitot's spots (Fig. 23.2b) is crucial. Treatment with high-dose vitamin A (200,000 IU orally × 3 doses—one dose each day for 2 days and then the third dose 2 weeks later) reverses early stages. Give topical eye antibiotic.
  - For children with severe PEM, acute lower respiratory tract infection and/or severe dehydration give one dose of vitamin A 200,000 IU orally. For children with measles, give a dose of vitamin A 200,000 IU orally for 2 consecutive days.
  - Prevention: Food fortification such as milk. Promoting yellow/orange fruits and vegetables, green leafy vegetables, meats where possible. Single high dose (200,000 IU orally) can be used every 6 months in children 6 months–5 years. Also important to provide supplementation to children with measles.
- Prognosis: Excellent if treated early. Once corneal changes occur, corneal transplant may be needed to restore vision. Vitamin A deficiency often occurs with iron deficiency, and supplementation of both micronutrients is often required to treat anemia more effectively.

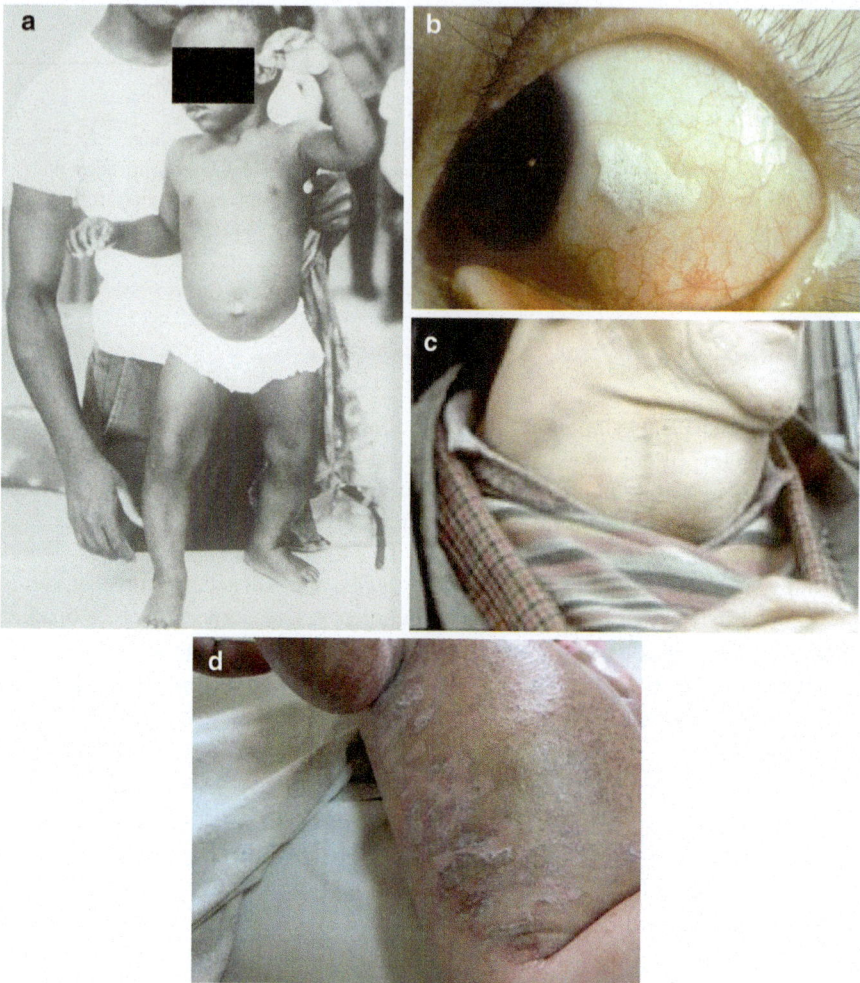

Fig. 23.2 Clinical findings in micronutrient deficiency. (**a**) Frontal bossing and bow legs seen in rickets. Source: Department of Health and Human Services, Centers for Disease Control and Prevention, Public Health Image Library (PHIL). (**b**) Bitot's spots seen in vitamin A deficiency. Source: Community Eye Health Journal. http://www.cehjournal.org/. (**c**) Goiter typical of severe iodine deficiency. Source: Robert Tyabji under Creative Commons License. Accessed at: http://www.flickr.com/photos/69751997@N00/123208739/. (**d**) Dermatitis seen in severe zinc deficiency. Source: Global Pediatrics Residents On Elective, Travel stories by Global Pediatrics residents on international elective. Creative Commons. Accessed at http://blog.lib.umn.edu/iac/electives/2012/04/vislisels-third-week-at-ahc.html

Iodine

- Clinical signs and symptoms: Spectrum includes stillbirth and spontaneous abortions; cretinism and severe mental retardation; reduced intellectual ability and low IQ. Stunted growth, dry skin and hair, fatigue, weight gain, depression, low body temperature and heart rate.
- Etiology/pathogenesis: Occurs in areas of the world where iodine is not present in diet. Thyroid hormone production is affected, leading to goiter or enlarged thyroid and symptoms of hypothyroidism.
- Diagnosis and testing: Clinical diagnosis based on prevalence of goiter (Fig. 23.2c). Median urine iodine is another method and <100 µg/l is considered low.
- Management:
  - Individual field management: Iodine supplementation resolves symptoms. Cognitive impairment in infants/preschool age can be permanent, leading to lower IQ scores.
  - Iodized oil: one oral dose—infants 100 mg, children 200–400 mg, pregnant women 400 mg, adults 400–1,000 mg—every 6–18 months. Can also make home-made supplement with potassium iodide solution (30 mg of potassium iodide in 20 ml of boiled water). Goiters may need surgery if large and in danger of compromising airway or other neck structures.
  - Prevention: Salt fortification is a cost-efficient strategy. 34 countries have reached the Universal Salt Iodization (USI) goal (whereby 90 % of the population consume iodized salt), and at least 28 more have 70–89 % of the population covered. 47 countries are at risk for iodine deficiency due to low coverage with iodized salt.
- Prognosis: Cognitive impairment at an early age cannot be reversed. Goiter and symptoms of hypothyroidism in adults will resolve completely with supplementation.

Zinc

- Clinical signs and symptoms: Growth retardation; poor immunity leading to chronic infections, especially diarrhea, and slow wound healing; inability to smell and taste, hair loss, hypogonadism, rash (Fig. 23.2d) and delayed sexual maturation. Poor pregnancy outcomes.
- Etiology/pathogenesis: Found in high protein foods—meats, nuts, legumes. Poor diet causes deficiency. Required for immune function, normal growth and development, wound healing, and catalyst for many enzymes involved in cell membrane stabilization and protein synthesis.
- Diagnosis and testing: Clinical diagnosis. Plasma zinc levels are unnecessary.
- Management:

- Individual field management: Most multivitamins have zinc. Oral zinc supplements are also available. Children <6 months 10 mg/day, >6 months to adult 20 mg/day orally for 10–14 days. Tablets can be chewed or dissolved. Malnourished children with chronic diarrhea and subsequent growth stunting have been shown to benefit from supplementation, with reduction in incidence of diarrhea and pneumonia, and improved growth.
- Prevention: Inclusion in infant formulas and multivitamin supplements. The WHO advocates widespread zinc supplementation for reduction of childhood diarrhea and pneumonia in developing countries. Better availability of high protein foods.
- Prognosis: Usually improves with overall improvement of nutritional status.

Folic Acid

- Deficiency in pregnant women leads to fetal neural tube defects. In children symptoms include loss of appetite, weakness, growth faltering, and anemia.
- Management:
  - Daily dose of 400 µg of folic acid to pregnant mothers along with iron is recommended. Use in first trimester is needed to prevent neural tube defects.
  - For children 1–11 months of age: 15 µg/kg/day, maximum dose 50 µg/day; for children 1–10 years old: 100–400 µg/day; for children >10 years old: 400 µg/day.
  - Prevention: Diet rich in fruit and vegetables.

Vitamin D

- Rickets: Seen between ages 6 months and 2 years, delayed closure of fontanelle, bone deformities: spinal scoliosis, pigeon chest, swollen costochondral joints ("rachitic rosary"), genu valgus/varum (bow legs, knock-knees), frontal bossing, and craniotabes. There is short stature. Dental deformities are also seen. In severe cases tetany (from hypocalcemia) or seizures are present Fig. 23.2a.
- Osteomalacia: Primarily women, often in pregnancy, resulting in painful bones and fractures. Dosing guidelines are still being evaluated in pregnant women.
- Diagnosis: Clinical signs as above. X-rays of wrists—metaphyses show typical cupping, and fraying.
- Management:
  - Oral vitamin D (calcitriol) weekly for 1 month, then monthly for 3 months. Children 100,000 IU/week, adults 300,000 IU/week. Also need to give calcium supplements.
  - Prevention: Vitamin D supplementation 400 IU per day.

Vitamin C

- Also known as "scurvy." In children associated with bleeding gums, limb pain (distal femur, proximal tibia) due to subperiosteal hemorrhage, costochondral bleeding, diarrhea.
- Management:
  - Ascorbic acid for 2 weeks: infants 50 mg/day PO, children 150 mg/day, adults 500 mg/day.
  - Prevention: Diet with plenty of fresh fruit, particularly citrus. Supplementation: 50 mg/day.

Vitamin B1 (Beriberi)

- Dry beriberi: mixed sensory and motor peripheral neuropathy. Gradual onset of weakness and muscle wasting starting at legs and spreading upwards. Loss of tendon reflexes and loss of sensation in "stocking and glove" distribution. Ataxia, incontinence in late stage and death from diaphragm paralysis.
- Wet beriberi: high output right heart failure with associated signs—raised jugular venous pressure, low blood pressure with wide pulse pressure, tricuspid regurgitation with systolic murmur, edema, oliguria, hepatomegaly. Infants of B1-deficient mothers can also develop heart failure.
- Management:
  - Severe neuropathy or cardiomyopathy: Thiamine 50–100 mg IV three times a day transitioning to PO 10 mg/day when symptoms improving. Fluid restriction with high-protein and low-salt diet.
    Infant: Thiamine 25 mg IV 1×, then 25 mg IM twice a day until improved, then 10 mg orally once a day. If breastfeeding, treat mother 10 mg/day PO for 4–6 weeks.
    Non-severe: Thiamine 10 mg/day PO for 4–6 weeks.
  - Prevention: Whole grain instead of white rice, milk, eggs, green vegetables, legumes and whole grain breads and cereals in diet.

Vitamin B2 (Riboflavin)

- Characterized by angular stomatitis, sore red lips, fissuring of lips, purple tongue with enlarged papillae, scrotal dermatitis, rough skin.
- Management:
  - Riboflavin 5 mg orally daily.
  - Prevention: Diet containing meat, vegetables, and milk.

Vitamin B12

- Developmental delay in infants/children, hypotonia, optic atrophy, subacute combined degeneration of spinal cord resulting in twitching, motor and sensory peripheral neuropathy, ataxia, dementia, psychiatric symptoms, hyperpigmentation of palmar and plantar skin and mucous membranes, diarrhea. megaloblastic anemia (also seen with folate deficiency, can occur together).
- Management:
    - Hydroxycobalamin 1 mg IM three times a week for 2 weeks. If due to malabsorption, 1 mg IM every 3–6 months. Neonates/infants: 10 µg/day PO for up to 6 weeks.
    - Diet containing B12-rich foods: eggs, milk, meat.
    - Anemia may need additional folate and iron.

Niacin (Pellagra)

- Multi-system involvement. Triad of diarrhea, dermatitis, dementia. Gingival swelling, dysphagia, skin lesions at sites of pressure, exposure. Red swollen, itchy, burning rash on back of hands and feet, worse with sunlight, peels after 2 weeks. Depression, psychosis, mania, neuropathy. Conjunctival edema and corneal dystrophy.
- Management:
    - Nicotinamide 150–250 mg PO twice a day for 3–4 weeks.
    - Prevention: Diet containing foods rich in B vitamins such as nuts, most whole grains, dairy, and meats. Maize and sorghum do not provide sufficient niacin in diet. Vitamin B complex supplementation.

Recommended Reading

1. WHO, UNICEF, World Bank, USAID, Flour Fortification Initiative (FFI), Micronutrient Initiative (MI), The Global Alliance for Improved Nutrition (GAIN). Investing in the future: a united call to action on vitamin and mineral deficiencies. 2009. http://www.unitedcalltoaction.org/documents/Investing_in_the_future.pdf
2. Black RE, Allen LH, Bhutta ZA, Caulfield LE, de Onis M, Ezzati M, Mathers C, Rivera J, Maternal and Child Undernutrition Study Group. Maternal and child undernutrition: global and regional exposures and health consequences. Lancet. 2008;371:243–60.
3. Grantham-McGregor S, Cheung YB, Cueto S, Glewwe P, Richter L, Strupp B, International Child Development Steering Group. Developmental potential in the first 5 years for children in developing countries. Lancet. 2007;369:60–70.
4. Micronutrient Initiative. Vitamin and mineral deficiency: a global damage assessment report. 2004. http://www.micronutrient.org/CMFiles/PubLib/Report-67-VMD-A-Global-Damage-Assessment-Report1KSB-3242008-9634.pdf
5. WHO, World Food Program, UNICEF. Preventing and controlling micronutrient deficiencies in populations affected by an emergency. 2006. http://www.unicef.org/nutrition/files/Joint_Statement_Micronutrients_March_2006.pdf

Chapter 24
Emergency Pediatric Care in Resource-Limited Settings

Sylvia Veronica Romm, Daniel P. Ryan, and Linda T. Wang

Keywords Pediatric • Trauma • Wounds • Injuries • Poisoning • Orthopedic • Fracture • Suture • Techniques

Overview

- Nearly 50 % of all child mortality (ages 5–17 years) is due to injury; globally, 11.5 % of deaths due to injury are intentional.
- For every child who dies of injuries, there are an estimated 30 children disabled, 300 hospitalized, and thousands treated emergently.
- The leading mechanisms of injury include road traffic accidents, self-induced injuries, violence between persons, war, poisoning, drowning, and fire-related injuries.

S.V. Romm, M.D., M.P.H.
Pediatrics Department, MassGeneral Hospital for Children, 5 Vinal Ave., #1, Somerville, Boston, MA 02143, USA
e-mail: svromm@partners.org

D.P. Ryan, M.D.
Pediatric Surgery Division, Department of Surgery, Massachusetts General Hospital, Boston, MA, USA

Harvard Medical School, Harvard University, Boston, MA, USA

L.T. Wang, M.D. (✉)
Pediatric Emergency Medicine, Division of Global Health, MassGeneral Hospital for Children, 100 Cambridge Street, 15th Floor, Boston, MA 02114, USA

Harvard Medical School, Harvard University, Boston, MA, USA
e-mail: ltwang@partners.org

Introduction

Injuries are a primary burden of disease for pediatric patients worldwide. Across the globe, nearly half of all non-infant deaths among children 5–17 years old are due to injury. The global disease burden from injuries extends far beyond mortality. Nonfatal injuries causing permanent and temporary disabilities affect not only the growth and the development of the injured children, but also have a significant impact on families and societies, including missed school and workdays, and decreased future earning potential.

Road traffic accidents, self-inflicted injuries, interpersonal violence, war injuries, drowning, poisoning, and injuries related to fires are among the ten most common mechanisms of mortality due to injury of children 5–17 years old. Poor infrastructure in lower-income countries is a primary contributor to the likelihood or severity of injury. Despite lower per capita rates of car ownership, developing countries account for 85 % of all deaths due to road traffic accidents, including 96 % of all pediatric motor vehicle-related mortality. Similarly, in many African and Central American countries, the incidence of drowning is 10–20 times higher than in the US. Ethnic minorities and rural populations are at even greater risk. Gender and age are significant factors in determining the incidence and extent of injury. For example, female children suffer greater mortality and morbidity from fire-related injuries, including inhalation injuries due to poor ventilation, likely due to gender normative roles such as cooking. Toddlers, meanwhile, are the primary victims of hot-water burns from inadvertent submersion. These variations in injury presentation by demographic should be considered in clinical screening and treatment Fig. 24.1.

This chapter discusses how to evaluate an injured child, and then focuses on presentation and management of the most common types of injuries seen in children worldwide: head trauma, abrasions, lacerations, and fractures. There is a brief discussion of how to manage pain in children. Following this, the authors present a basic approach to caring for children with burns, poisoning, drowning, and animal, snake, scorpion, and spider bites.

Primary Survey of the Injured Child

Although injuries present in a continuum of type and severity, all injuries are treated with an initial stabilization and survey before more in-depth treatment can be given Fig. 24.2 and Table 24.1.

Head Trauma

- *Minor head injury*: Normal mental status at initial exam, no abnormal or focal findings on neurologic exam, including pupillary exam. No physical evidence of skull fracture. Can be discharged to home with careful observation.

Distribution of global child injury deaths by cause, 0-17 years, World 2004

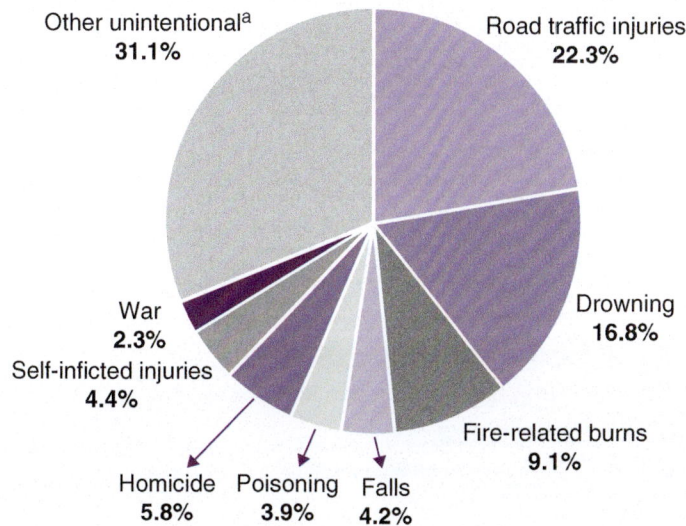

a "Other unintentional" includes categories such as smothering, asphyxiation, choking, animal and venomous bites, hypothermia and hyperthermia as well as natural disasters.

Source: WHO (2008), Global Burden of Disease: 2004 update.

Fig. 24.1 Distribution of global child injury by cause. Source: World Report on Child Injury Prevention. WHO 2008 Page 6, Fig. 1.1. Accessed at: http://www.unicef.org/eapro/World_report.pdf

- Age <2 years: may be asymptomatic despite intracranial injury; skull fractures can occur after minor head injury. Inflicted injuries occur more often in this age group.
- *Significant head injury*: Often associated with loss of consciousness, amnesia, change in mental status, seizure, vomiting, headache (post-concussive syndrome, also sign of increased intracranial pressure (ICP) [rare]), abnormal gait, weakness, and visual changes. *Physical exam findings* suggestive of intracranial injury include boggy scalp hematoma, step off on scalp palpation, bulging anterior fontanelle in infants, focal neurologic exam, cerebral spinal fluid(CSF) otorrhea/rhinorrhea, and signs of basilar skull fracture such as Battle's sign or ecchymosis behind the pinna, raccoon eye or periorbital ecchymosis, and hemotympanum.
- *Management*:
- Stabilize patient following ABC rules. Consider cervical spine immobilization if indicated.

Within 5 minutes....

Airway
- Obstruction → Open airway, suction secretions, administer 100% O2
- Difficult airway/direct airway injury → surgical airway

Breathing
- Tension Pneumothorax → Needle decompression
- Massive hemothorax → Place chest tube
- Open Pneumothorax → Apply 3 sided occlusive dressing
- Flail Chest → Perform bag-valve ventilation
- Impaired oxygen/ventilation → rapid sequence endotracheal intubation

Circulation
- Absent circulation → CPR
- External hemorrhage → Control bleeding
- Signs of shock → IV access, fluid resuscitation, lab studies
- Cardiac tamponade → Pericardiocentesis followed by thoracotomy
- Pelvic fracture → Wrap or bind pelvis

Disability
- GCS <9 or rapidly declining GCS → Endotracheal intubation
- Pupillary response → Elevate head of bed to 30° if no signs of shock
- Signs of impending herniation → Moderate hyperventilation, Neurosurgical consultation, Osmotic agents if normotensive
- Immobilize C-spine
- Immobilize/splint long bone fractures

Exposure
- Hypothermia → Remove clothing, initiate warming

Within 10 minutes....

Repeat vital signs every 5 minutes
Reassess response to interventions
Intubated patients
- Monitor End tidal Co2 → Gastric tube placement
- Obtain blood gas

Within 15 minutes....

Reassess response to interventions → Provide analgesia
Reassess level of consciousness
Examine head, neck, chest, abdomen, pelvis, and extremities → place urinary catheter if no signs of urethral disruption
Obtain screening radiographs (lateral C-spine, AP chest, AP pelvis) and FAST examination, if possible

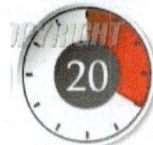

Within 20 minutes....

Reassess response to interventions → Provide analgesia, splint fractures
Reassess level of consciousness
Perform complete PE → Update tetanus immunization, antibiotics for open fractures, contaminated wounds, or suspected bowel perforation

Transition to definitive care at a regional pediatric trauma center

Fig. 24.2 Initial Trauma Management in Children. Data from Lee LK, Fleisher GR. Trauma management: Approach to the unstable child. In: Basow DS (Ed), UpToDate 2012, Waltham, MA. For more information visit www.uptodate.com

- *For Increased ICP:*
    - Consider oxygen or advanced airway if decreased mental status, GCS <9, marked respiratory distress, hemodynamic instability.
    - Elevate head of bed 30°, with head in neutral position. This helps to decrease ICP and optimize cerebral perfusion.
    - Consider seizure prophylaxis.
- *Refer to tertiary center* if possible, if the following are present: increased ICP, change in mental status, neurologic deficits, seizures, persistent headache,

Table 24.1 GCS-scale used to objectively follow a patient's level of consciousness

Modified pediatric Glasgow Coma Scale		
Eyes opening	Spontaneous	4
	To speech	3
	To pain	2
	None	1
Verbal	Oriented (coos, babbles)	5
	Confused (irritable)	4
	Inappropriate words (cries to pain)	3
	Nonspecific sounds (moans to pain)	2
	None	1
Motor	Follows commands (spontaneous movements)	6
	Localizes pain (withdraws to touch)	5
	Withdraws to pain	4
	Abnormal flexion	3
	Abnormal extension	2
	None	1

persistent vomiting, CSF otorrhea/rhinorrhea or hemotympanum, depressed skull fracture, basilar skull fracture, history of bleeding disorder.
- Minor head injury: can resume normal activities once completely asymptomatic for at least 1 week.

Approach to Child with Laceration/Abrasion

- To prevent wound infection, use clean irrigation fluid (i.e., free of debris); sufficient irrigation at adequate pressure is more effective than sterility of irrigation fluid to reduce the risk of infection. In resource-limited settings, using sterile technique for wound closure has not been shown to reduce infection rates when compared to non-sterile technique; non-suture (e.g., Steri-Strips) wound management is an acceptable alternative in *lacerations under* 2 cm. Once closed, if a wound appears *infected*, remove the stitches and irrigate wound, give antibiotics if needed and available. An infected wound should be left open to granulate and close.
- *Hair braids*: For scalp wounds, hair can be taken approximately one half inch on either side of the wound and tied together to approximate the wound edge.
- *Large lacerations*: Close if clean and less than 12 hours old. See below for animal bites.
- *Suture removal*: Cut the thread on one side of the knot and pull the knot until the thread comes out. *Timing for suture removal*:
  - Face: 4–5 days
  - Body and upper extremities: 8–10 days
  - Lower extremities: 11–14 days

Approach to Child with an Orthopedic Injury

General Overview of Treatment of Fractures and Dislocations

- Splinting or casting a broken bone can help tremendously with pain control and is appropriate for fractures that are non-displaced or minimally displaced. Do not use traction if the bones seem more or less in the right position.
- Treatment for displaced factures is closed reduction to realign the bones. Reducing a displaced fracture will optimize future use of that limb. Use traction to set bones before splinting or casting. Before performing closed reduction consider diazepam (0.1–0.3 mg/kg max 5 mg PO 45 min before procedure) to relax the muscles and codeine (0.5–1 mg/kg max 60 mg PO every 4–6 h) for pain control.
- Remember to splint/cast fracture in a position of function in order to minimize future contractures.
- The worse the break or the older the person, the longer healing takes. Length of immobilization: Arm: 1 month. Leg: 2 months.
- Treatment of open fractures.
  - All patients with open fractures should receive an antibiotic that has gram-positive coverage (first-generation cephalosporin); consider the addition of an aminoglycoside for gram-negative coverage of more severe fractures.
  - Consider the addition of penicillin or clindamycin for injuries at risk for anaerobic infections (e.g., farm injuries, severe tissue necrosis).
  - Administer tetanus toxoid if the last booster was given more than 10 years prior or if history is not reliable or available. Give tetanus immunoglobulin to patients with incomplete primary immunization or to patients for whom it has been longer than 10 years since their last booster dose.

Clavicular fractures: For closed fractures, place in sling and immobilize for 2–6 weeks, until repeat radiographs show callus formation and healing across the fracture site.

Dislocated Shoulder

- Have the injured person lie face down on a table or other firm surface with his arm hanging over the side. Pull down on the arm toward the floor, using a strong, steady force, for 15–20 min. Then gently let go. The shoulder should move back into correct placement.
- Alternatively, attach something to the arm that weighs 5–10 kg (start with 5 kg, increase weight as needed to maximum of 10 kg) and leave it there for 15–20 min.
- After the shoulder is in place, bandage the arm firmly against the body.
- To prevent frozen shoulder (the inability to move the shoulder due to shoulder capsule thickening and tightening), unbandage the arm for a few minutes three times a day and, with the arm hanging at its side, move it gently in small circles.

Dislocated (Nursemaid's) Elbow

- Hold affected arm with one hand on the radial head and the other grasping the hand.
- Applying compression between the two hands and gently supinate patients' forearm while flexing arm.

Fractures of the Upper Extremity

- Fracture/dislocation of the hands/fingers: Splint fingers as if in use, for example as if gripping a can.
- For a displaced wrist fracture, pull the hand with a slow, steady, increasing force for 5–10 min, to separate the bones.
- One person continues to hold the hand, while the other gently lines up and straightens the bones. Splint with wrist extended to 30° extension and fingers flexed to 60°.
- Fractured Radius/Ulna: Splint with wrist at 30° of extension, and the fingers at the mcetacarpal–phalangeal joints flexed to approximately 60°.
- A broken arm should be kept in a cast for about a month, and no force put on it for another month.

Injuries of the Lower Extremity

- In children >6 years of age, an ankle fracture is likely if the following are true:
  - There is pain in the midfoot zone PLUS any one of the following:
    - Bone tenderness at the base of the fifth metatarsal (for foot injuries)
    - Bone tenderness at the navicular bone (for foot injuries)
    - An inability to bear weight for four steps
- If suspicious of an ankle fracture, treat as if it were a tibia/fibula fracture.
- If the child has an ankle sprain, then rest, ice, wrap, and elevate the ankle and support with an ankle bandage.
- Tibia/Fibula fracture: splint the foot at 90°, after 2–4 weeks switch to a short leg cast or cast brace for a total of 12–16 weeks.

General Care of Amputations

- Wash hands thoroughly and wear protective barriers on hands and body, if available.
- Lie the patient down and elevate the amputation site.

- Remove foreign bodies in the wound that are easy to remove, and remove or cut clothing from around the wound.
- Apply direct pressure to the amputation site with a barrier for at least 15 min. Do not remove the barrier; if blood soaks through the barrier, place another on top of the first. If there is a foreign body in the wound, apply pressure around the foreign body, not directly over it.
- Do all you can to keep the wound clean and avoid further injury to the area.
- Refer immediately to tertiary care center.

Pain Control in Children

The World Health Organization has established a "pain ladder" for use of analgesics (Fig. 24.3).

The guidelines recommend for mild pain, starting with non-opioid drugs such as acetaminophen and NSAIDs. If desired pain relief is not reached, attempt adding a mild opioid such as codeine. If the pain is still not controlled, discontinue the mild opioid and start a stronger opioid (such as morphine, heroin, fentanyl, buprenorphine, oxymorphone, oxycodone, or hydromorphone), while continuing the non-opioid therapy, increasing the opioid dose until you have reached the goal pain control or the patient is unable to tolerate the side effects. If patient presents in severe pain, start with a strong opioid in combination with a non-opioid analgesic.

Evaluation and Treatment of Burns (Table 24.2)

- If electrical injury suspected, can have rhabdomyolysis with myoglobinuria, cardiac arrhythmias, and injury at distal sites.
- If there is altered mental status consider carbon monoxide poisoning and give 100 % oxygen.
- Consider acetaminophen, codeine, or morphine for pain.

Determining % Body Surface Area (BSA) of Burns

- *>12 years*: Rule of 9 s: Head 9 %, front and back of torso 18 % each, arms 9 % each, leg 18 % each.
- *<12 years*: Modified Rule of 9 s, head and neck 18 %, each lower extremity 15 %, each upper extremity 10 %, and anterior and posterior torsos each 16 %.
- Irregular, nonconfluent burns: Rule of palms: palmar surface of patient's hand ~1 % of BSA.

WHO'S Pain Relief Ladder

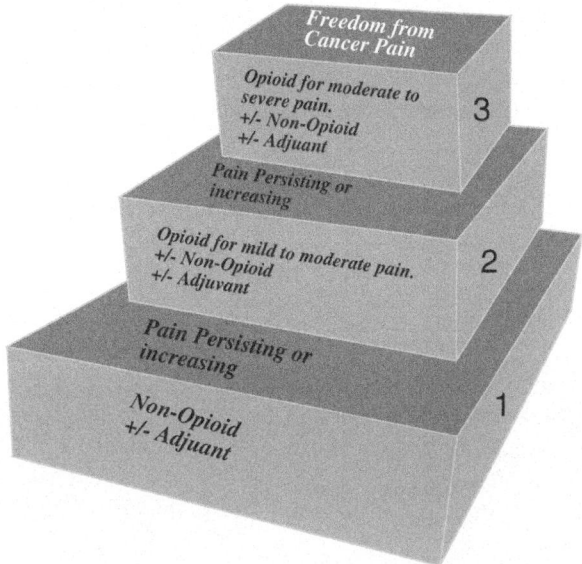

Fig. 24.3 WHO pain management pyramid. Source: World Health Organization (1998). Cancer pain relief and palliative care in children. Geneva. Accessed at: http://www.who.int/cancer/palliative/painladder/en/

Table 24.2 Degree of burns

Degree	Description
First degree	Only epidermis involved, painful and erythematous
Second degree	Epidermis and dermis involved, but dermal appendages spared; any blistering qualifies as second degree; deep second-degree burns may be white and painless, require grafting and progress to full thickness with wound infection
Third degree	Full-thickness burns involving epidermis and all of dermis, including dermal appendages; leathery and painless; require grafting
Fourth degree	Full thickness involving muscle, bone, or fascia; evaluate for compartment syndrome

Management of Minor Burns

- *Initial Stabilization*: ABCs and pain control.
- *Clean* with mild soap and water or saline.
- *Debride* only open blisters (closed blister is best bandage), devitalized tissue.
- *Topical antimicrobial agent* daily (silver sulfadiazine, combination antibiotic cream, and chlorhexidine.) Choice can be made based on cost, availability, and provider familiarity. Note: silver sulfadiazine with cerium or alone, and povidone–iodine are contraindicated in newborns, pregnancy, and lactation.

- Cool skin if within 30 min of injury to decrease damage.
- If burn <10 % BSA, apply clean towels soaked in cold water.
- If >10 % BSA, apply clean dry towels to avoid hypothermia.
- If chemical burn, wash with copious amounts of water for 20 min.
- Prophylactic oral antibiotics usually not indicated.
- Tetanus prophylaxis if none in the past 5 years.

Management of Severe Burns (as available)

- *Evaluate for other injuries* from fall or injuries with electrical burns or if concern for non-accidental trauma.
- *Oxygen or advanced airway* for facial burns, facial swelling, CO poisoning.
- *IV fluids*:
- If *hypotensive*, give NS or LR 20 ml/kg bolus, repeat if still hypotensive.
- If *normotensive*, use the Parkland Formula: give crystalloid 4 ml/kg/day/% BSA burned, plus maintenance rate ½ in first 8 h and ½ in next 16 h.
- *GI*: NPO, NGT, stress ulcer prophylaxis with H2 blockers (e.g., Ranitidine) and antacids (e.g., Maalox).
- *GU*: Place Foley catheter to monitor urine output (UOP), keep UOP = 0.5–2 ml/kg/h.
- *Eye*: Careful exam with fluorescein to check for abrasions. Topical antibiotics if needed.

When to Refer to Tertiary Center

- Concern for airway compromise.
- Burn >10 % of infant BSA or >15 % of child's BSA.
- Electrical or chemical burns, burns of face, hands, feet, perineum or joints, full thickness burns, circumferential burns; concern of abuse/neglect; burns in a child with underlying illness; smoke inhalation; CO poisoning or burns associated with life-threatening injuries.

Approach to Poisoning in a Child

Prevention

- Educate the community on the importance of keeping all poisons out of reach of children.
- Discourage families from storing poisons commonly kept in the home in used drinking containers, because children may try to drink from them.

Treatment

If you suspect poisoning, do the following *immediately*:

- Lay unconscious child on his/her side and monitor ABCs.
- If there is altered mental status consider carbon monoxide poisoning and give 100 % oxygen.
- For *skin decontamination*, remove contaminated clothing. Wash patient with soap and water. Remember to use protective clothing for yourself.
- For *eye decontamination*, irrigate with clean water or normal saline for 20 min.
- For *oral decontamination*, if the child is awake and alert, give ample PO fluids to dilute the poison (~250 ml of water every 15 min).
- *Caution:* Do not make a child vomit if he has swallowed kerosene, gasoline (petrol), bleach, paint thinner, or strong acids or corrosive substances, most hydrocarbons, or is unconscious.
- If available, the best oral decontamination is activated charcoal (AC). Dose for children is 1 g/kg PO and adolescents 50–100 g, mixed with water at a 1:4 ratio.

AC is contraindicated in patients with depressed mental status without airway protection, bowel obstruction, caustic ingestion, hydrocarbon ingestion, and foreign-body ingestion.

Approach to the Child with Near-Drowning

- Give rescue breathing while removing victim from the water.
- Pay attention to cervical spine precautions and remove victim in a prone position.
- If injury is suspected, move the individual the least amount possible and begin cardiopulmonary resuscitation (CPR).
- In the patient with an altered mental status, check airway for foreign material and vomitus. Debris visible in the oropharynx should be removed with a finger-sweep maneuver.
- Do not use the abdominal thrust (Heimlich) maneuver.
- If the patient is hypothermic because of cold water drowning, remove wet clothing and gently dry the skin to rewarm the patient slowly. Can use warm, humidified oxygen, blankets, and warm IV fluids. Avoid fast, active rewarming to avoid warming aftershock.

Approach to the Child with Animal, Snake, Scorpion or Spider Bites

Animal Bite Management

- Rabies is an important consideration as it occurs in 150 countries and territories worldwide. Rabid dogs cause the majority of human rabies deaths.

- Carefully explore wound to identify injury to underlying structures and any foreign body.

    Irrigate wound and debride devitalized tissue. If a possibly rabid animal bit the child, thoroughly flush the wound for a minimum of 15 min with soap and water, detergent, or povidone–iodine to kill the rabies virus.
- Close open lacerations in healthy patients with wounds that meet all of the following criteria: (1) cosmetically important (e.g., facial lacerations), (2) clinically uninfected, (3) less than 12 h old (24 h on the face), and (4) wounds NOT located on the hand or foot.
- Do NOT seal with tissue adhesive.
- Do NOT close wounds at high risk for infection: (1) crush injuries, (2) puncture wounds, (3) bites involving the hands or feet, (4) wounds more than 12 h old (24 h old on face), (5) cat or human bites (except those to the face), or (6) bite wounds in compromised hosts (e.g., immunocompromised, absent spleen or splenic dysfunction, venous stasis).
- Indications for antibiotics: (1) deep puncture wounds, (2) moderate to severe crush injuries, (3) wounds in areas with venous or lymph compromise, (4) wounds on hands or near joints, (5) wounds requiring surgical repair, or (6) wounds in immunocompromised hosts.
- Give tetanus and rabies prophylaxis if needed.

Snake Bite

- A significant proportion of snakebites do not result in envenomation, and patients can be discharged after observation.
- *Management:*
- Try to determine if the snake was poisonous:
    - Two prominent fang marks → likely poisonous.
    - Two rows of teeth marks, but no fang marks → likely not poisonous.
- Then, clean the wound, keep the limb immobile and below the level of the heart.
- Remove jewelry on the limb due to potential for rapid swelling.
- Clinically assess for sign of envenomation (neurotoxicity, coagulopathy, shock, rhabdomyolysis and renal failure). If signs of envenomation, give antivenom and take precautions for allergic shock. Treat other symptoms (e.g., infection, pain) appropriately based on local resources.
- Give tetanus antitoxin. If clinically well, maintain under close observation and discharge after 6–12 h.
- *Do not:*
    - Cut the skin or the flesh around the bite.
    - Tourniquet any area of the body.
    - Use ice directly on the skin as a cold compresses.
    - Try to mouth-suction the blood or the venom out of the bite.
    - Allow the patient to consume alcohol.

Scorpion Stings

Although normally painful but not dangerous for adults, for physically small children, scorpion stings on the head or body can have high morbidity and mortality. Management includes the following:

- Monitor ABCs and watch for respiratory depression.
- Immobilize the limb below the heart.
- Inject scorpion antivenom within 2 h of the sting.
- Hospitalize for priapism, vomiting, SBP >160, or hemodynamic instability.
- Acetaminophen for pain and benzodiazepines for muscle spasms.
- Give tetanus antitoxin.
- Abatement of symptoms and ability is dependent on species and variable.

Black Widow and Other Spider Bites

Most spider bites can cause significant pain but are not dangerous. However, bites from black widows and other *Latrodectus* spiders can be dangerous for a physically small child. A black widow bite can cause muscle cramps, including rigid abdominal muscles, which can be confused with appendicitis. Black widow bite management includes the following:

- Acetaminophen or ibuprofen for pain. Diazepam for muscle spasm.
- Treat signs of allergic shock. Take diphenhydramine 5 mg/kg/day PO divided every 6 h for itchiness.
- Give tetanus antitoxin. If available, give antivenom.

Recommended Reading

1. Pediatric surgery and medicine for hostile environments, Michael Fuenfer and Kevin Creamer editors. 2010.
2. Krug E, editor. Injury: a leading cause of the global burden of disease. Geneva: WHO; 1999.
3. Prasad P, editor. Massachusetts General Hospital for Children. Pocket pediatrics: The Massachusetts General Hospital for Children handbook of pediatrics. Philadelphia: Lippincott Williams & Wilkins; 2010
4. Werner D. Where there is no doctor: a village health care handbook. Palo Alto: Hesperian Foundation; 1994.
5. Fleisher GR, Ludwig S, Henretig FM, editors. Textbook of pediatric emergency medicine. 5th ed. Philadelphia: Lippincott Williams & Wilkins; 2006.
6. UpToDate, Rose BD (ed) UpToDate, Waltham, MA; 2012

Chapter 25
Child and Adolescent Mental Health

Giuseppe Raviola and Sarabeth Broder-Fingert

Keywords Mental health • Culture • Psychoeducation • Psychosocial • Nonpharmacologic interventions • Community-based support systems • Psychotherapy • Pharmacologic interventions • Internalizing problems • Anxiety • Depression • Trauma • Suicide • Psychosomatic • Externalizing problems • ADHD • Conduct • Substance use • Psychosis • Schizophrenia • Bipolar • Eating disorders

Overview

- Mental disorders are a significant cause of disability in children and adolescents, more prevalent than leukemia, diabetes and AIDS combined.
- Mental health services are greatly underfunded in most low-income countries, particularly for children and adolescents. There is a paucity of trained specialist providers in most of the world.

G. Raviola, M.D., M.P.H.
Psychiatry Quality Program, Department of Psychiatry, Boston Children's Hospital, Boston, MA, USA

Department of Psychiatry, Harvard Medical School, Boston, MA, USA

Program in Global Mental Health and Social Change, Department of Global Health and Social Medicine, Harvard Medical School, Boston, MA, USA

S. Broder-Fingert, M.D., M.A. (✉)
Department of Pediatrics, Center for Child and Adolescent Health Research and Policy, Massachusetts General Hospital, 100 Cambridge Street, 15th Floor, Boston, MA, USA

Department of Pediatrics, Harvard Medical School, Boston, MA, USA
e-mail: sbroderfingert@gmail.com

- While culture and local belief systems can inform how mental disorders are manifested, there exists a common set of broad mental health problems and disorders that can present across cultures.
- Basic skills in spoken communication, evaluation, and psychoeducation can be important interventions for children and families.
- Psychosocial approaches that include a range of nonpharmacologic interventions that engage the child, adolescent and family in the process of adaptive change should take precedence over a medical or pharmacologic approach. This requires familiarity with the range of local resources, formal (medical systems) and informal (community systems), as well as the variety of "talking" therapeutic techniques and their indication in context.

The Global Burden of Disease

- Neuropsychiatric disorders comprise at least 13 % of the total global burden of illness in Disability Adjusted Life Years (DALYs)—adults and children combined—and are the most economically costly set of non-communicable diseases to societies.
- It is estimated that at least 20 % of children aged 9–17 have a diagnosable mental disorder with impairment in functioning. Most do not receive treatment.
- Anxiety disorders are the most frequent condition in children, followed by behavior disorders, mood disorders and substance use disorders.
- Suicide is the third leading cause of death among adolescents worldwide, with unipolar depressive disorder becoming the leading cause of lifetime disability—adults and children combined—globally.

Scope of the Problem

- ~50 % of all adult mental disorders begin before the age of 14, with continuity from infancy into adulthood.
- Disproportionate allocation of economic resources exists, with governments spending an average of approximately 4 % of healthcare budgets on mental health across high- and low-income countries (2 % in low-income countries).
- Almost half of the world's population lives in a country where, on average, there is one psychiatrist or less to serve 200,000 people.

The Mental Health and Psychosocial Evaluation

- A balanced *bio-psycho-social* approach to case assessment and formulation is essential. This requires adequate evaluation.
- Stigma, including within the health care professions, is a significant barrier to safe and effective management of problems related to mental health. Rapport

- with and respect for parents as well as the child or adolescent is critical for reducing and managing stigma, and developing a trusting working alliance.
- While the Diagnostic and Statistical Manual of Mental Disorders (DSM 4, 1994) represents the official classification system of psychiatric conditions in the USA, it should be used with caution in other contexts and cultures. WHO endorses the International Statistical Classification of Diseases and Related Health Problems (ICD). In some circumstances, neither of these may capture particular clinical presentations in local context.
- Interviewing in the context of a pediatric assessment requires adequate time and privacy. The purpose of an evaluation should be explained to the child and parents (for example, "to make sure things are going OK at home, at school, and with friends"). Issues of confidentiality should be discussed across settings and cultures, with attention to the limits of confidentiality in context. This includes legal considerations. Adolescents in particular should be offered an interview separate from parents.
- Essential components include: medical history and differential with knowledge of potential contributors; family genogram and current supports; history of trauma, loss or displacement; assessment of risk (suicide, violence, sexual history, drugs and alcohol); knowledge of areas of strength; and collateral contact with family members or others close to the child/adolescent in the community.
- Because of high degree of comorbidity with medical problems, brief screening should be attempted in all major developmentally appropriate categories of cognitive, developmental, emotional, behavioral, and social disturbance, including problems with mood, anxiety, attention, behavior, thinking and perception, substance use, social relatedness, eating, elimination, development, language and learning.
- The "11 Mental Health Action Signs" (Action Signs Project, 2011) provide a useful guide for inquiry with older youth and adolescents and their parents, preceded by the transition statement, "Now I'd like to ask you about some other issues that I ask all parents and kids about":
    - Feeling very sad or withdrawn for more than 2 weeks
    - Seriously trying to harm or kill self, or making plans to do so
    - Sudden overwhelming fear for no reason, sometimes with a racing heart or fast breathing
    - Involvement in fights, using a weapon, or wanting to hurt others
    - Severe out-of-control behavior that can hurt self or others
    - Not eating, throwing up, or using other means to make yourself lose weight
    - Intense worries or fears that get in the way of daily activities
    - Extreme difficulty in concentrating or staying still that puts person in physical danger or causes school failure
    - Repeated use of drugs or alcohol
    - Severe mood swings that cause problems in relationships
    - Drastic changes in behavior or personality
- While sometimes difficult to obtain in contexts where formal psychiatric services are not common, a family history of psychiatric problems can be helpful in assessing a child's biological or social vulnerability. Recall that general categories of

illness in adults can include: suicide; depression; bipolar disorder; anxiety; panic disorder; obsessive-compulsive disorder (OCD); alcoholism; ADHD; schizophrenia; pervasive developmental disorder; and personality disorder.
- Functional impairment can be assessed by inquiring about symptoms and functioning in major life domains. These domains are included in the HEADSS (home, education, activities, drugs, sexuality, suicide/depression) interview guide (Cohen, MacKenzie, Yates 1991), for use in interviewing both parents and adolescents:
  - Home
    - "How do you get along with your parents/family?"
  - Education
    - "Do you go to school? If no, why not?"
    - "How do you like school and your teachers?"
    - "How well do you do in school?"
  - Activities
    - "What do you like to do?"
    - "Do you have a best friend or group of good friends?"
  - Drugs
    - "Have you ever used alcohol or drugs?"
  - Sexuality
    - "Are there any issues regarding sexuality or sexual activity that are of concern to you?"
  - Suicide/depression
    - "Everyone feels sad or angry some of the time. How about you?"
    - "Did you ever feel so upset that you wished you were not alive or so angry you wanted to hurt someone else badly?"
- General review of symptoms screening: "I'm now going to ask you some questions about how you feel most of the time. Over the past several weeks, how would you say you have felt most of the day? Over the past few months?"
- Always assess strengths and environmental resources, with focused consideration of how to enhance these while treating disabling symptoms.

Principles of Care and Management

- Local knowledge is critical to understanding presentation of mental disorders in context. Integration of Euro-American and local concepts of mental health in a globalized, rapidly changing world remain a real, but surmountable, challenge in global health.

- Addressing social determinants of poor health such as lack of basic needs or education, parental and environmental stressors and/or illness, or other major traumas, losses or displacements, is essential.
- Basic tools exist for delivering safe, effective, evidence-based, and culturally sound mental health services. An optimal approach integrates psychobiological and psychosocial perspectives; works to balance approaches that strengthen social and economic structures; enhances resilience and mobilization of innate individual and community resources; and, when resources are available, addresses acute forms of distress and illness based on rational clinical practice that is attuned to culture and local context.
- Given the lack of specialists, a range of people can potentially provide components of psychosocial and /or mental health services ("task sharing"): community members (leaders, religious figures, teachers), community health workers, nurses, social workers, psychologists, and physicians. Components include psychosocial assistance (such as financial, nutritional, and housing support or establishing a safe environment), psychoeducation, screening, triage and referral, psychotherapeutic treatments, and psychopharmacologic treatments.
- Utilizing basic skills in communication, evaluation, and psychoeducation are important initial interventions. These can include (adapted from Verdeli H, 2012):
  - Basic interview skills:
    - Speak with the person in a place that promotes confidentiality and makes the person feel safe.
    - Be sensitive and respect the person's emotional vulnerability.
    - Show empathy.
    - Use active listening.
    - Ask open-ended questions that will help you to understand the problems that the person is having in her or his life.
    - Learn the person's whole story.
    - Meet the person at her or his energy level.
    - Follow the person's lead about religion and spirituality.
  - Psychoeducation:
    - Letting the person know that she or he may have a mental health problem or disorder (naming the problem), and explaining to the child/adolescent and family members what that means in context.
    - Giving support. This includes giving the person and family hope, assigning the person the sick role if appropriate, and helping the person and the family to mobilize social supports.
- Psychotherapy in children can be effective in reducing symptomatology. Effect sizes in research studies range from 0.71 to 0.84, as large or larger than the effects of psychopharmacology and other medicines for many physical illnesses. Psychotherapy involves a series of discrete steps including: assessment; deciding

upon treatment with the patient; obtaining treatment assent and consent; a monitoring plan; and implementing treatment. Cognitive, emotional, and/or behavioral symptoms are identified that become the targets for evidence-based psychotherapeutic interventions, elements of which can be combined with other treatment approaches, including psychopharmacology. *The quality of the therapist-patient alliance is the strongest predictor of treatment outcome.* Psychotherapeutic approaches in rank order of comparative effectiveness include (adapted from Walter H, DeMaso D in Nelson Textbook of Pediatrics):

- Cognitive-behavioral therapy: First-line treatment for anxiety and mild depression. Based on the theory that antecedent events stimulate thoughts and beliefs that cause emotional consequences. Problem-oriented.
- Interpersonal therapy: Also effective for depression. Addressed relationships in the "here and now," with a focus on four areas: grief; role transitions; role disputes; and interpersonal deficits.
- Family Therapy: Problems exist in family interactions and not just in individuals. Solutions involve improving communication, reframing of behaviors and giving directives to disrupt dysfunctional patterns.
- Psychodynamic psychotherapy: Based on the belief that much of one's mental activity, including internal conflicts, occurs outside one's awareness.
- Supportive psychotherapy: Aims to minimize levels of emotional distress.
- Narrative therapy: Based on the principle that self-stories organize, interpret and assign meaning to events in a person's life.

• Medication should only be used for severe presentations of illness, when clearly indicated, sustainable, and when adequate follow-up is possible. To ensure safe and appropriate use, psychopharmacology prescription should involve best practice principles that include:

- Identification and assessment of clear target symptoms agreed upon with the child/adolescent and family.
- Search for medical factors that may be causing or exacerbating target symptoms.
- Completion of medical tests that have a bearing on treatment course.
- Evidence of: clear disturbance in functioning; research findings that support use of the medication for the specific target symptom; and suboptimal response to psychosocial interventions that may include environmental changes or psychotherapy, if available.
- Consideration of likely efficacy, potential adverse side effects, practical considerations such as formulations available and dosing schedules, and clearly articulated informed consent from parents with assent from patient.
- Establishment of a plan for monitoring of effects, including: outcomes measurement; time course of effects; follow-up; alternative plans if response suboptimal; and baseline laboratory data if necessary.
- Consideration of withdrawal of medication after 6–12 months to determine if still needed.

- A target symptom approach to management, emphasizing use of a single medication, single dose adjustments at a time:
  - Agitation
    - Atypical antipsychotics (ex: risperidone); monitor for sedation, weight gain, akathisia or dystonia (treat with anticholinergic), diabetes, prolonged QTc.
    - Typical antipsychotics (ex: haloperidol or chlorpromazine; avoid cotreatment); monitor for sedation, weight gain, akathisia or dystonia (treat with anticholinergic), tardive dyskinesia, diabetes, prolonged QTc.
    - Anxiolytic (ex: benzodiazepine such as diazepam); monitor for sedation, behavioral disinhibition.
  - Anxiety
    - Antidepressant (ex: fluoxetine or other selective serotonin reuptake inhibitor [SSRI]); monitor for suicidal ideation, stomach upset, poor sleep/activation.
    - Anxiolytic
  - Hyperactivity, inattention, impulsivity related to ADHD
    - Stimulant (ex: methylphenidate- or amphetamine-based medications); monitor for reduced appetite, poor sleep/activation.
    - Clonidine, an alpha-2 adrenergic agonist, for impulsivity; monitor blood pressure, used with caution at higher doses.
    - Bupropion, also an effective antidepressant, for inattention; monitor for seizures, use with caution in those with prior history of head trauma.
    - Atomoxetine, also effective for anxiety, for inattention; monitor for suicidal ideation.
  - Mania
    - Atypical antipsychotic
    - Mood stabilizer (ex: carbamazepine or lithium); monitor for reduced WBC count (carbamazepine), toxicity with dehydration (lithium).
  - Psychosis
    - Atypical antipsychotic
    - Typical antipsychotic
- Dosing of medication should generally be conservative, with attention to the specific clinical situation, indication and other medications the patient is taking.

List of Specific Disorders and Problems

Internalizing Problems

Anxiety

- Epidemiology: Prevalence approximately 5–18 %. Genetic susceptibility, psychosocial factors, often comorbid with depression and other disorders. Must differentiate between normal from abnormal anxiety across development.
- Screening questions:
  - "Are there things that you are afraid of?"
  - "Do you often feel nervous? Are there things that bring this on?"
  - "Do you have thoughts that you can't get out of your head, even though they really bother you? What are they?"
  - "Are there things that you feel you must do to help you feel less anxious—like washing your hands, checking on something, or counting things?"
- Clinical presentation (DSM-based criteria): Maintain broad differential and always consider anxiety and/or depression when meeting children or adolescents with new or unusual physiologic, perceptual or behavioral symptoms, somatic complaints, irritability and social withdrawal. Younger children may be less able to verbalize feeling states. Older children with anxiety may present with psychotic or melancholic symptoms or suicidal behavior.
  - GAD—most common (DSM 4: at least 6 months of symptoms.) Excessive worry and anxiety, more days than not, about multiple concerns. Child has trouble controlling them. At least 1/6 symptoms along with anxious feelings: restless/easily fatigued/concentration poor or mind blank/irritable or cranky/muscle tension/sleep disturbance.
  - Post-Traumatic Stress Disorder (DSM 4: duration >1 month)—Exposed to traumatic event; at time child was intensely scared, confused or horrified. Reexperiencing symptoms (1 symptom); avoidance, social detachment or emotional numbing (3 symptoms); hyper-arousal (2 symptoms).
  - Obsessive Compulsive Disorder (DSM 4: duration >1 h per day)—Presence of either obsessions (thoughts that happen over and over, cause anxiety or distress, come from within mind and are inappropriate/person tries to neutralize them or ignore them/thoughts are not just excessive worries about real life problems) or compulsions (repetitive behaviors, following a strict rule, child feels he or she must do to ward off a thought or dreaded occurrence; behaviors have no protective effect in reality); Person realizes that OCD symptoms are excessive or unreasonable; symptoms cause marked distress, are time consuming (at least 1 h per day), or cause significant interference with normal activities and routines. Refer to C-YBOCS for detailed history. 10 % with Beta-hemolytic streptococcal infection.

- Separation Anxiety Disorder (DSM 4: at least 3 symptoms for >4 weeks)—Child experiences excessive anxiety concerning separation from home or attachment figures. Separation anxiety is accompanied by at least 3 of: recurrent distress anticipating separation/worry about parent's safety/worry about losing or being separated from parent/reluctance to go to school or elsewhere because of fear of separation/reluctance to be alone at home/reluctance to go to sleep without parent/recurrent nightmares about being separated/repeated physical complaints when anticipating or thinking about separation. Duration of symptoms is at least 4 weeks and onset is before 18. Anxiety causes sign distress or interferes with school, relationships, and activities.
- Panic/agoraphobia: Discrete episodes of intense fear or discomfort in which anxiety symptoms began abruptly and peaked within about 10 min and accompanied by at least 4/13 symptoms (DSM 4): dizziness/palpitations/chest pain/sweating/chills/trembling/numbness or tingling/shortness of breath/choking/nausea/feelings of unreality/fear of losing control/fear of dying.
- Other: Selective mutism (consistent failure to speak in social situations >1 month); Social/specific phobia; acute stress disorder (due to trauma<1 month ago; do not diagnose PTSD).

- Differential diagnosis: Normal anxiety, anxiety due to a general medical condition, adjustment disorder, substance-induced, Pervasive Developmental Disorder (PDD), school refusal related to conduct disorder, delusional or psychotic disorder (rare).
- Management: Support coping and relaxation; refer for CBT by specialist if available; if severe, medication—1st line is fluoxetine or other SSRI; adjunct is diazepam or other benzodiazepine (also for severe distress), diphenhydramine for sleep (monitor additive sedation if concurrent with benzo). Monitor for disinhibition/dysregulation with benzodiazepine. Educate about seizure risk with sudden stopping of benzodiazepine. Additional interventions include support with (adapted from Patel V, Where There Is No Psychiatrist):
    - Coping with stress
        i. "Identify situations that make you feel stressed"
        ii. "Imagine how your friends would respond to these situations"
        iii. "List as many ways as you can think of to make these situations less stressful"
        iv. "Imagine yourself doing these things"
        v. "Rehearse a situation before you face it"
        vi. "Share your stress with others, such as friends, family or teachers"
        vii. "Do not be embarrassed to see a counselor"
    - Relaxation and breathing exercises: Relaxation is a very useful way of reducing the effects of stress on the human mind for some adolescents and children. It is used in traditional types of meditation as well as in modern psychology. Most methods of relaxation use some form of breathing exercise. Relaxation exercise can be done at any time of day. The person should devote at least 10 min a day to the exercise. It is best done in a room that is quiet and where the person will not be disturbed.

- Begin the exercise by lying down or sitting in a comfortable position. There is no special position; any position which the person finds comfortable is the right one.
- Close your eyes.
- After about 10 s, start concentrating your mind on your breathing rhythm.
- Concentrate on breathing slow, regular, steady breaths through the nose.
- If the person asks how slow the rhythm should be, you can suggest that she or he should breathe in until he can count slowly to 3, then breathe out to the count of 3 and then pause for the count of 3, until she breathes in again.
- You can suggest that each time the person breathes out, she could say in her mind the word "relax." People who are religious can use a word that has some importance to their faith. For example, a Christian might say "Praise the Lord."
- Demonstrate to the person how to breathe steady, deep breaths.
- The person should continue doing this for at least 10 min.
- Explain to the person that if she practices daily, she will begin to feel the benefits of relaxation within 2 weeks. With adequate experience, she may even be able to relax in a variety of situations, for example while sitting in a bus.

- Prognosis: most resolve but 50 % can develop other mental disorder.

Depression

- Epidemiology: Occurs in 2 % of children and 4–8 % in adolescents. 40–90 % with one co-occurring disorder and 50 % with 2 co-occurring disorders. Most common include anxiety, disruptive behavior, ADHD and substance use disorder.
- Screening questions:
  - "Would you say that you have been getting satisfaction from school and your friendships and the things you do every day? Have you been enjoying your favorite activities?"
  - "Would you say that you are very hard on yourself? Have you ever felt hopeless, as though life was not worth living anymore? Do you have plans for the future?"
  - "Have you felt sad, hopeless or empty for several days or weeks at a time? Have you felt irritable or tired most of the time for hardly any reason at all?"
  - "How long do these feelings last? What is the longest they have lasted?"
- Etiology: Multifactorial, highly familial with genetic and environmental influences including parental psychopathology, impaired parenting, loss, physical and sexual abuse, neglect, exposure to violence, other correlates of disadvantaged socioeconomic status.
- Clinical presentation: at least 5 symptoms >2 weeks with change from previous functioning (DSM 4). Must have depressed/irritable mood or loss interest/pleasure; also, weight gain or loss, sleep problems, psychomotor agitation or

retardation, poor energy, guilt/hopelessness/poor self-esteem, decreased concentration, thoughts of death.
- Differential diagnosis: Includes anxiety (also comorbid), substance abuse, adjustment disorder, ADHD, bipolar disorder, dysthymic disorder, medication side effects, failure to thrive, sleep disturbance, anemia, hypothyroid disease, HIV, mononucleosis, Addison's Disease, diabetes, epilepsy, Wilson's disease
- Diagnosis: Clinical diagnosis through interview and evaluation. Obtain a thorough medical, developmental, social and family history. Screening tools helpful but not sufficient alone. Consider adjunctive use of Pediatric Symptoms Checklist (6–12 years old). In adolescents consider use of PHQ-9. Screen parents for depression and anxiety.
- Management: Can include psychoeducation, problem-solving, behavioral activation, relaxation, psychotherapy/ cognitive-behavioral therapy (CBT), psychopharmacology.
  - Behavioral activation: The person identifies activities and relationships that she or he values and finds rewarding. Then the provider encourages the person to engage in the activity or relationship for a period of time each day. Over the course of the sessions, the provider and the person evaluate how the activities are affecting the person's symptoms.
  - SSRIs-fluoxetine or other (monitor for reduced appetite, poor sleep, suicidal ideation, worsening anxiety, "switching" to mania in those with family history of bipolar disorder).
- Prognosis: Median duration of episode 8 months for clinical referred youth. Recurrence of 70 % after 5 years. 20–40 % of those develop bipolar disorder. 60 % of youth with depression think about suicide, 30 % attempt.
- Distinguish from juvenile onset bipolar disorder: Lifetime prevalence of 1 %. Often begins with an episode of depression, not mania.
  - Criteria for diagnosis (DSM 4): Distinct period of excessively elevated, expansive, and/or irritable mood; has 3 of the following 7 symptoms: distractibility/increased reckless involvement in pleasurable activities/grandiosity/flight of ideas or racing thoughts/activity level increased/sleep decreased/talkative or pressured speech (DIGFAST).
  - Manic episode: lasts greater than 1 week, and associated with marked impairment, hospitalization, or psychotic symptoms.
  - Hypomanic episode: manic symptoms have lasted greater than 4 days and obvious changes observed by others, but no marked impairment.
  - Bipolar Disorder with psychotic features: history of psychotic symptoms and occurring only during the manic episode.
  - Bipolar I: at least 1 manic episode.
  - Bipolar II: at least 1 hypomanic episode plus 1 major depressive episode.
  - Bipolar NOS: no full blown Mania or Major Depression or insufficient duration.

Self-Harm/Suicide and Safety/Violence Assessment

- Suicide is the leading cause of injury and death worldwide. Each year 1 million people worldwide die by suicide. Most common in those with mood disorder.
- Screening questions:

    Self-Harm/Suicide

    - "I now want to ask you some questions about your safety. The most important thing we want to do here today is make sure that you feel safe here, and at home."
    - "Have things ever been so difficult/Have there been other times in your life that you wanted to die? Thought about taking your own life? Do you currently feel at risk in any way of harming yourself? Have you ever tried to harm yourself? When and how?"
    - "Has there been a time when you have thought about hurting someone else? How about currently?"

    Safety/Violence

    - "Do you currently feel safe at home? Are people nice to each other at home? Are there arguments? Do they ever turn into fights, with yelling or hitting?"
    - "Are there any guns or other weapons at home?"
    - "Have you ever been threatened or hurt physically by either a family member or someone else close to you? Does anyone ever say things to you at home or at school that hurt your feelings? Have you experienced any bullying at school? Either at home or at school, has anyone ever touched you inappropriately against your will? If yes: I am so sorry to hear that that happened. Do you know who it was? Do you know where they are now? Do you feel safe from them? Is there anything we can do here today, right now, to help with this?"

- Clinical presentation: Earliest onset is age 3–4 years, with sharp rise in adolescence. 65 % can name precipitating event.
- Risk factors: preexisting mental disorder (anxiety, depression, conduct disorder, substance use, psychosis, mania), negative self-attribution, stressful life events (academic or social problems, being bullied, trouble with law, family instability, questioning sexual orientation, newly diagnosed condition, recent loss), lower educational attainment.
- Identification: Ask screening questions, exploring intent, potential lethality past and present, written note or plan, altered mental status, supportiveness of family, home supervision, access to firearms/medication/alcohol/drugs at home; gather information from multiple sources; identify personal and household strengths.
- Management: High risk should be hospitalized if available although inpatient conditions should be assessed. Remove means of self-harm. Secure home environment. Set up frequent follow-up either at home or in clinic prior to departure from clinic. Develop plan involving patient and family supports. Consider medication for symptoms.

Psychosomatic Illness

- Medically unexplained physical symptoms causing distress and functional impairment. Somatoform disorders defined by predominantly psychologic factors contributing to the presentation of somatic symptoms.
  - Lack of child-specific diagnostic criteria.
  - 7 types: somatization, undifferentiated somatoform, conversion, pain, hypochondriasis, body dysmorphic disorder and somatoform disorder NOS.
- Epidemiology: Somatic complaints 4.5–10 % in boys, 10–15 % in girls. Conversion disorder between 0.5 and 10 %.
- Etiology: Stressful life events, local cultural ideas about acceptable expression of psychologic distress, genetic predisposition to depression/anxiety, lower socioeconomic status, family illness, medical illness, sensitive/anxious temperament, reinforced attention for complaints, comorbid mental disorder, prior history of somatization
- Clinical presentation: Recurrent abdominal pain and headaches most common.
  - Somatization (DSM 4): Many physical complaints including pain, gastrointestinal, sexual, pseudoneurological.
  - Conversion (DSM 4): One or more symptoms or deficits affecting voluntary motor or sensory function that suggest a neurologic or other medical condition. Examples include "nonelectrical" seizures and loss of limb function.
- Differential diagnosis: Physical illness, anxiety, depression, factitious disorder and factitious disorder by proxy, malingering.
- Diagnosis: Thorough physical examination may rule out other cause. Often there is overlap of psychologic and medical pathology, and one should be careful not to take an "either-or" position in formulation, or in discussing with patient and family.
- Management: Education of patient and family by first informing of medical evaluation findings without implied blame or judgment. Gently explore resistance, give time for adaptation to findings. Regular team meetings to reduce miscommunications that can promote mistrust and frustration. A rehabilitation model facilitates focus away from cure to normal adaptive functioning. CBT, individual supportive psychotherapy and family therapy can help adjustment of child to illness and learn new coping strategies. Psychopharmacology for comorbid depression and anxiety.
- Prognosis: 50–100 % have significant improvement or recovery.

Externalizing Problems/Behavioral Disorders

Attention Deficit Hyperactivity Disorder (ADHD)

- Epidemiology: Prevalence of 5–10 %; World Health Organization (WHO) uses the term "hyperkinetic disorder"
- Screening Questions:
  - "Do you have difficulty focusing? Feeling like you can't slow down? Could you tell me more about that?"
- Clinical presentation (DSM 4):
  - Hyperactive Type: At least 6 symptoms of difficulty with: hyperactivity and impulsivity/fidgeting/staying seated/running and climbing/playing quietly/always on the go/talks/blurting/waiting/interrupting
  - Inattentive Type: At least 6 symptoms of difficulty with: attention to details/sustaining attention/listening/finishing work/organization/avoiding tasks/losing.
  - Things/distractability/forgetting.
  - Combined Type: both present.
- Diagnosis: Careful history and evaluation required; started before age 7, lasting longer than 6 months; behavioral scales such as Vanderbilt, Conner or SNAP helpful but not sufficient alone.
- Differential diagnosis: Chronic illness (migraine headache, absence seizures, asthma, allergies), enlarged tonsils, sleep disorder, substance abuse, depression, anxiety, OCD, PDD.
- Comorbidity with learning disability, language disorder, mood and anxiety disorders.
- Management: Psychoeducation; behavioral management and targeting of specific skill areas (disruptive behavior, difficulty completing schoolwork, failure to obey home or school rules); parental guidance and support; if available, stimulant (methylphenidate- or amphetamine-based) or non-stimulant medications (atomoxetine, bupropion, alpha-blockers such as clonidine or guanfacine) with caution. Monitor for reduced appetite, growth pattern, sleep quality, worsening mood, anxiety, or mania.
- Prognosis: ADHD prevalence decreases to 2 % in adults. 40–60 % of childhood ADHD persists to adulthood. Increased risk-taking behavior, accidents, educational and occupational difficulty, and drug abuse.

Oppositional Defiant and Conduct Problems

- Persistent behavior in which basic rights of others or age-appropriate norms are violated.
- Prevalence: 1–10 %. More common in extreme poverty, boys.

- Clinical presentation (DSM 4):
  - Oppositional-Defiant Disorder (ODD): "Do you have difficulty when adults tell you 'no'?"; At least 6 months of negative, hostile, and defiant behavior; at least 4/8 symptoms including: loses temper/argues/defies rules/deliberately annoys others/easily annoyed/blames others for mistakes/angry and resentful/spiteful or vindictive; causes significant impairment in social, academic or occupational functioning. Note absence of physical aggression or other severe antisocial behavior.
  - Conduct Disorder (CD): "Have you had difficulty with the police? Have you been involved in fighting at home or outside the home?"; Repetitive persistent behavior that violates basic rights of others or societal rules; 4/16 symptoms over past 12 months and at least 1 over past 6 months, including: aggression—bullying/fighting/using weapons to steal/physically cruel to people/physically cruel to animals/stole while confronting victim/forcing someone to have sex; destruction—setting fires/destroying property; deceitful—breaking into others' property/lying to "con" or avoid obligations/stealing nontrivial things; and rule violation—repeated curfew violation (less than 13 y/o)/running away from home 2 different times, or 1 prolonged time/truancy from school. If meets criteria for both ODD and CD, CD takes precedence.
- Differential diagnosis: ADHD, bipolar disorder, developmental delay or disorder, communication disorder, psychoses, mood disorder, history of physical/sexual abuse, reactive attachment in response to prior trauma, substance abuse, seizure disorder.
- Diagnosis: Review detailed list of behaviors, inquire about head trauma, other trauma, sexual abuse
- Management: Parent management training, social–emotional skills training, multisystemic therapy, medication for comorbid conditions.
  - Parent management training:
    i. Developing warm, supportive relationship with child.
    ii. Providing predictable, structured household environment.
    iii. Setting clear and simple household rules.
    iv. Consistently praising and materially rewarding positive behavior.
    v. Consistently ignoring annoying behavior followed by praise when behavior ceases.
    vi. Consistently giving consequences such as time out or loss of privileges for dangerous or destructive behavior.
  - Social-emotional skills training:
    i. Introducing skill.
    ii. Verbally instructing the skill.
    iii. Modeling the skill.
    iv. Role-playing the skill.
    v. Coaching during skill practice by the child.

vi. Summarizing.
vii. Giving homework to practice the skill outside the training situation.

- Multisystemic therapy: A treatment that involves extensive contact between the therapist and the multiple life contexts of the patient, especially the family, school and peer group, with goal of developing competencies and rewarding adaptive behavior. Resource-intensive.
- Prognosis: Most disruptive symptoms peak between 8 and 11 years and decline in frequency. Earlier age at onset predicts worse prognosis. 30 % with ODD progress to CD, with higher progression with comorbid ADHD. Substantial fraction with CD develop antisocial personality disorder as adults.

Substance Use Disorders

Alcohol and Drug Abuse

- Epidemiology: More than 2 billion alcohol and 200 million illicit drug users worldwide. Alcohol contributes to 3.2 % of all deaths globally and 9 % in 15–29 year age group. Associated with negative outcomes (e.g., HIV, STI). More likely in men.
- Screening Questions:
  - "Have you ever tried cigarettes? Do you smoke currently? How much? Do you want to stop? Would you be open to trying?"
  - "Have you ever tried alcohol to make yourself feel good? How about (marijuana, mushrooms, speed, crack, cocaine, heroin, ecstasy, LSD) or any other drugs? Do you ever sniff glue of gasoline, or drink home brew?"
  - "CRAFFT Questionnaire (Boston Children's Hospital 2001): Has anyone ever expressed *concern* about your drinking or drug use? Have you ever driven in a *car (or on a scooter/motorcycle)* with someone who was drinking or high or when you were? Have you ever drank or used drugs to *relax*, feel better or fit in? Have you ever used drugs or alcohol when you were *alone*? Have you ever *forgotten* things you did while drinking alcohol or using drugs? Have your *family or friends* ever told you to cut down? Have you ever gotten into *trouble* while using drugs or drinking?" 2 or more yes responses are of concern.
- Clinical presentation: Impaired control over drinking, preoccupation with alcohol, use of alcohol despite adverse consequences, distortion of thinking/denial, continuous or periodic drinking.
- Differential diagnosis: Often comorbid with mood or anxiety disorders.
- Diagnosis—For severe alcohol use findings on physical exam include tremulousness, elevated blood pressure, rhinophyma, telangiectasias, tachycardia, hepatosplenomegaly, peripheral neuropathy, evidence of trauma. However, the physical exam can be normal. Lab analysis, when available, may reveal: 90 % with

macrocytosis (MCV between 100 and 110 fL). Serum (AST [SGOT] and ALT [SGPT]) and gammaglutamyl transferase (GGT) often abnormal. AST:ALT ratio ≥ 2:1.
- Management: Withdrawal from alcohol potentially fatal. Symptoms range from tremulousness, anxiety, headache, palpitations to delirium tremens and grand mal seizures. Psychosocial treatments include motivational interviewing, CBT, physiologic detoxification: inpatient, residential, day treatment, or outpatient. Pharmacological treatment for alcohol abuse includes Naltrexone, start at 25 mg and repeat in 1 hour if no signs of withdrawal (can be increased to 100 mg every other day) also available as depot preparation; acamprosate, 666 mg three times daily, or disulfiram initially dosed at 500 mg/day for 1–2 weeks, followed by an average maintenance dose of 250 mg/day with a range of 125–500 mg based on the severity of adverse effects. These medications may not be available in low-resource settings.
- Prognosis: Factors associated with higher rates of relapse include male gender, younger age, fewer social supports, greater alcohol consumption prior to treatment, poor compliance with drug therapy.

Psychotic Disorders

Schizophrenia

- Epidemiology: Childhood onset schizophrenia is a rare disorder, particularly before age 12, thought to have a prevalence of 1–2 per 1,000. Boys tend to be twice as affected as girls. 1 % of adults suffer from schizophrenia.
- Evaluation of hallucinations: Do not rush to a diagnosis of early onset schizophrenia. In children hallucinations can be part of normal development or can be associated with nonpsychotic psychopathology, psychosocial stressors, drug intoxication or physical illness. A medical evaluation is the first step in evaluating hallucinations. Delirium should be ruled out. Ask about substance experimentation.
- Screening for hallucinations:
  - "Have you ever had any experiences like dreaming when you're awake?"
  - "Do you ever hear or see things that other people can't hear or see?"
  - "Do you ever feel that your mind is playing tricks on you?"
- Differential diagnosis: Normal causes of hallucinations can include fantasy, cultural phenomena, grief, hypnogogic hallucinations, night terrors, acute phobic hallucinations, and fever. True delusions or psychosis can reflect brief psychotic disorder due to overwhelming stress, schizophrenia, bipolar disorder, major depressive disorder and can be substance-induced.
- Clinical presentation: "Positive symptoms" include symptoms that are actively experienced, such as florid hallucinations, delusions and thought disorder.

"Negative symptoms" describe a lack of normal experiences, including flat affect, anergia, and poverty of speech or thought.
- Diagnosis (DSM): Two symptoms for 1 month plus 5 months of prodromal or residual symptoms, including delusions, hallucinations, speech disorganization, behavior disorganization and negative symptoms (flat affect, paucity of speech, or avolition).
- Management: Psychoeducation with focus on need for treatment compliance, and provision of hope; psychosocial treatments including social skills training and supportive psychotherapy; school interventions to support learning; antipsychotic medications are a foundation of treatment. Potential longer-term side effects of medications (tardive dyskinesia, weight gain or diabetes, cognitive blunting) need to be weighed against medication effectiveness. Use of smallest possible amount of medication to control symptoms, exercise and nutrition plan, and close medication monitoring are required. Typical antipsychotics (ex: haloperidol, chlorpromazine) as effective as newer atypicals (ex: risperidone), but carry greater risk of DYSTONIA and tardive dyskinesia. Newer atypicals with risk of weight gain, hyperlipidemia, diabetes, prolonged QTc interval on EKG (assess that QTc < 460), neutropenia and agranulocytosis.
- Prognosis: Disorder likely present throughout life course. Outcome varies greatly. Some individuals function well with medication. Earlier onset is associated with poorer outcome. Earlier identification and treatment likely reduces decline in functioning and long-term impairments from schizophrenia.

Other Problems

Eating Disorders

- Epidemiology: Less common in low-income countries. Ten percent of some adolescent female populations have an eating disorder. Female-to-male ratio 10:1.
- Screening Questions:
  - "Have you ever lost so much weight on a diet that people started to seriously worry about you? Have you ever been afraid of getting fat even when other said you were thin enough?"
  - "Have you ever had a problem with binge eating, eating so much food so fast that it made you feel sick? Did you feel that urge was not really normal? Was the urge so strong that you couldn't stop? Did you feel depressed, ashamed or disgusted with yourself? Would you vomit after eating, use laxatives, or excessively exercise?"
- Clinical presentation: Overestimation of body size, shape or parts leading to weight control practices intended to reduce weight (anorexia nervosa) or prevent weight gain (bulimia). Denial of seriousness of illness, dental erosion, perioral dermatitis, metabolic alkalosis with hypokalemia, cardiac arrhythmia, renal failure, seizure, hypoproteinemia, decreased bone density.

- Differential diagnosis: Consider failure to thrive or pica, comorbid OCD, depression, anxiety and personality disorder.
- Diagnosis (DSM 4):
  - Anorexia: refusal to maintain body weight at >85 % of ideal, fear of gaining weight, altered body image, amenorrhea.
  - Bulimia: recurrent episodes of binge eating; compensatory behavior to prevent weight gain (e.g., purging, diuretic use); episodes occurring twice per week for >3 months; body weight >85 % of ideal.
- Management:
  - Anorexia: Difficult to treat. Management determined by severity of illness. Range from ICU to outpatient care. Monitor EKG, electrolytes, urinalysis. Increase calories slowly due to concern for refeeding syndrome/hypophosphatemia. Weight restoration, family therapy, may consider antidepressants. Family-based approach appears most effective.
  - Bulimia: CBT is first-line therapy. Antidepressants shown to be effective.
- Prognosis: 25 % recover fully. 20 % mortality over 30 years.

Recommended Reading

1. Walter H, DeMaso D et al. Behavioral and psychiatric disorders. In: Kliegman R, Stanton B, St. Geme J, Schor N, Behrman R, editors. Nelson's textbook of pediatrics, 19th ed. US: Elsevier Saunders; 2011.
2. Eapen V, Graham P, Shoba S. Where there is no child psychiatrist: a mental health care manual. UK: RCPsych; 2012.
3. Patel V. Where there is no psychiatrist: a mental health care manual. UK: Gaskell/RCPsych; 2002, 2008
4. Stubbe D. Practical guides in psychiatry: child and adolescent psychiatry. USA: Lippincott Williams and Wilkins; 2007.
5. World Health Organization. WHO mhGAP Intervention Guide for mental, neurological and substance use disorders in non-specialized health settings. 2010. Available at: http://www.who.int/mental_health/publications/mhGAP_intervention_guide/en/index.html

Chapter 26
Child and Adolescent Health and Human Rights

Ashkon Shaahinfar and Theresa S. Betancourt

Keywords Child and adolescent rights • UN Convention on the Rights of the Child • Right to health • Child protection • Legal mechanisms • Human rights-based approach • Vulnerability

Overview

- Human rights are universal, inalienable, indivisible, interrelated and interdependent, and treaty signatories are bound to "respect, protect, and fulfill" these rights, which includes a *progressive realization* of economic, social, and cultural rights.
- The Convention on the Rights of the Child (1989) incorporates social, economic, cultural, civil, and political rights and is the most widely ratified human rights treaty in the world.
- Fulfillment of the right to health depends on *availability, accessibility, acceptability, and quality* of health care and public health.

A. Shaahinfar, M.D., M.P.H. (✉)
Pediatrics Department, MassGeneral Hospital for Children,
175 Cambridge St., 5th Floor, Boston, MA 02114, USA
e-mail: ashaahinfar@partners.org

T.S. Betancourt, Sc.D., M.A.
Department of Global Health and Population, Francois-Xavier Bagnoud Center
for Health and Human Rights, Harvard School of Public Health, Boston, MA, USA

- Work in human rights can take the form of advocacy, application of legal mechanisms, and a human rights approach to health programming and service delivery.
- The concept of vulnerability can provide a human rights lens to analyze and minimize health risks.

Background

> We are children whose voices are not being heard: it is time we are taken into account.
> We want a world fit for children, because a world fit for us is a world fit for everyone.

So declared hundreds of children participating in the UN General Assembly's first Special Session on Children in 2002, which culminated in a commitment of more than 180 countries to "A World Fit for Children," a child rights compact and plan of action that drew from both the UN Convention on the Rights of the Child (CRC) and the Millennium Development Goals (MDGs). The CRC is the most widely ratified UN human rights treaty (only the USA, Somalia, and South Sudan have yet to ratify) and made history in 1989 by being the first such treaty to integrate economic, social, and cultural rights with civil and political rights. Now more than 20 years later, tremendous strides have been made towards the realization of child and adolescent rights, such as the decrease in under-5 mortality, improvement in school dropout and gender parity, higher rate of HIV treatment, and more holistic view of child protection in international legal instruments and national monitoring systems. However, overwhelming challenges and gross violations of child rights still remain:

- It has been estimated that more than one billion children are denied at least one of their rights to water and sanitation, nutrition, shelter, health care, education, and access to information.
- Despite efforts to date, progress has been particularly slow towards meeting MDG targets for sanitation, malnutrition, and maternal mortality.
- In the absence of adequate child-conscious safeguards for the most vulnerable, globalization and the global financial crisis have coincided with widened disparities, with sub-Saharan Africa/South Asia, girls/young women, the poor, minority/indigenous children, children with disabilities, and rural settings faring worse by many indicators.
- Child protection statistics are sobering: >1 billion children live in countries affected by armed conflict; 150 million children ages 5–14 are engaged in child labor; >64 million women aged 20–24 were married as children; 18 million children are made more vulnerable by displacement; and 1.2 million children are trafficked each year.

Clearly, children's rights should be at the forefront of the work of any health-care provider, public health practitioner, advocate, or researcher working to make the world more fit for children. This chapter arms the reader with an understanding of the legal framework and fundamental principles of child and adolescent rights, the close connections between child health and human rights, and the tenets of a human rights-based approach to health.

Human Rights Framework, Key Principles, and the CRC

Legal Framework, Principles, and Mechanisms

Grounded in the inherent dignity of every human being, human rights are freedoms and protections that are guaranteed by law and refer specifically to the relationship between the individual (rights-holder) and the State (duty-bearer). Fundamentally, all human rights are universal, inalienable, indivisible, interrelated, and interdependent. Human rights can be found in both legally binding and nonbinding instruments and documents:

- International human rights *treaties* (i.e., conventions/covenants) and associated *optional protocols*—binding on ratifying governments and often accompanied by nonbinding *general comments* that further clarify rights and government obligations.
- *Declarations* (e.g., UNDHR, 1944), *international conferences, consensus documents, plans of actions*—although legally nonbinding, may describe norms and standards reflective of binding *customary international law*.

In a divided Cold War world, these rights were enshrined separately in the first two legally binding international human rights treaties, the International Covenant on Economic, Social, and Cultural Rights (ICESCR) and the International Covenant on Civil and Political Rights (ICCPR), which entered into force in 1976. Treaty bodies monitor human rights by eliciting periodic reports from ratifying countries, which can be accompanied by *shadow reports* by local and international NGOs, and responding with *concluding comments and observations*. Furthermore, the UN High Commissioner of Human Rights tasks various country- and theme-specific *special rapporteurs* and working groups to examine and report on specific human rights issues (e.g., Special Representative of the Secretary-General on Children and Armed Conflict).

States are held accountable to "respect, protect, and fulfill" human rights, meaning that they must avoid direct infringement upon or violation of rights; protect individuals and groups from human rights abuses by non-State actors; and proactively facilitate the fulfillment of these rights, respectively. Under a standard of *progressive realization*, which acknowledges the constraints on developing countries and calls for international cooperation, States must make consistent and efficient forward progress towards the full realization of economic, social, and cultural rights by their incorporation into and the effective implementation of domestic law.

This fulfillment includes local mechanisms of recourse for individuals and groups facing human rights violations, such as judicial system or mediating *ombudspersons*. If these domestic mechanisms are exhausted, victims might be able to pursue regional mechanisms or, for certain international treaties, *individual complaints* procedures directly to the relevant treaty committee. In February 2012, the UN CRC Committee adopted and opened for State signature an optional protocol on an individual complaints mechanism for violations of children's rights.

The Convention on the Rights of the Child

Adopted in 1989, the CRC explicitly acknowledged that children have inherent human rights and that individuals under the age of 18 need special protection and care. The CRC was the first Convention that incorporated civil and political and social, economic, and cultural rights into one legally binding international document. Its *optional protocols on the involvement of children in armed conflict* and *on the sale of children, child prostitution and child pornography* followed in 2000. In addition to those described above, the CRC is based on the following guiding principles:

- *Nondiscrimination* (art. 2)—as with all human rights, a child's rights must be ensured regardless of that child's or his/her parent/guardian's "race, color, sex, language, religion, political or other opinion, national, ethnic or social origin, property, disability, birth or other status."
- Best interests of the child (art. 3)—the central concern underlying all actions by public and private social welfare institutions, courts, administrative and legislative groups; specifically relevant to issues of care and protection.
- Right to life, survival, and development (art. 6)—to the "maximum extent possible."
- Right to be heard (art. 12)—reflective of broader human rights principle of *participation*, children must be able to form and freely express their views and have them taken into consideration, including in judicial and administrative proceedings, according to their *evolving capacities* as they mature (UN General Assembly 1989).

It is important to recognize that while countries are signatories of the CRC and other human rights treaties, cultural norms, political ideology, social and economic constraints can impact the degree of child rights fulfillment on the ground. States can make *reservations* to specific provisions, thus limiting reflection of the treaty in domestic laws. Furthermore, effective implementation of even the most progressive laws requires political will, budget and resources, and governance that are often in short supply, particularly when nonvoting and non-taxpaying children are concerned. Reading the recent CRC country report, NGO shadow reports, and concluding observations is a great place to start when trying to gain an essential understanding of the local child rights context (visit http://www.crin.org/docs/).

The Right to Health, the CRC and Beyond

The Relationship Between Health and Human Rights

- The promotion or neglect/violation of human rights can have both positive and detrimental effects on health, respectively.
- Public health policies and programs can lead to promotion or violation of human rights based on how they are designed and implemented.
- An individual's state of health can impact his or her ability to enjoy other human rights, and poor health can make one more vulnerable to human rights violations.

The Right to Health

Article 24 of the CRC makes explicit the right of children to "the highest attainable standard of health" and access to "facilities for the treatment of illness and rehabilitation of health." Specifically, the treaty stipulates that States take measures to:

- Diminish infant and child mortality.
- Provide health care to all children, particularly developing primary health care.
- Fight disease and malnutrition through primary care, available technologies, nutritious foods, clean drinking water, and addressing risks of environmental pollution.
- Provide prenatal and postnatal care for mothers.
- Ensure education of and dissemination of health information to parents and children to support their application of knowledge of child health and nutrition, advantages of breastfeeding, hygiene and sanitation, and accident prevention.
- Develop preventive health care and family planning education/services.

The article further places particular emphasis on urging States to "take all effective and appropriate measures with a view of abolishing traditional practices prejudicial [i.e. detrimental and at times potentially life-threatening] to the health of children," such as female genital mutilation, sexual abuse, child marriage, and honor killings (UN General Assembly 1989).

"Triple A-Q"

General Comment 14 of the ICESCR provides additional guidelines towards the implementation of the right to health, including addressing the underlying determinants of health, working towards the realization of the other human rights upon which it is dependent, and fulfilling the *AAA-Q* criteria:

- *Availability*—"functioning public health and health-care facilities, goods and services, as well as programs, have to be available in sufficient quantity," including safe drinking water/sanitation, health-care providers, and essential drugs.
- *Accessibility*—"health facilities, goods and services must be accessible to everyone without discrimination," which includes nondiscrimination, (safe) physical accessibility, economic accessibility (affordability), and information accessibility.
- *Acceptability*—"health facilities, goods and services must be respectful of medical ethics and culturally appropriate," (i.e., sensitive to gender and age, respectful of confidentiality and local cultures, and effective in improving health status).
- *Quality*—"health facilities, goods and services must be scientifically and medically appropriate and of good quality," including skilled personnel, unexpired and approved drugs/equipment, safe and potable water, and adequate sanitation (WHO 2002).

Relevant CRC General Comments

The following health-related general comments of the CRC might prove to be helpful resources in work abroad. In each of the below contexts, the Committee provides countries with more detailed guidance in respecting, protecting, and fulfilling child rights, including health policy and strategy suggestions that may well overlap with one's own efforts or collaborations:

- General Comment No. 3—HIV/AIDS
- General Comment No. 4—Adolescent health and development
- General Comment No. 7—Early childhood
- General Comment No. 9—Children with disabilities
- General Comment No. 13—Freedom from all forms of violence
- Upcoming General Comment—Children and the business sector

Rights-Based Approach to Health

Human rights might play any of the following roles in global health work: advocacy, legal mechanisms, and a human rights approach to programming and service delivery.

Advocacy (e.g., Advocacy-Related Research, Human Rights NGOs)

- Witnessing and documenting human rights violations, assessing the contribution of both government action and inaction, and proposing solutions to fulfill rights in a public arena is integral to the work of many nongovernmental and civil society organizations.

- For those focused on health-care delivery, such sensitive efforts must be balanced with remaining safe and sustainably providing health services.

Legal Mechanisms (e.g., Changing Policy, Seeking Legal Redress)

- Improvements can be made in local laws relevant to the health of children through the persuasion of policymakers to comply with national and international legal obligations.
- If one witnesses gross violation of children's rights while undertaking service delivery or public health work, local mechanisms of redress can be undertaken (e.g., judicial system, ombudsperson, children's commissioner or Child Protective Services Office of local government, local child welfare committee).
- NGOs can be essential resources in accessing these modes of redress (e.g., Save the Children, ECPAT, and Human Rights Watch). For a broader list of child rights-minded NGOs: http://www.crin.org/NGOGroupforCRC/about.asp.
- For more information on leveraging the law to advance child rights: http://www.crin.org/law/index.asp.

Human Rights-Based Approach to Programming

A human rights-based approach (HRBA) can be applied across the life cycle of care delivery and public health programming, from needs assessment, intervention/program design, implementation, to monitoring and evaluation. The key components have been described as follows:

- Consider the interdependence/interrelations among rights and the implications of the legal and policy context in which the program will be or is currently placed.
- Incorporate key health and human rights principles (i.e., nondiscrimination, participation and inclusion of children/marginalized communities/affected rights-bearers, transparency, and accountability).
- Pay close attention to and aim to maximize the central components of the right to health (see above; *availability, accessibility, acceptability, and quality*).

Vulnerability Analysis: A Health and Human Rights Tool

Certain problems intuitively call for a human rights approach. For example, one might imagine developing an intervention to diminish the risk of early pregnancy among migrant girls living and even working at a construction site in urban India.

Guided by the frameworks and concepts above, the program developer might first attempt to gain an understanding of the human rights and policy contexts surrounding these children. Conducting focus groups with the girls and their families might be an important component of the intervention design. However, it might be a struggle to grasp a starting point for this complex problem. The concept of vulnerability can be a helpful human rights lens through which to view situations like these:

- Individual vulnerability refers to one's lack of autonomy over his or her destiny and thus makes an individual more prone to health risks (e.g., via high-risk behaviors/situations).
- Vulnerability is determined by three sets of factors that mutually impact one another—individual vulnerability (e.g., lack of information, economic/educational opportunity), program-related vulnerability (e.g., discrimination), and societal vulnerability (e.g., cultural norms regarding gender, implementation of child labor/child marriage laws).
- Interventions should thus aim to reduce these various aspects of vulnerability and address the related human rights shortcomings and violations rather than focusing purely on risk reduction (e.g., condom use for early pregnancy prevention).
- Furthermore, youth and community participation can play a tremendous role in holding the State and other parties accountable for rights violations and in working with both advocates and health service providers to enact sustainable improvements in protecting, respecting, and fulfilling child rights.

Recommended Reading

Gruskin S, Tarantola D. HIV/AIDS, health and human rights. In: Lamptey PR, Gayle HD, editors. HIV/AIDS prevention and care in resource constrained settings: a handbook for design and management of programs. Arlington, VA: Family Health International; 2001. p. 659–78.

Gruskin S, Mill EJ, Tarantola D. History, principles, and practice of health and human rights. Lancet. 2007;370(9585):449–55.

UN General Assembly. Convention on the Rights of the Child. United Nations, Treaty Series. 1989 Nov 20; 1577:3. http://www.unhcr.org/refworld/docid/3ae6b38f0.html.

UNICEF. State of the World's children: celebrating 20 years of the convention on the rights of the child. New York, NY: UNICEF; 2009.

World Health Organization. 25 Questions and answers on health and human rights, Health and human rights publication series, vol. 1. Geneva: World Health Organization; 2002.

Chapter 27
Pediatric Preventive and Clinical Oral Health Care

Brittany Seymour, Michele Nations Martin, and Grace J. Kim

Keywords Normal oral anatomy • Pediatric oral anatomy • Common pediatric oral diseases and conditions • Management of common pediatric oral conditions

Overview

- Healthy normal oral anatomy is important for eating, speaking, and healthy development and well being in children and adolescents.
- Common oral conditions affecting infants, children, and adolescents, particularly in low resources settings, include dental caries, gingivitis, pulpitis, retained primary teeth, trauma, herpes simplex, and oral candidiasis.
- Other oral conditions affecting infants and children include cleft lip and palate and noma.
- Children and adolescents with HIV/AIDS are at risk for specific oral conditions, which can be an indicator of HIV status.
- Commonly used oral health interventions in resource-limited regions include oral hygiene, fluoride varnish, and extraction of primary teeth.

B. Seymour, D.D.S., M.P.H. (✉) • M.N. Martin, D.D.S., D.M.D. • G.J. Kim, D.M.D.
Harvard School of Dental Medicine, 188 Longwood Ave., REB204, Boston, MA 02115, USA
e-mail: brittany_seymour@hsdm.harvard.edu

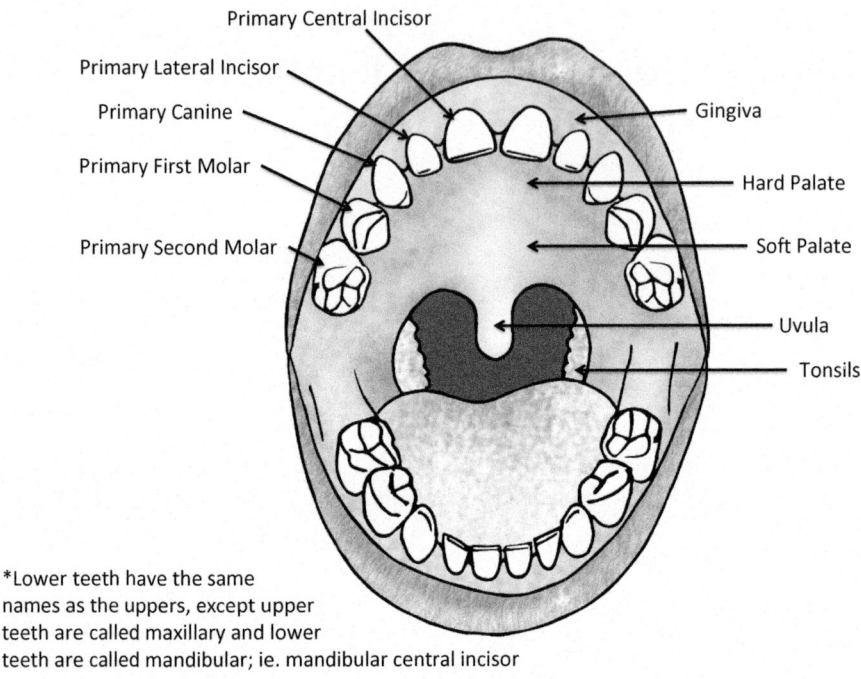

Fig. 27.1 Some basic pediatric oral anatomy (Artist credit: Alison Seliger)

Normal Anatomy

Good oral health is vital for children to eat, speak, learn, and grow normally. Oral health refers to more than just teeth; it includes the jaws, muscles of mastication (chewing), hard and soft palate, and the lining of the throat. Normal oral anatomy is illustrated in Fig. 27.1.

The importance of primary teeth: Baby teeth are called primary teeth, and adult teeth are called permanent teeth. The period when children exfoliate their primary teeth while their permanent teeth erupt is called "mixed dentition." Unhealthy primary teeth mean significantly higher risk for lifelong problems with permanent dentition, including but not limited to dental caries (cavities) and malocclusion (bite and jaw problems). Typical eruption and exfoliation patterns are outlined in Fig. 27.2.

Baby teeth are essential for the following:

- Speaking: Teeth assist in the formation of words and proper speech.
- Eating: Teeth are needed for chewing and eating all foods in a healthy diet.

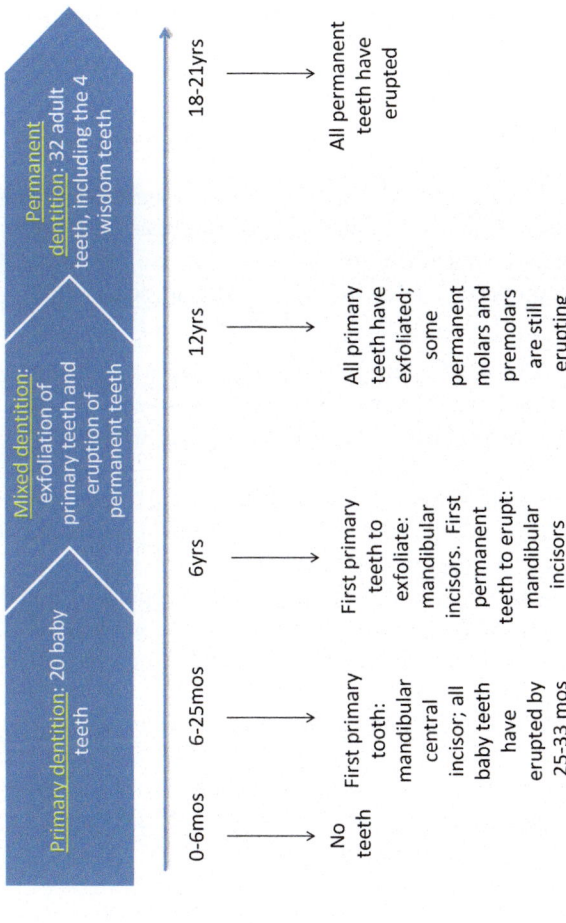

Fig. 27.2 Timeline for primary, mixed, and permanent dentition (Credit: Brittany Seymour)

- Development of the oral cavity: Chewing and speaking provide exercise to the muscles and bones of the oral cavity.
- Smiling and building self-esteem: The appearance of healthy teeth and smile contributes to high self-esteem and positive relationships with others.
- Guiding the eruption of permanent teeth: Baby teeth provide a path for erupting adult teeth to follow.

Common Oral Conditions Affecting Infants, Children, and Adolescents

Dental Caries (Cavities)

- *Etiology*: Oral bacteria found in plaque metabolize sugar from foods and beverages; this produces acid that demineralizes enamel, causing a cavity.
- *Prevalence*: Most common chronic childhood disease worldwide; 60–90 % of children have experienced decay by the time they are school-aged.
- *Prevention*:
  - Keep teeth clean and remove plaque daily with a brush, chewing stick, or cloth; fluoridated toothpaste or baking powder mixed with water can be used but is not necessary. Floss in between teeth daily with dental floss (if available) or use string or strong fibers from leaves.
  - Limit the frequency of sugar intake each day; the pH of the mouth drops every time sugar is ingested, and this drop in pH increases the risk for developing a cavity. Remove plaque after sugar ingestion.
  - Do not allow the child to sleep with any bottles containing liquids other than water (primary cause of early childhood caries, see below); salivary flow decreases during sleep, allowing more rapid demineralization of teeth if plaque and sugar are present.
  - When available, topical fluorides such as fluoride varnish can be placed; Atraumatic Restorative Treatment (ART) sealants (see below under Management of Primary Caries) or pit and fissure sealants can be painted into the grooves of the molars. (Armamentarium is often not available to place pit and fissure sealants in resource-limited settings.)
- *Diagnosis*:
  - Visual diagnosis is possible for many cavities (see clinical presentation).
  - Tactile sensation using a sharp/pointy instrument, placing the end of the instrument into the suspected carious lesion in the tooth and feeling for "sticky" surface.
  - Radiographic diagnosis for demineralization of enamel (often not possible in resource-limited settings).

Fig. 27.3 A 3-year-old boy with severe early childhood caries (Photo credit: Brittany Seymour)

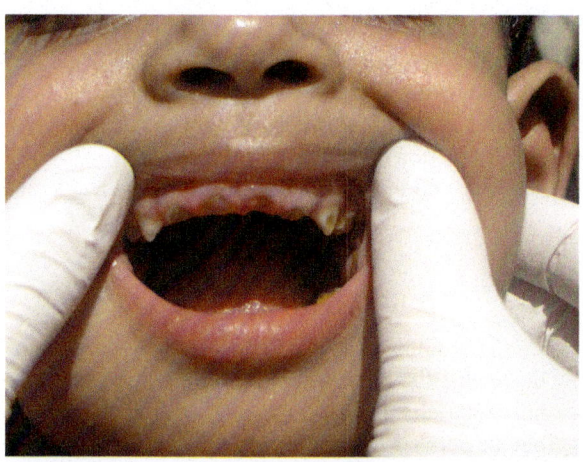

- *Clinical presentation*:
    - Incipient caries: Chalky white surface, not shiny like surrounding enamel.
    - Primary caries: Brown or yellow "hole" in the enamel, missing tooth structure.
    - Secondary caries: Same as primary but occurs around the margins of a filling or dental restoration.
    - Severe caries: 50 % or more of the tooth has decayed.
    - Early childhood caries (ECC)/rampant caries: Earliest clinical signs of ECC can begin as early as 1 year of age, involve multiple teeth, and often, without treatment, the front teeth will decay to the gums by age 3 (Fig. 27.3).
- *Management* (*including referral*):
    - Incipient: Keep tooth surface plaque-free daily, place fluoride varnish when available.
    - Primary caries: ART (Atraumatic Restorative Treatment)—manual removal of soft tooth structure using a small spoon-shaped excavator hand instrument; then placement of an auto-cure glass ionomer restorative material, which contains fluoride; this material can be placed in the grooves of molars as sealants to prevent caries. These materials are economical and prevent unnecessary loss of teeth; they are not always readily available in low-resource areas but are affordable and should be procured along with other essential medical supplies.

- Secondary caries: ART method; however, if the cavity extends underneath the filling, referral to a dental practitioner is necessary for complete removal of both restoration and cavity.
- Severe caries: Extraction. (For details on extraction method, see section "Extraction of Primary Teeth".)
- Early childhood caries/rampant caries: Extraction.

Gingivitis

- *Etiology*: Gingivitis is inflammation that occurs in the soft tissues surrounding the teeth—the gingiva. This inflammation can be caused by several factors (HIV, hormonal changes, and medications), but the most common cause is excessive plaque deposited around the teeth *due to poor oral hygiene*.
- *Prevalence*: Gingivitis has a high prevalence in all ages. However, around the time of puberty, there is an increased vulnerability to gingivitis. Peak prevalence occurs between 11 and 17 years of age (puberty) and then frequency declines as long as adequate oral hygiene is maintained.
- *Prevention*: Adequate hygiene and plaque removal, brush twice a day and floss once a day.
- *Diagnosis/clinical presentation*: The easiest method of diagnosis is bleeding after gentle probing on the gingiva immediately adjacent to the tooth. Healthy gingiva is light pink; when gingivitis is present, the gums become light red and as the condition worsens, become redder, edematous, painful, and spontaneously bleed.
- *Management*: Improve oral hygiene to decrease plaque that is responsible for the inflammation. Gingivitis begins to reverse within 24–48 h after adequate plaque removal. There is no indication for oral antibiotics when gingivitis is present.

Pulpitis Leading to Dental Infection

- *Etiology*: Most often untreated dental caries, followed by tooth trauma.
- *Prevalence*: If caries remains untreated, progression to a form of pulpitis and/or infection is very likely over time. Pulpitis is highly prevalent in resource-limited regions and provider-shortage areas.
- *Prevention*: Prevent dental caries or trauma; treat caries that is present or extract a carious tooth.
- *Diagnosis/clinical presentation*:
    - Reversible pulpitis: Temperature or chewing sensitivity.
    - Irreversible pulpitis/acute infection: Spontaneous sensitivity for no reason; lingering discomfort after eating or drinking; pain upon chewing; facial or intraoral swelling with moderate to severe pain; patient may have a fever.

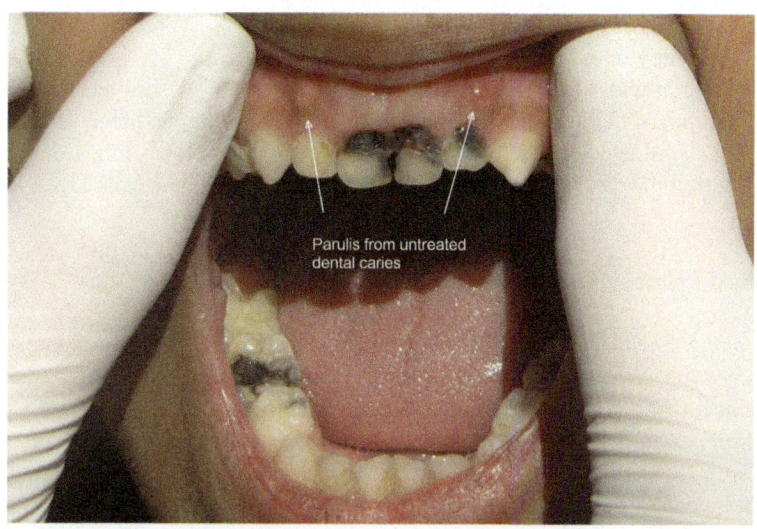

Fig. 27.4 A parulis is present above both maxillary primary lateral incisors due to a chronic infection from untreated caries (Photo credit: Brittany Seymour)

- ○ Necrotic tooth/chronic infection: History of caries and/or pain and/or swelling; radiograph (if available) shows a periapical radiolucency at the root of the tooth; tooth does not respond to temperature but pain to chewing may be present; a draining fistula or parulis may be present at or near the necrotic tooth (Fig. 27.4).
- *Urgent and life-threatening facial space infections*:
    - ○ Ludwig's Angina: Bilateral submandibular swelling, risk of airway obstruction.
    - ○ Cavernous sinus thrombosis: Can result from a severe dental infection in any facial space.
    - ○ Periorbital and infraorbital space infections: Risk of infection from severe untreated dental caries leading to loss of vision, meningitis, or brain abscess.
- *Management*:
    - ○ Reversible pulpitis: Treat caries and observe, symptoms should resolve.
    - ○ Irreversible pulpitis: Referral for endodontic therapy (root canal) or extraction is necessary; drainage of swelling can be done by injecting a needle into the area until it hits bone and pressing to allow for drainage of the pus; analgesic pain medication (i.e., Ibuprofen 400 mg, take one tablet by mouth every 4 h for pain, or liquid Ibuprofen take 4–10 mg/kg every 6 h as needed, maximum 40 mg/kg/24 h); if child has a fever, administer antibiotics (e.g., Penicillin V potassium liquid, 125 mg/5 ml, children should take one teaspoon by mouth every 6 h for 14 days).

- Necrotic tooth: Extraction if a primary tooth; otherwise, referral for endodontic therapy or extraction is necessary.
- Children with life-threatening facial space infections described above should be referred to the nearest hospital or healthcare facility and receive IV antibiotics immediately (e.g., Benzyl-Penicillin 1 g four times daily and Metronidazole 500 mg three times a day until infection is cleared).

Retained Primary Tooth

- *Etiology*: Severe caries, ankylosis (roots are fused to the bone), or unknown.
- *Prevention*: When tooth becomes mobile, assist child in "wiggling" tooth over the next few days to a week until he/she is able to remove it.
- *Diagnosis/clinical presentation*: Visual diagnosis, the permanent tooth has begun to erupt, is visible in the mouth, and the primary tooth has not become mobile or exfoliated; when a primary tooth has severe caries, the permanent tooth may erupt right through the retained roots and coronal structure of the primary tooth.
- *Management*: Extraction of retained structure or primary tooth, or referral for surgery if ankylosed; ankylosed teeth will have no mobility or movement at all due to absence of the periodontal ligament (PDL); surgical sectioning and possible bone removal is necessary.

Trauma

- *Etiology*: Sports, injury to the face, fall, unsafe environments (playgrounds), traffic accidents, domestic violence, or abuse.
- *Prevalence*: An estimated 5–18 % of children and adolescents experience trauma to their orofacial region; the most common dental injury is to the two maxillary central incisors.
- *Prevention*: Mouth guard when playing sports, seat belt, proper supervision during play.
- *Clinical presentation*: Pain may be present, along with bleeding.
    - Subluxation: Tooth is slightly mobile with bleeding in the gingival sulcus surrounding the tooth.
    - Lateral luxation: Crown is pushed back toward the hard palate or tongue.
    - Intrusive luxation: Tooth is pushed into the socket.
    - Avulsion: Tooth is completely knocked out of the mouth.
- *Management*:
    - Subluxation
        - Primary tooth: Observe, if tooth becomes discolored or dark over a period of a few months and pain does not reside or new symptoms develop, the tooth is likely necrotic, and extraction is needed.

- Permanent tooth: Observe; if tooth becomes discolored or dark over a period of a few months and pain does not reside or new symptoms develop, extract or refer for endodontic therapy.

- Lateral luxation
- Primary tooth: Apply local anesthetic (see section "Extraction of Primary Teeth"); position tooth back into socket by gently pushing forward and upward into socket; then observe and manage like subluxation.
- Permanent tooth: Apply local anesthetic and position tooth back into socket; if tooth is mobile, splint with a wire and a composite bonding material if available or refer to the nearest dental provider if materials are not available; instruct patient not to eat or bite on tooth for several days; observe and manage as with subluxation.

- Intrusive luxation
- Primary and permanent tooth: Prognosis is poor for both primary and permanent teeth and risk for infection or ankylosis is high; refer for extraction for both cases; an exception is young permanent teeth in someone around the age of 8–10, which may erupt back into position in a matter of several days: if this does not occur, refer for extraction.

- Avulsion
- Primary tooth: Do nothing; the permanent tooth should erupt in time, although it may be delayed.
- Permanent tooth: Immediately place the tooth in milk to preserve the cells on the roots (milk can preserve the tooth for up to 3 h; without milk, the cells will die within 15–20 min and the tooth cannot be saved); then wash the tooth with clean water or saline if available and gently place the tooth back into the socket, splint with a wire and a composite or glass ionomer bonding material if available and instruct patient to avoid biting or chewing on the tooth; prognosis is still fair to poor even if these steps are taken; if these steps are not possible in the time specified, do nothing.

Herpes Simplex

- *Etiology*: Also known as HSV-1, the herpes simplex virus spreads through infected saliva or active perioral lesions. Typically asymptomatic, the primary infection most often occurs during the first couple of years of life. The most common sites are the pharynx, intraoral sites, lips, eyes, and skin above the waist. The herpes simplex inoculates within individuals without antibodies. This causes what is known as the primary infection. Nearly all primary infections are the result of contact with an infected individual. Once localized, the virus is taken up by the sensory nerves and then goes into a latent state. The most frequent site of latency is the trigeminal ganglion. In symptomatic cases, individuals exposed to

HSV-1 at an early age tend to exhibit gingivostomatitis—acute phase of primary infection.
- *Prevalence*: Many reports suggest that nearly 90 % of the population worldwide has had prior infection. In developing countries, over half the population is exposed by 5 years of age, 95 % by 15 years of age, and nearly 100 % exposure by 30 years of age. Individuals could be exposed to the virus and not know it since 90 % of the first time infections are asymptomatic.
- *Prevention*: Avoid sharing dishes or utensils, use lip sunscreen and avoid direct contact with a lesion, e.g., kissing.
- *Diagnosis/clinical presentation*: Most cases of acute herpetic gingivostomatitis (primary herpes) occur between 6 months and 5 years of age with peak prevalence between 2 and 3 years of age. The initial onset is quick and can also cause anterior cervical lymphadenopathy, chills, fever (103–105 F; 39–40 °C), nausea, anorexia, irritability, and sore mouth lesions.

Diagnosis includes painful blisters on lip or outer edges of mouth; blister can be crusted over with a scab; tingling sensations may occur before blister becomes visible. The manifestations of the virus range from mild to extremely debilitating. Mild cases usually resolve within 5–7 days. Severe cases may extend to 2 weeks.

At first the affected mucosa develops several vesicles that rapidly collapse to form numerous small, red lesions. It is not unusual for the involvement of the labial mucosa to extend past the wet line to include the adjacent vermilion border of the lips.

- *Management*: Patients should be instructed to restrict contact with others when they have active lesions in order to prevent the spread to other sites on the body or to other people. If the infection is diagnosed early (i.e., during the first 3 symptomatic days), acyclovir 200 mg/5 ml oral suspension five times per day for 5 days can significantly accelerate resolution.

Pain control with topical antiviral medication such as topical acyclovir (Acyclovir ointment, apply to oral lesion with a cotton tip applicator five times daily until lesion resolves) and nonsteroidal anti-inflammatory drugs (i.e., Ibuprofen 400 mg, take one tablet by mouth every 4 h for pain, or liquid Ibuprofen take 4–10 mg/kg every 6 h as needed, maximum 40 mg/kg/24 h) is very important. Keep the child hydrated.

Oral Candidiasis/Oral Thrush

- *Etiology*: Candidiasis is an infection caused by the fungal organism *Candida albicans*. The three most important factors responsible for clinical symptoms are the immune status of the individual, the strain of *C. albicans*, and the oral mucosa environment. Patients with leukemia or HIV or who have taken long courses of antibiotics that disrupt the normal balance of oral microorganisms are more susceptible to exhibiting candidiasis (details on HIV are presented in section "Oral Conditions Affecting Children and Adolescents with HIV/AIDS").

- *Prevalence*: Candidiasis is by far the most common oral fungal infection worldwide. Up to 50 % of people carry the organism in their mouth but do not necessarily exhibit symptoms of infection.
- *Prevention*: Proper hygiene is the best method of prevention, allowing for a healthy balance of the normal oral flora.
- *Diagnosis*: In addition to the clinical presentation, patients may experience burning sensations or unpleasant taste in the mouth. Sometimes patients complain of irregular texture on the oral mucosa that can be misinterpreted as blisters when they are actually elevated plaques. The diagnosis is usually established by clinical signs and if available, cytologic examination and culture.
- *Clinical presentation*: The most well known form of candida infection is the pseudomembranous candidiasis also known as thrush. (Other less common forms are erythematous candidiasis, chronic multifocal, angular cheilitis, and hyperplastic). Thrush is characterized by white plaques that look similar to cottage cheese or curdled milk, commonly located on the inside of cheeks or lips, tongue, and palate. To better determine if a lesion is candidiasis, scrape with gauze exposing the underlying mucosa and see if patches could easily be wiped away revealing a red area.

Candida infection can range from mild mucosa involvement, which is the most common, to fatal, which is seen in patients with severely compromised immune systems.

- *Management*: Nystatin (Oral suspension, 30 ml, one teaspoonful for 2 min 4–5 times per day for 14 days), Clotrimazole (Mycelex Troche 10 mg dissolve one troche in mouth five times per day for 14 days), Fluconazole (Diflucan 100 mg, take two tablets the first day and one tablet each day thereafter until resolved), and Ketoconazole (Nizoral 200 mg, take one tablet per day for 10 days). Clinicians should advise caregivers to clean bottles, pacifiers, etc. It is also important to explain the importance of oral health and nutrition.

Other Oral Conditions Affecting Infants and Children

Cleft Lip/Cleft Palate

- *Etiology*: Unclear but possible causes include genetic factors, associated syndromes, maternal smoking, maternal alcohol consumption, inadequate folic acid intake, and certain infections during pregnancy.
- *Prevalence*: Most common congenital defect worldwide, affecting approximately 1 in 1,000 newborns; Asians and Native Americans have the highest incidence, and Africans having the lowest incidence; cleft lip and palate more common in males, cleft palate more common in females.
- *Prevention*: Take multivitamins before pregnancy (prenatal vitamins during pregnancy), abstain from smoking or drinking alcohol during pregnancy, receive early and regular prenatal care.

- *Diagnosis*: Physical examination of mouth, nose, and palate shows a cleft lip or palate.
- *Clinical presentation*: Cleft lip—small notch in lip that may continue into base of nose, cleft palate—fissure on roof of mouth that may extend to lip.
- *Management*: Surgical closure of lip at around 10–12 weeks of age, closure of palate between 9 and 18 months, additional surgery and follow-up treatment may be needed with plastic surgeon, ear, nose, and throat specialist, pediatric dentist, orthodontists, speech therapists, etc. If surgical management is not possible, education and assistance with bonding and feeding challenges that may occur between mother and child are necessary at birth.

Noma (Disfiguring Orofacial Gangrene)

- *Etiology*: *Fusobacterium necrophorum* and *Prevotella intermedia* are major causes, but may be polymicrobial; due to poor oral hygiene.
- *Other predisposing factors*: Poverty, malnutrition or dehydration, immunodeficiency, lack of sanitation or clean drinking water, recent infection (e.g., measles, malaria, chicken pox, scarlet fever), close proximity to livestock.
- *Prevalence*: Approximately 100,000 new cases a year in Africa, Asia, and South America. Children aged 2–6 are at greatest risk. Untreated, noma is fatal in 80 % of cases and leaves survivors with intolerable mutilations.
- *Prevention*: Awareness and early detection by primary health-care workers, adequate hygiene, and sanitation.
- *Diagnosis*: Physical examination shows inflammation of soft tissues in oral cavity with ulcers that may have purulent drainage, presence of necrotic tissues over time.
- *Clinical presentation*: Gingiva and lining of the mouth become very inflamed and ulcers prevalent; gangrene spreads further to skin with soft tissue of lips and cheeks dying; infection can destroy soft and hard tissue.
- *Management*: Complex interventions involving improved nutrition, rehydration, antibiotics, surgical removal of affected tissues, and plastic surgery.

Oral Conditions Affecting Children and Adolescents with HIV/AIDS

- Common oral infections and conditions that are often the earliest signs of progression from HIV to AIDS. Nearly 80 % of AIDS patients will exhibit one or more of these conditions:
    - Candidiasis/Angular cheilitis: Manage as described previously; one of the early signs of an immune-compromised child.
    - Acute Necrotizing Ulcerative Gingivitis: A very severe form of gingivitis causing painful, inflamed and ulcerated gingiva; administer topical anesthetic

and remove plaque, with continued optimal oral hygiene practice for reversal; analgesic pain medications can assist until symptoms resolve; administer antibiotics if fever is present (i.e., Children: Penicillin V potassium liquid, 125 mg/5 ml, take one teaspoon by mouth every 6 h for 14 days; Adolescents: Penicillin V 500 mg tablets, take two tablets immediately, then one tablet every 6 h for 14 days).
- ○ Necrotic tooth: Extraction if a primary tooth; referral for endodontic.
- ○ Herpes simplex: Same as previously described.
- ○ Recurrent aphthous ulcerations: Also known as canker sores, appear as a burning white plaque with an erythematous border on the soft palate or intra-oral mucosa (movable tissue as opposed to fixed tissue with herpes); level of pain often does not match the size, meaning a small ulcer can cause great discomfort; size can be 1 cm or larger; usually resolve in 10–14 days; pain can be eased by applying topical anesthetic (Xylocaine 2 % viscous solution, rinse with one teaspoon as needed for pain, expectorate after rinsing) or topical corticosteroids (Hydrocortisone acetate ointment 0.5 %, apply to oral lesion after meals and before bedtime), and analgesic pain medication (i.e., Ibuprofen 400 mg, take one tablet by mouth every 4 h for pain, or liquid Ibuprofen take 4–10 mg/kg every 6 h as needed, maximum 40 mg/kg/24 h).
- ○ Kaposi's sarcoma: Most common cancer associated with HIV/AIDS; vascular tumor, bluish purple in color that appears on the oral mucosal tissues, most often the hard palate, followed by the gingiva; radiation and/or chemotherapy are necessary.
- ○ Xerostomia: Otherwise known as dry mouth; leads to increased risk of caries due to salivary inhibition. Hydration is extremely important, and xylitol rinses or xylitol gum can assist with stimulating saliva.
- ○ Parotid enlargement: Swelling of the major salivary glands anterior to the ears, and superior to the jaw line; clinically, unilateral or bilateral swelling occurs in the cheeks or at or below the chin depending on the child's anatomy; not to be confused with an acute odontogenic swelling cause by dental infection with accompanying pain.

- Optimal oral hygiene and healthy diet are particularly important for people with HIV/AIDS to minimize risk of the above conditions. *Oral screenings are an easy and valid way to identify progression of HIV to AIDS through early detection of the above conditions.*

Instructions for Oral Hygiene, Fluoride Varnish Application, and Extraction of a Primary Tooth

Oral Hygiene

- *Healthy diet*: Give only water or milk in baby's bottle, do not put baby to bed with a bottle with anything in it but water; wean child from bottle by 1 year of age; avoid sugary, starchy snacks or drinks especially in between meals, especially sodas. Prepare healthy snacks for your child, such as whole grain breads and fruits and vegetables, and encourage more water consumption.

- *Tooth brushing*:

    – *Infants and toddlers*: Wipe infant's gingiva after feeding with a clean cloth; when teeth start to erupt, brush the gingiva with a small soft bristled brush or soft stick with frayed ends, or continue wiping clean after meals with a cloth; brush toddlers teeth with a pea size drop of fluoride toothpaste, if available, or make a paste with baking soda and water and brush for at least 2 min twice a day; teach children to spit out tooth paste and not swallow; always clean children's teeth before going to bed.

    – *Young children*: Place brush or soft stick with frayed ends to the teeth at a 45° angle and gently brush in circular motions, clean the outside surfaces of upper and lower teeth; clean the inner surface of the upper and lower teeth; clean the chewing surfaces of upper and lower teeth, also brush the tongue; parents and caregivers should brush their children's teeth twice a day.

- *Dentist visits*: First dentist visit by age 1; at least once a year for checkups. If no dentist is available, ask the primary care provider or community health worker to check the teeth and oral cavity for optimal health.

Fluoride Varnish (FV) Application (Fig. 27.5)

- Fluoride varnish is a sticky gel with a high concentration of fluoride that is painted onto all the enamel surfaces of teeth; it is economical and effective in preventing cavities (along with proper oral hygiene) for up to 6 months after one application.
- Apply: Dry teeth by wiping them with a piece of clean, dry cotton or cloth. The teeth must stay dry throughout the FV application. Apply a thin layer of varnish on all surfaces of teeth according to manufacture's direction. Do not apply on large cavities; do not worry about saliva getting to teeth after application, the varnish dries very quickly.
- Advise: Do not drink for at least 30 min. The teeth may appear to have a yellow sticky surface for the day, this is normal. Have the child avoid hard, sticky, or crunchy snacks for the rest of the day. Do not let the child brush, floss, or use mouth rinse until the next morning.

Extraction of Primary Teeth

Step 1: Administer local anesthetic, typically 0.9–1.8 ml 2 % lidocaine in 1: 100,000 epinephrine. For maxillary teeth and mandibular canines and incisors inject in the buccal vestibule near the apex of the tooth first, this will anesthetize the buccal

Fig. 27.5 Fluoride varnish (Photo credit: Brittany Seymour)

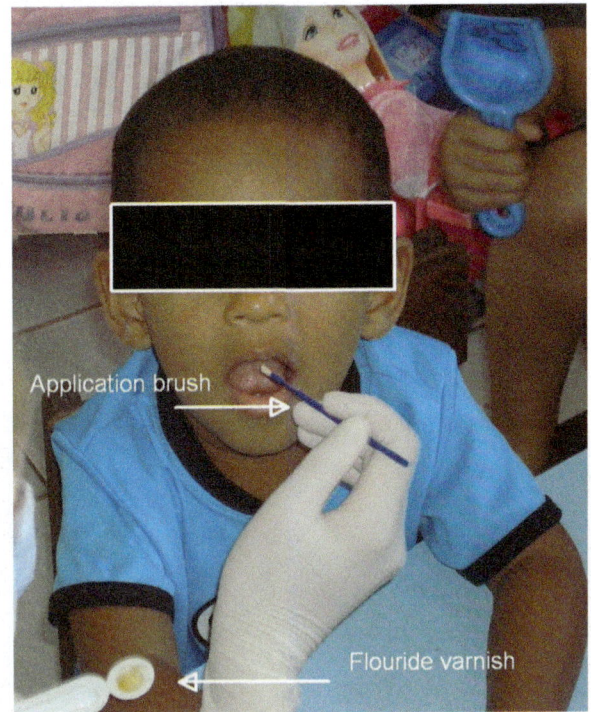

tissue and the tooth. For mandibular molars, use an Inferior Alveolar Block in addition to the above technique; manually find the ramus of the mandible-place thumb on the anterior ramus and forefinger on the posterior angle of the jaw. Aim for the lingual, just before the nerve enters the mandibular foramen (see Fig. 27.6).

After administering the above injections, wait about 30–60 s, and inject only a slight amount into the lingual/palatal gingiva until you see blanching; if you begin the procedure and the tooth does not appear to be fully anesthetized (i.e., patient exhibits pain), you can insert the needle into the PDL space between the root of the tooth and the bone and inject a slight amount until you see blanching—you will feel a great amount of "push-back" due to very limited room to inject the anesthetic (see Fig. 27.7).

Step 2: Use a sterilized periosteal elevator (or a spoon-shaped instrument with a slightly pointed end). Place it between the tooth and the gingiva and twist; repeat this all the way around the tooth to break the soft tissue fibers and loosen the gingiva adequately (see Fig. 27.8).

Step 3: Use a sterilized elevator (or another spoon-shaped instrument with a more blunted end) and place it under the gingival tissue, between the tooth to be extracted and the tooth next to it; be sure that the elevator is between the tooth and its own gingiva, not the neighboring tooth. Twist the elevator slightly from side to side to

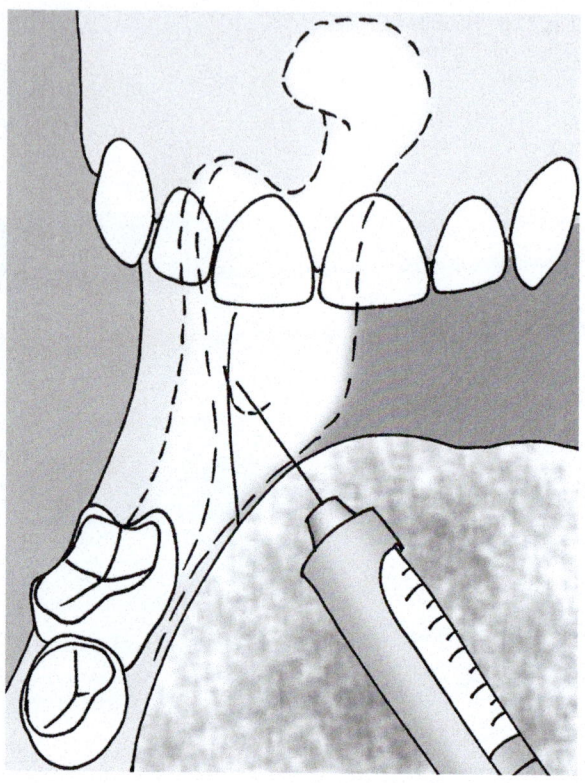

Fig. 27.6 Inferior alveolar block (Artist Credit: Alison Seliger)

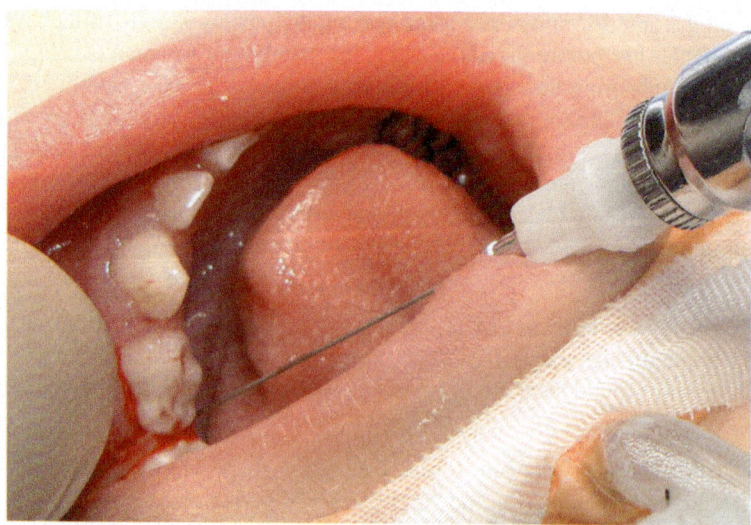

Fig. 27.7 Periodontal ligament injection (Photo credit: The Children's Hospital Boston)

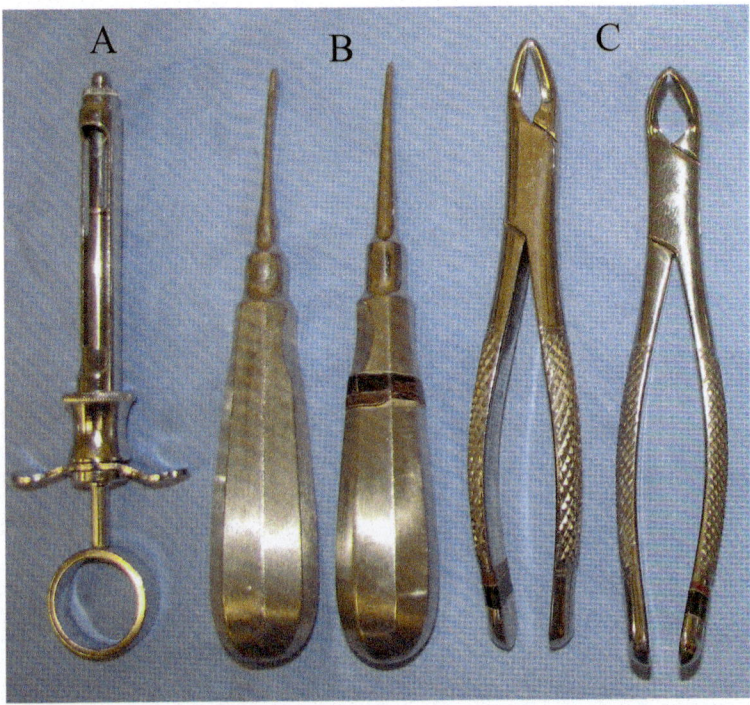

Fig. 27.8 Example of extraction instruments. (**a**) Anesthetic syringe. (**b**) Elevators. (**c**) Forceps (Photo credit: The Children's Hospital Boston)

break the PDL from the bone. The tooth should begin to lift and move slightly with each twist. Again, be sure that you are elevating only the tooth to be extracting by applying pressure again the tooth and supporting bone only, and not on the neighboring tooth. Repeat for the other side of the tooth (see Figs. 27.8 and 27.9).

Step 4: Use sterilized extraction forceps (or pliers with serrated edges that will grab the tooth without slipping), and grab the tooth at the base of the crown near the gingiva. Apply apical pressure to the tooth while slowly rocking the tooth front to back (if a molar) or twisting the tooth around side to side (if an incisor or canine). Apical pressure toward the roots helps to prevent a root from breaking off in the socket during extraction. If the tooth is not moving in a range of at least several millimeters during this step, repeat Step 3. Continue to apply apical pressure and slowly rocking the tooth until you hear the PDL breaking and the tooth begins to lift with ease out of the socket (see Figs. 27.8, 27.10, and 27.11).

Tip: Take your time. Extractions are a matter of proper technique, not strength or force. Once the tooth lifts with ease, pull it out completely from the socket. Be careful and keep in mind that a permanent tooth is likely directly below, and you do not want to disturb it. Primary molars have flared roots to accommodate the developing permanent tooth below, so use extra care not to break a root when extracting a primary molar (see Fig. 27.12).

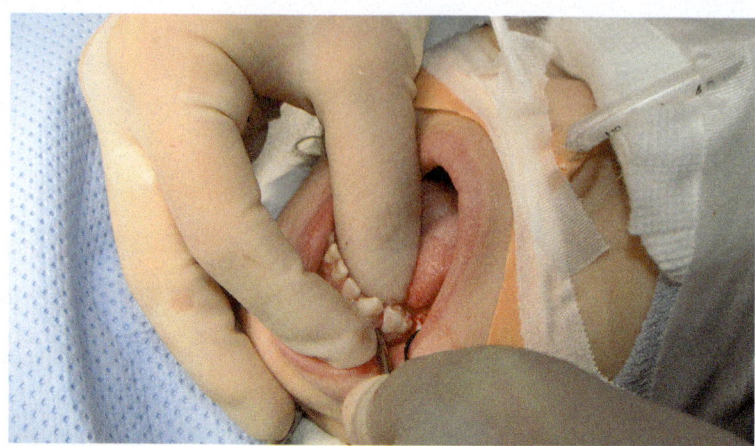

Fig. 27.9 Elevation of a tooth for extraction (Photo credit: The Children's Hospital Boston)

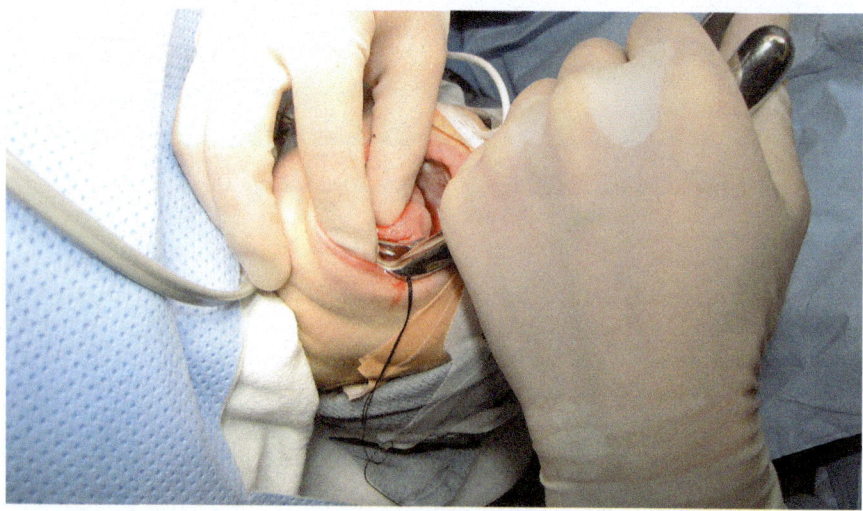

Fig. 27.10 Hand positioning of the extraction forceps. Note the string tied around the tooth so the child does not swallow it (Photo credit: The Children's Hospital Boston)

Step 5: Apply pressure to the socket with cotton or cloth; have the patient bite on it for several minutes to control bleeding. Prescribe pain medications as needed.

Postoperative instructions: Have the patient continue to bite on the cotton for about 10–20 min. Oozing throughout the rest of the day and even into night is normal but continued bleeding is not. Parents should report uncontrolled bleeding the same day. The anesthetic will wear off in about 1–2 h; parents should watch to be sure their child does not bite or chew his lips or cheeks while he is still numb, causing

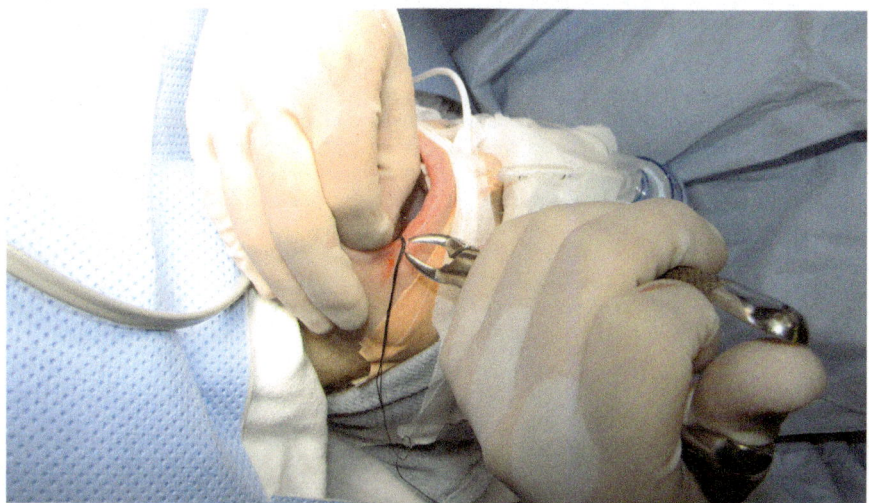

Fig. 27.11 Forceps positioned over tooth, apical pressure applied (Photo credit: The Children's Hospital Boston)

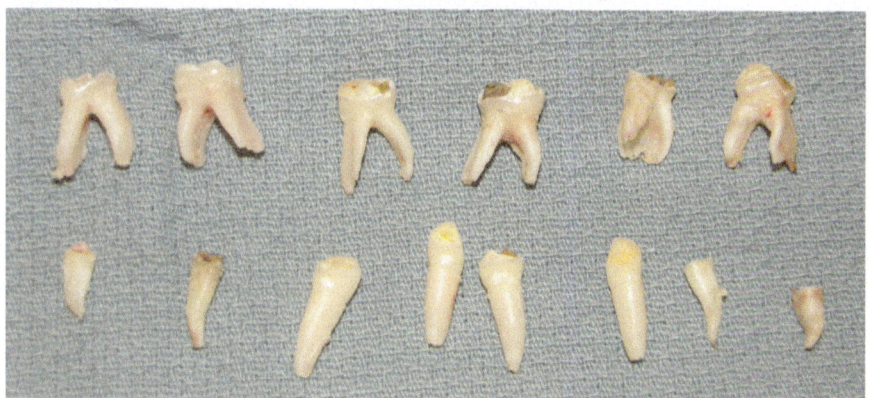

Fig. 27.12 Examples of primary teeth. Note the flared roots of the molars in the *top row*; maxillary molars have three roots, mandibular molars have two roots. Rounded roots of the canines and incisors, *bottom row*, allow for twisting during extraction (Photo credit: The Children's Hospital Boston)

trauma unknowingly. Tell parents to give the child a soft or liquid diet for the next 2 days and do not allow the child to drink soda or carbonated beverages. This increases the chances of "dry socket," where there is not adequate blood supply for healing, leading to painful bone exposure in the extraction site. Have the parent assist the child to maintain normal hygiene and rinse daily for the next 7 days to remove any food particles trapped in the extraction site.

Recommended Reading

Beaglehole R, Benzian H, Crail J, Mackay J. The oral health atlas: mapping a neglected global health issue. Cointrin: FDI World Dental Education and Myriad Editions; 2009.

Dickson M. Where there is no dentist. Berkeley, CA: Hesperian Foundation; 2006.

Langlais RP, Miller CS. Color atlas of common oral diseases. 2nd ed. Philadelphia, PA: Williams and Wilkins; 1998.

Frencken JE, Holmgren C, van Palenstein Helderman WH. Basic package of oral care. Nijmegen: World Health Organization Collaborating Center for Oral Health Care Planning and Future Scenarios and College of Dental Science, University of Nijmegen; 2002.

Association of State and Territorial Dental Directors. Basic screening surveys: an approach to monitoring community oral health of preschool and school children. Revised; 2008.

Chapter 28
Neurological Issues and Epilepsy in Children and Adolescents in the Developing World

Amy C. Lee

Keywords Global neurology • Epilepsy • Hydrocephalus • Motor impairment • Traumatic brain injury

Overview

- Epilepsy can often be diagnosed clinically without the need for ancillary testing.
- Epilepsy treatment is highly cost-effective and 70 % of epilepsy patients can become seizure free with antiepileptic drugs (AEDs).
- Early recognition of hydrocephalus is important as a potentially treatable cause of cognitive and motor impairment, but treatment remains challenging in low- and middle-income countries (LMICs).
- In patients presenting with motor impairment, a good clinical history and physical examination can help localize the lesion and narrow the differential diagnosis.
- Traumatic brain injury (TBI), especially from road traffic accidents, is a significant cause of morbidity and mortality in children in LMICs.

A.C. Lee, M.D., M.P.H. (✉)
Neurology Department, Palo Alto Medical Foundation, 701 E El Camino Real, Mountain View, CA 94040, USA
e-mail: amylee@gmail.com; leea9@sutterhealth.org

Neurological Burden in Children

Data on neurological diseases and disability in children in LMICs is scarce. A population-based study in Kilifi, Kenya surveying children age 6–9 for disability or epilepsy demonstrated a prevalence of 6.1 %, with the majority suffering from epilepsy (epilepsy 4.1 %, cognitive impairment 3.1 %, hearing loss 1.4 %, motor impairment 0.5 %, and visual deficits 0.2 %). In children attending a tertiary neurological clinic in Mulago, Uganda, the main presenting problems were epileptic seizures (45 %), motor deficits (28 %), mental handicap (17 %), behavior problems (3.9 %), movement disorder (2.0 %), hydrocephalus (1.8 %), and other (2.3 %). Similar findings have been described in other studies from LMICs. Using data from the Global Burden of Disease study (2004), epilepsy accounts for 1.6 % of total disability adjusted life years (DALYs) for children ages 5–14 in LMICs.[1] This chapter discusses evaluation and treatment of common neurological diseases in resource limited settings, particularly epilepsy. Central nervous system (CNS) infections such as meningitis, encephalitis, and cerebral malaria are discussed elsewhere in this handbook.

Epilepsy and Seizures

Definitions: *Epilepsy* is a chronic condition characterized by recurrent seizures not provoked by an acute brain insult or metabolic disturbance. *Active epilepsy* is defined as more than two unprovoked seizures in the past year. *Seizures* occur due to abnormal excess electrical discharges in the brain. *Status epilepticus* is a prolonged seizure lasting more than 30 min or recurrent seizures without return to consciousness in between.

Epidemiology: Eighty percent of the 50 million people with epilepsy (PWE) live in LMICs, and even though highly cost-effective treatment exists, the majority does not receive or have access to it. Studies suggest a higher incidence and prevalence of epilepsy in LMICs compared to developed countries, presumably due to increase exposure to risk factors: perinatal brain injury, intracranial infections (e.g., meningitis, encephalitis, cerebral malaria, cysticercosis, tuberculosis), TBI, and toxic exposures (e.g., lead, pesticides).

Clinical history/presentation: Table 28.1 describes the most common seizure types. PWE may have multiple seizure types. *The diagnosis of seizures and epilepsy can usually be made from a thorough clinical history*:

- Description of clinical event: aura/prodrome, evolution, post-ictal phase, duration and frequency, triggers

---

[1] World Health Organization. Global Burden of Disease Statistics. http://www.who.int/healthinfo/global_burden_disease/estimates_regional/en/index.html. Accessed October 15, 2012.

Table 28.1 Clinical presentation of most common seizure types[a]

Generalized tonic clonic seizures (convulsions)	• Loss of consciousness with period of stiffening, followed by shaking from alternating contraction and relaxation movements. May be associated with tongue biting, bowel or bladder incontinence • May be primarily generalized or may start out as focal seizures that secondarily generalize • Most common presenting seizure type
Absence seizures	• Change in awareness with blank stare, eyes usually roll up with frequent blinking, lasting a few seconds and many times over course of a day • Typically in children
Complex partial seizures	Change in awareness with automatisms such as lip smacking and repeated aimless movements
Simple partial seizures	Ranges from rhythmic shaking of one side of the body; tingling and numbness of one side of the body; altered taste, small, vision, or hearing

[a]Myoclonic, tonic, and atonic seizures are rare

- Symptoms to suggest a seizure provoking factor: fever, recent malaise, headache
- Risk factors for and family history of epilepsy
- Prior AED trials

Febrile seizures, due to fever without evidence of an intracranial infection, are common in children 6 months to 6 years, usually present as brief generalized convulsions, and do not require AED treatment. Complex febrile seizures that are focal, more than 15 min, or repetitive, should raise suspicion for intracranial infection, especially cerebral malaria.

Physical examination: *Fever, hypertension, head injury, or meningismus* may be signs of a provoking factor. *Hypotension or cardiac abnormalities* may suggest syncope rather than seizure. *Developmental delay or focal neurological deficits* may indicate an underlying risk factor. *Unequal or unreactive pupils* may signal cerebral edema in unconscious patients.

Diagnostic testing: May not be needed. For acute or first time seizures, consider tests (if available) to rule out provoking factors: complete blood count, sodium, glucose, calcium, urea/creatinine, liver function, malaria smear, HIV, RPR, lumbar puncture.

Electroencephalogram (EEG) and neuroimaging, even when available, are prohibitively expensive and obtained judiciously. An EEG is unlikely to change management in patients with a clinical history clearly consistent with epilepsy, but may be helpful when the diagnosis is unclear or seizures are refractory. Brain imaging evaluates for underlying etiologies such as tumors, focal infections/abscesses, strokes, and hemorrhages, and should be considered for children presenting with focal onset seizures with an unexplained cause, HIV and new onset seizures, and frequent and severe headaches.

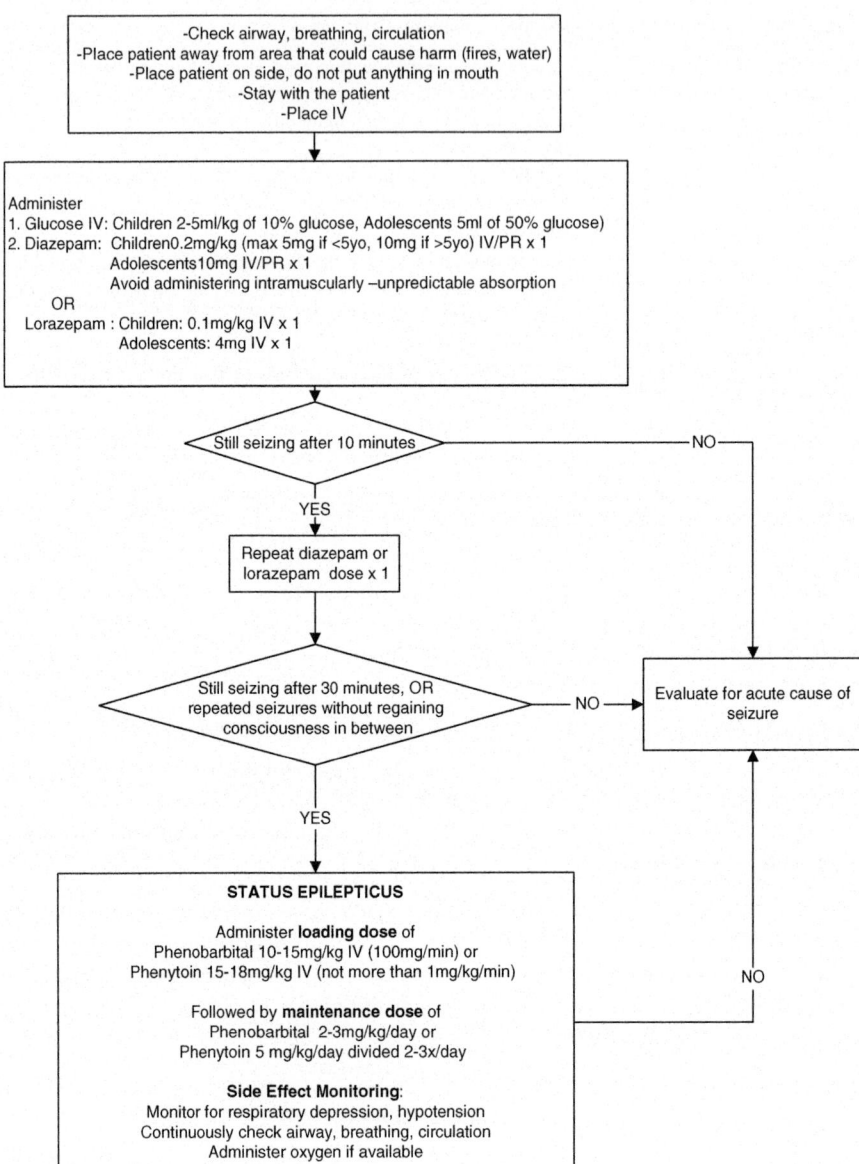

Fig 28.1 Management of acute seizures and status epilepticus

Treatment: See Fig. 28.1 for management of acute seizures and status epilepticus. In children diagnosed with active epilepsy, start AEDs (Tables 28.2 and 28.3).

AED choice: Phenobarbital, phenytoin, carbamazepine, and valproic acid are all on the WHO core list of essential medicines for children. Availability and cost are highly variable in resource limited settings, and usually the major determinant of AED choice. Phenobarbital remains the most widely available due to its low cost

Table 28.2 Dosing of most commonly available antiepileptic drugs in resource limited settings

	Starting dose	Increments	Maintenance dose
Carbamazepine			
Children	5 mg/kg/day divided 2×/day	5 mg/kg/day every week	10–30 mg/kg/day divided 2–3×/day
Adolescents	100–200 mg divided 2×/day	200 mg every week	400–1,400 mg divided 2–3×/day
Phenobarbital			
Children	2–3 mg/kg/day at bedtime	1 mg/kg/day every month	2–6 mg/kg/day at bedtime
Adolescents	60 mg at bedtime	60 mg every month	60–180 mg at bedtime
Phenytoin			
Children	3–4 mg/kg/day divided 2×/day	1 mg/kg/day every week	3–8 mg/kg/day divided 2–3×/day
Adolescents	150–200 mg daily	50 mg every week	200–400 mg daily
Valproic acid			
Children	15–20 mg/kg/day divided 2×/day	5–10 mg/kg/day every week	15–30 mg/kg/day divided 2–3×/day
Adolescents	400 mg divided 2×/day	200 mg every week	400–2,000 mg divided 2–3×/day

Table 28.3 Side effects of most commonly available antiepileptic drugs in resource limited settings

	Dose dependent	Idiosyncratic
Carbamazepine	Blurry vision, double vision, dizziness, nausea, ataxia	Hyponatremia, skin rash, bone marrow suppression, hepatitis
Phenobarbital	Drowsiness, behavioral disturbance, hyperactivity	Skin rash, bone marrow suppression, hepatitis
Phenytoin	Drowsiness, ataxia. Long term: gum hyperplasia, coarse face, hirsutism	Skin rash, bone marrow suppression, hepatitis
Valproic acid	Drowsiness, tremor, weight gain, transient hair loss	Pancreatitis, thrombocytopenia, highest risk of hepatic failure

and is a first-line agent in many countries. All four are effective for partial and generalized seizures aside from absence seizures; only valproic acid is effective for absence seizures. In children with cognitive or behavioral disorders, carbamazepine or valproic acid may be preferred due to concerns that phenobarbital and phenytoin may have cognitive and behavioral side effects. In children with coexisting epilepsy and HIV, valproic acid may be preferred due to concerns that enzyme inducing AEDs may lower antiretroviral drug levels.

AED principles: Monotherapy generally provides better seizure control and less side effects than polytherapy, and polytherapy should not be tried until at least two attempts at monotherapy. Aim for the lowest dose that achieves seizure control without intolerable side effects. Drug failure is defined as continued seizures despite maximal dosage, and/or unacceptable side effects. If one drug fails, switch to a second drug, slowly tapering the first drug only after the second drug has reached a therapeutic dose. If two monotherapies fail, consider treatment adherence, switching to a third drug, using a combination of two drugs, or reviewing the diagnosis. Stopping AEDs may be considered after 2 years of seizure freedom, slowly tapering the drug by about 25 % every month.

Efficacy: About 30 % of PWE will not become seizure free with AEDs, but half of them will have a substantial decrease in frequency. Refractory seizures are more common in children with coexisting developmental delay.

Follow-up: Every month in patients who continue to have seizures. Every 3–6 months in children with controlled epilepsy; intervals may be dependent on how much medication can be dispensed with each visit/prescription.

Education: Patient, family, and community education are critical to dispel misconceptions and social stigma surrounding epilepsy. Family should be counseled on the following:

- What epilepsy is: a *treatable* medical condition that is not contagious.
- Proper medication use: medications must be taken every day; seizures may continue initially until sufficient blood levels of medication are reached; abrupt discontinuation can be dangerous; and each medication has potential side effects.
- Lifestyle factors: children can attend school and do most things, but should avoid being near open fires, at high heights, or swimming alone, where having a seizure can cause significant injury.
- The importance of regular follow-up.

Hydrocephalus

Definition: Increase in cerebrospinal fluid (CSF) volume, usually due to obstruction of CSF flow or abnormal CSF absorption.

Epidemiology: Risk factors include prematurity, meningitis/ventriculitis, spina bifida, and maternal toxoplasmosis. Prevention includes proper antenatal care such as folate supplementation and prompt treatment of CNS infections.

Clinical symptoms/presentation: Macrocephaly/accelerated head growth if hydrocephalus develops prior to fontanel closure (<2 years old). Other symptoms include poor feeding, irritability, vomiting, lethargy, cognitive slowing or regression, visual disturbance, headache, seizures, and difficulty walking.

Physical examination: Follow head circumference monthly in infants with risk factors. Look for downward gaze deviation (setting sun sign); signs of increased intracranial pressure (ICP) such as bulging fontanel, scalp vein distension, papilledema, and lateral gaze impairment (sixth nerve palsy); lower extremity spasticity.

Diagnostic studies: Cranial ultrasound (if fontanels are not closed) or head CT scan to evaluate ventricular size. Skull X-ray may show separation of the cranial sutures. If focal neurological deficit is not present to suggest a mass lesion, consider lumbar puncture to measure CSF pressure in children with closed fontanels.

Treatment: Refer to surgeon for definitive management, usually ventriculoperitoneal shunt (VPS) placement. Endoscopic third ventriculostomy, in which an opening is created in the floor of the third ventricle for CSF drainage to the subarachnoid space, is under evaluation in some LMICs as an alternative to avoid shunt dependence. Use acetazolamide (100 mg/kg/day) and furosemide (1 mg/kg/day) only as temporizing measures. Management remains challenging due to late presentation to medical attention and lack of access to surgical care.

Follow-up: Regular surgical follow-up is needed due to high rates of shunt complications, which is especially dangerous in resource limited settings where urgent evaluation may not be available. Shunt malfunction manifests with recurrent symptoms of hydrocephalus, and shunt infection presents with signs of meningitis, abdominal pain, and surgical site erythema/swelling.

Motor Deficits

The differential diagnosis of motor deficits is broad and a detailed discussion is beyond the scope of this handbook (please see relevant chapters in Fenichel (2009) for more information). This section briefly discusses basic diagnostic and treatment considerations. While definitive diagnoses may not be possible without advanced diagnostic studies and especially neuroimaging, a good clinical history and physical examination can help narrow the differential diagnosis (Table 28.4). Clinical history should elicit whether the deficits are congenital, acute, or progressive in onset; physical examination should focus on localizing the process to the brain, spinal cord, or peripheral nervous system.

If deficits are acute in onset and a stroke is suspected, obtain available tests to look for common causes of childhood stroke (connective tissue disorders/vasculopathy, congenital heart disease, rheumatic heart disease, infectious complications, and sickle cell disease). If fever is present and CNS infection is suspected (e.g., abscess, tuberculosis, or opportunistic infections in HIV patients) initiate empiric treatment promptly. Lumbar puncture is contraindicated without imaging due to the presence of focal neurological deficits. Signs of increased ICP, discussed in the previous section, may indicate mass lesions (e.g., tumors, CNS infections) or hydrocephalus. High-dose steroids (dexamethasone 0.1–0.3 mg/kg intravenous every 6 h or equivalent) may temporarily reduce cerebral edema from these causes, but will only be a temporizing measure for mass lesions without definitive treatment, and could worsen CNS infections if appropriate antibiotic therapy has not been initiated.

Table 28.4 Clinical evaluation of motor impairment

Localization	Physical examination		Differential diagnosis (common diseases)
	Typical pattern of weakness	Associated findings	
Brain	Hemiparesis ± face weakness	Hyperreflexia Spasticity ± sensory loss	Congenital: cerebral palsy Acute: stroke Trauma: traumatic brain injury/hematoma Fever: encephalitis, abscess, tuberculosis, opportunistic infections in HIV patient Signs of increased ICP: mass lesions from tumor or CNS infections, hydrocephalus
	Ataxia[a]	Cranial nerve palsies	Posterior fossa tumor
Spinal cord (myelopathy)	Paraparesis or quadriparesis	Hyperreflexia Spasticity ± sensory level Urinary retention or incontinence	Back pain: compressive etiologies such as Pott's disease, epidural abscess, trauma/epidural hematoma, tumor Other: infectious or inflammatory transverse myelitis, nutritional deficiency (e.g., B12), tropical spastic paraparesis
Peripheral nervous system	Variable	Hyporeflexia Flaccid ± sensory loss	Rapidly ascending: Guillain Barre Syndrome Fever, not vaccinated: poliomyelitis

[a] Patients with impairment from ataxia often present with the clinical complaint of weakness

Patients presenting with spastic paraplegia or quadriplegia consistent with a spinal cord process (i.e., myelopathy) should obtain spine X-rays to evaluate for findings that might suggest a compressive cause (e.g., Pott's disease, epidural abscess, trauma/epidural hematoma, tumor). A high ESR and/or positive blood cultures may point to an epidural abscess. If a structural cause is found, the patient should be promptly referred for surgical intervention. A complete blood count may reveal macrocytosis to suggest B12 deficiency. Lumbar puncture for cell count, glucose, protein, gram stain and culture, AFB stain and culture should be considered to evaluate for an infectious etiology of transverse myelitis, a demyelinating disorder of the spinal cord. If studies are unrevealing, a trial of high-dose steroids (prednisone 2 mg/kg/day not to exceed 100 mg or equivalent, followed by 4 week taper) may be considered to empirically treat for an inflammatory transverse myelitis. A syndrome of tropical spastic paraparesis has been described in a number of LMICs, especially in Africa, and is thought to be due to neurotoxic substances from cassava-based diets or grass pea; unfortunately no treatment is available.

Developmental Disorders

Developmental disorders may occur as a result of genetic syndromes, metabolic disease, or maternal/perinatal injury/infection. Reversible causes associated with malnutrition (e.g., iodine or folate deficiency) or hydrocephalus should be sought. Epilepsy, depression, and behavioral disorders are common coexisting conditions that should be properly treated when present (see Chap. 25). Education and support of family members, as well as community-based rehabilitation, can improve the quality of life of family and children with developmental disorders.

Traumatic Brain Injury

Epidemiology: Mechanisms include road traffic accidents, falls, and violence. Road traffic accidents are the major cause globally, with higher incidence and six times higher fatality rate among children in LMICs than high income countries, and can be prevented by use of seat belts, traffic helmets, improved road conditions, and traffic laws.

Physical examination: ABCs; signs of skull fracture (raccoon eyes, hemotympanum, otorrhea/rhinorrhea, Battle's sign/mastoid ecchymoses); signs of other trauma (chest, abdomen, spine, skin); level of consciousness; pupil asymmetry indicating increased ICP from cerebral edema; eye deviation or nystagmus to suggest ongoing seizure; focal neurological deficits. Severity can be classified by the Glasgow Coma Scale (mild 13–15, moderate 9–12, and severe 3–8).

Diagnostic tests: Skull X-rays or head CT, cervical spine X-rays.

Table 28.5 Medical management of moderate or severe TBI

Fluids	• Aim for euvolemia with normal saline
	• Glucose or hypotonic saline can exacerbate cerebral edema
Gastric ulcer prophylaxis	• Sucralfate, H2 antagonist, or proton pump inhibitor
Antiepileptic drugs	• Prophylaxis for 7 days in cases of traumatic intracranial hemorrhage
	• Treatment if concern for ongoing seizure—may be non-convulsive (look for gaze deviation, nystagmus)
	• Phenobarbital 10–15 mg/kg IV/IM followed by 2–3 mg/kg/day *or* Phenytoin 15–18 mg/kg IV followed by 5 mg/kg/day
	• Monitor for respiratory depression, hypotension
Decrease ICP	• Initiate measures in unresponsive patients or for worsening exam (2 point GCS decline)
	• Elevate head of bed 45°
	• Hyperventilation if bag mask or other ventilatory assistance is available, only acutely temporizing and prolonged hyperventilation can lead to rebound increase in ICP
	• Mannitol 0.25–2 g/kg IV bolus followed by 0.25–0.5 g/kg IV q4–6 h, monitor renal function/urinary output
	• Treat fever, avoid aspirin or nonsteroidal anti-inflammatory drugs

Treatment: Patients should undergo cervical spine precautions until they can be clinically cleared. About 2 % of patients presenting clinically with mild TBI will deteriorate. Observe for 24 h patients at the greatest risk: worsening level of consciousness, focal neurological deficit, seizure, or fracture on skull X-ray. For patients with moderate or severe TBI, transfer, if possible, to higher level care where intensive care and neurosurgical capabilities are available. Medical management is shown in Table 28.5.

Recommended Reading

Bauman N, Poenaru D. Hydrocephalus in Africa: a surgical perspective. Surgery in Africa. The Ptolemy Project-Office of International Surgery-University of Toronto Web site. April 2008. http://ptolemy.library.utoronto.ca/surgery-in-africa. Accessed 18 Oct 2012.

Dekker PA. Epilepsy: A manual for Medical and Clinical Officers in Africa [Internet]. Revised ed. Geneva: World Health Organization; 2002. Available from: http://www.who.int/mental_health/publications/epilepsy_neurological_disorders/en/index.html.

Fenichel GM. Clinical pediatric neurology: a signs and symptoms approach. 6th ed. Philadelphia, PA: Elsevier Saunders; 2009.

Howlett W. Neurology in Africa. Bergen, Norway: BRIC; 2012. Available from: http://www.uib.no/cih/en/resources/neurology-in-africa.

Idro R, Newton C, Kiguli S, Kakooza-Mwesige A. Child neurology practice and neurological disorders in East Africa. J Child Neurol. 2010;25:518–24.

World Health Organization. mhGAP Intervention Guide. Geneva: World Health Organization; 2010: p. 32–43. Available from: http://www.who.int/mental_health/publications/mhGAP_intervention_guide/en/index.html.

Chapter 29
Care of the Child Immigrant

Jennifer Kasper, Nupur Gupta, Andrea J. Hunter, and Brett D. Nelson

Keywords Child immigrant • Public assistance programs • Screening • Immunizations • Preventive care

Overview

- Children of immigrants are the fastest-growing segment of the US population under age 18.
- Taking a complete history can be challenging due to language and cultural barriers and lack of written information on the child's prior health status and health care interventions in the child's country of origin.
- Children who arrive from other countries may have a host of nutritional deficiencies, physical ailments and disabilities, developmental/cognitive delays, and mental

J. Kasper, M.D., M.P.H.
Division of Global Health, MassGeneral Hospital for Children, 100 Cambridge St., 15th Floor, Boston, MA 02114, USA
e-mail: jkasper1@partners.org

N. Gupta, M.D., M.P.H.
MassGeneral Hospital for Children, Harvard Medical School,
55 Fruit Street, Boston, MA 02114, USA
e-mail: ngupta3@partners.org

A.J. Hunter, M.D., F.R.C.P.C., F.A.A.P., D.T.M.&H.
Division of General Pediatrics, Pediatrics Department, McMaster Children's Hospital, McMaster University, Hamilton, ON, Canada

B.D. Nelson, M.D., M.P.H., D.T.M.&H. (✉)
Division of Global Health, MassGeneral Hospital for Children, 100 Cambridge St., 15th Floor, Boston, MA 02114, USA
e-mail: brett.d.nelson@gmail.com

health issues. Therefore, screening tests and referrals to subspecialists (e.g., oral health, cardiology, development) should be tailored to the disease(s) of concern.
- An immigrant or refugee child faces many challenges in adjusting to life in the USA. It is important to be familiar with national and state policies regarding immigrant eligibility for public assistance programs (e.g., health insurance, TANF, food stamps, WIC) to ensure that a child receives appropriate health, nutrition, and educational services for optimal health and development.

Introduction

One in five children in the USA is a child of an immigrant, and the majority of them live in mixed-status households (i.e., a mix of people with documented and undocumented immigration statuses). Furthermore, three-quarters of children in immigrant families are US citizens. One in four low-income children (i.e., in families with incomes below 200 % of the federal poverty level) is the child of an immigrant; a subset of these children are refugees or children of refugees. In 2011, 56,424 refugees from around the world arrived in the USA and settled in all 50 states. The majority of refugees come from Afghanistan, Iraq, Sudan, Somalia, Democratic Republic of Congo, Burundi, Vietnam, Turkey, Angola, and Myanmar.

Public assistance programs provide economic support. However, health care providers need to understand who is eligible for which programs. Federal Welfare Reform (Enacted August 22, 1996) imposed new restrictions on Medicaid eligibility for legally present noncitizens in the USA and persons residing under color of law (PRUCOL, e.g., a person with temporary protected status). Most legal permanent residents (green card holders) who entered the USA after August 22, 1996 are barred from Medicaid for 5 years after obtaining their status. However, certain groups are eligible for Medicaid: refugees, asylum seekers, persons with deportation withheld, veterans (and spouses, widows, children of veterans), certain victims of domestic violence, certain Cuban/Haitians, all Native Americans born outside the USA, and certain Amerasians from Vietnam, victims of severe forms of trafficking (and dependent children); special immigrants from Iraq for first 6 months, and special immigrants from Afghanistan for first 8 months.

Immigrants fear accessing public assistance because they think that there may be negative consequences. Current information about immigrant eligibility for public assistance programs and other immigrant issues can be found at the National Immigration Law Center, www.nilc.org, Massachusetts Law Reform Institute, www.mlri.org, Massachusetts Immigrant and Refugee Association, www.mira.org.

Taking a History

With few exceptions, health care providers should use an interpreter and be mindful of age and gender cultural differences. For example, it may not be appropriate for a male health care provider to perform a physical exam on a female patient, or the mother or the patient may not be allowed to answer certain questions. Ask parents' permission prior to removing clothing or examining certain parts of the body. A comprehensive history contains the following elements:

- Current concerns, questions
- Past medical history: includes age, date of birth, perinatal and birth history, history of infectious diseases, and gynecological/sexual history/history of STIs/female cutting in children and adolescents aged 10–21
- Medications, traditional remedies, allergies
- Immunization record
- Family history
- Review of systems: pay close attention to signs and symptoms of abuse, PTSD, depression, anxiety, adjustment disorders
- Social history: country of origin; language spoken; religious beliefs; prior living conditions: housing, sanitation, access to food/water, exposure to violence/abuse, health care access; transit/time spent in detention centers; and current social/housing situation (e.g., is the child living with one/both biological parents and/or other family members, and are there family members in country of origin), immigration status of household members
- Developmental milestones and concerns, school integration/expectations for school and work in adolescents

Physical Examination

- Vital signs including temperature
- Anthropometrics: weight-for-age, height-for-age, weight-for-height, head circumference-for-age, BMI
- Nutritional status: signs/symptoms of micronutrient deficiency (e.g., Bitot's spots, rachitic changes)
- Hearing, vision
- Oral health assessment
- Thyroid exam: evidence of goiter
- Signs of congenital infection: microcephaly, rash, dental changes
- Scoliosis, other vertebral malformations: signs of Pott's disease
- Heart murmurs, clubbing, clicks: undiagnosed congenital heart disease, rheumatic heart disease, pulmonary disease
- BCG scar
- Scars suggestive of present or past physical abuse
- Lymphadenopathy
- Hepatosplenomegaly
- Signs of female genital mutilation/sexual abuse/STIs including condyloma

Screening Tests

Children who arrive from other countries may have a host of nutritional deficiencies, physical ailments and disabilities, developmental/cognitive delays, and mental health issues. Prevalence of infectious diseases such as intestinal parasites, latent tuberculosis, HIV, Hepatitis B and C, and malaria may range between 15 and 40 %, depending on country of origin. Therefore, screening tests and referrals to subspecialists (e.g., dentist, cardiologist, developmental) should be tailored to the disease of concern (Table 29.1). Evidence-based guidelines for screening child immigrant are an evolving field.

Immunizations

In most countries throughout the world, the vaccine schedule follows the WHO recommendations (please see the Chap. 21 for more information); hence, most immigrant and refugee children arrive in the USA lacking protection from some vaccine-preventable diseases. For children who arrive in the USA without vaccine records, recommendations are as follows: revaccinate all children <13 years of age according to the AAP/CDC guidelines for catch-up immunizations, and check serology for children >13 years of age and give vaccines if the child does not have antibodies to vaccine-preventable illnesses. Giving vaccines to children less than 13 years of age is more cost-effective than checking serology in this age group. Two important categories of children deserve special attention: immunocompromised children (e.g., HIV-infected children with CD4+ T-lymphocyte percentages ≤ 15 % or ≤ 200 cells/µL) should not receive live vaccines; and patients with Hgb SS disease are at high risk of infection with encapsulated bacteria and, therefore, should receive pneumococcal (conjugate and polysaccharide), meningococcal (C conjugate and quadrivalent polysaccharide), Hemophilus influenzae, and yearly influenza vaccines.

Psychosocial Assessment

Research suggests that immigrant status confers increased risk of psychological and behavioral disorders. Immigrant children may have been victims of abuse or exposed to violence and torture (e.g., in their native country, while migrating to the USA). It is important to monitor for PTSD, depression, anxiety, adjustment disorder, substance abuse. See Chap. 25 for an extensive review of the most common mental health disorders in children and adolescents.

Table 29.1 Screening tests as dictated by clinical presentation or risk factors

Disease of concern	Screening test(s)	Reference values
Infectious		
Gastritis due to *H. pylori*	Stool	± *H. pylori* Ag
Gonorrhea, Chlamydia	Urine for gonorrhea and chlamydia	±
Hepatitis	Hepatitis A, B, and C serology, liver enzymes, albumin, PT/PTT	HBsAb = immune HBsAg = carrier state, current or chronic infection HBcAg = current or past infection Hep A and Hep C ± AST/SGOT infants 18–74 U/L, children 15–46 U/L ALT/SGPT 0–2 months old 8–78 U/L, >2 months old 8–36 U/L Albumin 0–1 year old 2–4 g/dL, >1 year old 3.5–5.5 g/dL PT 11–15 s PTT 42–54 s
HIV	HIV PCR (if <18 months old) or HIV Ab (if >18 months old)	±
Intestinal parasitic infection	Stool (one sample) for ova/parasite	±; presence of trophozoites and/or cysts on wet prep or ± Ag (Giardia)
Malaria	Thick and thin smears	Falciparum, Ovale, Vivax, Malariae
Pertussis	Nasal swab for Bordetella Pertussis if high suspicion due to age and lack of immunization	± PCR
Schistosomiasis	Urinalysis and serology	Hematuria, + serology
Syphilis	Enzyme immunoassay (EIA)	± (if +, must be confirmed with nontreponemal test such as VDRL, which becomes reactive 4–6 weeks after infection and titers peak in secondary to early latent stage, or RPR)
Skin infection—fungal, bacterial	Incision and drainage, culture, skin scrapings for microscopic evaluation	±

(continued)

Table 29.1 (continued)

Disease of concern	Screening test(s)	Reference values
Tuberculosis	PPD ± chest X-ray upon arrival and consider repeat 6 months later, gamma interferon	>10 mm (if past receipt of BCG less than 1 year ago; if BCG placed greater than 1 year ago, it should not be factored in PPD reading). >5 mm if from endemic/high risk area, known contact with adult with active TB, abnormal CXR, signs and symptoms of TB, or immunocompromised
Varicella and measles	Varicella and measles serology (or give vaccination)	±
Noninfectious		
Anemia	CBC, ferritin (±CRP), iron, hemoglobin electrophoresis, G6PD assay	Hemoglobin <11 mg/dL Ferritin males 24–336 μg/L, females 11–307 μg/L Iron 50–120 μg/dL G6PD 150–215 U/dL Normal hemoglobin electrophoresis (for >3 months of age): >96 % Hgb A1, 1.5–4 % HgbA2, 0–2 % Hgb F
Developmental delay	TSH, lead level, newborn metabolic screen (for infants), karyotype, fragile X	TSH 0–10 μIU/mL Lead <10 μg/dL Newborn screen as per individual diseases
Heart murmur	Echocardiogram, four limb blood pressures, ECG; Antistreptolysin O (ASO) if there is murmur suggestive of regurgitation	ASO <200 IU/ml
Mental health	SIGECAPS (Sleep disturbance, Interest reduced, guilt and self-blame, energy loss/fatigue, concentration problems, appetite changes, psychomotor changes, suicidal thoughts)	Depressed or sad mood + four other symptoms most of the time, most days, for at least 2 weeks

Micronutrient deficiency	25-OH Vitamin D or alkaline phosphatase Vitamin A Zinc	>20 ng/dL (50 nmol/L) Alkaline phosphatase newborns 60–130 U/L 1–16 year old 85–400 U/L >16 year old 30–115 U/L Retinol <20 μg/dL Albumin 0–1 year old 2–4 g/dL, >1 year old 3.5–5.5 g/dL
Poor growth (wasting, stunting)	Weight-for-age, height-for-age, BMI, MUAC, albumin	
Vision and hearing and oral health	Allen cards, stereopsis, hearing screening, screen for dental pain	

Recommended Reading

American Academy of Pediatrics. Health care for children of immigrant families. Pediatrics. 1997;100(1):153–6.

Centers for Disease Control and Prevention (CDC). Travel health. Available at: http://www.cdc.gov/travel

Davidson N, Skull S, Chaney G, Frydenberg A, Jones C, Isaacs D, Kelly P, Lampropoulos B, Raman S, Silove D, Buttery J, Smith M, Steel Z, Burgner D. Comprehensive health assessment for newly arrived refugee children in Australia. J Paediatr Child Health. 2004;40(9–10):562–8.

Gavagan T, Brodyaga L. Medical care for immigrants and refugees. Am Fam Physician. 1998;57(5):1061–8. Available at: http://www.aafp.org/afp/1998/0301/p1061.html

Jenista JA. The immigrant, refugee, or internationally adopted child. Pediatr Rev. 2001;22(12):419–29.

Appendix A
WHO Integrated Management of Childhood Illness for High HIV Settings

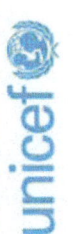

INTEGRATED MANAGEMENT OF CHILDHOOD ILLNESS FOR HIGH HIV SETTINGS

Department of Child and Adolescent Health and Development (CAH)

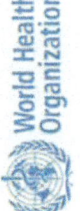

CHILD AGED 2 MONTHS UP TO 5 YEARS
ASSESS AND CLASSIFY THE SICK CHILD
Assess, Classify and Identify Treatment

- Check for General Danger Signs ... 2
- Then Ask About Main Symptoms:
  - Does the child have cough or difficult breathing? ... 2
  - Does the child have diarrhoea? ... 3
  - Does the child have fever? ... 4
  - Does the child have an ear problem? ... 5
- Then Check for Malnutrition and Anaemia ... 6
- Then Check for HIV Infection ... 7
- Then Check for Mouth and Gum Conditions ... 8
- Then Check the Child's Immunization Status ... 9
- Assess Other Problems ... 9
- Then Establish HIV Infection Status ... 10
- WHO Paediatric clinical staging for HIV ... 11
- HIV testing for the exposed child ... 10

TREAT THE CHILD
Teach the mother to give oral drugs at home:

- Oral Antibiotic ... 12
- Ciprofloxacin ... 12
- Co-trimoxazole ... 11
- Pain Relief ... 13
- Iron ... 13
- Co-artemether ... 13
- Bronchodilator ... 13

Teach the Mother to Treat Local Infections at Home

- Clear the ear by dry wicking and give eardrops ... 14
- Treat for mouth ulcers and thrush ... 14
- Soothe throat, relieve cough with safe remedy ... 14
- Treat eye infection ... 14

Give Preventive Treatments in Clinic

- Vitamin A ... 15
- Mebendazole ... 15

Give Emergency Treatment in Clinic only

- Quinine for severe malaria ... 16
- Intramuscular Antibiotic ... 16
- Diazepam for convulsions ... 16
- Treat low blood sugar ... 17

TREAT THE CHILD, continued
Give Extra Fluid for Diarrhoea and Continue Feeding

- Plan A: Treat for Diarrhoea at Home ... 18
- Plan B: Treat for Some Dehydration with ORS ... 18
- Plan C: Treat for Severe Dehydration Quickly ... 19

Give Follow-up Care

- Pneumonia ... 20
- Dysentery ... 20
- Persistent diarrhoea ... 20
- Malaria ... 21
- Fever – malaria unlikely ... 21
- Measles with eye or mouth complications ... 21
- Ear Infection ... 22
- Feeding problem ... 22
- Anaemia ... 22
- Very Low Weight ... 22
- Follow up care for child with possible HIV infection / suspected symptomatic /confirmed HIV ... 23

COUNSEL THE MOTHER

- Assess the feeding of sick infants ... 24
- Feeding Recommendations ... 25
- Counsel the mother about feeding and HIV:
  - Feeding advice for the HIV confirmed ... 26
  - Stopping breastfeeding for HIV exposed ... 26
  - AFASS criteria for stopping breastfeeding ... 27
  - Counsel the mother about feeding Problems ... 28
  - Feeding Recommendations for HIV exposed child ... 29
  - Counsel the mother about her own health ... 30
- Advise mother to increase fluids during illness ... 30
- Advise mother when to return to health worker ... 30
- Advise mother when to return immediately ... 30

SICK YOUNG INFANT AGED UP TO 2 MONTHS
ASSESS, CLASSIFY AND TREAT THE SICK YOUNG INFANT
Assess, Classify and Identify Treatment

- Check for Severe Disease and Local Infection ... 31
- Then check for Jaundice ... 32
- Then ask: Does the young infant have diarrhoea? ... 33
- Then check the young infant for HIV Infection ... 34
- Then check for Feeding Problem or Low Weight for Age in breastfed ... 35
- Then check for Feeding Problem or Low Weight for Age in non-breastfed ... 36
- Then check the young infant's immunization status ... 37
- Assess Other Problems ... 37

Treat the Young Infant and Counsel the Mother

- Intramuscular antibiotics ... 38
- Treat the young infant to prevent low blood sugar ... 38
- Keep the young infant warm on the way to hospital ... 39
- Oral antibiotic ... 39
- Treat local infections at home ... 40
- Correct positioning and attachment for breastfeeding ... 41
- Teach mother how to express breast milk ... 41
- Teach mother how to feed by cup ... 42
- How to prepare commercial formula milk ... 42
- Teach the mother to keep the low weight infant warm at home ... 43
- Advice mother to give home care to the young infant ... 44

Give Follow-up Care for the Sick Young Infant

- Local Bacterial Infection ... 45
- Jaundice ... 45
- Diarrhoea ... 46
- Possible HIV/HIV exposed ... 46
- Feeding Problem ... 47
- Low Weight for age ... 47
- Thrush ... 47

Recording Forms: Sick Child ... 48
Sick young Infant ... 49

- ANNEX A: Skin and mouth conditions ... 51
- ANNEX B: Antiretroviral therapy: Dosages ... 56
- ANNEX C: Antiretroviral therapy: Side effects ... 60
- ANNEX D: Drug dosages for opportunistic infections ... 61

Appendix A

ASSESS AND CLASSIFY THE SICK CHILD AGED 2 MONTHS UP TO 5 YEARS

ASSESS   CLASSIFY   IDENTIFY TREATMENT

ASK THE MOTHER WHAT THE CHILD'S PROBLEMS ARE
- Determine whether this is an initial or follow-up visit for this problem.
  - if follow-up visit, use the follow-up instructions on *TREAT THE CHILD* chart
  - if initial visit, assess the child as follows:

CHECK FOR GENERAL DANGER SIGNS

ASK:
- Is the child able to drink or breastfeed?
- Does the child vomit everything?
- Has the child had convulsions?

LOOK:
- See if the child is lethargic or unconscious.
- Is the child convulsing now?

A child with any general danger sign needs *URGENT* attention; complete the assessment and any pre-referral treatment immediately so that referral is not delayed.

THEN ASK ABOUT MAIN SYMPTOMS:
Does the child have cough or difficult breathing?

IF YES, ASK:
- For how long?

LOOK, LISTEN, FEEL:
- Count the breaths in one minute.
- Look for chest indrawing.
- Look and listen for stridor.
- Look and listen for wheezing.

If wheezing and either fast breathing or chest indrawing:
Give a trial of rapid acting bronchodilator for up to three times 15–20 minutes apart. Count the breaths and look for chest indrawing again, and then classify.

CHILD MUST BE CALM

Classify COUGH or DIFFICULT BREATHING

If the child is:	Fast breathing is:
2 months up to 12 months	50 breaths per minute or more
12 months up to 5 years	40 breaths per minute or more

USE ALL BOXES THAT MATCH THE CHILD'S SYMPTOMS AND PROBLEMS TO CLASSIFY THE ILLNESS.

SIGNS	CLASSIFY AS	TREATMENT (Urgent pre-referral treatments are in bold print)
• Any general danger sign or • Chest indrawing or • Stridor in calm child	SEVERE PNEUMONIA OR VERY SEVERE DISEASE	➤ **Give first dose of an appropriate antibiotic** ➤ **Refer URGENTLY to hospital**
• Fast breathing	PNEUMONIA	➤ *Give oral antibiotic for 5 days* ➤ If wheezing (even if it disappeared after rapidly acting bronchodilator) give an inhaled bronchodilator for five days* ➤ Soothe the throat and relieve the cough with a safe remedy ➤ If coughing for more than 3 weeks or if having recurrent wheezing, refer for assessment for TB or asthma ➤ Advise the mother when to return immediately ➤ Follow-up in 2 days
• No signs of pneumonia or very severe disease	COUGH OR COLD	➤ If wheezing (even if it disappeared after rapidly acting bronchodilator) give an inhaled bronchodilator for 5 days* ➤ Soothe the throat and relieve cough with a safe remedy ➤ If coughing for more than 3 weeks or if having recurrent wheezing, refer for assessment for TB or asthma ➤ Advise mother when to return immediately ➤ Follow up in 5 days if not improving

* In settings where inhaled bronchodilator is not available, oral salbutamol may be the second choice

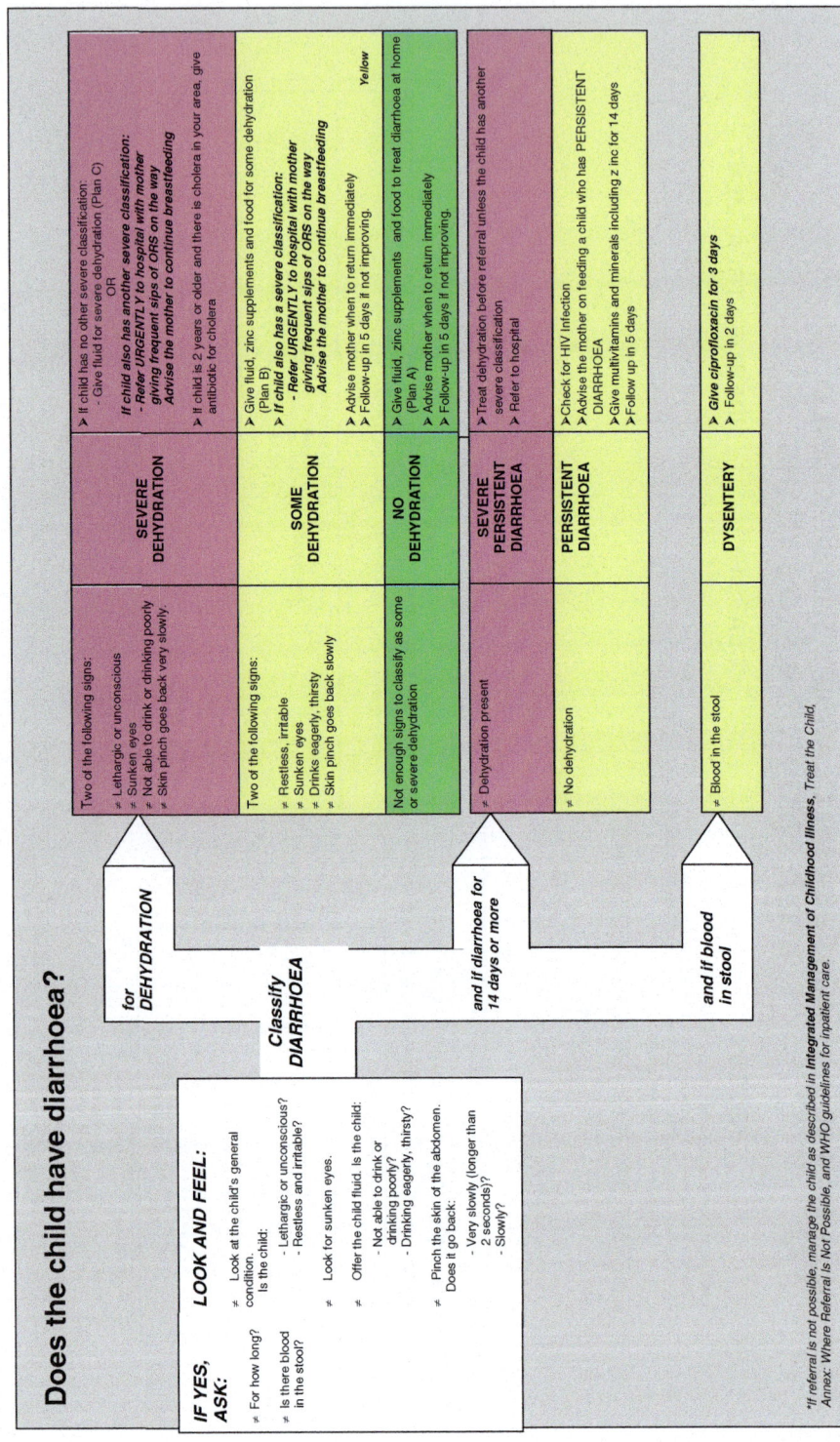

Appendix A

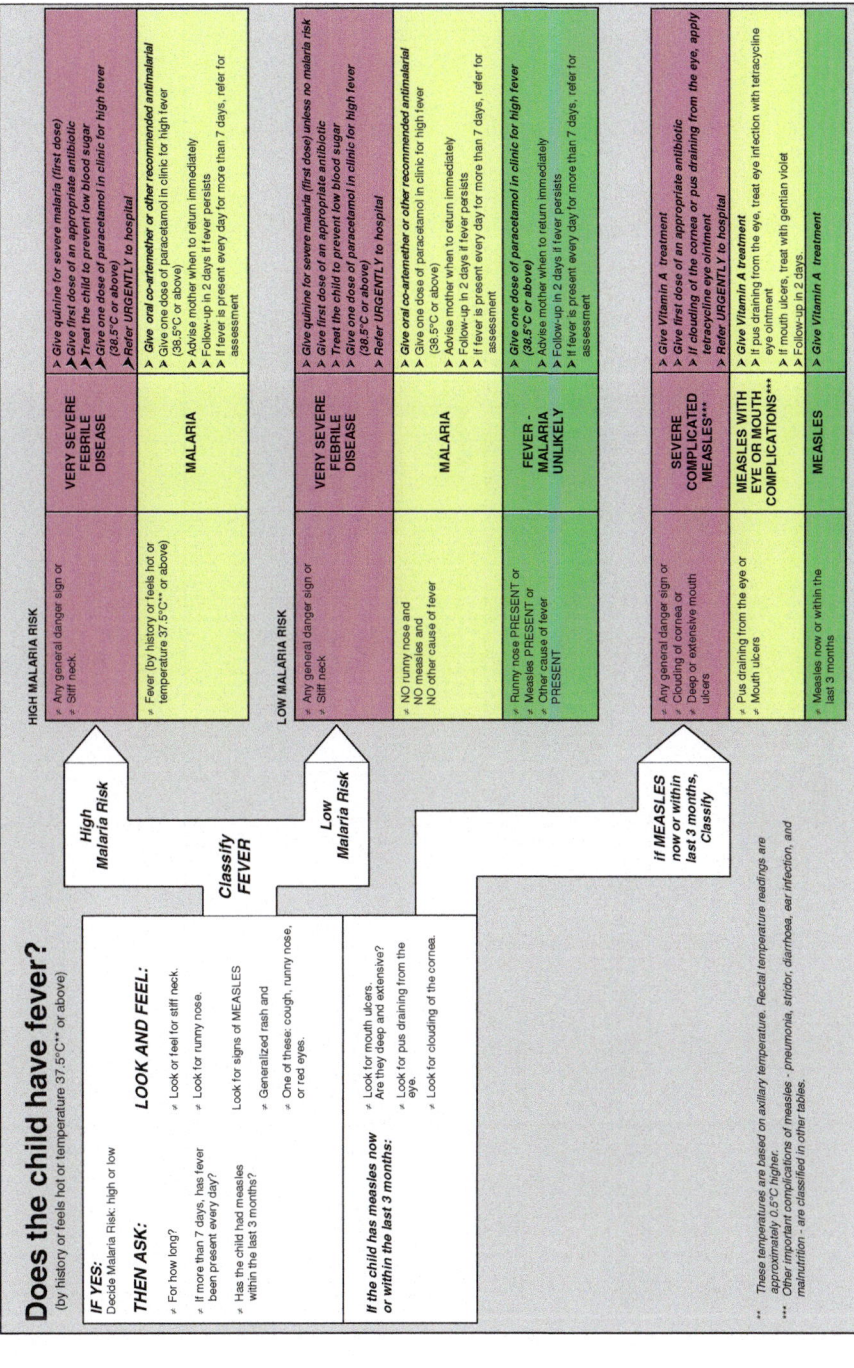

Does the child have an ear problem?

IF YES, ASK:
- Is there ear pain?
- Is there ear discharge? If yes, for how long?

LOOK AND FEEL:
- Look for pus draining from the ear.
- Feel for tender swelling behind the ear.

Classify
EAR PROBLEM

Signs	Classify as	Treatment
• Tender swelling behind the ear.	**MASTOIDITIS**	➤ *Give first dose of an appropriate antibiotic.* ➤ *Give first dose of paracetamol for pain.* ➤ *Refer URGENTLY to hospital.*
• Pus is seen draining from the ear and discharge is reported for less than 14 days, or • Ear pain.	**ACUTE EAR INFECTION**	➤ *Give an antibiotic for 5 days.* ➤ Give paracetamol for pain. ➤ Dry the ear by wicking. ➤ If ear discharge, check for HIV infection ➤ Follow-up in 5 days.
• Pus is seen draining from the ear and discharge is reported for 14 days or more.	**CHRONIC EAR INFECTION**	➤ Dry the ear by wicking. ➤ Treat with topical quinolone eardrops for 2 weeks ➤ Check for HIV infection ➤ Follow-up in 5 days.
• No ear pain and • No pus seen draining from the ear.	**NO EAR INFECTION**	➤ No treatment.

Appendix A

THEN CHECK FOR MALNUTRITION AND ANAEMIA

CHECK FOR MALNUTRITION

LOOK AND FEEL:

- Look for visible severe wasting
- Look for oedema of both feet
- Determine weight for age

CLASSIFY NUTRITIONAL STATUS

Signs	Classify as	Treatment
• Visible severe wasting or • Oedema of both feet	**SEVERE MALNUTRITION**	➤ *Treat the child to prevent low sugar* ➤ *Refer URGENTLY to a hospital*

• Very low weight for age	**VERY LOW WEIGHT**	➤ Assess the child's feeding and counsel the mother on feeding according to the feeding recommendations
		  ➤ If feeding problem, follow-up in 5 days
		  ➤ Check for HIV infection
		  ➤ Advise mother when to return immediately
		  ➤ Follow-up in 30 days

• Not very low weight for age and no other signs of malnutrition	**NOT VERY LOW WEIGHT**	➤ If child is less than 2 years old, assess the child's feeding and counsel the mother on feeding according to the feeding recommendations - If feeding problem, follow-up in 5 days ➤ Advise mother when to return immediately

CHECK FOR ANAEMIA

LOOK and FEEL:

- Look for palmar pallor. Is it:
  o Severe palmar pallor?
  o Some palmar pallor?

CLASSIFY ANAEMIA

Signs	Classify as	Treatment
• Severe palmar pallor	**SEVERE ANAEMIA**	➤ *Refer URGENTLY to hospital*
• Some palmar pallor	**ANAEMIA**	➤ Give iron ➤ Give oral antimalarial if high malaria risk ➤ Check for HIV infection ➤ Give mebendazole if child is 1 year or older and has not had a dose in the previous six months ➤ If child is less than 2 years old, assess the child's feeding and counsel the mother on feeding according to the feeding recommendations - If feeding problem, follow-up in 5 days ➤ Advise mother when to return immediately ➤ Follow up in 14 days
• No palmar pallor	**NO ANAEMIA**	If child is less than 2 years old, assess the child's feeding and counsel the mother on feeding according to the feeding recommendations - If feeding problem, follow-up in 5 days

THEN ASSESS FOR HIV INFECTION**

- ☑ Has the mother or child had an HIV test?
  OR
- ☑ Does the child have one or more of the following

  ≠ Pneumonia **
  ≠ Persistent diarrhoea **
  ≠ Ear discharge (acute or chronic)
  ≠ Very low weight for age**

If yes to one of the two questions above, enter the box below and look for the following conditions suggesting HIV infection:

NOTE OR ASK:

≠ PNEUMONIA ?
≠ PERSISTENT DIARRHOEA?
≠ EAR DISCHARGE?
≠ VERY LOW WEIGHT?

LOOK and FEEL:

≠ Oral thrush
≠ Parotid enlargement
≠ Generalized persistent lymphadenopathy

HIV test result available for mother/child?

CLASSIFY

** A child who is on ART does not need to enter this HIV box.
* Includes severe forms such as severe pneumonia. In the case of severe forms, complete assessment quickly and refer child URGENTLY.
^A child with these classifications or on ART, assess for mouth and gum conditions as in next page.

HIV status of mother and child unknown

Signs	Classify	Treatment
≠ 2 or more conditions AND ≠ No test results for child or mother	**SUSPECTED SYMPTOMATIC HIV INFECTION**	▸ If the child also has a severe classification give appropriate pre referral treatment and refer urgently ▸ Treat, counsel and follow-up existing infection ▸ Give co-trimoxazole prophylaxis ▸ Give Vitamin A supplements ▸ Assess the child's feeding and provide appropriate counselling to the mother ▸ Test to confirm HIV infection ▸ Refer for further assessment including HIV care/ART ▸ Advise the mother on home care ▸ Follow up in 14 days, then monthly for 3 months and then every 3 months
≠ Less than 2 conditions AND ≠ No test result for child or mother	**SYMPTOMATIC HIV INFECTION UNLIKELY**	▸ Treat, counsel and follow-up existing infection ▸ Advise the mother about feeding and about her own health ▸ Encourage HIV testing

HIV status of mother and/or child known

Signs	Classify	Treatment
≠ Positive HIV antibody test for child 18 months and above OR ≠ Positive HIV virological test	**CONFIRMED HIV INFECTION***	▸ If the child also has a severe classification give appropriate pre referral treatment and refer urgently ▸ Treat, counsel and follow-up existing infection ▸ Give co-trimoxazole prophylaxis ▸ Check immunization status ▸ Give Vitamin A supplements ▸ Assess the child's feeding and provide appropriate counselling to the mother ▸ Refer for further assessment including HIV care/ART ▸ Advise the mother on home care ▸ Follow up in 14 days, then monthly for 3 months and then every 3 months
One or both of the following: ≠ Mother HIV positive and no test result for child OR ≠ Child less than 18 months with positive antibody test	**HIV EXPOSED: POSSIBLE HIV INFECTION***	▸ Treat, counsel and follow-up existing infection ▸ Give co-trimoxazole prophylaxis ▸ Give Vitamin A supplements ▸ Refer/do PCR to confirm infant's HIV with best available test ▸ Assess the child's feeding and provide appropriate counselling to the mother ▸ Refer for further assessment including HIV care/ART ▸ Confirm HIV infection status of child as soon as possible with best available test ▸ Follow up in 14 days, then monthly or as per national guidelines**
≠ Negative HIV test in mother or child AND not enough signs to classify as suspected sympto-	**HIV INFECTION UNLIKELY**	▸ Treat, counsel and follow-up existing infections ▸ Advise the mother about feeding and about her own health

ASSESS MOUTH AND GUM CONDITIONS
(FOR CHILDREN ON ART OR CLASSIFIED FOR HIV INFECTION)

Look
- Deep or extensive ulcers or outh or gums
- Ulcers of mouth or gums

Classify **MOUTH or GUM CONDITIONS**

• Deep or extensive ulcers of mouth or gums or • Not able to eat	**SEVERE GUM OR MOUTH INFECTION**	■ Refer URGENTLY to hospital ■ If possible, give first dose acyclovir pre-referral. ■ Start metronidazole if referral not possible ■ If child is on antiretroviral therapy this may be a drug reaction so refer to second level for assessment.
• Ulcers of mouth or gums	**GUM OR MOUTH ULCERS**	■ Show mother how to clean the ulcers with saline or peroxide or sodium bicarbonate. ■ If lips or anterior gums involved, give acyclovir, if possible. If not possible, refer. ■ If child receiving cotrimoxazole or antiretroviral drugs or isoniazid (INH) prophylaxis (for TB) within the last month, this may be a drug rash, especially of the child also has a skin rash, so refer. ■ Provide pain relief. ■ Follow up in 7 days.
• No ulcers of the mouth or gums	**NO GUM OR MOUTH ULCERS**	■ Treat, counsel and follow up existing infections. ■ Advise the mother about feeding and about her own health.

THEN CHECK THE CHILD'S IMMUNIZATION, VITAMIN A SUPPLEMENTATION

VITAMIN A SUPPLEMENTS	
AGE*	VITAMIN A
9-12 months	dose 1
15-18 months	dose 2
21-24 months	dose 3
27-30 months	dose 4
33-36 months	dose 5
39-42 months	dose 6
45-48 months	dose 7
51-54 months	dose 8
57-60 months	dose 9
*Give vitamin A only if no dose in last six months has been given	

ASSESS OTHER PROBLEMS

ASSESS MOTHER'S OWN HEALTH

CHILD'S IMMUNIZATION, VITAMIN A AND DEWORMING STATUS

IMMUNIZATION SCHEDULE: Follow national guidelines

Age	VACCINE			HIV-EXPOSED	HIV-INFECTED
Birth	BCG	OPV-0		BCG*	NO BCG
6 weeks	DPT+HIB-1	OPV-1	Hep B1	Same	Same
10 weeks	DPT+HIB-2	OPV-2	Hep B2	Same	Same
14 weeks	DPT+HIB-3	OPV-3	Hep B3	Same	Same
9 months	Measles**			Measles at 6 months	Same***
				Repeat at or after 9 months	Same***

*****BCG should NOT be given** any time after birth to infants known to be HIV infected or born to HIV infected women and HIV status unknown but who have signs or reported symptoms suggestive of HIV infection
****** Second dose of measles vaccine may be given at any opportunistic moment during periodic supplementary immunisation activities as early as one month following the first dose..
******* Measles vaccine is NOT given if child is severely immunocompromised due to HIV infection.

MAKE SURE CHILD WITH ANY GENERAL DANGER SIGN IS REFERRED after first dose of an appropriate antibiotic and other urgent treatments.

VITAMIN A SUPPLEMENTATION
Give every child a dose of Vitamin A every six months from the age of 6 months. Record the dose on the child's card
Same protocol for HIV-exposed and infected children

ROUTINE WORM TREATMENT
Give every child mebendazole every 6 months from the age of one year. Record the dose on the child's card.
Same protocol for HIV exposed and infected children

ASSESS OTHER PROBLEMS:

ESTABLISH HIV INFECTION STATUS

RECOMMEND HIV testing for:
- **All children born to an HIV positive mother**
- **All sick children with symptomatic suspected HIV infection**
- **All children brought for child health service in a generalized epidemic setting**

For children > 18 months, a positive HIV antibody test result means the child is infected.

For HIV exposed children <18 months of age,
- If PCR or other virological test is available, test from 6 weeks of age
  - A positive result means the child is infected
  - A negative result means the child is not infected, but could become infected if they are still breastfeeding
- If PCR or other virological test not available, use HIV antibody test.
  - A positive result is consistent with the fact that the child has been exposed to HIV, but does not tell us if the child is definitely infected.

If PCR or other virological test is not available, use HIV antibody test.
- If the child becomes sick, recommend HIV antibody test.
- If the child remains well, recommend HIV antibody test at 9–12 months.
- If child > 12 month has not yet been tested, recommend HIV antibody test.

Interpreting the HIV antibody test results in a child < 18 months of age

Test result	HIV antibody test is positive	HIV antibody test is negative
Not breastfeeding or not breastfed in last 6 weeks	HIV exposed and /or HIV infected Manage as if they could be infected. Repeat test at 18 months	**HIV negative** Child is not HIV infected
Breast feeding	HIV exposed and /or HIV infected Manage as if they could be infected. Repeat test at 18 months or once breastfeeding has been discontinued for more than 6 weeks	**Child can still be infected by breastfeeding.** Repeat test once breastfeeding has been discontinued for more than 6 weeks.

1. The older the child is the more likely the HIV antibody is due to their own infection and not due to maternal antibody
2. Very exceptionally a very severely sick child who is HIV infected will have HIV antibody test results that are negative. If the clinical picture strongly suggests HIV, then virological testing will be needed.

WHO PAEDIATRIC CLINICAL STAGING OF HIV

Has the child been confirmed HIV Infected?

(If yes, perform clinical staging: any one condition in the highest staging determines stage. If no, you cannot stage the patient)[1]

	WHO Paediatric Clinical Stage 1 - Asymptomatic	WHO Paediatric Clinical Stage 2 - Mild Disease	WHO Paediatric Clinical Stage 3 - Moderate Disease	WHO Paediatric Clinical Stage 4 - Severe Disease (AIDS)
Growth	-	-	Moderate unexplained malnutrition not responding to standard therapy	Severe unexplained wasting or stunting or Severe malnutrition not responding to standard therapy
Symptoms/ signs	No symptoms or only: ≠ Persistent Generalized Lymphadenopathy (PGL)	➤ Unexplained persistent enlarged liver and/or spleen ➤ Unexplained persistent enlarged parotid ➤ Skin conditions (prurigo, seborrhoeic dermatitis, extensive molluscum contagiosum or warts, fungal nail infections, herpes zoster) ➤ Mouth conditions (recurrent mouth ulcerations, angular cheilitis, lineal gingival Erythema) ➤ Recurrent or chronic upper RTI (sinusitis, ear infections, otorrhoea)	➤ Oral thrush (outside neonatal period) ➤ Oral hairy leukoplakia ➤ Unexplained and unresponsive to standard therapy: ≠ Diarrhoea >14 days ≠ Fever >1 month ≠ Thrombocytopenia* (<50,000/mm3 for > 1 month) ≠ Neutropenia (<500/mm³ for 1 month) ≠ Anaemia for >1 month (haemoglobin < 8 g/dl)* ➤ Recurrent severe bacterial pneumonia ➤ Pulmonary TB ➤ TB lymphadenopathy ➤ Symptomatic LIP* ➤ Acute necrotizing ulcerative gingivitis/ periodontitis ➤ Chronic HIV associated lung disease including bronchiectasis*	➤ Oesophageal thrush ➤ More than one month of herpes simplex ulcerations ➤ Severe multiple or recurrent bacterial infections ≥ 2 episodes in a year (not including pneumonia) ➤ *Pneumocystis* pneumonia (PCP)* ➤ Kaposi sarcoma ➤ Extrapulmonary tuberculosis ➤ Toxoplasma* ➤ cryptococcal meningitis* ➤ Acquired HIV-associated rectal fistula ➤ HIV encephalopathy* ART is indicated: Irrespective of the CD4 count, and should be started as soon as possible NB[1] If HIV infection is NOT confirmed in infants <18 months, presumptive diagnosis of severe HIV disease can be made on the basis of: ** ➤ HIV antibody positive AND ➤ One of the following: ρ AIDS defining condition OR ρ Symptomatic with two or more of: ≠ Oral thrush ≠ Severe pneumonia ≠ Severe sepsis
ARV Therapy	Indicated: ο All infants below 12 mo irrespective of CD4 ο 12-35 mo and CD4 ≤ 20% (or ∞750 cells) ο 36-59 mo and CD4≤20% (or ∞350 cells) ο 5 yrs and CD4 ≤15% (< 200 cells/mm3)	Indicated: Same as stage 1	ART is indicated: ≠ Child is over 12 months—usually regardless of CD4 but if LIP/TB/ oral hairy leukoplakia—ART Initiation may be delayed if CD4 above age related threshold for advanced or severe immunodeficiency	

* conditions requiring diagnosis by a doctor or medical official (should be referred for appropriate diagnosis and treatment).
** In a child with presumptive diagnosis of severe HIV disease and ART initiated, HIV infection should be confirmed as soon as possible.

[1] Note that these are interim recommendations and may be subject to change.

Appendix A

TREAT THE CHILD
CARRY OUT THE TREATMENT STEPS IDENTIFIED ON THE ASSESS AND CLASSIFY CHART

TEACH THE MOTHER TO GIVE ORAL DRUGS AT HOME

Follow the instructions below for every oral drug to be given at home.
Also follow the instructions listed with each drug's dosage table.

▲ Determine the appropriate drugs and dosage for the child's age or weight
▲ Tell the mother the reason for giving the drug to the child
▲ Demonstrate how to measure a dose
▲ Watch the mother practise measuring a dose by herself
▲ Ask the mother to give the first dose to her child
▲ Explain carefully how to give the drug, then label and package the drug. If more than one drug will be given, collect, count and package each drug separately
▲ Explain that all the tablets or syrup must be used to finish the course of treatment, even if the child gets better
▲ Check the mother's understanding before she leaves the clinic

▲ Give Co-trimoxazole to Children with Confirmed or Suspected HIV Infection or Children who are HIV Exposed

▲ Co-trimoxazole should be given starting at 4- 6 weeks of age to :
  ≈ All infants born to mothers who are HIV infected until HIV is definitively ruled out
  ≈ All infants with confirmed HIV infection aged <12 months or those with stage 2,3 or 4 disease or
  ≈ Asymptomatic infants or children (stage 1) if CD4 <25%.
▲ Give co-trimoxazole once daily.

Age	CO-TRIMOXAZOLE dosage—single dose per day		
	5 ml syrup 40 mg / 200 mg	Single strength adult tablet 80 mg / 400 mg	Single strength paediatric tablet 20 mg / 100 mg
Less than 6 months	2.5 ml	1/4 tablet	1 tablet
6 months up to 5 years	5 ml	1/2 tablet	2 tablets
5 - 14 years	10 ml	1 tablet	4 tablets
> 15 years	NIL	2 tablets	-

▲ Give an Appropriate Oral Antibiotic
> FOR PNEUMONIA, ACUTE EAR INFECTION:

FIRST-LINE ANTIBIOTIC:
SECOND-LINE ANTIBIOTIC:

	CO-TRIMOXAZOLE (trimethoprim / sulphamethoxazole) Give two times daily for 5 days			AMOXYCILLIN* Give two times daily for 5 days	
AGE or WEIGHT	ADULT TABLET (80/400mg)	PAEDIATRIC TABLET (20/100 mg)	SYRUP (40/200 mg/5ml)	TABLET (250 mg)	SYRUP (125 mg /5 ml)
2 months up to 12 months (4 - <10 kg)	1/2	2	5.0 ml	3/4	7.5 ml
12 months up to 5 years (10 - 19 kg)	1	3	7.5 ml	1 1/2	15 ml

*Amoxycillin should be used if there is high co-trimoxazole resistance.

▲ FOR CHOLERA:
First-line antibiotic for cholera

	TETRACYCLINE Give 4 times daily for 3 days	ERYTHROMYCIN Give 4 times daily for 3 days
AGE or WEIGHT	TABLET 250 mg	TABLET 250 mg
2 years up to 5 years (10-19 kg)	1	1

▲ For dysentery give ciprofloxacin
15mg/kg/day—2 times a day for 3 days
Second-line antibiotic for dysentery

	250 mg TABLET	500 mg TABLET
AGE	DOSE/ tabs	DOSE/ tabs
Less than 6 months	1/2 tablet	1/4 tablet
6 months up to 5 years	1 tablet	1/2 tablet

TEACH THE MOTHER
TO GIVE ORAL DRUGS AT HOME

Give pain relief

- Safe doses of paracetamol can be slightly higher for pain. Use the table and teach mother to measure the right dose
- Give paracetamol every 6 hours if pain persists
- **Stage 2 pain** is chronic severe pain as might happen in illnesses such as AIDS:
  - Start treating Stage 2 pain with regular paracetamol
  - In older children, ½ paracetamol tablet can replace 10 ml syrup
  - If the pain is not controlled, **add** regular codeine 4 hourly
  - For severe pain, morphine syrup can be given

WEIGHT	AGE (if you do not know the weight)	PARACETAMOL 120mg / 5mls	Add CODEINE 30mg tablet	ORAL MORPHINE 5mg/5ml
4 - <6kg	2 months up to 4months	2 ml	1/4	0.5ml
6 - <10 kg	4 months up to 12 months	2.5 ml	1/4	2ml
10 - <12 kg	12 up to 2 years	5 ml	1/2	3ml
12 - <14 kg	2 years up to 3 years	7.5 ml	1/2	4ml
14 - 19 kg	3 to 5 years	10 ml	3/4	5ml

Give Iron

- Give one dose daily for 14 days

AGE or WEIGHT	IRON/FOLATE TABLET Ferrous sulfate 200 mg + 250 μg Folate (60 mg elemental iron)	IRON SYRUP Ferrous fumarate 100 mg per 5 ml (20 mg elemental iron per ml)
2 months up to 4 months (4 - <6 kg)		1.0 ml (< 1/4 tsp)
4 months up to 12 months (6 - <10kg)		1.25 ml (1/4 tsp)
12 months up to 3 years (10 - <14 kg)	1/2 tablet	2.0 ml (<1/2 tsp)
3 years up to 5 years (14 - 19 kg)	1/2 tablet	2.5 ml (1/2 tsp)

► GIVE INHALED SALBUTAMOL for WHEEZING

USE OF A SPACER*

A spacer is a way of delivering the bronchodilator drugs effectively into the lungs. No child under 5 years should be given an inhaler without a spacer. A spacer works as well as a nebuliser if correctly used.

- From salbutamol metered dose inhaler (100μg/puff) give 2 puffs.
- Repeat up to 3 times every 15 minutes before classifying pneumonia.

Spacers can be made in the following way:
- Use a 500ml drink bottle or similar.
- Cut a hole in the bottle base in the same shape as the mouthpiece of the inhaler. This can be done using a sharp knife.
- Cut the bottle between the upper quarter and the lower 3/4 and disregard the upper quarter of the bottle.
- Cut a small V in the border of the large open part of the bottle to fit to the child's nose and be used as a mask.
- Flame the edge of the cut bottle with a candle or a lighter to soften it.
- In a small baby, a mask can be made by making a similar hole in a plastic (not polystyrene) cup.
- Alternatively commercial spacers can be used if available.

To use an inhaler with a spacer:
- Remove the inhaler cap. Shake the inhaler well.
- Insert mouthpiece of the inhaler through the hole in the bottle or plastic cup.
- The child should put the opening of the bottle into his mouth and breath in and out through the mouth.
- A carer then presses down the inhaler and sprays into the bottle while the child continues to breath normally.
- Wait for three to four breaths and repeat for total of five sprays.
- For younger children place the cup over the child's mouth and use as a spacer in the same way.

*If a spacer is being used for the first time, it should be primed by 4-5 extra puffs from the inhaler.

Give Oral Co-artemether

- Give the first dose of co-artemether in the clinic and observe for one hour
  If child vomits within an hour repeat the dose. **2nd** dose at home after 8 hours
- Then twice daily for further two days as shown below

	Co-artemether tablets (20mg artemether and 120 mg lumefantrine)						
WEIGHT (age)	0h	8h	24h	36h	48h	60h	
5-15kg (2 mo -<3 years)	1	1	1	1	1	1	
15-24kg (4-8 years)	2	2	2	2	2	2	
25-34 kg (9-14 years)	3	3	3	3	3	3	
>34 kg (>14 years)	4	4	4	4	4	4	

Appendix A 441

TEACH THE MOTHER TO TREAT LOCAL INFECTIONS AT HOME

- ➤ Explain to the mother what the treatment is and why it should be given
- ➤ Describe the treatment steps listed in the appropriate box
- ➤ Watch the mother as she gives the first treatment in the clinic (except for remedy for cough or sore throat)
- ➤ Tell her how often to do the treatment at home
- ➤ If needed for treatment at home, give mother a tube of tetracycline ointment or a small bottle of gentian violet or nystatin
- ➤ Check the mother's understanding before she leaves the clinic

➤ **Clear the Ear by Dry Wicking and Give Eardrops***

> Do the following 3 times daily

  - Roll clean absorbent cloth or soft, strong tissue paper into a wick
  - Place the wick in the child's ear
  - Remove the wick when wet
  - Replace the wick with a clean one and repeat these steps until the ear is dry
  - Instil quinolone eardrops for two weeks

➤ **Soothe the Throat, Relieve the Cough with a Safe Remedy**

- Safe remedies to recommend:
  - Breast milk for a breastfed infant
  _____
  _____

- Harmful remedies to discourage:
  _____
  _____

➤ **Treat Eye Infection with Tetracycline Eye Ointment**

➤ Clean both eyes 4 times daily.
  - Wash hands.
  - Use clean cloth and water to gently wipe away pus.
➤ Then apply tetracycline eye ointment in both eyes 4 times daily.
  - Squirt a small amount of ointment on the inside of the lower lid.
  - Wash hands again.
➤ Treat until there is no pus discharge.
➤ Do not put anything else in the eye.

➤ **Treat Mouth Ulcers with Gentian Violet (GV)**

> Treat for mouth ulcers twice daily

  - Wash hands
  - Wash the child's mouth with a clean soft cloth wrapped around the finger and wet with salt water
  - Paint the mouth with 1/2 strength gentian violet (0.25% dilution)
  - Wash hands again
  - Continue using GV for 48 hours after the ulcers have been cured
  - Give paracetamol for pain relief

➤ **Treat for Thrush with Nystatin**

> Treat for thrush four times daily for 7 days

  - Wash hands
  - Wet a clean soft cloth with salt water and use it to wash the child's mouth
  - Instill nystatin 1ml four times a day
  - Avoid feeding for 20 minutes after medication
  - If breastfed check mother's breasts for thrush. If present treat with nystatin
  - Advise mother to wash breasts after feeds. If bottle fed advise change to cup and spoon
  - If severe, recurrent or pharyngeal thrush consider symptomatic HIV (p. 7)
  - Give paracetamol if needed for pain (p.12)

* Quinolone eardrops may contain ciprofloxacin, norfloxacin, or ofloxacin eardrops

GIVE VITAMIN A AND MEBENDAZOLE IN CLINIC

➢ **Explain to the mother why the drug is given**
➢ **Determine the dose appropriate for the child's weight (or age)**
➢ **Measure the dose accurately**

➢ Give Vitamin A

VITAMIN A SUPPLEMENTATION:

➢ Give Vitamin A first dose any time after 6 months of age
➢ Thereafter give vitamin A **every six months** to ALL CHILDREN

VITAMIN A TREATMENT:

➢ Give an extra dose of Vitamin A (same dose) for *treatment* if the child has MEASLES or PERSISTENT DIARRHOEA. If the child has had a dose of Vitamin A within the past month, DO NOT GIVE.

➢ Always record the dose of Vitamin A given on the child's chart

Age	VITAMIN A DOSE
6 up to 12 months	100 000 IU
One year and older	200 000 IU

➢ Give Mebendazole

➢ Give 500 mg mebendazole as a single dose in clinic if:
- hookworm/ whipworm is a problem in your area
- the child is 1 year of age or older, and
- has not had a dose in the previous 6 months

Appendix A

GIVE THESE TREATMENTS IN THE CLINIC ONLY

- Explain to the mother why the drug is given
- Determine the dose appropriate for the child's weight (or age)
- Use a sterile needle and sterile syringe when giving an injection
- Measure the dose accurately
- Give the drug as an intramuscular injection
- If the child cannot be referred, follow the instructions provided

▶ Give Diazepam to Stop a Convulsion

- Turn the child to his/her side and clear the airway. Avoid putting things in the mouth
- Give 0.5mg/kg diazepam injection solution per rectum using a small syringe without a needle (like a tuberculin syringe) or using a catheter
- Check for low blood sugar, then treat or prevent
- Give oxygen and REFER
- If convulsions have not stopped after 10 minutes repeat diazepam dose

WEIGHT	AGE	DOSE OF DIAZEPAM (10mg/2mls)
<5kg	<6 months	0.5 ml
5 - <10kg	6 - <12 months	1.0 ml
10 - <15kg	1 - <3 years	1.5ml
15 - 19 kg	4 - <5years	2.0 ml

▶ Give An Intramuscular Antibiotic

- GIVE TO CHILDREN BEING REFERRED URGENTLY
- Where there is a strong suspicion of meningitis the dose of ampicillin can be increased 4 times
- Give Ampicillin (50 mg/kg) and Gentamicin (7.5mg/kg)

AMPICILLIN
- Dilute 500mg vial with 2.1ml of sterile water (500mg/2.5ml)

AGE	WEIGHT	AMPICILLIN 500 mg vial	Gentamicin 2ml vial with 40 mg/ml
2 up to 4 months	4 y <6kg	1 ml	0.5 - 1.0 ml*
4 up to 12 months	6 y <10kg	2 ml	1.1 - 1.8 ml
1 up to 3 years	10 y <15kg	3 ml	1.9 - 2.7 ml
3 up to 5 years	15 y 20kg	5 ml	2.8 - 3.5 ml

- IF REFERRAL IS NOT POSSIBLE OR DELAYED, repeat the ampicillin injection every 6 hours and gentamicin once per day
- * Lower value for lower range of age and weight

▶ Give Quinine for Severe Malaria

FOR CHILDREN BEING REFERRED WITH VERY SEVERE FEBRILE DISEASE:
- Check which quinine formulation is available in your clinic
- Give first dose of intramuscular quinine and refer child urgently to hospital

IF REFERRAL IS NOT POSSIBLE:
- Give first dose of intramuscular quinine
- The child should remain lying down for one hour
- Repeat the quinine injection at 4 and 8 hours later, and then every 12 hours until the child is able to take an oral antimalarial. Do not continue quinine injections for more than 1 week
- If low risk of malaria, do not give quinine to a child less than 4 months of age

AGE or WEIGHT	INTRAMUSCULAR QUININE	
	150 mg /ml* (in 2 ml)	300 mg /ml* (in 2 ml)
2 months up to 4 months (4 - <6 kg)	0.4 ml	0.2 ml
4 months up to 12 months (6 - <10 kg)	0.6 ml	0.3 ml
12 months up to 2 years (10 - <12 kg)	0.8 ml	0.4 ml
2 years up to 3 years (12 - <14 kg)	1.0 ml	0.5 ml
3 years up to 5 years (14 - 19 kg)	1.2 ml	0.6 ml

*quinine salt

Treat the Child to Prevent Low Blood Sugar

▲ **If the child is able to breastfeed:**

   Ask the mother to breastfeed the child

▲ **If the child is not able to breastfeed but is able to swallow:**

   ∗ Give expressed breast milk or breast-milk substitute
   ∗ If neither of these is available give sugar water
   ∗ Give 30-50 ml of milk or sugar water before departure

   To make sugar water: Dissolve 4 level teaspoons of sugar (20 grams) in a 200-ml cup of clean water

▲ **If the child is not able to swallow:**

   ∗ Give 50ml of milk or sugar water by nasogastric tube

Appendix A 445

GIVE EXTRA FLUID FOR DIARRHOEA AND CONTINUE FEEDING
(See FOOD advice on COUNSEL THE MOTHER chart)

Plan A: Treat for Diarrhoea at Home

Counsel the mother on the 4 Rules of Home Treatment:
1. Give Extra Fluid 2. Give Zinc Supplements (age 2 months up to 5 years)
3. Continue Feeding 4. When to Return

> **TELL THE MOTHER:**

1. GIVE EXTRA FLUID (as much as the child will take)

> **TELL THE MOTHER:**
  - Breastfeed frequently and for longer at each feed
  - If the child is exclusively breastfed, give ORS or clean water in addition to breast milk
  - If the child is not exclusively breastfed, give one or more of the following: food-based fluids (such as soup, rice water, and yoghurt drinks), or ORS

It is especially important to give ORS at home when:
  - the child has been treated with Plan B or Plan C during this visit
  - the child cannot return to a clinic if the diarrhoea gets worse

> **TEACH THE MOTHER HOW TO MIX AND GIVE ORS. GIVE THE MOTHER 2 PACKETS OF ORS TO USE AT HOME.**

> **SHOW THE MOTHER HOW MUCH FLUID TO GIVE IN ADDITION TO THE USUAL FLUID INTAKE:**

  Up to 2 years: 50 to 100 ml after each loose stool
  2 years or more: 100 to 200 ml after each loose stool

Tell the mother to:
  - Give frequent small sips from a cup.
  - If the child vomits, wait 10 minutes then continue - but more slowly
  - Continue giving extra fluid until the diarrhoea stops

2. GIVE ZINC (age 2 months up to 5 years)

> **TELL THE MOTHER HOW MUCH ZINC TO GIVE (20 mg tab):**

  2 months up to 6 months —— 1/2 tablet daily for 14 days
  6 months or more —— 1 tablet daily for 14 days

> **SHOW THE MOTHER HOW TO GIVE ZINC SUPPLEMENTS**
  - Infants—dissolve tablet in a small amount of expressed breast milk, ORS or clean water in a cup
  - Older children - tablets can be chewed or dissolved in a small amount of clean water in a cup

3. CONTINUE FEEDING (exclusive breastfeeding if age less than 6 months)

4. WHEN TO RETURN

Plan B: Treat for Some Dehydration with ORS

In the clinic, give recommended amount of ORS over 4-hour period

> **DETERMINE AMOUNT OF ORS TO GIVE DURING FIRST 4 HOURS**
  Use the child's age only when you do not know the weight. The approximate amount of ORS required (in ml) can also be calculated by multiplying the child's weight in kg times 75.

AGE*	Up to 4 months	4 months up to 12 months	12 months up to 2 years	2 years up to 5 years
WEIGHT	< 6 kg	6 - < 10 kg	10 - < 12 kg	12 - <20kg
Amount of fluid (ml) over 4 hours	200 - 450	450 - 800	800 - 960	960 - 1600

  - If the child wants more ORS than shown, give more
  - For infants below 6 months who are not breastfed, also give 100-200ml clean water during this period

> **SHOW THE MOTHER HOW TO GIVE ORS SOLUTION:**
  - Give frequent small sips from a cup
  - If the child vomits, wait 10 minutes then continue - but more slowly
  - Continue breastfeeding whenever the child wants

> **AFTER 4 HOURS:**
  - Reassess the child and classify the child for dehydration
  - Select the appropriate plan to continue treatment
  - Begin feeding the child in clinic

> **IF THE MOTHER MUST LEAVE BEFORE COMPLETING TREATMENT:**
  - Show her how to prepare ORS solution at home
  - Show her how much ORS to give to finish 4-hour treatment at home
  - Give her instructions how to prepare salt and sugar solution for use at home
  - Explain the 4 Rules of Home Treatment:

1. GIVE EXTRA FLUID
2. GIVE ZINC (age 2 months up to 5 years)
3. CONTINUE FEEDING (exclusive breastfeeding if age less than 6 months)
4. WHEN TO RETURN

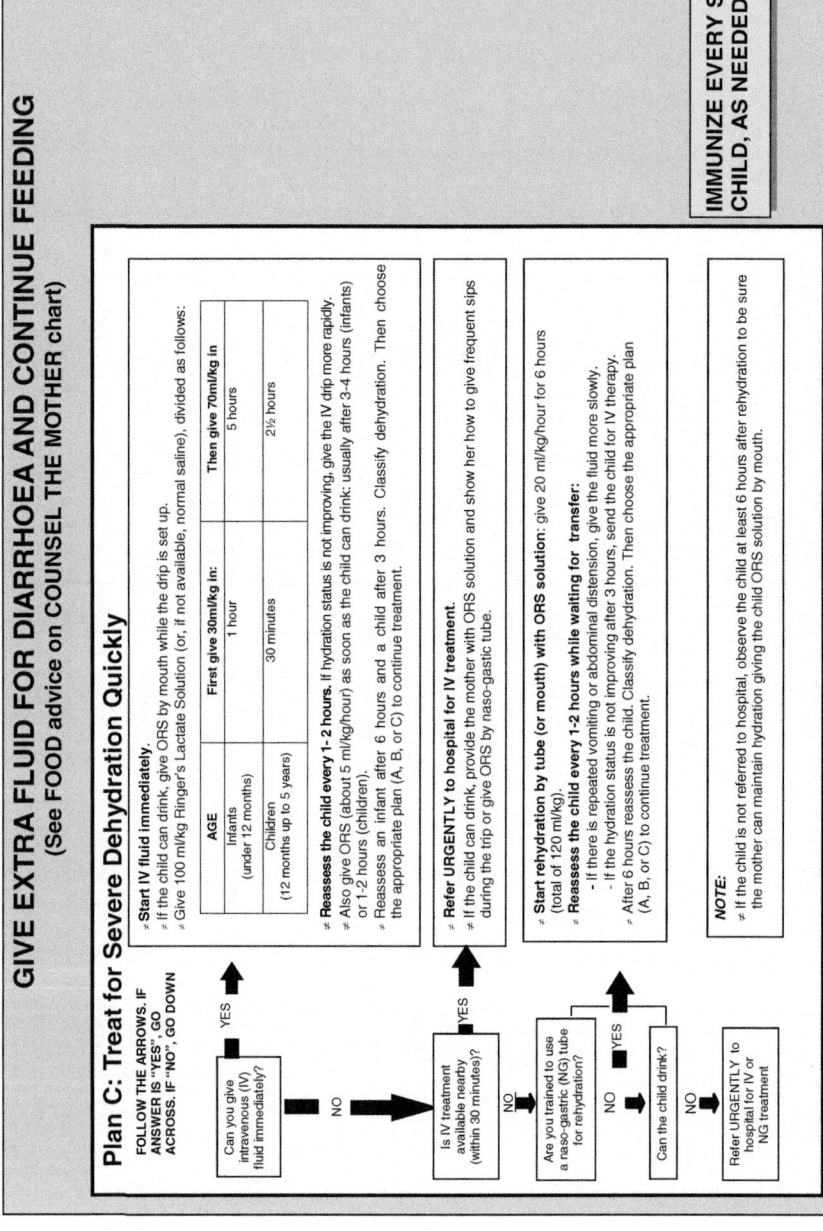

Appendix A

GIVE FOLLOW-UP CARE

Care for the child who returns for follow-up using all the boxes that match the child's previous classification
If the child has any new problems, assess, classify and treat the new problem as on the *ASSESS AND CLASSIFY* chart

➤ PNEUMONIA

After 2 days:
Check the child for general danger signs.
Assess the child for cough or difficult breathing. } *See ASSESS & CLASSIFY chart.*

Ask:
- Is the child breathing slower?
- Is there less fever?
- Is the child eating better?

Assess for HIV infection

Treatment:

➤ If *chest indrawing or a general danger sign*, give a dose of second-line antibiotic or intramuscular chloramphenicol. Then refer URGENTLY to hospital.

➤ If *breathing rate, fever and eating are the same*, change to the second-line antibiotic and advise the mother to return in 2 days or refer. (If this child had measles within the last 3 months or is known or suspected to have Symptomatic HIV Infection, refer.)

➤ If *breathing slower, less fever, or eating better*, complete the 5 days of antibiotic.

➤ PERSISTENT DIARRHOEA

After 5 days:
Ask:
- Has the diarrhoea stopped?
- How many loose stools is the child having per day?

Assess for HIV infection

Treatment:

➤ If **the diarrhoea has not stopped** (child is still having 3 or more loose stools per day) do a full assessment of the child. Treat for dehydration if present. Then **REFER** to hospital including for assessment for ART.

➤ If **the diarrhoea has stopped** (child having less than 3 loose stools per day), tell the mother to follow the usual feeding recommendations for the child's age.

➤ DYSENTERY:

After 2 days:
Assess the child for diarrhoea   *> See ASSESS & CLASSIFY chart*

Ask:
- Are there fewer stools?
- Is there less blood in the stool?
- Is there less fever?
- Is there less abdominal pain?
- Is the child eating better?

Treatment:

➤ If the child is *dehydrated*, treat for dehydration.

➤ If *number of stools, blood in the stools, fever, abdominal pain, or eating is worse or the same*

Change to second-line oral antibiotic recommended for shigella in your area. Give it for 5 days. Advise the mother to return in 2 days. If you do not have the second line antibiotic, refer to hospital.

Exceptions: if the child is less than 12 months old or was dehydrated on the first visit, or if he had measles within the last 3 months, REFER TO HOSPITAL.

➤ If *fewer stools, less fever, less abdominal pain, and eating better*, continue giving ciprofloxacin until finished.

Ensure that the mother understands the oral rehydration method fully and that she also understands the need for an extra meal each day for a week.

GIVE FOLLOW-UP CARE

> Care for the child who returns for follow-up using all the boxes that match the child's previous classification

> If the child has any new problems, assess, classify and treat the new problem as on the ASSESS AND CLASSIFY chart

➢ MALARIA (Low or High Malaria Risk)

If fever persists after 2 days, or returns within 14 days:

Do a full reassessment of the child > *See ASSESS & CLASSIFY chart.* Assess for other causes of fever.

Treatment:

➢ If the child has *any general danger sign or stiff neck,* treat as VERY SEVERE FEBRILE DISEASE.

➢ If the child has any *cause of fever other than malaria,* provide treatment.

➢ If *malaria is the only apparent cause of fever:*

- Treat with the second-line oral antimalarial (If no second-line antimalarial is available, refer to hospital). Advise the mother to return again in 2 days if the fever persists.

- If fever has been present for 7 days, refer for assessment.

➢ FEVER-MALARIA UNLIKELY (Low Malaria Risk)

If fever persists after 2 days:

Do a full reassessment of the child > *See ASSESS & CLASSIFY chart.* Assess for other causes of fever.

Treatment:

➢ If the child has *any general danger sign or stiff neck,* treat as VERY SEVERE FEBRILE DISEASE.

➢ If the child has any *cause of fever other than malaria,* provide treatment.

➢ If *malaria is the only apparent cause of fever:*

- Treat with the first-line oral antimalarial. Advise the mother to return again in 2 days if the fever persists.

- If fever has been present for 7 days, refer for assessment.

➢ MEASLES WITH EYE OR MOUTH COMPLICATIONS

After 2 days:

Look for red eyes and pus draining from the eyes.
Look at mouth ulcers.
Smell the mouth.

Treatment for Eye Infection:

➢ If *pus is draining from the eye,* ask the mother to describe how she has treated the eye infection. If treatment has been correct, refer to hospital. If treatment has not been correct, teach mother correct treatment.

➢ If *the pus is gone but redness remains,* continue the treatment.

➢ If *no pus or redness,* stop the treatment.

Treatment for Mouth Ulcers:

➢ If *mouth ulcers are worse, or there is a very foul smell coming from the mouth,* refer to hospital.

➢ If *mouth ulcers are the same or better,* continue using half-strength gentian violet for a total of 5 days.

Appendix A   449

GIVE FOLLOW-UP CARE

➤ Care for the child who returns for follow-up using all the boxes that match the child's previous classification
➤ If the child has any new problems, assess, classify and treat the new problem as on the *ASSESS AND CLASSIFY* chart

➤ EAR INFECTION

After 5 days:

Reassess for ear problem. > See *ASSESS & CLASSIFY chart*. Measure the child's temperature.

Check for HIV infection.

Treatment:

➤ If there is *tender swelling behind the ear or high fever (38.5°C or above)*, refer URGENTLY to hospital.
➤ *Acute ear Infection*: if *ear pain or discharge* persists, treat with 5 more days of the same antibiotic. Continue wicking to dry the ear. Follow-up in 5 days.
➤ *Chronic ear Infection*: Check that the mother is wicking the ear correctly. Encourage her to continue.
➤ If *no ear pain or discharge*, praise the mother for her careful treatment. If she has not yet finished the 5 days of antibiotic, tell her to use all of it before stopping.

➤ FEEDING PROBLEM

After 5 days:

Reassess feeding. > See *questions at the top of the COUNSEL chart*. Ask about any feeding problems found on the initial visit.

➤ Counsel the mother about any new or continuing feeding problems. If you counsel the mother to make significant changes in feeding, ask her to bring the child back again.
➤ If the child is very low weight for age, ask the mother to return 30 days after the initial visit to measure the child's weight gain.

➤ VERY LOW WEIGHT

After 30 days:

Weigh the child and determine if the child is still very low weight for age. Reassess feeding. > See *questions at the top of the COUNSEL chart*.

Check for HIV infection.

Treatment:

➤ If the child is *no longer very low weight for age*, praise the mother and encourage her to continue.
➤ If the child is still *very low weight for age*, counsel the mother about any feeding problem found. Ask the mother to return again in one month. Continue to see the child monthly until the child is feeding well and gaining weight regularly or is no longer very low weight for age.

Exception:

If you do not think that feeding will improve, or if the child has *lost weight*, refer the child.

➤ ANAEMIA

After 14 days:

➤ Give iron. Advise mother to return in 14 days for more iron.
➤ Continue giving iron every 14 days for 2 months.
➤ If the child has palmar pallor after 2 months, refer for assessment.

GIVE FOLLOW-UP CARE FOR THE CHILD WITH POSSIBLE HIV INFECTION / HIV EXPOSED OR SUSPECTED SYMPTOMATIC OR CONFIRMED HIV INFECTION

GENERAL PRINCIPLES OF GOOD CHRONIC CARE FOR HIV-INFECTED CHILDREN

- ➤ Develop a treatment partnership with the mother and infant or child
- ➤ Focus on the mother and child's concerns and priorities
- ➤ Use the "5 As" : Assess, Advise, Agree, Assist, Arrange to guide you the steps on chronic care consultation. Use the 5As at every patient consultation
- ➤ Support the mother and child's self-management
- ➤ Organize proactive follow-up
- ➤ Involve "expert patients", peer educators and support staff in your health facility
- ➤ Link the mother and child to community-based resources and support
- ➤ Use written information – registers, Treatment Plan and treatment cards - to document, monitor and remind
- ➤ Work as a clinical team
- ➤ Assure continuity of care

IF POSSIBLE HIV INFECTION / HIV EXPOSED

- ➤ Follow-up in 14 days, monthly or as per national guidelines.
- ➤ Do a full re-assessment at each follow-up visit and reclassify for HIV on each follow-up visit
- ➤ Counsel about feeding practices (page 25 in chart booklet and according to the recommendations in Module 3)
- ➤ Follow **co-trimoxazole prophylaxis** as per national guidelines
- ➤ Follow national immunization schedule
- ➤ Follow Vitamin A supplements from 6 months of age every 6 months
- ➤ Monitor growth and development
- ➤ Virological Testing for HIV infection as early as possible from 6 weeks of age
- ➤ Refer for ARVs if infant develops severe signs suggestive of HIV
- ➤ Counsel the mother about her own HIV status and arrange counselling and testing for her if required

IF SUSPECTED SYMPTOMATIC HIV INFECTION

- ➤ Follow-up in 14 days, monthly or as per national guidelines.
- ➤ Do a full assessment ÿ classify for common childhood illnesses, for malnutrition and feeding, skin and mouth conditions and for HIV on each visit
- ➤ Check if diagnostic HIV test has been done and if not, test for HIV as soon as possible
- ➤ Assess feeding and check weight and weight gain
- ➤ Encourage breastfeeding - mothers to continue exclusive breastfeeding
- ➤ Advise on any new or continuing feeding problems
- ➤ Initiate or follow up **co-trimoxazole prophylaxis** according to national guidelines
- ➤ Give immunizations according to schedule. Do not give BCG
- ➤ Give Vitamin A according to schedule
- ➤ Provide pain relief if needed
- ➤ Refer for confirmation of HIV infection and ART, if not yet confirmed

IF CHILD IS CONFIRMED HIV INFECTED*

- ➤ Follow-up in 14 days, monthly or as per national guidelines.
- ➤ Continue **co-trimoxazole prophylaxis**
- ➤ Follow-up on feeding
- ➤ Home care:
  - ≠ Counsel the mother about any new or continuing problems
  - ≠ If appropriate, put the family in touch with organizations or people who could provide support
  - ≠ Explain the importance of early treatment of infections or refer
  - ≠ Advise the mother about hygiene in the home, in particular when preparing food
- ➤ Reassess for eligibility for ART or REFER
- ➤ Check mother's health and advise on safe sexual practices and family planning

IF CHILD CONFIRMED UNINFECTED

- ➤ Stop co-trimoxazole only if no longer breastfeeding and more than 12 months of age
- ➤ Counsel mother on preventing HIV infection and about her own health

IF HIV TESTING HAS NOT BEEN DONE

- ➤ Re-discuss the benefits of HIV testing
- ➤ Identify where and when HIV testing including virological testing can be done
- ➤ If mother consents arrange HIV testing and follow-up visit

IF MOTHER REFUSES TESTING

- ➤ Provide ongoing care for the child, including routine monthly follow-up
- ➤ Discuss and provide **co-trimoxazole prophylaxis**
- ➤ On subsequent visits, re-counsel the mother on preventing HIV and on benefits of HIV testing

---

* Any child with confirmed HIV infection should be enrolled in chronic HIV care, including assessment for eligibility of ART ÿ refer to subsequent sections of the chart booklet.

Appendix A

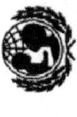

COUNSEL THE MOTHER

➤ Assess the Feeding of Sick Infants under 2 years (or if child has very low weight for age)

Ask questions about the child's usual feeding and feeding during this illness. Note whether the mother is HIV infected, uninfected, or does not know her status. Compare the mother's answers to the *Feeding Recommendations* for the child's age.

ASK — How are you feeding your child?

If the infant is receiving *any* breast milk, ASK:
- How many times during the day?
- Do you also breastfeed during the night?

If infant is receiving replacement milk, ASK:
- What replacement milk are you giving?
- How many times during the day and night?
- How much is given at each feed?
- How is the milk prepared?
- How is the milk being given? Cup or bottle?
- How are you cleaning the utensils?
- If still breastfeeding as well as giving replacement milk could the mother give extra breast milk instead of replacement milk (especially if the baby is below 6 months)

Does the infant take any other food or fluids?
- What food or fluids?
- How many times per day?
- What do you use to feed the child?

If low weight for age, ASK:
- How large are servings?
- Does the child receive his own serving?
- Who feeds the child and how?

During this illness, has the infant's feeding changed?
- If yes, how?

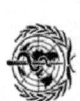

FEEDING RECOMMENDATIONS DURING SICKNESS AND HEALTH

NOTE: These feeding recommendations should be followed for infants of **HIV negative** mothers. Mothers who DO NOT KNOW their HIV status should be advised to breastfeed but also to be HIV tested so that they can make an informed choice about feeding

Up to 6 Months of Age	6 Months up to 12 Months	12 Months up to 2 Years	2 Years and Older
	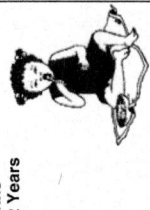	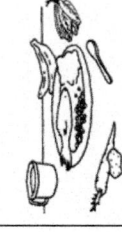	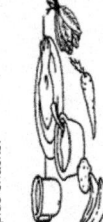
≠ Breastfeed as often as the child wants, day and night, at least 8 times in 24 hours. ≠ Do not give other foods or fluids.	≠ Breastfeed as often as the child wants. ≠ Give adequate servings of: _____ _____ _____ - 3 times per day if breastfed plus snacks - 5 times per day if not breastfed.	≠ Breastfeed as often as the child wants. ≠ Give adequate servings of: _____ _____ _____ or family foods 3 or 4 times per day plus snacks.	≠ Give family foods at 3 meals each day. Also, twice daily, give nutritious food between meals, such as: _____ _____ _____

Feeding Recommendations for a child who has PERSISTENT DIARRHOEA

≠ If still breastfeeding, give more frequent, longer breastfeeds, day and night.
≠ If taking other milk:
  - replace with increased breastfeeding OR
  - replace with fermented milk products, such as yoghurt OR
  - replace half the milk with nutrient-rich semisolid food

COUNSEL THE MOTHER

▶ Feeding advice for the mother of a child with CONFIRMED HIV INFECTION

- ▸ The child with confirmed HIV infection needs the benefits of breastfeeding and should be encouraged to breastfeed. S/he is already HIV infected therefore there is no reason for stopping breastfeeding or using replacement feeding.
- ▸ The child should be fed according to the feeding recommendations for his age.
- ▸ Children with confirmed HIV infection often suffer from poor appetite and mouth sores, give appropriate advice.
- ▸ If the child is being fed with a bottle encourage the mother to use a clean cup as this is more hygienic and will reduce episodes of diarrhoea.
- ▸ Inform the mother about the importance of hygiene when preparing food because her child can easily get sick. She should wash her hands after going to the toilet and before preparing food. If the child is not gaining weight well, the child can be given an extra meal each day and the mother can encourage him

"AFASS" CRITERIA FOR STOPPING BREASTFEEDING for HIV exposed

Acceptable:
Mother perceives no problem in replacement feeding.

Feasible:
Mother has adequate time, knowledge, skills, resources, and support to correctly mix formula or milk and feed the infant up to 12 times in 24 hours.

Affordable:
Mother and family, with community can pay the cost of replacement feeding without harming the health and nutrition of the family.

Sustainable:
Availability of a continuous supply of all ingredients needed for safe replacement feeding for up to one year of age or longer.

Safe:
Replacement foods are correctly and hygienically prepared and stored.

▶ Counsel the mother about Stopping Breastfeeding (for HIV exposed)

- ▸ While you are breastfeeding teach your infant to drink expressed breast milk from a cup. This milk may be heat-treated to destroy HIV.
- ▸ Once the infant is drinking comfortably, replace one breastfeed with one cup feed using expressed breast milk.
- ▸ Increase the number of cup-feeds every few days and reduce the number of breastfeeds. Ask an adult family member to help with cup feeding.
- ▸ Stop putting your infant to your breast completely as soon as your baby is accustomed to frequent cup feeding. From this point on it is best to heat-treat your breast milk.
- ▸ If your infant is receiving milk only check that your baby has at least 6 wet nappies in a 24 hour period. This means he is getting enough milk.
- ▸ Gradually replace the expressed breast milk with commercial infant formula or another milk after 6 months.
- ▸ If your infant needs to suck, give him/her one of your clean fingers instead of the breast.
- ▸ To avoid breast engorgement (swelling) express a little milk whenever your breasts feel full. This will help you feel more comfortable. Use cold compresses to reduce inflammation. Wear a firm bra to prevent discomfort.
- ▸ Do not begin breastfeeding again once you have stopped. If you do you can increase the chances of passing HIV to your infant. If your breasts become engorged express breast milk by hand.
- ▸ Begin using a family planning method of your choice, if you have not already done so, as soon as you start reducing breastfeeds.

COUNSEL THE MOTHER ABOUT FEEDING PROBLEMS

If the child is not being fed as described in the above recommendations, counsel the mother accordingly. In addition:

➤ **If the mother reports difficulty with breastfeeding, assess breastfeeding (see *YOUNG INFANT* chart). As needed, show the mother correct positioning and attachment for breastfeeding.**

➤ **If the child is less than 6 months old and is taking other milk or foods*:**
  - Build mother's confidence that she can produce all the breast milk that the child needs.
  - Suggest giving more frequent, longer breastfeeds day or night, and gradually reducing other milk or foods.

If other milk needs to be continued, counsel the mother to:
  - Breastfeed as much as possible, including at night.
  - Make sure that other milk is a locally appropriate breast milk substitute.
  - Make sure other milk is correctly and hygienically prepared and given in adequate amounts.
  - Finish prepared milk within an hour.

➤ **If the mother is using a bottle to feed the child:**
  - Recommend substituting a cup for bottle.
  - Show the mother how to feed the child with a cup.

➤ **If the child is not feeding well during illness, counsel the mother to:**
  - Breastfeed more frequently and for longer if possible.
  - Use soft, varied, appetizing, favourite foods to encourage the child to eat as much as possible, and offer frequent small feeds.
  - Clear a blocked nose if it interferes with feeding.
  - Expect that appetite will improve as child gets better.

➤ **If the child has a poor appetite:**
  - Plan small, frequent meals.
  - Give milk rather than other fluids except where there is diarrhoea with some dehydration.
  - Give snacks between meals.
  - Give high energy foods.
  - Check regularly.

➤ **If the child has sore mouth or ulcers:**
  - Give soft foods that will not burn the mouth, such as eggs, mashed potatoes, pumpkin or avocado.
  - Avoid spicy, salty or acid foods.
  - Chop foods finely.
  - Give cold drinks or ice, if available.

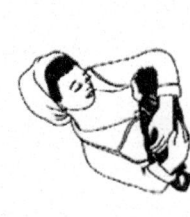

* *if child is HIV exposed, counsel the mother about the importance of not mixing breastfeeding with replacement feeding.*

FEEDING RECOMMENDATIONS: Child classified as HIV exposed

Up to 6 Months of Age

Breastfeed exclusively as often as the child wants, day and night. Feed at least 8 times in 24 hours.

Do not give other foods or fluids (mixed feeding increases the risk of HIV transmission from mother to child when compared with exclusive breastfeeding).

Stop breastfeeding as soon as this is AFASS.

OR (if feasible and safe)

Formula feed exclusively (no breast milk at all) Give formula. Other foods or fluids are not necessary.

Prepare correct strength and amount just before use. Use milk within two hours and discard any left over (a fridge can store formula for 24 hours)
Cup feeding is safer than bottle feeding
Clean the cup and utensils with hot soapy water
Give these amounts of formula 6 to 8 times per day

* **Exception: heat-treated breast milk can be given**

Age months	Amount and times per day
0 up to 1	60 ml x 8
1 up to 2	90 ml x 7
2 up to 3	120 ml x 6
3 up to 4	120 ml x 6
4 up to 5	150 ml x 6
5 up to 6	150 ml x 6

6 Months up to 12 Months

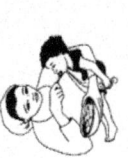

If still breast feeding, breastfeed as often as the child wants

Give 3 adequate servings of nutritious complementary foods plus one snack per day (to include protein, mashed fruit and vegetables).
Each meal should be 3/4 cup*. If possible, give an additional animal-source food, such as liver or meat

If an infant is not breastfeeding, give about 1-2 cups (500 ml) of full cream milk or infant formula per day

Give milk with a cup, not a bottle
If no milk is available, give 4-5 feeds per day
* one cup= 250 ml

12 Months up to 2 Years

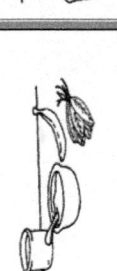

⋆ If still breastfeeding, breastfeed as often as the child wants.

⋆ Give adequate servings of:
_____
_____
_____
_____
or family foods 5 times per day.
If breastfed, give adequate servings 3 times per day plus snacks

If an infant is not breastfeeding, give about 1-2 cups* (500 ml) of full cream milk or infant formula per day

Give milk with a cup, not a bottle
If no milk is available, give 4-5 feeds per day
* one cup = 250 ml

Stopping breastfeeding

Stopping breastfeeding means changing from all breast milk to no breast milk (over a period of 2-3 days to 2-3 weeks). Plan in advance to have a safe transition.

Stop breastfeeding as soon as this is AFASS (see page 27). This would usually be at the age of 6 months but some women may have to continue longer.

Help mother prepare for stopping breastfeeding:

⋆ Mother should discuss and plan in advance stopping breastfeeding with her family if possible
⋆ Express milk and give by cup
⋆ Find a regular supply of formula or other milk, e.g. full cream cows milk
⋆ Learn how to prepare and store milk safely at home

Help mother make the transition:

⋆ Teach mother to cup feed her baby
⋆ Clean all utensils with soap and water
⋆ Start giving only formula or cows milk once the baby takes all feeds by cup

Stop breastfeeding completely:

⋆ Express and discard enough breast milk to keep comfortable until lactation stops

COUNSEL THE MOTHER ABOUT HER OWN HEALTH

➤ If the mother is sick, provide care for her, or refer her for help.

➤ If she has a breast problem (such as engorgement, sore nipples, breast infection), provide care for her or refer her for help.

➤ Advise her to eat well to keep up her own strength and health.

➤ Check the mother's immunization status and give her tetanus toxoid if needed.

➤ Make sure she has access to:
  - Family planning
  - Counselling on STD and AIDS prevention.

➤ Encourage every mother to be sure to know her own HIV status and to seek HIV testing if she does not know her status or is concerned about the possibility of HIV in herself or her family.

Appendix A   457

FLUID

Advise the Mother to Increase Fluid During Illness

FOR ANY SICK CHILD:
- If child is breastfed, breastfeed more frequently and for longer at each feed. If child is taking breast-milk substitutes, increase the amount of milk given
- Increase other fluids. For example, give soup, rice water, yoghurt drinks or clean water.

FOR CHILD WITH DIARRHOEA:
- Giving extra fluid can be lifesaving. Give fluid according to Plan A or Plan B on the *TREAT THE CHILD* chart

WHEN TO RETURN

Advise the Mother When to Return to Health Worker

FOLLOW-UP VISIT

If the child has:	Return for first follow-up in:
≠ PNEUMONIA ≠ DYSENTERY ≠ MALARIA, if fever persists ≠ FEVER-MALARIA UNLIKELY, if fever persists ≠ MEASLES WITH EYE OR MOUTH COMPLICATIONS	2 days
≠ PERSISTENT DIARRHOEA ≠ ACUTE EAR INFECTION ≠ CHRONIC EAR INFECTION ≠ FEEDING PROBLEM ≠ COUGH OR COLD, if not improving	5 days
≠ ANAEMIA ≠ CONFIRMED HIV INFECTION ≠ SUSPECTED SYMPTOMATIC HIV INFECTION ≠ HIV EXPOSED/ POSSIBLE HIV	14 days
≠ VERY LOW WEIGHT FOR AGE	30 days

Advise the mother to come for follow-up at the earliest time listed for the child's problems.

WHEN TO RETURN IMMEDIATELY

Advise mother to return immediately if the child has any of these signs:

Any sick child	≠ Not able to drink or breastfeed ≠ Becomes sicker ≠ Develops a fever
If child has NO PNEUMONIA: COUGH OR COLD, also return if:	≠ Fast breathing ≠ Difficult breathing
If child has Diarrhoea, also return if:	≠ Blood in stool ≠ Drinking poorly

ASSESS, CLASSIFY AND TREAT THE SICK YOUNG INFANT AGED UP TO 2 MONTHS

DO A RAPID APPRAISAL OF ALL WAITING INFANTS

ASK THE MOTHER WHAT THE YOUNG INFANT'S PROBLEMS ARE

- Determine if this is an initial or follow-up visit for this problem.
  - if follow-up visit, use the follow-up instructions
  - if initial visit, assess the young infant as follows:

CHECK FOR VERY SEVERE DISEASE AND LOCAL INFECTION

ASK:
- Is the infant having difficulty in feeding?
- Has the infant had convulsions (fits)?

LOOK AND FEEL:
- Count the breaths in one minute. Repeat the count if 60 or more breaths per minute.
- Look for severe chest indrawing.
- Measure axillary temperature.
- Look at the umbilicus. Is it red or draining pus?
- Look for skin pustules.
- Look at the young infant's movements. *If infant is sleeping, ask the mother to wake him/her.*
  - Does the infant move on his/her own?

  If the infant is not moving, gently stimulate him/her.
  - Does the infant move only when stimulated but then stops?
  - Does the infant not move at all?

YOUNG INFANT MUST BE CALM

Classify ALL YOUNG INFANTS

USE ALL BOXES THAT MATCH INFANT'S SYMPTOMS AND PROBLEMS TO CLASSIFY THE ILLNESS.

SIGNS	CLASSIFY AS	TREATMENT (Urgent pre-referral treatments are in bold print)
Any one of the following signs • Not feeding well or • Convulsions or • Fast breathing (60 breaths per minute or more) or • Severe chest indrawing or • Fever (37.5°C or above) or • Low body temperature (less than 35.5°C*) or • Movement only when stimulated or no movement at all	**VERY SEVERE DISEASE**	➤ *Give first dose of intramuscular antibiotic.* ➤ *Treat to prevent low blood sugar.* ➤ *Refer URGENTLY to hospital.*** ➤ *Advise mother how to keep the infant warm on the way to the hospital.*
• Umbilicus red or draining pus • Skin pustules	**LOCAL BACTERIAL INFECTION**	➤ *Give an appropriate oral antibiotic.* ➤ Teach mother to treat local infections at home. ➤ Advise mother to give home care for the young infant. ➤ Follow up in 2 days.
• None of the signs of very severe disease or local bacterial infection	**SEVERE DISEASE OR LOCAL INFECTION UNLIKELY**	➤ Advise mother to give home care for the young infant.

* *These thresholds are based on axillary temperature. The thresholds for rectal temperature readings are approximately 0.5°C higher.*
** *If referral is not possible, see* Integrated Management of Childhood Illness, Management of the sick young infant module, *Annex 2 "Where referral is not possible"*

Appendix A

THEN CHECK FOR JAUNDICE

ASK:
- When did jaundice first appear?

LOOK AND FEEL:
- Look for jaundice (yellow eyes or skin).
- Look at the young infant's palms and soles. Are they yellow?

Classify Jaundice

SIGNS	CLASSIFY AS	TREATMENT *(Urgent pre-referral treatments are in bold print)*
≠ Any jaundice if age less than 24 hours **or** ≠ Yellow palms and soles at any age	**SEVERE JAUNDICE**	➤ ***Treat to prevent low blood sugar.*** ➤ ***Refer URGENTLY to hospital.*** ➤ ***Advise mother how to keep the infant warm on the way to the hospital.***
≠ Jaundice appearing after 24 hours of age **and** ≠ Palms and soles not yellow	**JAUNDICE**	➤ Advise the mother to give home care for the young infant ➤ Advise mother to return immediately if palms and soles appear yellow. ➤ If the young infant is older than 3 weeks, refer to a hospital for assessment. ➤ Follow-up in 1 day.
≠ No jaundice	**NO JAUNDICE**	➤ Advise the mother to give home care for the young infant.

THEN ASK: Does the young infant have diarrhoea*?

IF YES, LOOK AND FEEL:

- Look at the young infant's general condition:
  - Infant's movements
    - Does the infant move on his/her own?
    - Does the infant move only when stimulated but then stops?
    - Does the infant not move at all?
  - Is the infant restless and irritable?
- Look for sunken eyes.
- Pinch the skin of the abdomen.
  Does it go back:
  - Very slowly (longer than 2 seconds)?
  - or slowly?

Classify DIARRHOEA FOR DEHYDRATION

SIGNS	CLASSIFY AS	TREATMENT (Urgent pre-referral treatments are in bold print)
Two of the following signs: ≠ Movement only when stimulated or no movement at all ≠ Sunken eyes ≠ Skin pinch goes back very slowly.	**SEVERE DEHYDRATION**	➤ If infant has no other severe classification: - Give fluid for severe dehydration (Plan C). OR ➤ *If infant also has another severe classification:* *- Refer URGENTLY to hospital with mother giving frequent sips of ORS on the way.* *- Advise mother to continue breastfeeding.*
Two of the following signs: ≠ Restless, irritable ≠ Sunken eyes ≠ Skin pinch goes back slowly.	**SOME DEHYDRATION**	➤ Give fluid and breast milk for some dehydration (Plan B). OR ➤ *If infant also has another severe classification:* *- Refer URGENTLY to hospital with mother giving frequent sips of ORS on the way.* *- Advise mother to continue breastfeeding.* ➤ Advise mother when to return immediately ➤ Follow-up in 2 days if not improving
≠ Not enough signs to classify as some or severe dehydration.	**NO DEHYDRATION**	➤ Give fluids and breast milk to treat for diarrhoea at home (Plan A) ➤ Advise mother when to return immediately ➤ Follow up in 2 days if not improving

---

* **What is diarrhoea in a young infant?**

A young infant has diarrhoea if the stools have changed from usual pattern and are many and watery (more water than fecal matter).

The normally frequent or semi-solid stools of a breastfed baby are not diarrhoea.

Appendix A

THEN CHECK THE YOUNG INFANT FOR HIV INFECTION

ASK:

Has the mother or the infant had an HIV test?

What was the result?

→ Classify by test result

SIGNS	CLASSIFY AS	TREATMENT (Urgent pre-referral treatments are in bold print)
≠ Child has positive virological test	**CONFIRMED HIV INFECTION**	➤ Give cotrimoxazole prophylaxis from age 4-6 weeks ➤ Assess the child's feeding and counsel as necessary ➤ Refer for staging and assessment for ART ➤ Advise the mother on home care ➤ Follow-up in 14 days
One or both of the following conditions: ≠ Mother HIV positive ≠ Child has positive HIV antibody test (sero-positive)	**POSSIBLE HIV INFECTION/ HIV EXPOSED**	➤ Give co-trimoxazole prophylaxis from age 4-6 weeks ➤ Assess the child's feeding and give appropriate feeding advice ➤ Refer/ do virological test to confirm infant's HIV status at least 6 weeks after breastfeeding has stopped ➤ Consider presumptive severe HIV disease ➤ Follow-up in one month
Negative HIV test for mother or child	**HIV INFECTION UNLIKELY**	➤ Treat, counsel and follow-up existing infections ➤ Advise the mother about feeding and about her own health

THEN CHECK FOR FEEDING PROBLEM OR LOW WEIGHT FOR AGE IN BREASTFED INFANTS*

If an infant has no indications to refer urgently to hospital

ASK:
- Is the infant breastfed? If yes, how many times in 24 hours?
- Does the infant usually receive any other foods or drinks? If yes, how often?
- If yes, what do you use to feed the infant?

ASSESS BREASTFEEDING:
- Has the infant breastfed in the previous hour?

If the infant has not fed in the previous hour, ask the mother to put her infant to the breast. Observe the breastfeed for 4 minutes.

(If the infant was fed during the last hour, ask the mother if she can wait and tell you when the infant is willing to feed again.)

- Is the infant well attached?

  not well attached   *good attachment*

  TO CHECK ATTACHMENT, LOOK FOR:
  - More areola seen above infant's top lip than below bottom lip
  - Mouth wide open
  - Lower lip turned outwards
  - Chin touching breast

  (All of these signs should be present if the attachment is good).

- Is the infant suckling effectively (that is, slow deep sucks, sometimes pausing)?

  not suckling effectively   *suckling effectively*

  Clear a blocked nose if it interferes with breastfeeding.

LOOK AND FEEL:
- Determine weight for age.
- Look for ulcers or white patches in the mouth (thrush).

Classify FEEDING

SIGNS	CLASSIFY AS	TREATMENT (Urgent pre-referral treatments are in bold print)

≠ Not well attached to breast **or**
 ≠ Not suckling effectively, **or**
 ≠ Less than 8 breastfeeds in 24 hours, **or**
 ≠ Receives other foods or drinks, **or**
 ≠ Low weight for age, **or**
 ≠ Thrush (ulcers or white patches in mouth)
	FEEDING PROBLEM OR LOW WEIGHT FOR AGE	➤ If not well attached or not suckling effectively, teach correct positioning and attachment.
		 ➤ If not able to attach well immediately, teach the mother to express breast milk and feed by a cup
		 ➤ If breastfeeding less than 8 times in 24 hours, advise to increase frequency of feeding. Advise her to breastfeed as often and for as long as the infant wants, day and night.
		 ➤ If receiving other foods or drinks, counsel mother about breastfeeding more, reducing other foods or drinks, and using a cup.
		   - Refer for breastfeeding counselling and possible relactation.
		   - Advise about correctly preparing breast-milk substitutes and using a cup.
		 ➤ Advise the mother how to feed and keep the low weight infant warm at home
		 ➤ If thrush, teach the mother to treat thrush at home.
		 ➤ Advise mother to give home care for the young infant.
		 ➤ Follow up any feeding problem or thrush in 2 days.
		 ➤ Follow-up low weight for age in 14 days.

≠ Not low weight for age and no other signs of inadequate feeding.	**NO FEEDING PROBLEM**	➤ Advise mother to give home care for the young infant ➤ Praise the mother for feeding the infant well.

35

Appendix A

THEN CHECK FOR FEEDING PROBLEM OR LOW WEIGHT FOR AGE IN INFANTS RECEIVING NO BREAST MILK

(use this chart when an HIV positive mother has chosen not to breastfeed)

ASK:

- What milk are you giving?
- How many times during the day and night?
- How much is given at each feed?
- How are you preparing the milk?
  o Let mother demonstrate or explain how a feed is prepared, and how it is given to the infant.
- Are you giving any breast milk at all?
- What foods and fluids in addition to replacement feeds is given?
- How is the milk being given? Cup or bottle?
- How are you cleaning the feeding utensils?

LOOK, LISTEN, FEEL:

- Determine the weight for age.
- Look for ulcers or white patches in the mouth (thrush).

Classify **FEEDING**

SIGNS	CLASSIFY AS	TREATMENT (Urgent pre-referral treatments are in bold)
• Milk incorrectly or unhygienically prepared Or • Giving inappropriate replacement feeds Or • Giving insufficient replacement feeds Or • An HIV positive mother mixing breast and other feeds before 6 months Or • Using a feeding bottle Or • Thrush Or • Low weight for age	**FEEDING PROBLEM OR LOW WEIGHT FOR AGE**	➤ Counsel about feeding ➤ Explain the guidelines for safe replacement feeding ➤ Identify concerns of mother and family about feeding. ➤ If mother is using a bottle, teach cup feeding ➤ If thrush, teach the mother to treat it at home ➤ Follow-up FEEDING PROBLEM or THRUSH in 2 days ➤ Follow up LOW WEIGHT FOR AGE in 7 days
• Not low weight for age and no other signs of inadequate feeding	**NO FEEDING PROBLEM**	➤ Advise mother to continue feeding, and ensure good hygiene ➤ Praise the mother for feeding the infant

THEN CHECK THE YOUNG INFANT'S IMMUNIZATION AND VITAMIN A STATUS:

IMMUNIZATION SCHEDULE:	AGE	VACCINE		
	Birth	BCG	OPV-0	
	6 weeks	DPT+HIB-1	OPV-1	Hepatitis 1
	10 weeks	DPT+HIB-2	OPV-2	Hepatitis 2

VITAMIN A

200 000 IU to the mother within 6 weeks of delivery

➤ **Give all missed doses on this visit.**
➤ Immunize sick infants unless being referred.
➤ Advise the caretaker when to return for the next dose.

ASSESS OTHER PROBLEMS

Appendix A

TREAT THE YOUNG INFANT AND COUNSEL THE MOTHER

▸ Give First Dose of Intramuscular Antibiotics

▸ Give first dose of ampicillin intramuscularly <u>and</u>
▸ Give first dose of Gentamicin intramuscularly.

	AMPICILLIN Dose: 50 mg per kg To a vial of 250 mg Add 1.3 ml sterile water = 250 mg/1.5 ml	GENTAMICIN	
		Undiluted 2 ml vial containing 20 mg= 2 ml at 10 mg/ml OR Add 6 ml sterile water to 2 ml vial containing 80 mg* = 8 ml at 10 mg/ml	
WEIGHT		AGE <7 days Dose: 5 mg per kg	AGE ≥7 days Dose: 7.5 mg per kg
1–<1.5 kg	0.4 ml	0.6 ml*	0.9 ml*
1.5–<2 kg	0.5 ml	0.9 ml*	1.3 ml*
2–<2.5 kg	0.7 ml	1.1 ml*	1.7 ml*
2.5–<3 kg	0.8 ml	1.4 ml*	2.0 ml*
3–<3.5 kg	1.0 ml	1.6 ml*	2.4 ml*
3.5–<4 kg	1.1 ml	1.9 ml*	2.8 ml*
4–<4.5 kg	1.3 ml	2.1 ml*	3.2 ml*

*Avoid using undiluted 40 mg/ml gentamicin.

▸ Referral is the best option for a young infant classified as VERY SEVERE DISEASE. If referral is not possible, continue to give ampicillin <u>and</u> gentamicin for at least 5 days. Give ampicillin two times daily to infants less than one week of age and 3 times daily to infants one week or older. Give gentamicin once daily.

▸ Treat the Young Infant to Prevent Low Blood Sugar

▸ **If the young infant is able to breastfeed:**
Ask the mother to breastfeed the young infant.

▸ **If the young infant is not able to breastfeed but is able to swallow:**
Give 20-50 ml (10 ml/kg) expressed breastmilk before departure. If not possible to give expressed breastmilk, give 20-50 ml (10 ml/kg) sugar water (*To make sugar water: Dissolve 4 level teaspoons of sugar (20 grams) in a 200-ml cup of clean water*).

▸ **If the young infant is not able to swallow:**
Give 20-50 ml (10 ml/kg) of expressed breastmilk or sugar water by nasogastric tube.

TREAT THE YOUNG INFANT

➤ Teach the Mother How to Keep the Young Infant Warm on the Way to the Hospital

➤ Provide skin to skin contact, OR
➤ Keep the young infant clothed or covered as much as possible all the time. Dress the young infant with extra clothing including hat, gloves, socks and wrap the infant in a soft dry cloth and cover with a blanket.

➤ Give an Appropriate Oral Antibiotic for local infection

For local bacterial infection:

First-line antibiotic: _____
Second-line antibiotic: _____

AGE or WEIGHT	COTRIMOXAZOLE (trimethoprim + sulphamethoxazole) ➤ Give two times daily for 5 days			AMOXICILLIN ➤ Give two times daily for 5 days	
	Adult Tablet single strength (80 mg trimethoprim + 400 mg sulphamethoxazole)	Paediatric Tablet (20 mg trimethoprim + 100 mg sulphamethoxazole)	Syrup (40 mg trimethoprim + 200 mg sulphamethoxazole)	Tablet 250 mg	Syrup 125 mg in 5 ml
Birth up to 1 month (<4 kg)		1/2*	1.25 ml* 1/4		2.5 ml
1 month up to 2 months (4-<6 kg)	1/4	1	2.5 ml	1/2	5 ml

* Avoid cotrimoxazole in infants less than 1 month of age who are premature or jaundiced.

TREAT THE YOUNG INFANT AND COUNSEL THE MOTHER

➤ Teach the Mother How to Treat Local Infections at Home

➤ Explain how the treatment is given.
➤ Watch her as she does the first treatment in the clinic.
➤ Tell her to return to the clinic if the infection worsens.

To Treat Skin Pustules or Umbilical Infection

The mother should do the treatment twice daily for 5 days:

➤ Wash hands
➤ Gently wash off pus and crusts with soap and water
➤ Dry the area
➤ Paint the skin or umbilicus/cord with full strength gentian violet (0.5%)
➤ Wash hands again

To Treat Thrush (ulcers or white patches in mouth)

The mother should do the treatment 4 times daily for 7 days:

➤ Wash hands
➤ Paint the mouth with half-strength gentian violet (0.25%) using a clean soft cloth wrapped around the finger
➤ Wash hands again

➤ To Treat Diarrhoea, See TREAT THE CHILD CHART.

➤ Immunize Every Sick Young Infant, as needed.

COUNSEL THE MOTHER

➤ Teach Correct Positioning and Attachment for Breastfeeding

➤ Show the mother how to hold her infant
  - with the infant's head and body in line
  - with the infant approaching breast with nose opposite to the nipple
  - with the infant held close to the mother's body
  - with the infant's whole body supported, not just neck and shoulders.

➤ Show her how to help the infant to attach. She should:
  - touch her infant's lips with her nipple
  - wait until her infant's mouth is opening wide
  - move her infant quickly onto her breast, aiming the infant's lower lip well below the nipple.

➤ Look for signs of good attachment and effective suckling. If the attachment or suckling is not good, try again.

➤ Teach the Mother How to Express Breast Milk

Ask the mother to:

➤ Wash her hands thoroughly.
➤ Make herself comfortable.
➤ Hold a wide necked container under her nipple and areola.
➤ Place her thumb on top of the breast and the first finger on the under side of the breast so they are opposite each other (at least 4 cm from the tip of the nipple).
➤ Compress and release the breast tissue between her finger and thumb a few times.
➤ If the milk does not appear she should re-position her thumb and finger closer to the nipple and compress and release the breast as before.
➤ Compress and release all the way around the breast, keeping her fingers the same distance from the nipple. Be careful not to squeeze the nipple or to rub the skin or move her thumb or finger on the skin.
➤ Express one breast until the milk just drips, then express the other breast until the milk just drips.
➤ Alternate between breasts 5 or 6 times, for at least 20 to 30 minutes.
➤ Stop expressing when the milk no longer flows but drips from the start.

Appendix A   469

COUNSEL THE MOTHER

▶ **Counsel the HIV-positive mother who has chosen not to breastfeed (or the caretaker of a child who cannot be breastfed)**

The mother or caretaker should have received full counselling before making this decision

▵ Ensure that the mother or caretaker has an adequate supply of appropriate breast milk substitute replacement feed.
▵ Ensure that the mother or caretaker knows how to prepare milk correctly and hygienically and has the facilities and resources to do so.
▵ Demonstrate how to feed with a cup and spoon rather than a bottle.
▵ Make sure that the mother or caretaker understands that prepared feed must be finished within an hour after preparation.
▵ Make sure that the mother or caretaker understands that mixing breastfeeding with replacement feeding may increase the risk of HIV infection and should not be done.

HOW TO PREPARE COMMERCIAL FORMULA MILK

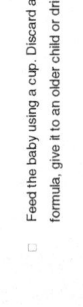

☐ Wash your hands before preparing the formula.
☐ Make ____ ml for each feed. Feed the baby ____ times every 24 hours.
☐ Always use the marked cup or glass to measure water and the scoop to measure formula powder. Your baby needs ____ scoops.
☐ Measure the exact amount of powder that you will need for one feed.
☐ Boil enough water vigorously for 1 or 2 seconds.
☐ Add the hot water to the powdered formula. The water should be added while it is still hot and not after it has cooled down. Stir well.
☐ Only make enough formula for one feed at a time. Do not keep milk in a thermos flask because it will become contaminated quickly.
☐ Feed the baby using a cup. Discard any unused formula, give it to an older child or drink it yourself.
☐ Wash the utensils.
☐ Come back to see me on ____.

▶ *Teach the Mother How to Feed by a Cup*

▵ Put a cloth on the infant's front to protect his clothes as some milk can spill
▵ Hold the infant semi-upright on the lap.
▵ Put a measured amount of milk in the cup.
▵ Hold the cup so that it rests lightly on the infant's lower lip.
▵ Tip the cup so that the milk just reaches the infant's lips.
▵ Allow the infant to take the milk himself. DO NOT pour the milk into the infant's mouth.

42

COUNSEL THE MOTHER

▸ *Teach the Mother How to Keep the Low Weight Infant Warm at Home*

- Keep the young infant in the same bed with the mother.
- Keep the room warm (at least 25°C) with home heating device and make sure that there is no draught of cold air.
- Avoid bathing the low weight infant. When washing or bathing, do it in a very warm room with warm water, dry immediately and thoroughly after bathing and clothe the young infant immediately.
- Change clothes (e.g. nappies) whenever they are wet.
- Provide skin to skin contact as much as possible, day and night. For skin to skin contact:
    - ➢ Dress the infant in a warm shirt open at the front, a nappy, hat and socks.
    - ➢ Place the infant in skin to skin contact on the mother's chest between the mother's breasts. Keep the infant's head turned to one side
    - ➢ Cover the infant with mother's clothes (and an additional warm blanket in cold weather)
- When not in skin to skin contact, keep the young infant clothed or covered as much as possible at all times. Dress the young infant with extra clothing including hat and socks, loosely wrap the young infant in a soft dry cloth and cover with a blanket.
- Check frequently if the hands and feet are warm. If cold, re-warm the baby using skin to skin contact.
- Breastfeed (or give expressed breast milk by cup) the infant frequently

COUNSEL THE MOTHER

➤ Advise the Mother to Give Home Care for the Young Infant

1. **EXCLUSIVELY BREASTFEED THE YOUNG INFANT**
   Give only breastfeeds to the young infant
   Breastfeed frequently, as often and for as long as the infant wants.

2. **MAKE SURE THAT THE YOUNG INFANT IS KEPT WARM AT ALL TIMES.**
   In cool weather cover the infant's head and feet and dress the infant with extra clothing.

3. **WHEN TO RETURN:**

Follow up visit	
If the infant has:	**Return for first follow-up in:**
⁂ JAUNDICE	1 day
⁂ LOCAL BACTERIAL INFECTION ⁂ FEEDING PROBLEM ⁂ THRUSH ⁂ DIARRHOEA	2 days
⁂ LOW WEIGHT FOR AGE	14 days
⁂ CONFIRMED HIV INFECTION or POSSIBLE HIV INFECTION/ HIV EXPOSED	14 days

WHEN TO RETURN IMMEDIATELY:

Advise the caretaker to return immediately if the young infant has any of these signs:

- ➤ Breastfeeding poorly
- ➤ Reduced activity
- ➤ Becomes sicker
- ➤ Develops a fever
- ➤ Feels unusually cold
- ➤ Fast breathing
- ➤ Difficult breathing
- ➤ Palms and soles appear yellow

GIVE FOLLOW-UP CARE FOR THE YOUNG INFANT

ASSESS EVERY YOUNG INFANT FOR "VERY SEVERE DISEASE" DURING FOLLOW UP VISIT.

➤ LOCAL BACTERIAL INFECTION

After 2 days:
Look at the umbilicus. Is it red or draining pus?
Look for skin pustules.

Treatment:
- ➤ If umbilical *pus or redness remains same or is worse,* refer to hospital. If *pus and redness are improved,* tell the mother to continue giving the 5 days of antibiotic and continue treating the local infection at home.
- ➤ If skin pustules are *same or worse,* refer to hospital. If *improved,* tell the mother to continue giving the 5 days of antibiotic and continue treating the local infection at home.

➤ JAUNDICE

After 1 day:
Look for jaundice. Are palms and soles yellow?

- ➤ If palms and soles are yellow, refer to hospital.
- ➤ If palms and soles are not yellow, but jaundice has not decreased, advise the mother home care and ask her to return for follow up in 1 day.
- ➤ If jaundice has started decreasing, reassure the mother and ask her to continue home care. Ask her to return for follow up at 3 weeks of age. If jaundice continues beyond three weeks of age, refer the young infant to a hospital for further assessment.

➤ DIARRHOEA

After 2 days:
Ask: Has the diarrhoea stopped ?

Treatment:
- ➤ If the diarrhoea has not stopped, assess and treat the young infant for diarrhoea. >SEE "Does the Young Infant Have Diarrhoea ?"
- ➤ If the diarrhoea has stopped, tell the mother to continue exclusive breastfeeding.

GIVE FOLLOW-UP CARE FOR THE YOUNG INFANT

➤ POSSIBLE HIV/HIV EXPOSED

- ➤ Follow-up after 14 days and then monthly or according to immunization programme.
- ➤ Counsel about feeding practices. Avoid giving both breast milk and formula milk (mixed feeding).
- ➤ Start **co-trimoxazole prophylaxis** at 4-6 weeks, if not started already and check compliance.
- ➤ Test for HIV infection as early as possible, if not already done so.
- ➤ Refer for ART if presumptive severe HIV infection as per definition above.
- ➤ Counsel the mother about her HIV status and arrange counselling and testing for her if required.

➤ FEEDING PROBLEM

After 2 days:

Reassess feeding. ➤ See "Then Check for Feeding Problem or Low Weight" above.
Ask about any feeding problems found on the initial visit.

- ➤ Counsel the mother about any new or continuing feeding problems. If you counsel the mother to make significant changes in feeding, ask her to bring the young infant back again.
- ➤ If the young infant is low weight for age, ask the mother to return 14 days after the initial visit to measure the young infant's weight gain.

Exception:
If you do not think that feeding will improve, or if the young infant has *lost weight*, refer to HOSPITAL.

GIVE FOLLOW-UP CARE FOR THE YOUNG INFANT

➤ LOW WEIGHT FOR AGE

After 14 days:
Weigh the young infant and determine if the infant is still low weight for age.
Reassess feeding. > See "Then Check for Feeding Problem or Low Weight" above.

➤ If the infant is *no longer low weight for age*, praise the mother and encourage her to continue.

➤ If the infant is *still low weight for age, but is feeding well*, praise the mother. Ask her to have her infant weighed again within a month or when she returns for immunization.

➤ If the infant is *still low weight for age and still has a feeding problem*, counsel the mother about the feeding problem. Ask the mother to return again in 14 days (or when she returns for immunization, if this is within 14 days). Continue to see the young infant every few weeks until the infant is feeding well and gaining weight regularly or is no longer low weight for age.

Exception:
If you do not think that feeding will improve, or if the young infant has *lost weight*, refer to hospital.

➤ THRUSH

After 2 days:
Look for ulcers or white patches in the mouth (thrush).
Reassess feeding. > See "Then Check for Feeding Problem or Low Weight" above.

➤ If *thrush is worse*, or the infant has *problems with attachment or suckling*, refer to hospital.

➤ If *thrush is the same or better*, and if the infant is *feeding well*, continue half-strength gentian violet for a total of 7 days.

Appendix A

MANAGEMENT OF THE SICK CHILD AGED 2 MONTHS UP TO 5 YEARS

Name: _____ Age: _____ Weight: _____ kg Temperature: _____ °C

ASK: What are the child's problems? _____ Initial visit? ___ Follow-up Visit? ___
ASSESS (Circle all signs present) **CLASSIFY**

CHECK FOR GENERAL DANGER SIGNS
  NOT ABLE TO DRINK OR BREASTFEED LETHARGIC OR UNCONSCIOUS
  VOMITS EVERYTHING   CONVULSING NOW
  CONVULSIONS
	General danger signs present?
	Yes___ No___
	Remember to use danger sign when selecting classifications

DOES THE CHILD HAVE COUGH OR DIFFICULT BREATHING? Yes___ No___	

≠ For how long? ____ Days   ≠ Count the breaths in one minute.
                          _____ breaths per minute. Fast breathing?
                          ≠ Look for chest indrawing.
                          ≠ Look and listen for stridor/wheeze.	

DOES THE CHILD HAVE DIARRHOEA? Yes ___ No ___	

≠ For how long? _____ Days   ≠ Look at the child's general condition. Is the child:
≠ Is there blood in the stools?   Lethargic or unconscious?
                                         Restless or irritable?
                          ≠ Look for sunken eyes.
                          ≠ Offer the child fluid. Is the child:
                                         Not able to drink or drinking poorly?
                                         Drinking eagerly, thirsty?
                          ≠ Pinch the skin of the abdomen. Does it go back:
                                         Very slowly (longer than 2 seconds)? Slowly?	

DOES THE CHILD HAVE FEVER? (by history/feels hot/temperature 37.5°C or above) Yes___ No___	

Decide Malaria Risk: High   Low
≠ For how long? _____ Days   ≠ Look or feel for stiff neck.
≠ If more than 7 days, has fever been   ≠ Look for runny nose.
   present every day?   Look for signs of MEASLES:
≠ Has child had measles within   ≠ Generalized rash and
   the last three months?   ≠ One of these: cough, runny nose, or red eyes.
If the child has measles now
or within the last 3 months: ≠ Look for mouth ulcers.
                                         If Yes, are they deep and extensive?
                                      ≠ Look for pus draining from the eye.
                                      ≠ Look for clouding of the cornea.	

DOES THE CHILD HAVE AN EAR PROBLEM? Yes___ No___	
≠ Is there ear pain? ≠ Look for pus draining from the ear. ≠ Is there ear discharge? ≠ Feel for tender swelling behind the ear. If Yes, for how long? ___ Days	
THEN CHECK FOR MALNUTRITION AND ANAEMIA	

≠ Look visible severe wasting.
                          ≠ Look for palmar pallor.
                              Severe palmar pallor? Some palmar pallor?
                          ≠ Look for oedema of both feet.
                          ≠ Determine weight for age.
                                Very Low ___ Not Very Low ___	

CHECK FOR HIV INFECTION	
HIV tested before (confidential): <u>Mother</u> o positive o negative o unknown <u>Child</u> o positive o negative o unknown <u>pneumonia</u> or <u>Very low weight</u> or <u>persistent diarrhoea</u> or <u>ear discharge or mother or child HIV status known</u>: Yes __NO __ ⇔ Pneumonia ⇔ Parotid enlargement ⇔ Very Low weight for age ⇔ Oral thrush ⇔ Ear discharge ⇔ Generalized persistent lymphadenopathy ⇔ Persistent diarrhoea If mother is HIV infected, and child less than 24 months old, decide on infant feeding counselling needs	
CHECK THE CHILD'S IMMUNIZATION STATUS Circle immunizations needed today.	Return for next immunization on:
____ ____ ____ ____ ____ ____ BCG DPT1 +HIB1 DPT2 +HIB2 DPT3+HIB3 Vitamin A Mebendazole ____ ____ ____ ____ ____ ____ OPV 0 OPV 1 OPV 2 OPV 3 Measles1 Measles2	_____ (Date)
ASSESS CHILD'S FEEDING if child has ANAEMIA OR VERY LOW WEIGHT or is less than 2 years old.	

≠ Do you breastfeed your child? Yes____ No ____
    If Yes, how many times in 24 hours? ___ times. Do you breastfeed during the night? Yes___ No___
≠ Does the child take any other food or fluids? Yes___ No ___
    If Yes, what food or fluids? _____
       How many times per day? ___ times. What do you use to feed the child? _____
       If very low weight for age: How large are servings? _____
       Does the child receive how own serving? ___ Who feeds the child and how? _____
≠   During the illness, has the child's feeding changed? Yes _____ No _____ If Yes, how?
	FEEDING PROBLEMS

ASSESS OTHER PROBLEMS Ask about mother's own health	

MANAGEMENT OF THE SICK YOUNG INFANT AGED UP TO 2 MONTHS

Name: _____ Age: _____ Weight: _____ kg Temperature: _____ °C

ASK: What are the infant's problems? _____ Initial visit? ___ Follow-up visit? ___

ASSESS (Circle all signs present)   **CLASSIFY**

CHECK FOR VERY SEVERE DISEASE AND LOCAL BACTERIAL INFECTION	Classify all young infants

≠ Is the infant having difficulty in feeding?
≠ Has the infant had convulsions (fits)?
                 ≠ Count the breaths in one minute. _____ breaths per minute
                           Repeat if 60 breaths or more _____ Fast breathing?
                 ≠ Look for severe chest indrawing.
                 ≠ Fever (temperature 37.5°C or above).
                 ≠ Low body temperature (less than 35.5°C)
                 ≠ Look at the umbilicus. Is it red or draining pus?
                 ≠ Look for skin pustules.
                 ≠ Look at the young infant's movements.
                     Does the infant move only when stimulated?
                     Does the infant not move at all?	

THEN CHECK FOR JAUNDICE ≠ If jaundice "yes", when did it first appear? ≠ Look for jaundice (yellow eyes or skin) ≠ Look at the young infant's palms and soles. Are they yellow?	

DOES THE YOUNG INFANT HAVE DIARRHOEA?   Yes _____ No _____
 	
                                         ≠ Look at the young infant's general condition.
 	
                                         Does the infant move only when stimulated?
                                         Does the infant not move at all?
 	
                                         Is the infant restless or irritable?
 	
                                         ≠ Look for sunken eyes.
 	
                                         ≠ Pinch the skin of the abdomen. Does it go back:
                                           Very slowly (longer than 2 seconds)?
                                           Slowly?	

IF AN INFANT HAS NO INDICATION FOR REFERRAL:
THEN CHECK FOR FEEDING PROBLEM OR LOW WEIGHT IN A BREASTFED INFANT
 	
≠ Is the infant breastfed? Yes _____ No _____   ≠ Determine weight for age. Low ___ Not Low _____
   If Yes, how many times in 24 hours? _____ times
                                              ≠ Look for ulcers or white patches in the mouth (thrush).
≠ Does the infant usually receive any
   other foods or drinks? Yes _____ No _____
   If Yes, how often?
 	
≠ If yes, what do you use to feed the infant?	

ASSESS BREASTFEEDING:
≠ Has the infant breastfed in the previous hour?   If infant has not fed in the previous hour, ask the mother to put her
                                                          infant to the breast. Observe the breastfeed for 4 minutes.
 	
                                            ≠ Is the infant able to attach? To check attachment, look for:
                                                - More areola seen above infant's top lip   Yes ___ No ___
                                                     than below bottom lip
                                                   - Mouth wide open   Yes ___   No ___
                                                   - Lower lip turned outwards   Yes ___   No ___
                                                   - Chin touching breast   Yes ___   No ___
 	
                                            not well attached   *good attachment*
 	
                                            ≠ Is the infant suckling effectively (that is, slow deep sucks, some-
                                               times pausing)?
 	
                                                 not suckling effectively *suckling effectively*	

THEN CHECK FOR HIV INFECTION ≠ Has the mother or infant had an HIV test? ≠ What was the result?	
THEN CHECK FOR FEEDING PROBLEM OR LOW WEIGHT IN AN INFANT WHO RECEIVES NO BREAST MILK ≠ Determine weight for age. Low ___ Not Low _____ Which breast-milk substitute? _____ Is enough milk being given in 24 hrs? •• yes ••no ≠ Look for ulcers or white patches in the mouth (thrush). Correct feed preparation? •• yes •• no Any food or fluids other than milk? •• yes •• no How is the milk being given? •• cup •• bottle Utensils cleaned adequately? •• yes •• no	

CHECK THE YOUNG INFANT'S IMMUNIZATION STATUS   Circle immunizations needed today.
 	
     ___   ___
    BCG   OPV 0
 	
     ___   ___   ___
    OPV 1   DPT1 + HIB1   Hepatitis B1
 	
     ___   ___   ___
    OPV 2   DPT2 + HIB2   Hepatitis B2
	Return for next immunization on:
	
	_____
	(Date)

ASSESS OTHER PROBLEMS ASK ABOUT MOTHER'S OWN HEALTH	

ANNEX A: SKIN AND MOUTH CONDITIONS*
Identify skin problem if skin is itching

	SIGNS	CLASSIFY AS:	TREATMENT	Unique features in HIV
	Itching rash with small papules and scratch marks. Dark spots with pale centres	PAPULAR ITCHING RASH (PRURIGO)	**Treat itching:** -calamine lotion -Antihistamine by mouth - If not improved, 1% hydrocortisone Can be an early sign of HIV and needs assessment for HIV	**Is a Clinical stage 2 defining disease**
	An itchy circular lesion with a raised edge and fine scaly area in centre with loss of hair. May also be found on body or web of feet.	RINGWORM (TINEA)	Zkwflogh#rl#wkh#vnlq#hitvkluz# anti-fungal cream if few patches If extensive Refer, if not give: ketoconazole for 2 up to 12 months (6-10 kg) 40 mg per day. For 12 up to 5 years give 60 mg per day . Or give griseofulvin 10 mg/kg/day. If in hairline, shave hair Treat itching as above	Extensive : There is a high incidence of coexisting nail infection which has to be treated adequately, to prevent recurrences of tinea infection of skin **Fungal nail infection is a Clinical stage 2 defining disease**
	Rash and excoriations on torso; burrows in web space and wrist. Face spared.	SCABIES	Treat itching as above Manage with anti-scabies: 25% topical benzyl benzoate at night , repeat for 3 days after washing 1% topical lindane cream or lotion once wash off after 12 hours	In HIV positive individuals scabies may manifest as crusted scabies. Crusted scabies presents as extensive areas of crusting mainly on the scalp face, back, and feet. Patients may not complain of itch but the scales will be teeming with mites.

* IMAI acute care module gives more information

ANNEX A cont/d

Identify skin problem if skin has blisters/sores/pustules

SIGNS	CLASSIFY AS:	TREATMENT	Unique features in HIV
Vesicles over body. Vesicles appear progressively over days and form scabs after they rupture	Chicken pox	Treat itching as above. Refer URGENTLY if pneumonia or jaundice appear	Presentation atypical only if child is immunocompromised. Duration of disease longer. Complications more frequent. Chronic infection with continued appearance of new lesions for >1 month; typical vesicles evolve into nonhealing ulcers that become necrotic, crusted, and hyperkeratotic.
Vesicles in one area on oneside of body with intense pain or scars plus shooting pain. Herpes zoster is uncommon in children except where they are immuno-compromised, for example if infected with HIV	HERPES ZOSTER	Keep lesions clean and dry. Use local anti septic. If eye involved give acyclovir 20 mg /kg (max 800 mg) 4 times daily for 5 days. Give pain relief. Follow-up in 7 days	Duration of disease longer. Hemorrhagic vesicles, necrotic ulceration. Rarely recurrent, disseminated or multidermatomal. **Is a Clinical stage 2 defining disease**
Vesicular lesion or sores, also involving lips and / or mouth	HERPES SIMPLEX	If child unable to feed, refer. If first episode or severe ulceration, give acyclovir as above	Extensive area of involvement. Large ulcers. Delayed healing (often greater than a month). Resistance to Acyclovir common. Therefore continue treatment till complete healing of ulcer. **Chronic HSV infection (>1 month) is a Clinical stage 4 defining disease**
Red, tender, warm crusts or small lesions	IMPETIGO OR FOLLICULITIS	Clean sores with antiseptic. Drain pus if fluctuant. Start cloxacillin if size >4cm or red streaks or tender nodes or multiple abscesses for 5 days (25-50 mg/kg every 6 hours). Refer URGENTLY if child has fever and / or if infection extends to the muscle	

See below for more information about drug reactions

Appendix A 479

ANNEX A cont'd

IDENTIFY PAPULAR LESIONS: NON-ITCHY

	Presenting signs & symptoms	Classify	Management & treatment	Unique features in HIV
	Skin colored pearly white papules with a central umblication. It is most commonly seen on the face and trunk in children.	**Molluscum contagiosum**	can be treated by various modalities: Leave them alone unless superinfected Use of phenol: pricking each lesion with a needle or sharpened orange stick and dabbing the lesion with phenol Electrodesiccaton Liquid nitrogen application (using orange stick) Curettage	Incidence is higher Giant molluscum (>1cm in size), or coalescent double or triple lesions may be seen More than 100 lesions may be seen. Lesions often chronic and difficult to eradicate **Extensive molluscum contagiosum is a Clinical stage 2 defining disease**
	The **common wart** appears as papules or nodules with a rough (verrucous) surface.	**Warts**	**Treatment:** Topical salicylic acid preparations (eg. Duofilm). Liquid nitrogen cryotherapy. Electrocautery	Lesions more numerous and recalcitrant to therapy. **Extensive viral warts is a Clinical stage 2 defining disease**
	Greasy scales and redness on central face, body folds	**Sebbhorrea**	Ketoconazole shampoo If severe, refer or provide tropical steroids. For seborrheic dermatitis: 1% hyrdocortison cream X2 daily. If severe, refer.	Seborrheic dermatitis may be severe in HIV infection. Secondary infection may be common

ANNEX A: ASSESS, CLASSIFY AND TREAT SKIN AND MOUTH

Mouth problems : Thrush

Presenting signs	CLASSIFY:	TREATMENTS
Not able to swallow	SEVERE OESOPHAGEAL THRUSH	Refer URGENTLY to hospital. If not able to refer, give fluconazole. If mother is breastfeeding check and treat the mother for breast thrush. (Stage 4 disease)
Pain or difficulty swallowing	OESOPHAGEAL THRUSH	Give fluconazole. Give oral care to young infant or child. If mother is breastfeeding check and treat the mother for breast thrush. Follow up in 2 days. Tell the mother when to come back immediately. Once stabilized, refer for **ART** initiation (Stage 4 disease)
White patches in mouth which can be scraped off.	ORAL THRUSH	Counsel the mother on home care for oral thrush. The mother should: Wash her hands Zdvk wkh |rxuj lqjidqw 2 fklogtiv prxwk zlwk d vriw fohdq forwk zudsshg durxqg khu ilcjhu dqg zhw ziwk salt water Instill 1ml nystatin four times per day or paint the mouth with half strength gentian violet for 7 days Wash her hands after providing treatment for the young infant or child Avoid feeding for 20 minutes after medication Li euhdvwihg/ fkhfn prwkhutiv euhdvwv iru wkuxvkl Li suhvhqw +gu|/ vklq| vfdohv rq qlssoh dqg duhrod,/ wuhdw with nystatin or GV Advise the mother to wash breasts after feeds. If bottle fed, advise to change to cup and spoon If severe, recurrent or pharyngeal thrush, consider symptomatic HIV Give paracetamol if needed for pain (Stage 3 disease)
most frequently seen on the sides of the tongue, a white plaque with a corrugated appearance.	ORAL HAIRY LEU-COPLAKIA	Does not independently require treatment, but resolve with ART and Acyclovir (Stage 2 disease)

ANNEX A: ASSESS, CLASSIFY AND TREAT SKIN AND MOUTH CONDITIONS

DRUG /ALLERGIC REACTIONS

Pictures	Signs	CLASSIFY	Treatment	Unique features o in HIV
	Generalized red, widespread with small bumps or blisters; or one or more dark skin areas (fixed drug reactions)	Fixed drug reactions	Stop medications Give oral antihistamines If peeling rash refer	Could be a sign of reaction to DUYüv#
	Wet, oozing sores or excoriated, thick patches	ECZEMA	Soak sores with clean water to remove crusts (no soap) Dry skin gently Short-term use of topical steroid cream not on face. Treat itching	
	Severe reaction due to co-trimoxazole or NVP involving the skin as well as the eyes and/mouth. Might cause difficulty breathing	Steven-Johnson syndrome	Stop medication Refer Urgently	The most lethal reaction to NVP, co-trimoxazole or even efafiretz .

ANNEX B: PAEDIATRIC ART

RECOMMENDED FIRST LINE ARV REGIMENS FOR CHILDREN

The following regimens are recommended by WHO as first line ART for children. The choice of regimen at the country level will be determined by the National ART guidelines.

AZT or d4T + 3TC + NVP or EFV1:	ABC +3TC + NVP or EFV1:
AZT + 3TC + NVP	ABC + 3TC + NVP
AZT + 3TC + EFV	ABC + 3TC + EFV
d4T + 3TC + NVP	
d4T + 3TC + EFV	

* If <3 years or <10 kg, use NVP. EFV cannot be used in these children.

Recommendations - When to Start ART

POPULATION	< 12 mo Confirmed HIV	≤ 12 mo Presumptive*	1-4 yrs	≥ 5yrs
START ART	All with confirmed HIV regardless of clinical/CD4	All	clinical or immunological criteria	clinical or immunological criteria
Strength of Recommendation	Strong	Strong (Time limited based on performance of algorithms)	Strong	Strong

*If lack ability for viral test, use WHO presumptive diagnosis of HIV allows initiation ART based on presumptive dx and stop if found uninfected. – with clinical sxor low CD4 TEXT ONLY -Well infant diagnose late may defer initiation base don CD4/VL

Recommendations – What to start ART

POPULATION	Up to 12 months	1-4 yrs	≥ 5
START ART	•PMTCT/NVP exposure : PI-regimen * •No PMTCT exposure : NVP-regimen	NVP/EFV+ 2NRTI	NVP/EFV+ 2NRTI
Strength of recommendation	Strong	Strong	Strong

TEXT
– * 3NRTI +NVP, other approaches need data before can be recommended, what to do where NO PI or no cold chain, i.e., no choice, use standard NVP
Need for research on new strategies for ART in MTCT exposed infants
Risks of NVP resistance from any NVP containing ART or MTCT regimens, esp. in BF mothers

Appendix A

ANNEX B: ARV DOSAGES

≠ Give for children 6 weeks of age and above
≠ 0.75 Twice daily means 1 tablet AM and 0.5 (half) tablet PM
≠ 1.5 twice daily means 2 tablets AM and 1 tablet PM

Lamivudine (3TC) - Give 4 mg/kg per dose twice daily

Weight	Syrup 10 mg/ml	Or	30 mg tablet	Or	150 mg tablet
3-3.9	3 ml		1		
4-5.9	3 ml		1		
6-9.9	4 ml		1.5		
10-13.9	6 ml		2		
14-19.9			2.5		0.5
20-24.9			3		0.75

Abacavir (ABC) - Give 8 mg/per dose twice daily

Weight	Syrup 20 mg/ml	Or	60 mg tablet	Or	300 mg tablet
3-3.9	3 ml		1		
4-5.9	3 ml		1		
6-9.9	4 ml		1.5		
10-13.9	6 ml		2		
14-19.9			2.5		0.5
20-24.9			3		0.75

Zidovudine (AZT or ZDV) - Give 180-240 mg/m² per dose twice daily

Weight	Syrup 10 mg/ml	Or	30 mg tablet	Or	150 mg tablet
3-3.9	6 ml		1		
4-5.9	6 ml		1		
6-9.9	9 ml		1.5		
10-13.9	12 ml		2		
14-19.9			2.5		
20-24.9			3		

Stavudine (d4T) - Give 1 mg/kg per dose twice daily

Weight	Syrup 10 mg/ml	Or	6 mg tablet	Or	15 mg tablet	Or	20 mg tablet
3-3.9	6 ml		1				
4-5.9	6 ml		1				
6-9.9	9 ml		1.5				
10-13.9			2				
14-19.9			2.5		1		1
20-24.9			3				1

ANNEX B: ARV DOSAGES cont/d

Nevirapine (NVP) - Give maintenance dose 160-200 mg/m² per dose twice daily. Lead-in dose during week 1 and 2, give only AM dose

Weight	Syrup 10 mg/ml	Or	30 mg tablet	Or	150 mg tablet
3-3.9	5 ml		1		
4-5.9	5 ml		1		
6-9.9	8 ml		1.5		
10-13.9	10 ml		2		
14-19.9			2.5		0.75
20-24.9			3		0.75

Lopinavir/ritonavir (lop/rit) - Give 230/75.5 mg/m² twice daily and increase to 300/75 mg/m² if taken with nevirapine

Weight	Syrup 80/20 mg/ml	Or	100/25 mg tablet
3-3.9	1 ml		
4-5.9	1.5 ml		
6-9.9	1.5 ml		
10-13.9	2 ml		1.5
14-19.9	2.5 ml		2
20-24.9	3 ml		2.5

Efavirenz (EFV) - Give 15 mg/kg/day if capsule or tablet once daily.

Weight	Combinations of 200, 100 and 50 mg capsules	Or	600 mg tablet
10-13.9	One 200 mg		
14-19.9	One 200 mg + one 50 mg		
20-24.9	One 200 mg + one 100 mg		

ANNEX B: ARV DOSAGES cont/d

lamivudine for PMTCT prophylaxis in newborns
Give 2 mg/kg/dose twice daily for 1 week

Weight unknown	AM	PM
1 – 1.9	0.4	0.4
2 – 2.9	0.8	0.8
3 – 3.9	1.2	1.2
4 – 4.9	1.6	1.6

nevirapine for PMTCT prophylaxis in newborns
2 mg/kg within 72 hours of birth - once only

Unknown weight	
1 – 1.9	0.2
2 – 2.9	0.4
3 – 3.9	0.6
4 – 4.9	0.8

Zidovudine 10mg/ml syrup for PMTCT prophylaxis in newborns. Give 4 mg/kg/ twice daily

Weight in kg	1-1.9	2-2.9	3-3.9	4-4.9
AM	0.4 ml	0.8 ml	1.2 ml	1.6 ml
PM	0.4 ml	0.8 ml	1.2 ml	1.6 ml

COMBINATION ARV

Weight	3-3.9	4-4.5	6-9.9	10-13.9	14-19.9	20-24.9
AZT/3TC 60/30 mg	1	1	1.5	2	2.5	3
AZT/3TC/NVP 60/30/50/mg	1	1	1.5	2	2.5	3
d4T/3TC 6/30 mg	1	1	1.5	2	2.5	3
d4T/3TC/NVP 6/30/50 mg	1	1	1.5	2	2.5	3
ABC/3TC 60/30	1	1	1.5	2	2.5	3
ABC/3TC/NVP 60/30/50 mg	1	1	1.5	2	2.5	3
ABC/AZT/3TC 60/60/30	1	1	1.5	2	2.5	3

Annex C : ARV side effects*

	Very common side-effects: warn patients and suggest ways patients can manage; also be prepared to manage when patients seek care	Potentially serious side effects: warn patients and tell them to seek care	Side effects occurring later during treatment: discuss with patients
d4T stavudine	Nausea Diarrhoea	Seek care urgently: Severe abdominal pain Fatigue AND shortness of breath Seek advice soon: Tingling, numb or painful feet or legs or hands	Changes in fat distribution: Arms, legs, buttocks, cheeks become THIN Breasts, belly, back of neck become FAT
3TC lamivudine	Nausea Diarrhoea		
NVP nevirapine	Nausea Diarrhoea	Seek care urgently: Yellow eyes Severe Skin rash Fatigue AND shortness of breath Fever	
ZDV zidovudine (also known as AZT)	Nausea Diarrhoea Headache Fatigue Muscle pain	Seek care urgently: Pallor (anaemia)	
EFV efavirenz	Nausea Diarrhoea Strange dreams Difficulty sleeping Memory problems Headache Dizziness	Seek care urgently: Yellow eyes Psychosis or confusion Severe Skin rash	

* for more guidance, refer to IMAI chronic care guideline module

ANNEX D: DRUG DOSAGES FOR OPPORTUNISTIC INFECTIONS

Fluconazole dosage

Weight of child	50mg/5ml oral suspension	50 mg capsule
3-<6kg	-	-
6-<10kg	-	-
10-<15kg	5 ml once a day	1
15-<20kg	7.5 ml once a day	1-2
20-<29kg	12.5 ml once a day	2-3

Nystatin oral suspension 100,000 units per ml given 1-2 ml four times daily for all age groups

Recommended dosages for acyclovir:

Age of child	Dose, frequency and duration
<2 years	200mg 8 hourly for 5 days
>2 years	400mg 8 hourly for 5 days

Recommended dosages for ketoconazole:

Age of child	Weight	Dose, frequency and duration
2 months up to 12 months	3-<6kg	20 mg once daily
	6-<10kg	40 mg once daily
12 months up to 5 years	10-19 kg	60 mg once daily

Recommended dosages for griseofulvin 10 mg per Kg per day

Recommended dosages for cloxacillin / flucloxacillin:

Weight of child	Form	Dose, every 6 hours for 5 days
3-<6kg	250mg capsule	1/2 tablet
6-<10kg		1
10-<15kg		1
15-<20kg		2

Integrated Management of Childhood Illness Chart booklet for high HIV settings

Process of updating the IMCI chart booklet for high HIV settings

The generic IMCI chart booklet was developed and published in 1995 based on evidence existing at that time (*Reference: Integrated management of Childhood Illness Adaptation Guide: C. Technical basis for adapting clinical guidelines, 1998*). New evidence on the management of acute respiratory infections, diarrhoeal diseases, malaria, ear infections and infant feeding, published between 1995 and 2004, was summarized in the document "*Technical updates of the guidelines on IMCI : evidence and recommendations for further adaptations, 2005*".

Evidence reviews supported the formulation of recommendations in each of these areas (see document and the references). Reviews were usually followed by technical consultations where the recommendations and their technical bases were discussed and consensus reached. Similarly, a review and several expert meetings were held to update the young infant section of IMCI to include "care of the newborn in the first week of life". More recently, findings of a multi-centre study (Lancet, 2008) led to the development of simplified recommendations for the assessment of severe infections in the newborn.

The chart booklet for high HIV settings is different because it includes sections on paediatric HIV care. The changes made in this edition are based on the new recommendations for paediatric ART following a technical consultation " Report of the WHO Technical Reference Group. Paediatric HIV/ART Care Guideline Group Meeting WHO Headquarters, Geneva, Switzerland,10-11 April 2008; as well as several meetings of the WHO paediatric ART Working Group.

Who was involved and their declaration of interests

The following experts were involved in the development of the updated newborn recommendations: Z. Bhutta, A. Blaise, W. Carlo, R. Cerezo, M.Omar, P. Mazmanyan, MK Bhan, H.Taylor, G.Darmstadt, V. Paul, A. Rimoin, L.Wright and WHO staff from Regional and Headquarter offices. Dr. Gul Rehman and a team of CAH staff members drafted the updated chart booklet based on the above. Dr Antonio Pio did the technical editing of the draft IMCI chart booklet, in addition to participating in its peer-review. Other persons who reviewed the draft chart booklet and provided comments include A. Deorari, T. Desta,. A.Kassie, D.P. Hoa, H.Kumar, V. Paul and S. Ramzi.. Their contributions are acknowledged.

The experts involved in making new paediatric ART recommendations were E. Abrams, NE Ata Alla, G. Anabwani, S. Bhakeecheep, S.Benchekroun, M.F.Bwakura-Dangarembizi.E. Capparelli R. DeLhomme, D. Clarke, M. Cotton, F. Dabis, B. Eley, S. Essajee, R. Ferris, L.Frigati, C. Giaquinto, D. Gibb, T.A. Jacobs, D.N.El Hoda, R. Lodha, P.Humblet, A.Z.Kabore, A.Kekitiinwa, P.N. Kazembe, I.Kalyesubula, C. Luo, V.Leroy, T.Meyers, M. Mirochnick, L.Mofenson, H.Moultrie, P.Msellati, J.S. Mukherjee, R.Nduaati, T.Nunn, A.Mutiti, N.Z. Nyazema, A.Ojoo, R.Pierre, J.Pinto, .A.Prendergast, E.Rivadeneira, M. Schaefer, P.Vaz, U. Vibol, Catherine M. Wilfert, P.Weidle, Agnes Mahomva, Zhao Yan, Martina Penazzato & Sally Girvin as well as WHO regional and HQ staff. Their contributions are acknowledged.

None of the above experts declared any conflict of interest.

The Department plans to review the need for an update of this chart booklet by 2011.

WHO Library Cataloguing-in-Publication Data

Integrated Management of Childhood Illness Complementary Course on HIV/AIDS.

8 v.

Contents: Facilitator guide -- Introduction -- Module 1. Recap and technical updates on IMCI -- Module 2. Assess, classify and manage the child for HIV/AIDS -- Module 3. Counsel the HIV positive mother -- Module 4. Follow-up and chronic care of HIV exposed and infected children -- Chart booklet -- Photo booklet.

1. HIV infections - diagnosis. 2. HIV infections - therapy. 3. Acquired immunodeficiency syndrome - diagnosis. 4. Acquired immunodeficiency syndrome - therapy. 5. Infant. 6. Child. 7. Disease management. 8. Teaching materials. I. World Health Organization. II. Title: IMCI complementary course on HIV/AIDS. III. Title: Complementary course on HIV/AIDS.

ISBN 92 4 159437 3   (NLM classification: WC 503.2)
ISBN 978 92 4 159437 0

© **World Health Organization 2008**

All rights reserved. Publications of the World Health Organization can be obtained from WHO Press, World Health Organization, 20 Avenue Appia, 1211 Geneva 27, Switzerland (tel.: +41 22 791 3264; fax: +41 22 791 4857; e-mail: bookorders@who.int). Requests for permission to reproduce or translate WHO publications – whether for sale or for non-commercial distribution – should be addressed to WHO Press, at the above address (fax: +41 22 791 4806; e-mail: permissions@who.int).

The designations employed and the presentation of the material in this publication do not imply the expression of any opinion whatsoever on the part of the World Health Organization concerning the legal status of any country, territory, city or area or of its authorities, or concerning the delimitation of its frontiers or boundaries. Dotted lines on maps represent approximate border lines for which there may not yet be full agreement.

The mention of specific companies or of certain manufacturers' products does not imply that they are endorsed or recommended by the World Health Organization in preference to others of a similar nature that are not mentioned. Errors and omissions excepted, the names of proprietary products are distinguished by initial capital letters.

All reasonable precautions have been taken by the World Health Organization to verify the information contained in this publication. However, the published material is being distributed without warranty of any kind, either expressed or implied. The responsibility for the interpretation and use of the material lies with the reader. In no event shall the World Health Organization be liable for damages arising from its use.

Printed by the WHO Document Production Services, Geneva, Switzerland.

For further information please contact:
Department of Child and Adolescent Health and Development (CAH)
World Health Organization
20 Avenue Appia
1211 Geneva 27
Switzerland
Tel: +41-22 791 3281   email: cah@who.int
Fax: +41-22 791 4853   http://www.who.int/child-adolescent-health

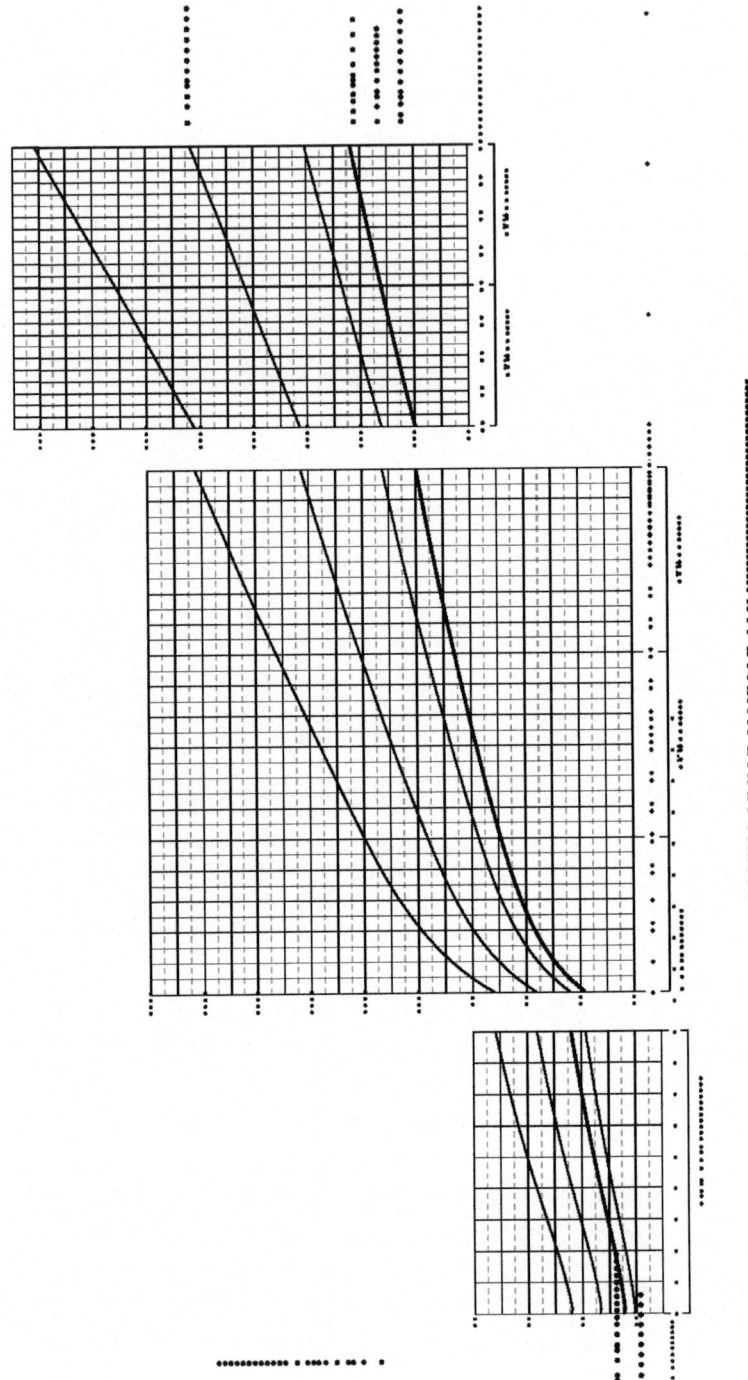

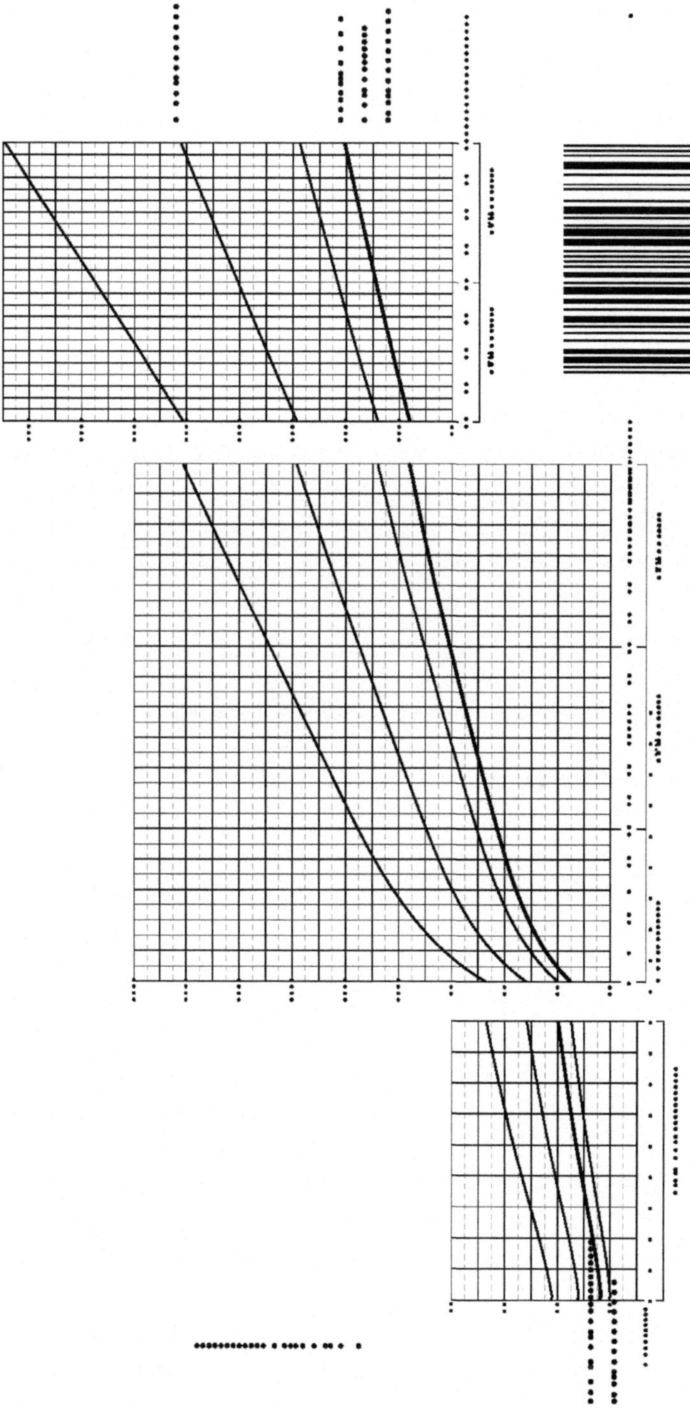

Appendix A

Appendix B
WHO Growth Charts Head Circumference Boys

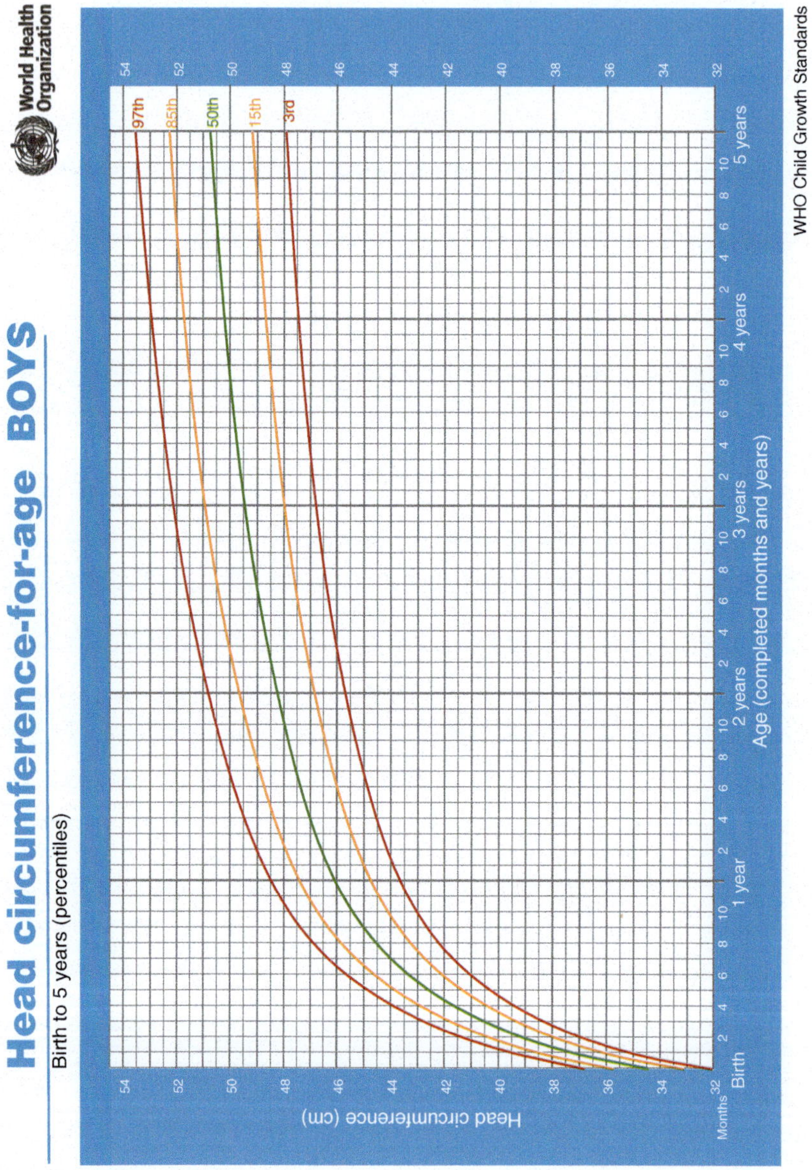
Head circumference-for-age BOYS
Birth to 5 years (percentiles)
World Health Organization
Head circumference (cm)
Months
Birth
1 year
2 years
3 years
4 years
5 years
Age (completed months and years)
97th
85th
50th
15th
3rd
32
34
36
38
40
42
44
46
48
50
52
54
2
4
6
8
10
WHO Child Growth Standards

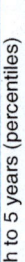

Appendix C
WHO Growth Charts Head Circumference for Girls

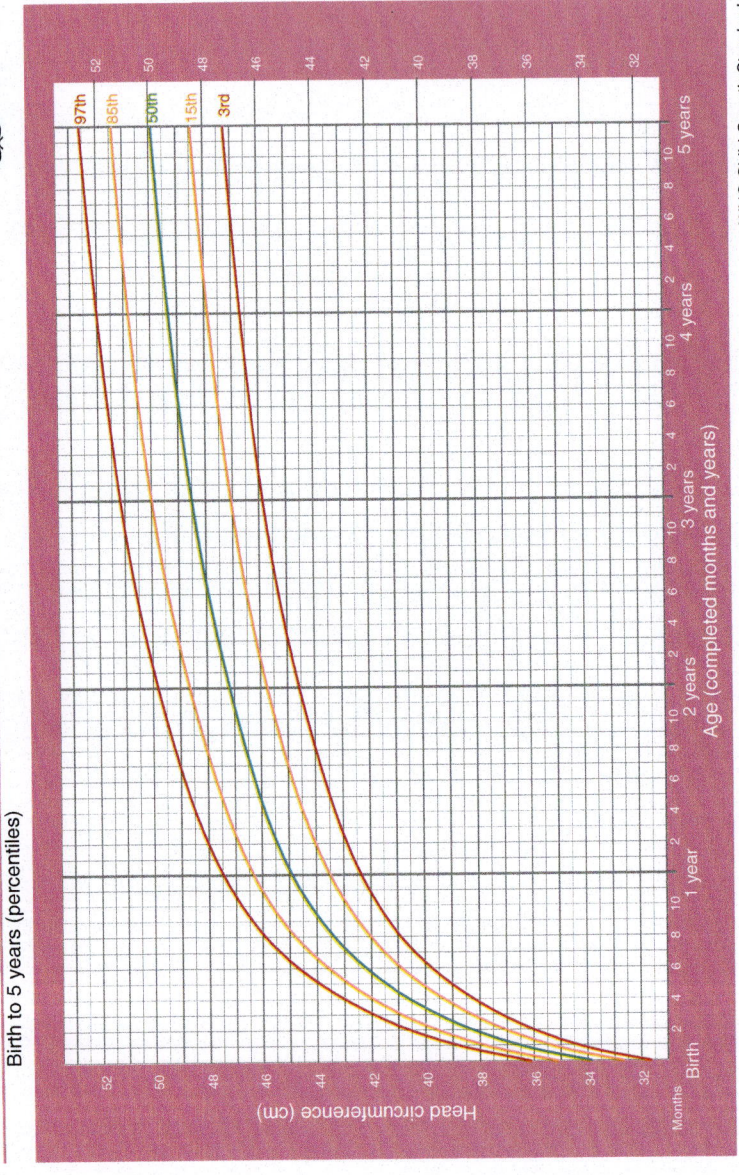

Appendix D
WHO Growth Charts Weight for Age Boys 0–5

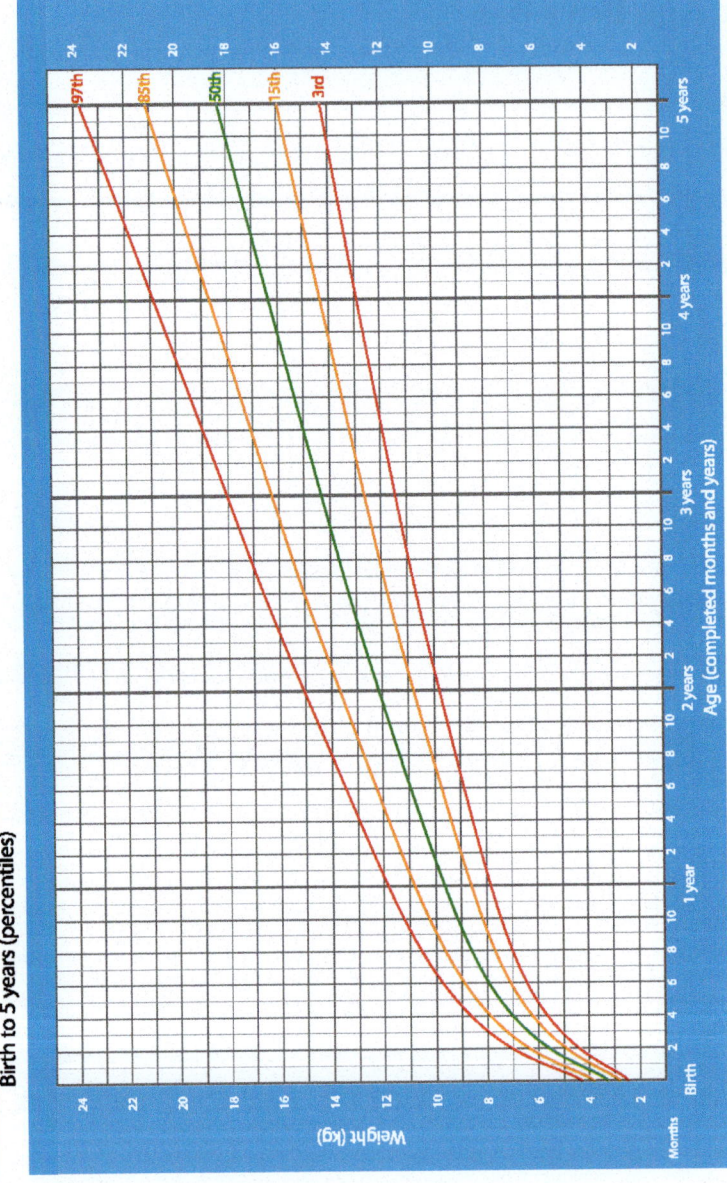

Appendix E
WHO Growth Charts Weight for Age Girls 0–5

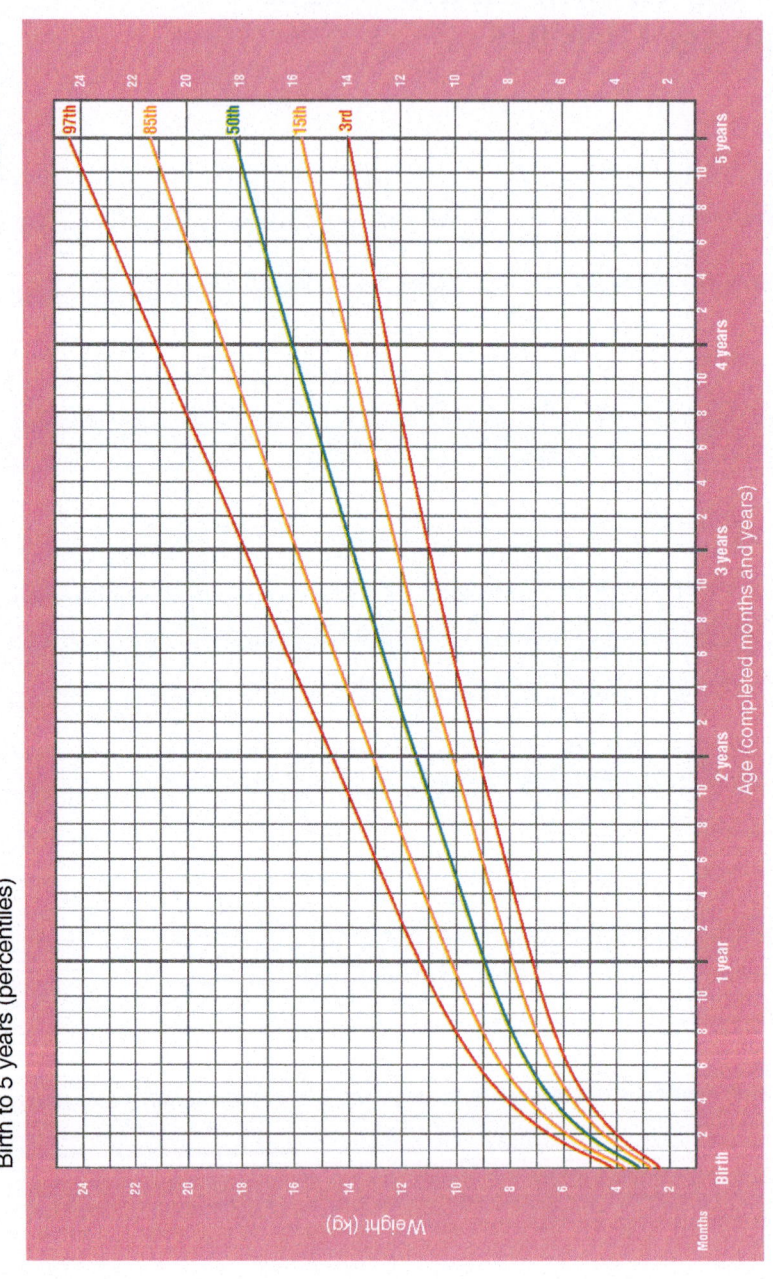

Appendix F
WHO Growth Charts Weight for Height Boys 2–5

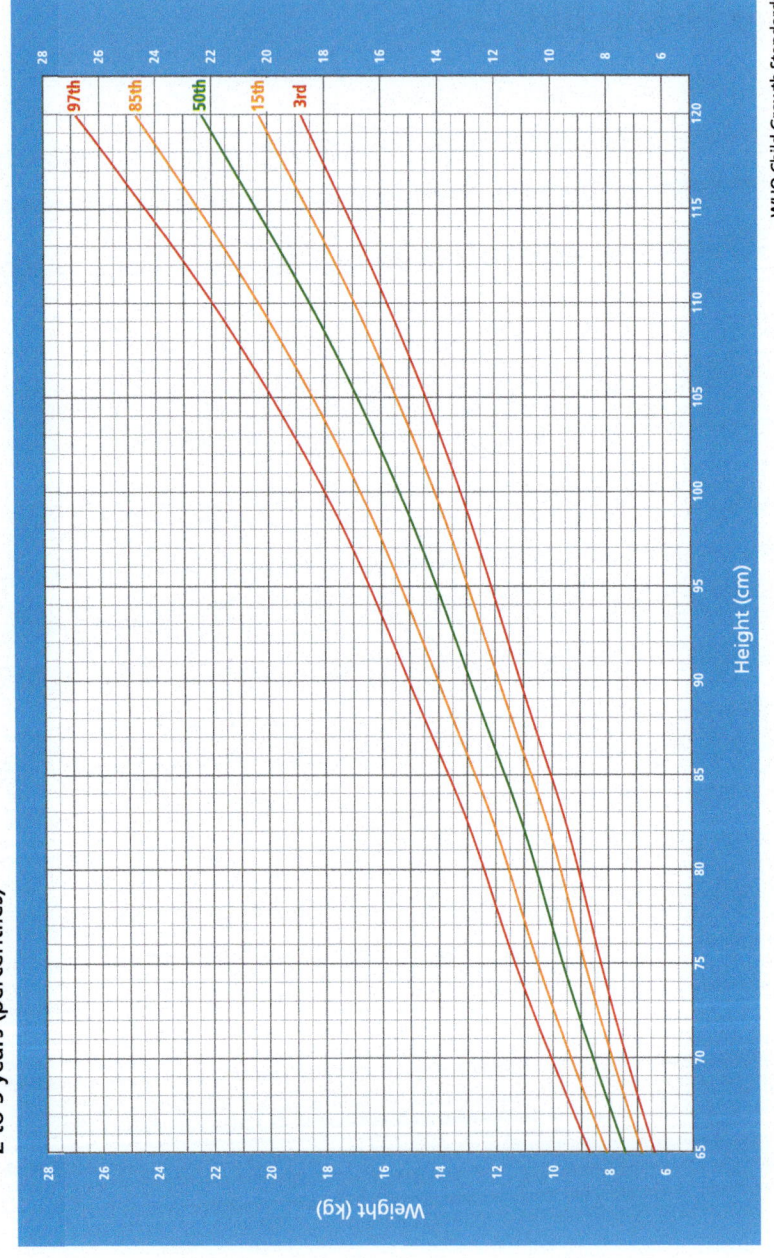

Appendix G
WHO Growth Charts Weight for Height Girls 0–5

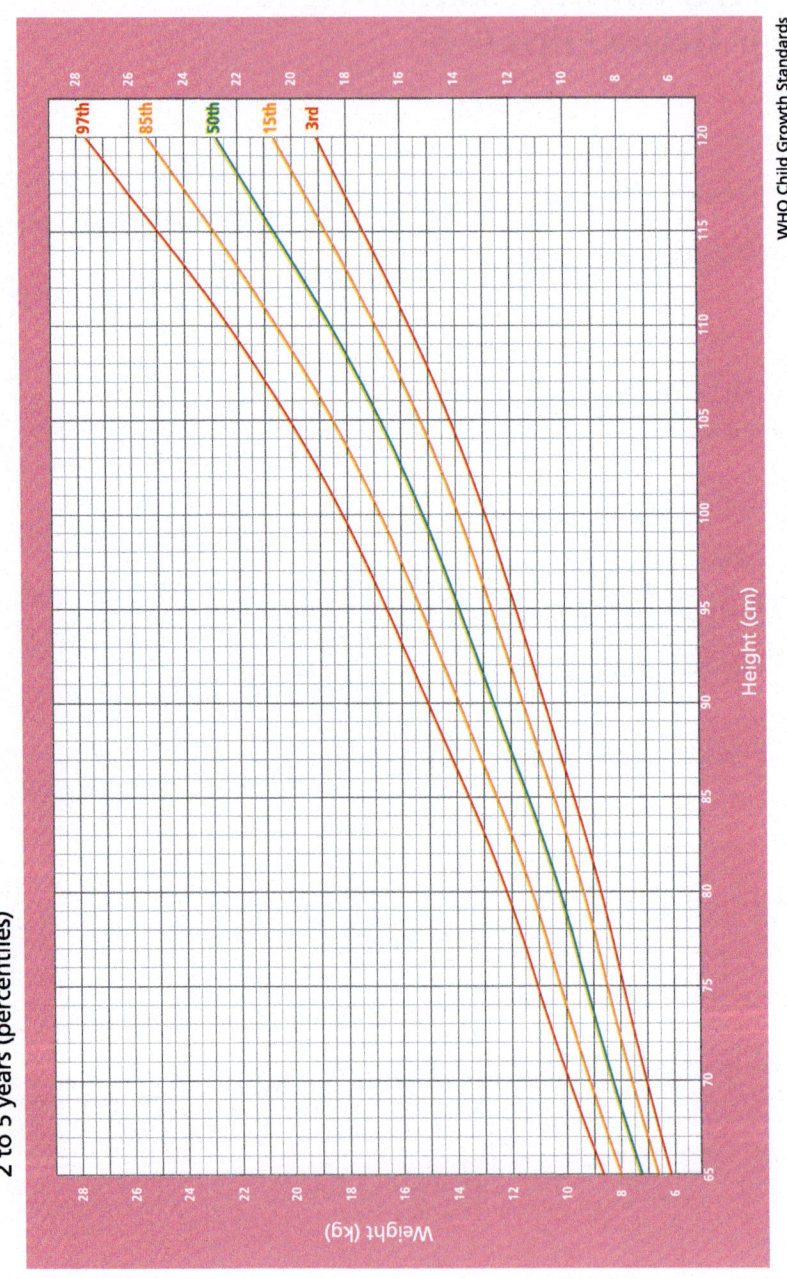

Appendix H
WHO Growth Charts Weight for Length Boys 0–2

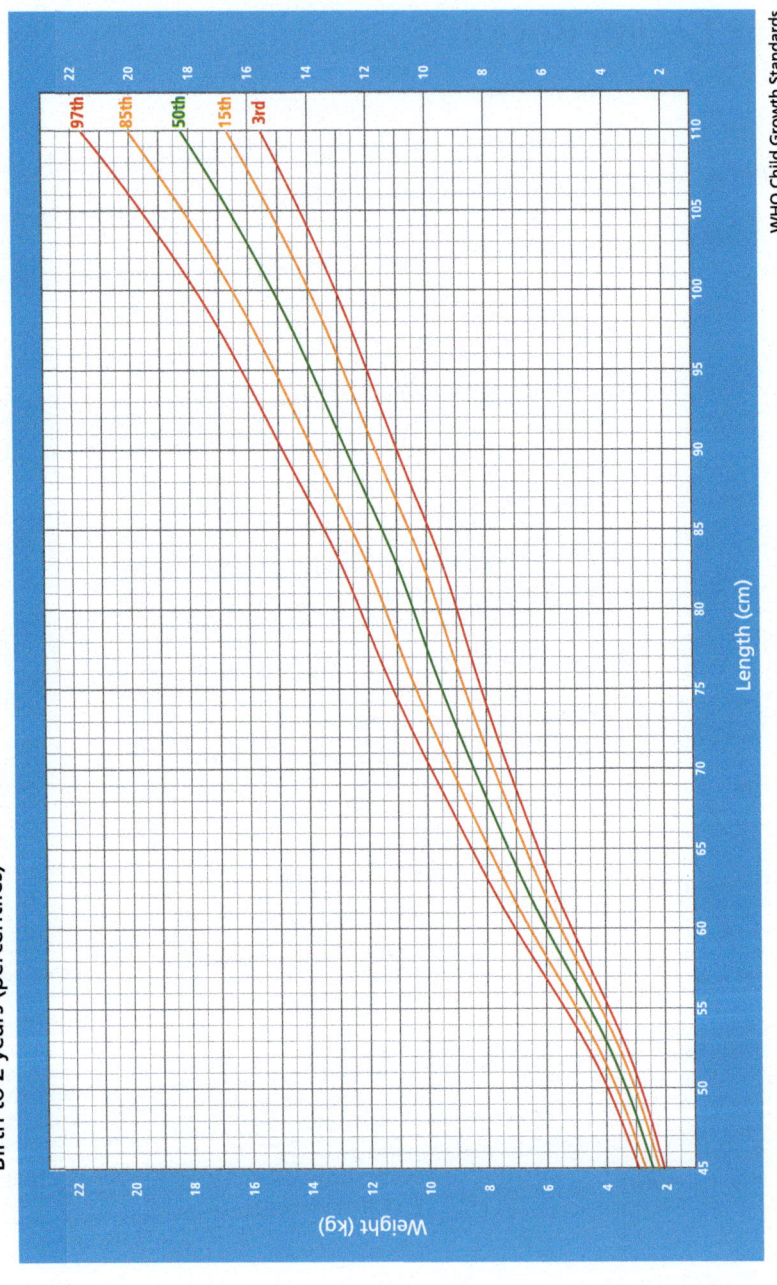

Appendix I
WHO Growth Charts Weight for Length Girls 0–2

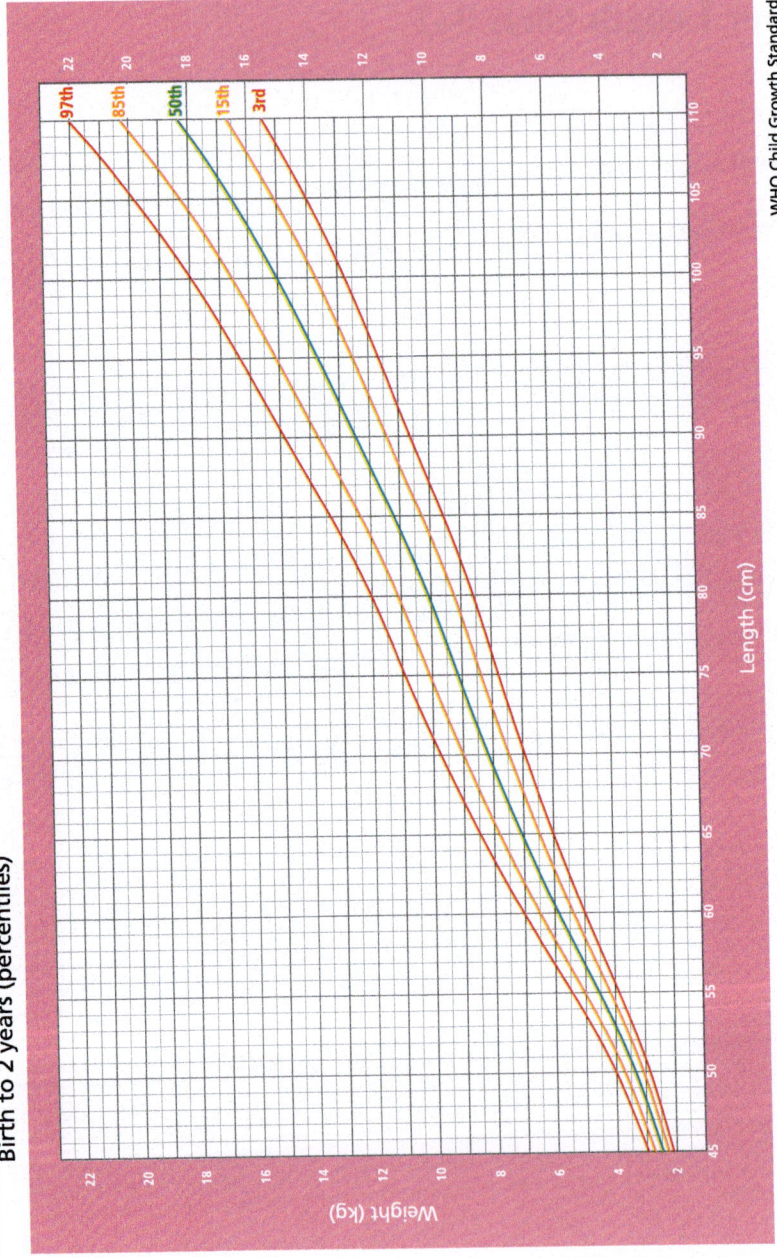

Appendix J
Essential Medications for RLS

Essential Medications for Resource-Limited Settings

Drug Class/Use	Drug Name
Anesthetics-inhalational medicines	Halothane, Isoflurane, Nitrous oxide, Oxygen
Anesthetics-injectable medications	Ketamine, Propofol
Anesthetics (local)	Bupivacaine, Lidocaine, Lidocaine+Epinephrine
Perioperative medication and sedation for short-term procedures	Atropine, Midazolam, Morphine
Muscle relaxants and cholinesterase inhibitors	Neostigmine, Suxamethonium, Vecuronium
Migraine	Ibuprofen, Paracetamol
Migraine prophylaxis	Propanolol
Medicines used in palliative care	Amitriptyline, Cyclizine, Dexamethasone, Diazepam, Docusate Sodium, Fluoxetine, Hyoscine Hydrobromide, Ibuprofen, Lactulose, Midazolam, Morphine, Ondansetron, Senna
Anti-inflammatory medicines (non-opioids and non-steroidal)	Ibuprofen, Paracetamol
Analgesic (opioid)	Morphine
Anti-allergics and medicines used in anaphylaxis	Chlorphenamine, Dexamethasone, Epinephrine, Prednisone, Hydrocortisone
Antidote (non-specific) for poisoning	Activated charcoal
Antidotes (specific) for poisoning	Acetylcysteine, Atropine, Calcium Gluconate, Naloxone
Anticonvulsants	Carbamazepine, Diazepam, Lorazepam, Phenobarbital, Phenytoin, Valproic Acid
Anti-helminthics	Albendazole, Mebendazole, Praziquantal, Pyrantel
Anti-filarials	Albendazole, Diethylcarbamazine, Ivermectin
Anti-schistosomals and other anti-trematode medicines	Praziquantal, Triclabendazole

(continued)

(continued)

Drug Class/Use	Drug Name
Anti-bacterials	Amoxicillin, Amoxicillin + Clavulanic Acid, Ampicillin, Benzathine Benzylpenicillin, Benzylpenicillin, Cefalexin, Cefazolin, Ceftriaxone, Cloxacillin, Phenoxymethylpenicillin, Procaine Benzylpenicillin, Azithromycin, Chloramphenicol, Ciprofloxacin, Doxycycline, Erythromycin, Gentamicin, Metronidazole, Nitrofurantoin, Trimethoprim + Sulfamethoxazole
Anti-leprosy medicines	Clofazimine, Dapsone, Rifampicin
Anti-tuberculosis medicines	Ethambutol, Isoniazid, Rifampin, Pyrazinamide, Streptomycin
Anti-fungal medicines	Fluconazole, Griseofulvin, Nystatin
Anti-herpes medicines	Acyclovir
Anti-retroviral medications-Nucleoside/ Nucleotide reverse transcriptase inhibitors	Abacavir, Didanosine, Emtricitabine, Lamivudine, Stavudine, Zidovudine
Anti-retroviral medications-Non-nucleoside reverse transcriptase inhibitors	Efavirenz, Nevirapine
Anti-retroviral medications-Protease inhibitors	Atazanavir, Lopinavir + Ritonavir, Saquinavir
Anti-retroviral medications-Fixed-dose combinations	Lamivudine + Nevirapine + Stavudine Lamivudine + Nevirapine + Zidovudine Lamivudine + Zidovudine
Anti-virals	Oseltamivir, Ribavirin
Anti-amoebic and anti-giardiasis medicines	Diloxanide, Metronidazole
Anti-leishmaniasis medicines	Amphotericin B, Miltefosine, Paromomycin,
Anti-malarial medicines	Amodiaquine, Artemether (+/− Lumefantrine, Artesunate (+/− Amodiaquine), Chloroquine, Doxycycline, Mefloquin, Primaquine, Quinine, Sulfadoxine + Pyrimethamine
Anti-malarial prophylaxis	Chloroquine, Doxycycline, Mefloquine, Proguanil
Anti-pneumocystosis and anti-toxoplasmosis medicines	Pyrimethamine, Sulfadiazine, Sulfamethoxazole + Trimethoprim
African trypanosomiasis	Pentamidine, Suramin Sodium, Eflornithine
American trypanosomiasis	Benznidazole, Nifurtimox
Anti-anemia medicines	Ferrous salt, Folic Acid, Hydroxocobalamin, Phytomenadione
Anti-hypertensive medications	Enalapril, Digoxin, Furosemide
Anti-fungal creams	Miconazole, Terbinafine
Anti-infective creams	Mupirocin, Potassium Permanganate, Silver Sulfadiazine
Anti-inflammatory/antipruritic creams	Betamethasone, Calamine, Hydrocortisone
Creams affecting skin differentiation and proliferation	Benzoyl Peroxide, Coal tar, Podophyllum, Salicylic Acid, Urea
Scabicides and pediculicides	Benzyl Benzoate, Permethrin
Antiulcer medications	Omeprazole, Ranitidine
Antiemetic medications	Dexamethasone, Metaclopramide, Ondansetron
Medicines used in diarrhea	Oral rehydration salts, Zinc Sulfate

(continued)

Drug Class/Use	Drug Name
Medications used for diabetes	Glucagon, Insulin
Adrenal hormones	Fludrocortisone, Hydrocortisone
Thyroid hormones	Levothyroxine
Sera and immunoglobulin	Antitetanus Immunoglobulin (human), Antivenom Immunoglobulin, Diphtheria Antitoxin, Rabies Immunoglobulin
Ophthalmic medications—anti-infective	Acyclovir, Gentamicin, Tetracycline
Ophthalmic medications—anti-inflammatory	Prednisolone
Ophthalmic medications—local anesthetic	Tetracaine
Ophthalmic medications—midriatics	Atropine
Ear, nose and throat medications	Acetic acid, Budesonide (nasal), Ciprofloxacin, Xylometazoline (nasal)
Respiratory—antiasthma medications	Budesonide, Epinephrine, Salbutamol
Neonatal care	Caffeine Citrate
Vitamins and minerals	Ascorbic Acid, Cholecalciferol, Iodine, Pyridoxine, Retinol, Riboflavin, Sodium Fluoride, Thiamine

Adapted from the WHO Model List of Essential Medications for Children, 3rd List, March 2011
Source: http://www.who.int/medicines/publications/essentialmedicines/en/index.html

Appendix K
GAPS Monograph

Several tools have been designed to support implementing the American Medical Association's (AMA) Guidelines for Adolescent Preventive Services (GAPS) program in your clinical setting. The six forms include the Younger Adolescent Questionnaire in English and Spanish, Middle-Older Adolescent Questionnaire in English and Spanish, and the Parent/Guardian Questionnaire in English and Spanish. The GAPS Recommendations Monograph is also included for your information and reference. The questionnaires and monograph are considered master copies that you can reproduce but not alter, modify, or revise without the expressed written consent of the Child and Adolescent Health Program at the American Medical Association.

American Medical Association
Physicians dedicated to the health of America

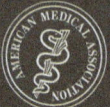

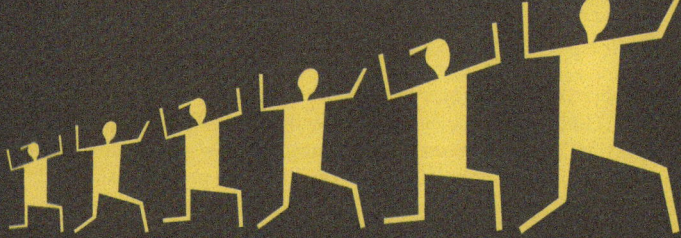

Guidelines for Adolescent Preventive Services (GAPS)

Recommendations Monograph

Department of Adolescent Health
American Medical Association
515 North State Street
Chicago, Illinois 60610

No part of this publication may be reproduced, stored in a retrieval system, or transmitted, in any form or by any means—electronic, mechanical, photocopying, recording, or otherwise—without the prior written permission of the American Medical Association.

Additional copies maybe ordered by calling the
American Medical Association at 800-621-8335.
Ask for product no. OP020997

©1997 American Medical Association
Printed in the USA
All Rights Reserved

Visit the AMA web site at http://www.ama-assn.org

ISBN: 0-89970-920-X
AA61:96-9810:7M:10/96

Acknowledgments

The authors gratefully acknowledge the guidance and critical contributions of the GAPS Executive Committee. Members of the Executive Committee are Beth Alexander, MD, David Kaplan, MD, Jonathan D. Klein, MD, MPH, Susan G. Millstein, PhD, and members of the AMA staff.

The members of the Scientific Advisory Board deserve special thanks for their thoughtful reviews and contributions throughout the project. Members of the board include Alfred O. Berg, MD, MPH, American Academy of Family Physicians; Robert Wm. Blum, MD, PhD, University of Minnesota; Lawrence D'Angelo, MD, American College of Physicians; A. Robert Davies, MD, Nationwide Insurance; E. Harvey Estes, Jr, MD, AMA Council on Scientific Affairs; Brian R. Flay, D. Phil., Prevention Research Center, University of Illinois-Chicago; Phillip J. Goldstein, MD, American College of Obstetricians and Gynecologists; Michael D. Klitzner, PhD, Pacific Institute; Jonathan D. Klein, MD, MPH, University of Rochester Medical Center; James F. Leckman, MD, American Psychiatric Association; Andrea Marks, MD, Society for Adolescent Medicine; Susan G. Millstein, PhD, University of California-San Francisco; Dan R.Offord, MD, Chedoke-McMaster Hospital, Hamilton, Ontario, Canada; Guy S. Parcel, PhD, Center for Health Promotion Research and Development, University of Texas, Houston Health Sciences Center; Anne C. Petersen, PhD, University of Minnesota; Joe M. Sanders, Jr, MD, American Academy of Pediatrics; John E. Schowalter, MD, American Academy of Child and Adolescent Psychiatry; Howard Schubiner, MD, Wayne State University; and Richard M. Steinhilber, MD, AMA Council on Scientific Affairs.

Many people, some of whom were anonymous, reviewed GAPS and provided helpful advice and suggestions. Special thanks go to Lloyd Kolbe, PhD, Mary E. Vernon, MD, MPH, and the other staff of the Division of Adolescent and School Health at the Centers for Disease Control; Gary Strokosch, MD, and Katherine Joyce, MD, of Rush-Presbyterian-St. Luke's Medical Center; Angela Mickalaide, PhD, of the National Safe Kids Campaign; Elizabeth R. McAnarney, MD and the adolescent panel of the Maternal and Child Health Bureau Bright Futures Project; and the organizational representatives of the American Medical Association National Coalition on Adolescent Health. Thanks also to John H. Himes, PhD, and Mary T. Story, PhD, RD, for convening a working group to assist in the development of the screening recommendations for weight and stature.

AMA staff assistance was provided by Arthur Elster, MD, Janet Gans Epner, PhD, Missy Fleming, PhD, Patricia B. Levenberg, PhD, and Patricia Watson, MBA. Additional support was provided by Todd Bake, Linda B. Bresolin, PhD, John J. Henning, PhD, Thomas P. Houston, MD, and Robert Rinaldi, PhD. Mary Kizer provided secretarial support.

Guidelines for Adolescent Preventive Services

Introduction

Changes in adolescent morbidity and mortality during the past several decades have created a health crisis for today's youth. Unintended pregnancy, STDs including HIV, alcohol and drug abuse, and eating disorders are just some of the health problems faced by an increasing number of adolescents from all sectors of society. This health crisis requires a fundamental change in the emphasis of adolescent services – a change whereby a greater number of services are directed at the primary and secondary prevention of the major health threats facing today's youth. School and community organizations have responded to the need for change by increasing health education programming. Primary care physicians and other health providers must respond by making preventive services a greater component of their clinical practice. *Guidelines for Adolescent Preventive Services (GAPS)* can direct providers in how to deliver these services.

GAPS is a comprehensive set of recommendations that provides a framework for the organization and content of preventive health services.

GAPS recommendations are organized into four types of services that address 14 separate topics or health conditions.

- Three recommendations pertain to the delivery of health care services.

- Seven recommendations pertain to the use of health guidance to promote the health and well-being of adolescents and their parents or guardians.

- Thirteen recommendations describe the need to screen for specific conditions that are relatively common to adolescents and that cause significant suffering either during adolescence or later in life.

- One recommendation pertains to the use of immunizations for the primary prevention of selected infectious diseases.

The topics or health conditions addressed by GAPS are:

- promoting parents' ability to respond to the health needs of their adolescents;
- promoting adjustment to puberty and adolescence;
- promoting safety and injury prevention;
- promoting physical fitness;
- promoting healthy dietary habits and preventing eating disorders and obesity;
- promoting healthy psychosexual adjustment and preventing the negative health consequences of sexual behaviors;
- preventing hypertension;
- preventing hyperlipidemia;
- preventing the use of tobacco products;
- preventing the use and abuse of alcohol and other drugs;
- preventing severe or recurrent depression and suicide;
- preventing physical, sexual, and emotional abuse;
- preventing learning problems;
- preventing infectious diseases.

A complete description of how GAPS recommendations were developed, the clinical approach to a comprehensive preventive services visit, and the scientific justification for each recommendation are contained in *Guidelines for Adolescent Preventive Services*, by Arthur B. Elster, MD and Naomi J. Kuznets, PhD, (1994) Williams and Wilkins: Baltimore.

GAPS recommendations are designed to be delivered ideally as a preventive services package during a series of annual health visits between the ages of 11 and 21. The recommended frequency of specific GAPS preventive services are presented in the table on the following page. Annual visits offer the opportunity to reinforce health promotion messages for both adolescents and their parents, identify adolescents who have initiated health risk behaviors or who are at early stages of physical or emotional disorders, provide immunizations, and develop relationships with the adolescents that will foster an open disclosure of future health information.

GAPS is a comprehensive set of recommendations developed to provide a framework for the organization and content of clinical preventive health services.

Recommendations for delivery of health services

The periodicity and manner in which services are delivered to adolescents can be important determinants of the effectiveness of preventive services. The rapid behavioral changes that occur during adolescence require frequent visits to screen for health risk behaviors and to provide health guidance. To ensure that providers obtain accurate information and deliver health guidance appropriate for each adolescent, GAPS recommends that services be tailored to the individual and that information shared by the adolescent during the medical visit remain confidential.

Recommendation 1: From ages 11 to 21, all adolescents should have an annual preventive services visit.

- These visits should address both the biomedical and psychosocial aspects of health, and should focus on preventive services.

Appendix K

Preventive health services by age and procedure

Adolescents and young adults have a unique set of health care needs. The recommendations for *Guidelines for Adolescent Preventive Services (GAPS)* emphasize annual clinical preventive services visits that address both the developmental and psychosocial aspects of health, in addition to traditional biomedical conditions. These recommendations were developed by the American Medical Association with contributions from a Scientific Advisory Panel, comprised of national experts, as well as representatives of primary care medical organizations and the health insurance industry. The body of scientific evidence indicated that the periodicity and content of preventive services can be important in promoting the health and well-being of adolescents.

Age of adolescent

Procedure	Early				Middle			Late			
	11	12	13	14	15	16	17	18	19	20	21
Health guidance											
Parenting*	————●————				————●————						
Development	■	■	■	■	■	■	■	■	■	■	■
Diet & physical activity	■	■	■	■	■	■	■	■	■	■	■
Healthy lifestyles**	■	■	■	■	■	■	■	■	■	■	■
Injury prevention	■	■	■	■	■	■	■	■	■	■	■
Screening history											
Eating disorders	■	■	■	■	■	■	■	■	■	■	■
Sexual activity***	■	■	■	■	■	■	■	■	■	■	■
Alcohol & other drug use	■	■	■	■	■	■	■	■	■	■	■
Tobacco use	■	■	■	■	■	■	■	■	■	■	■
Abuse	■	■	■	■	■	■	■	■	■	■	■
School performance	■	■	■	■	■	■	■	■	■	■	■
Depression	■	■	■	■	■	■	■	■	■	■	■
Risk for suicide	■	■	■	■	■	■	■	■	■	■	■
Physical assessment											
Blood pressure	■	■	■	■	■	■	■	■	■	■	■
BMI	■	■	■	■	■	■	■	■	■	■	■
Comprehensive exam	————●————				————●————			————●————			
Tests											
Cholesterol	——1——				——1——			——1——			
TB	——2——				——2——			——2——			
GC, Chlamydia, Syphilis & HPV	——3——				——3——			——3——			
HIV	——4——				——4——			——4——			
Pap smear	——5——				——5——			——5——			
Immunizations											
MMR	■										
Td	■				○						
Hep B	■				——6——			——6——			
Hep A	——7——				——7——			——7——			
Varicella	——8——				——8——			——8——			

1. Screening test performed once if family history is positive for early cardiovascular disease or hyperlipidemia.
2. Screen if positive for exposure to active TB or lives/works in high-risk situation, eg, homeless shelter, health care facility.
3. Screen at least annually if sexually active.
4. Screen if high-risk for infection.
5. Screen annually if sexually active or if 18 years or older.
6. Vaccinate if high risk for hepatitis B infection.
7. Vaccinate if at risk for hepatitis A infection.
8. Vaccinate if no reliable history of chicken pox.

* A parent health guidance visit is recommended during early and middle adolescence.
** Includes counseling regarding sexual behavior and avoidance of tobacco, alcohol, and other drug use.
*** Includes history of unintended pregnancy and STD.
○ Do not give if administered in last five years.

- Adolescents should have a complete physical examination during three of these preventive services visits. One should be performed during early adolescence (age 11-14), one during middle adolescence (age 15-17), and one during late adolescence (age 18-21), unless more frequent examinations are warranted by clinical signs or symptoms.

Recommendation 2: Preventive services should be age and developmentally appropriate, and should be sensitive to individual and sociocultural differences.

Recommendation 3: Physicians should establish office policies regarding confidential care for adolescents and how parents will be involved in that care. These policies should be made clear to adolescents and their parents.

Recommendations for health guidance

Adolescence is a time of experimentation and risk taking. Developmentally, adolescents are at a crossroads of health. Emerging cognitive abilities and social experiences lead adolescents to question adult values and experiment with health risk behaviors. Some behaviors threaten current health, while other behaviors may have long-term health consequences. The changes in cognitive abilities, however, also offer an opportunity to develop attitudes and lifestyles that enhance health and well-being. GAPS recommends that adolescents receive health guidance annually to help them cope with developmental challenges, develop and maintain healthy lifestyles, improve diet and fitness, and prevent injury. In addition, GAPS recommends health guidance be given to parents and guardians of adolescents to help them respond appropriately to the health needs of their adolescent.

Recommendation 4: Parents or other adult caregivers should receive health guidance at least once during their child's early adolescence, once during middle adolescence and, preferably, once during late adolescence.

This includes providing information about:

- normative adolescent development, including information about physical, sexual, and emotional development;
- signs and symptoms of disease and emotional distress;
- parenting behaviors that promote healthy adolescent adjustment;
- why parents should discuss health-related behaviors with their adolescents, plan family activities, and act as role models for health-related behaviors;
- methods for helping their adolescent avoid potentially harmful behaviors, such as:
  - monitoring and managing the adolescent's use of motor vehicles, especially for new drivers;
  - avoiding having weapons in the home. Parents who have weapons in the home should be advised to make them inaccessible to adolescents. If adolescents have weapons, parents and other adult caregivers should ensure that adolescents follow weapon safety procedures;
  - removing weapons and potentially lethal medications from the homes of adolescents who have suicidal intent;
  - monitoring their adolescent's social and recreational activities for the use of tobacco, alcohol and other drugs, and sexual behavior.

Recommendation 5: All adolescents should receive health guidance annually to promote a better understanding of their physical growth, psychosocial and psychosexual development, and the importance of becoming actively involved in decisions regarding their health care.

Recommendation 6: All adolescents should receive health guidance annually to promote the reduction of injuries.

Health guidance for injury prevention includes the following:

- counseling to avoid the use of alcohol or other substances while using motor or recreational vehicles, or where impaired judgment may lead to injury;
- counseling to use safety devices, including seat belts, motorcycle and bicycle helmets, and appropriate athletic protective devices;
- counseling to resolve interpersonal conflicts without violence;
- counseling to avoid the use of weapons and/or promote weapon safety;
- counseling to promote appropriate physical conditioning before exercise.

Recommendation 7: All adolescents should receive health guidance annually about dietary habits, including the benefits of a healthy diet, and ways to achieve a healthy diet and safe weight management.

Recommendation 8: All adolescents should receive health guidance annually about the benefits of physical activity and should be encouraged to engage in safe physical activities on a regular basis.

From ages 11 to 21, all adolescents should have preventive services visits that address both the biomedical and psychosocial aspects of health.

Appendix K

Clinics and offices should establish policies to deliver confidential care to adolescents and define how parents will be involved in that care.

Recommendation 9: All adolescents should receive health guidance annually regarding responsible sexual behaviors, including abstinence. Latex condoms to prevent STDs, including HIV infection, and appropriate methods of birth control should be made available, as should instructions on how to use them effectively.

Health guidance for sexual responsibility includes the following:

- counseling that abstinence from sexual intercourse is the most effective way to prevent pregnancy and sexually transmissible diseases (STDs), including HIV infection;
- counseling on how HIV infection is transmitted, the dangers of the disease, and the fact that latex condoms are effective in preventing STDs, including HIV infection;
- reinforcement of responsible sexual behavior for adolescents who are not currently sexually active and for those who are using birth control and condoms appropriately;
- counseling on the need to protect themselves and their partners from pregnancy; STDs, including HIV infection; and sexual exploitation.

Recommendation 10: All adolescents should receive health guidance annually to promote avoidance of tobacco, alcohol and other abusable substances, and anabolic steroids.

Recommendations for screening

GAPS includes recommendations for the screening of biomedical, behavioral, and emotional conditions. Some GAPS recommendations lead to a definitive diagnosis (eg, cervical culture in females to diagnose gonorrhea). Other recommendations lead to a presumptive diagnosis (eg, urine test for leukocyte esterase in males to screen for gonorrhea or asking about use of alcohol or other drugs during the past six months to screen for substance use) that must be confirmed with additional assessment. Physicians can use information from the initial screening to decide whether to continue the assessment themselves or to refer the adolescent elsewhere. Health risk behaviors may, in some adolescents, be interrelated and co-occur. Adolescents who are found to engage in one health risk behavior, therefore, should be asked about involvement in others.

Recommendation 11: All adolescents should be screened annually for hypertension according to the protocol developed by the National Heart, Lung, and Blood Institute Second Task Force on Blood Pressure Control in Children.

- Adolescents with either systolic or diastolic pressures at or above the 90th percentile for gender and age should have blood pressure (BP) measurements repeated at three different times within one month, under similar physical conditions, to confirm baseline values.
- Adolescents with baseline BP values greater than the 95th percentile for gender and age should have a complete biomedical evaluation to establish treatment options. Adolescents with BP values between the 90th and 95th percentile should be assessed for obesity and their blood pressure monitored every six months.

Recommendation 12: Selected adolescents should be screened to determine their risk of developing hyperlipidemia and adult coronary heart disease, following the protocol developed by the Expert Panel on Blood Cholesterol Levels in Children and Adolescents.

- Adolescents whose parents have a serum cholesterol level greater than 240 mg/dl and adolescents who are over 19 years of age should be screened for total blood cholesterol level (nonfasting) at least once.
- Adolescents with an unknown family history or who have multiple risk factors for future cardiovascular disease (eg, smoking, hypertension, obesity, diabetes mellitus, excessive consumption of dietary saturated fats and cholesterol) may be screened for total serum cholesterol level (nonfasting) at least once at the discretion of the physician.
- Adolescents with blood cholesterol values less than 170 mg/dl should have the test repeated within five years. Those with values between 170 and 199 mg/dl should have a repeated test. If the average of the two tests is below 170 mg/dl, total blood cholesterol level should be reassessed within five years. A lipoprotein analysis should be done if the average cholesterol value from the two tests is 170 mg/dl or higher, or if the result of the initial test was 200 mg/dl or greater.
- Adolescents who have a parent or grandparent with coronary artery disease, peripheral vascular disease, cerebrovascular disease, or sudden cardiac death at age 55 or younger should be screened with a fasting lipoprotein analysis.
- Treatment options are based on the average of two assessments of low-density lipoprotein cholesterol. Values below 110 mg/dl are acceptable; values between 110 and 129 mg/dl are borderline, and the lipoprotein status should be reevaluated in one year. Adolescents with values of 130 mg/dl or greater should be referred for further medical evaluation and treatment.

Recommendation 13: All adolescents should be screened annually for eating disorders and obesity by determining weight and stature, and asking about body image and dieting patterns.

- Adolescents should be assessed for organic disease, anorexia nervosa, or bulimia if any of the following are found: weight loss greater than 10% of previous weight; recurrent dieting when not overweight; use of self-induced emesis, laxatives, starvation, or diuretics to lose weight; distorted body image; or body mass index (weight/height^2) below the fifth percentile.
- Adolescents with a body mass index (BMI) equal to or greater than the 95th percentile for age and gender are overweight and should have an in-depth dietary and health assessment to determine psychosocial morbidity and risk for future cardiovascular disease.
- Adolescents with a BMI between the 85th and 94th percentile are at risk for becoming overweight. A dietary and health assessment to determine psychosocial morbidity and risk for future cardiovascular disease should be performed on these youth if:
  - their BMI has increased by two or more units during the previous 12 months;
  - there is a family history of premature heart disease, obesity, hypertension, or diabetes mellitus;
  - they express concern about their weight;
  - they have elevated serum cholesterol levels or blood pressure.

If this assessment is negative, these adolescents should be provided general dietary and exercise counseling and should be monitored annually.

Recommendation 14: All adolescents should be asked annually about their use of tobacco products including cigarettes and smokeless tobacco.

- Adolescents who use tobacco products should be assessed further to determine their patterns of use.
- A cessation plan should be provided for adolescents who use tobacco products.

Recommendation 15: All adolescents should be asked annually about their use of alcohol and other abusable substances, and about their use of over-the-counter or prescription drugs for nonmedical purposes, including anabolic steroids.

- Adolescents who report any use of alcohol or other drugs or inappropriate use of medicines during the past year should be assessed further regarding family history; circumstances surrounding use; amount and frequency of use; attitudes and motivation about use; use of other drugs; and the adequacy of physical, psychosocial, and school functioning.
- Adolescents whose substance use endangers their health should receive counseling and mental health treatment, as appropriate.
- Adolescents who use anabolic steroids should be counseled to stop.
- The use of urine toxicology for the routine screening of adolescents is not recommended.
- Adolescents who use alcohol or other drugs should also be asked about their sexual behavior and their use of tobacco products.

Recommendation 16: All adolescents should be asked annually about involvement in sexual behaviors that may result in unintended pregnancy and STDs, including HIV infection.

- Sexually active adolescents should be asked about their use and motivation to use condoms and contraceptive methods, their sexual orientation, the number of sexual partners they have had in the past six months, if they have exchanged sex for money or drugs, and their history of prior pregnancy or STDs.
- Adolescents at risk for pregnancy, STDs (including HIV), or sexual exploitation should be counseled on how to reduce this risk.
- Sexually active adolescents should also be asked about their use of tobacco products, alcohol, and other drugs.

Recommendation 17: Sexually active adolescents should be screened for STDs.

STD screening includes the following:

- a cervical culture (females) or urine leukocyte esterase analysis (males) to screen for gonorrhea;
- an immunologic test of cervical fluid (female) or urine leukocyte esterase analysis (male) to screen for genital chlamydia;
- a serologic test for syphilis if they have lived in an area endemic for syphilis, have had other STDs, have had more than one sexual partner within the last six months, have exchanged sex for drugs or money, or are males who have engaged in sex with other males;
- evaluation for human papilloma virus by visual inspection (males and females) and by Pap test.

GAPS recommends that physicians and other health care providers give health guidance to parents and guardians to help them respond appropriately to the health needs of their adolescent.

- If a presumptive test for STDs is positive, tests to make a definitive diagnosis should be performed, a treatment plan instituted according to guidelines developed by the Centers for Disease Control and Prevention, and the use of condoms encouraged.
- The frequency of screening for STDs depends on the sexual practices of the individual and the history of previous STDs.

Recommendation 18: Adolescents at risk for HIV infection should be offered confidential HIV screening with the ELISA and confirmatory test.

- Risk status includes having used intravenous drugs, having had other STD infections, having lived in an area with a high prevalence of STDs and HIV infection, having had more than one sexual partner in the last six months, having exchanged sex for drugs or money, being male and having engaged in sex with other males, or having had a sexual partner who is at risk for HIV infection.
- Testing should be performed only after informed consent is obtained from the adolescent.

GAPS recommends that health guidance be given annually to all adolescents to help them cope with developmental challenges, develop and maintain healthy lifestyles, and prevent injury.

- Testing should be performed only in conjunction with both pre- and post-test counseling.
- The frequency of screening for HIV infection should be determined by the risk factors of the individual.

Recommendation 19: Female adolescents who are sexually active or any female 18 or older should be screened annually for cervical cancer by use of a Pap test.

Adolescents with a positive Pap test should be referred for further diagnostic assessment and management.

Recommendation 20: All adolescents should be asked annually about behaviors or emotions that indicate recurrent or severe depression or risk of suicide.

- Screening for depression or suicidal risk should be performed on adolescents who exhibit cumulative risk as determined by declining school grades, chronic melancholy, family dysfunction, homosexual orientation, physical or sexual abuse, alcohol or other drug use, previous suicide attempt, and suicidal plans.
- If suicidal risk is suspected, adolescents should be evaluated immediately and referred to a psychiatrist or other mental health professional, or else should be hospitalized.
- Nonsuicidal adolescents with symptoms of severe or recurrent depression should be evaluated and referred to a psychiatrist or other mental health professional for treatment.

Recommendation 21: All adolescents should be asked annually about a history of emotional, physical, and sexual abuse.

- If abuse is suspected, adolescents should be assessed to determine the circumstances surrounding abuse and the presence of physical, emotional, and psychosocial consequences, including involvement in health risk behaviors.
- Health providers should be aware of local laws about the reporting of abuse to appropriate state officials, in addition to ethical and legal issues regarding how to protect the confidentiality of the adolescent patient.
- Adolescents who report emotional or psychosocial sequelae should be referred to a psychiatrist or other mental health professional for evaluation and treatment.

Recommendation 22: All adolescents should be asked annually about learning or school problems.

- Adolescents with a history of truancy, repeated absences, or poor or declining performance should be assessed for the presence of conditions that could interfere with school success. These include learning disability, attention deficit hyperactivity disorder, medical problems, abuse, family dysfunction, mental disorder, or alcohol or other drug use.
- This assessment, and the subsequent management plan, should be coordinated with school personnel and with the adolescent's parents or caregivers.

Recommendation 23: Adolescents should receive a tuberculin skin test if they have been exposed to active tuberculosis, have lived in a homeless shelter, have been incarcerated, have lived in or come from an area with a high prevalence of tuberculosis, or currently work in a health care setting.

- Adolescents with a positive tuberculin test should be treated according to CDC treatment guidelines.
- The frequency of testing depends on risk factors of the individual adolescent.

Recommendations for immunizations

The fourth set of recommendations involves the use of vaccinations to prevent infectious disease. National immunization policies have changed recently with the development of the vaccination against Hepatitis B virus and the resurgence of measles and rubella among adolescent and adult populations. Providers will need to determine the number and type of previous vaccinations to assess the immunization needs of the adolescent.

Recommendation 24: All adolescents should receive prophylactic immunizations according to the guidelines established by the federally convened Advisory Committee on Immunization Practices.

- Adolescents should receive a bivalent Td vaccine booster at the 11-12 year visit if not previously vaccinated within 5 years. With the exception of the Td booster at 11-12 years, routine boosters should be administered every 10 years.
- Adolescents should receive a second dose of MMR at age 11-12 years, unless there is documentation of two vaccinations earlier during childhood. MMR should not be administered to pregnant adolescents.
- Adolescents, 11-12 years of age, who have not been immunized as part of a routine childhood schedule and who do not have a reliable history of chickenpox should be offered varicella vaccine.
- Hepatitis B immunization should be initiated at 11-12 years of age. Older unvaccinated adolescents with identified risk factors for HBV infection should also be vaccinated. Major risk factors for acquisition of HBV infection in adolescents include multiple sex partners, intravenous drug abuse, living in areas where increased rates of parenteral drug abuse, teenage pregnancy, and/or sexually transmitted diseases. Widespread use of Hepatitis B vaccination is encouraged because risk factors are not always easily identifiable among adolescents.
- Hepatitis A should be given to adolescents who are traveling or living in countries with high or intermediate endemicity of hepatitis A virus(HAV), live in communities with high endemic rates of HAV, have chronic liver disease, are injecting drug users or are males who have sex with males.
- Ideally all vaccinations should be administered at the scheduled 11-12 year visit.

Clinical application

GAPS provides a strategy to organize the content and delivery of care within a clinical setting to address the health issues of adolescents. Most primary care providers offer some preventive services to adolescents but GAPS suggests a comprehensive approach that includes screening and health guidance on an annual basis. All adolescents should be scheduled for an initial GAPS visit at the 11-12 year visit.

Differences between GAPS and traditional approaches to health care

The major differences between GAPS services and the traditional approaches to health care are the emphasis on comprehensive rather than categorical services for adolescents, visits for their parents or guardians, and the orientation to preventive care. These differences are summarized in the following table.

For some adolescents, health risk behaviors may be interrelated. Adolescents who are found to engage in one health risk behavior, consequently, should be asked about involvement in others.

GAPS recommendations compared with traditional approaches to adolescent health care

GAPS recommendations	Traditional health care
Provider plays an important role in coordinating adolescent health promotion. This role complements health guidance that adolescents receive from their family, school, and community.	Provider role is considered to be independent of health education programs offered by schools, family, and the community.
Preventive interventions target social morbidities such as alcohol and other drug use, suicide, STDs (including HIV), unintended pregnancy, and eating disorders.	Emphasis is on biomedical problems alone, such as the medical consequences of health risk behaviors (eg, STDs, unintended pregnancy).
Provider emphasizes screening for comorbidities, ie, adolescent participation in clusters of specific health risk behaviors.	Emphasis is on the diagnosis and treatment of categorical health conditions.
Annual visits permit early detection of health problems and offer an opportunity to provide health education and develop a therapeutic relationship.	Visits are scheduled only as needed for acute care episodes or for other specific purposes (eg, immunizations or an examination prior to participating in sports).
Provider performs three comprehensive physical examinations: one during early, middle and late adolescence.	Current standards vary from as necessary to examinations every two years during adolescence.
It is recommended that all parents receive education about adolescent health care at least twice during their child's adolescence.	Parents are included in the health care of the adolescent solely at the discretion of the provider, who also serves as the sole decision maker of what health education topics should be addressed with parents.

Appendix K

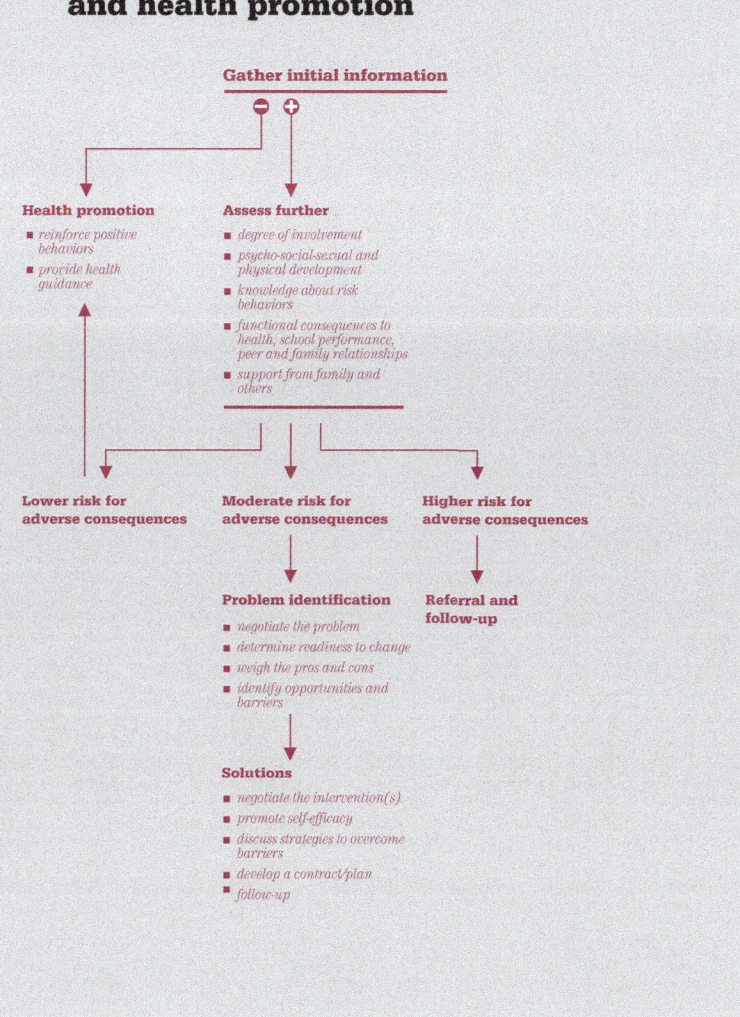

American Medical Association
515 North State Street
Chicago, Illinois 60610

OP020997
ISBN: 0-89970-929-X
AA61:98-1209:3M:9/98

Appendix L
GAPS Periodic Questionnaire

Several tools have been designed to support implementing the American Medical Association's (AMA) Guidelines for Adolescent Preventive Services (GAPS) program in your clinical setting. The six forms include the Younger Adolescent Questionnaire in English and Spanish, Middle-Older Adolescent Questionnaire in English and Spanish, and the Parent/Guardian Questionnaire in English and Spanish. The GAPS Recommendations Monograph is also included for your information and reference. The questionnaires and monograph are considered master copies that you can reproduce but not alter, modify, or revise without the expressed written consent of the Child and Adolescent Health Program at the American Medical Association.

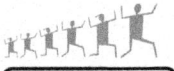

Guidelines for Adolescent Preventive Services
Middle-Older Adolescent Questionnaire

Confidential (Your answers will not be given out.) Chart # _____

Name _____ Date _____
         Last   First   Middle Initial

Date of Birth _____ Grade in School _____ Year in college _____ Sex: Male Female Age ___

Address _____ City _____ Zip _____

Phone number where you can be reached _____ Pager/beeper number _____

What languages are spoken where you live? _____ Race _____

Medical History

1. Why did you come to the clinic/office today? _____
2. Do you have any health problems? ☐ Yes ☐ No Problem(s) _____
3. Did you have any health problems in the past 12 months? ☐ Yes ☐ No Problem(s) _____
4. Are you taking any medicine now? ☐ Yes ☐ No Name of medicine _____

For Girls

5. Date when last period started _____ Are your periods regular (monthly)? .... ☐ No ☐ Yes
                                    Month   Date
6. Have you had a miscarriage, an abortion, or live birth in the past 12 months? .... ☐ Yes ☐ No

Specific Health Issues

7. Please check whether you have questions or are worried about any of the following:

   ☐ Height/weight   ☐ Mouth/teeth/breath   ☐ Frequent or   ☐ Trouble sleeping
   ☐ Blood pressure   ☐ Neck/back   painful urination   ☐ Feeling tired a lot
   ☐ Diet/food/appetite   ☐ Chest pain/trouble   ☐ Discharge from penis   ☐ Cancer
   ☐ Future plans/job   breathing   or vagina   ☐ Dying
   ☐ Skin (rash, acne)   ☐ Coughing/wheezing   ☐ Wetting the bed   ☐ Sad or crying a lot
   ☐ Headaches/migraines   ☐ Breasts   ☐ Sexual organs/genitals   ☐ Stress
   ☐ Dizziness/fainting   ☐ Heart   ☐ Menstruation/periods   ☐ Anger/temper
   ☐ Eyes/vision   ☐ Stomach ache   ☐ Wet dreams   ☐ Violence/personal safety
   ☐ Ears/hearing/ear aches ☐ Nausea/vomiting   ☐ Physical or sexual abuse ☐ Other (explain)
   ☐ Nose   ☐ Diarrhea/constipation   ☐ Masturbation   _____
   ☐ Lots of colds   ☐ Muscle or joint pain   ☐ HIV/AIDS   _____
                               in arms/legs

Health Profile

These questions will help us get to know you better. Choose the answer that best describes what you feel or do.
Your answers will be seen only by your health care provider and his/her assistant.

Eating/Weight

8. Are you satisfied with your eating habits? .... ☐ No ☐ Yes
9. Do you ever eat in secret? .... ☐ Yes ☐ No
10. Do you spend a lot of time thinking about ways to be thin? .... ☐ Yes ☐ No
11. In the past year, have you tried to lose weight or control your weight by vomiting,
    taking diet pills or laxatives, or starving yourself? .... ☐ Yes ☐ No
12. Do you exercise or participate in sport activities that make you sweat and breathe hard for
    20 minutes or more at a time at least three or more times during the week? .... ☐ No ☐ Yes

School

13. Are your grades this year worse than last year? .... ☐ Yes ☐ No ☐ Not in school
14. Have you either been told you have a learning problem or do you think you have a learning problem? ... ☐ Yes ☐ No
15. Have you been suspended from school this year? .... ☐ Yes ☐ No ☐ Not in school

Friends & Family

16. Do you have at least one friend who you really like and feel you can talk to? .... ☐ No ☐ Yes
17. Do you think that your parent(s) or guardian(s) *usually* listen to you and take your feelings seriously? ... ☐ No ☐ Yes
18. Have you ever thought seriously about running away from home? .... ☐ Yes ☐ No ☐ Not sure

Turn page

Appendix L

Weapons/Violence/Safety

19. Do you or anyone you live with have a gun, rifle, or other firearm? .... ☐ Yes ☐ No ☐ Not sure
20. In the past year, have you carried a gun, knife, club, or other weapon for protection? .... ☐ Yes ☐ No
21. Have you been in a physical fight during the *past 3 months*? .... ☐ Yes ☐ No
22. Have you ever been in trouble with the law? .... ☐ Yes ☐ No
23. Are you worried about violence or your safety? .... ☐ Yes ☐ No ☐ Not sure
24. Do you usually wear a helmet when you rollerblade, skateboard, ride a bicycle, motorcycle, minibike, or ride in an all-terrain vehicle (ATV)? .... ☐ No ☐ Yes
25. Do you usually wear a seat belt when you ride in or drive a car, truck, or van? .... ☐ No ☐ Yes

Tobacco

26. Do you ever smoke cigarettes/cigars, use snuff or chew tobacco? .... ☐ Yes ☐ No
26. Do any of your close friends ever smoke cigarettes/cigars, use snuff or chew tobacco? .... ☐ Yes ☐ No
28. Does anyone you live with smoke cigarettes/cigars, use snuff or chew tobacco? .... ☐ Yes ☐ No

Alcohol

29. In the past month, did you get drunk or very high on beer, wine, or other alcohol? .... ☐ Yes ☐ No
30. In the past month, did any of your close friends get drunk or very high on beer, wine, or other alcohol? ... ☐ Yes ☐ No
31. Have you ever been criticized or gotten into trouble because of drinking? .... ☐ Yes ☐ No ☐ Not sure
32. In the past year have you used alcohol and then driven a car/truck/van/motorcycle? .... ☐ Yes ☐ No ☐ Does not apply
33. In the past year, have you been in a car or other motor vehicle when the driver has been drinking alcohol or using drugs? .... ☐ Yes ☐ No
34. Does anyone in your family drink or take drugs so much that it worries you? .... ☐ Yes ☐ No

Drugs

35. Do you ever use marijuana or other drugs, or sniff inhalants? .... ☐ Yes ☐ No ☐ Not sure
36. Do any of your close friends ever use marijuana or other drugs, or sniff inhalants? .... ☐ Yes ☐ No ☐ Not sure
37. Do you ever use non-prescription drugs to get to sleep, stay awake, calm down, or get high? (These drugs can be bought at a store without a doctor's prescription.) .... ☐ Yes ☐ No
38. Have you ever used steroid pills or shots without a doctor telling you to? .... ☐ Yes ☐ No ☐ Not sure

Development

39. Do you have any concerns or questions about the size or shape of your body, or your physical appearance? .... ☐ Yes ☐ No ☐ Not sure
40. Do you think you may be gay, lesbian, or bisexual? .... ☐ Yes ☐ No ☐ Not sure
41. Have you ever had sexual intercourse? (How old were you the first time? _____) .... ☐ Yes ☐ No ☐ Not sure
42. Are you using a method to prevent pregnancy? (Which: _____) .... ☐ No ☐ Yes ☐ Not active
43. Do you and your partner(s) *always* use condoms when you have sex? .... ☐ No ☐ Yes ☐ Not active
44. Have any of your close friends ever had sexual intercourse? .... ☐ Yes ☐ No ☐ Not sure
45. Have you ever been told by a doctor or nurse that you had a sexually transmitted infection or disease? ... ☐ Yes ☐ No ☐ Not sure
46. Have you ever been pregnant or gotten someone pregnant? .... ☐ Yes ☐ No ☐ Not sure
47. Would you like to receive information or supplies to prevent pregnancy or sexually transmitted infections? ... ☐ Yes ☐ No ☐ Not sure
48. Would you like to know how to avoid getting HIV/AIDS? .... ☐ Yes ☐ No ☐ Not sure
49. Have you pierced your body (not including ears) or gotten a tattoo? .... ☐ Yes ☐ No ☐ Thinking about it

Emotions

50. Have you had fun during the past two weeks? .... ☐ No ☐ Yes
51. During the past few weeks, have you *often* felt sad or down or as though you have nothing to look forward to? .... ☐ Yes ☐ No
52. Have you ever *seriously* thought about killing yourself, made a plan or actually tried to kill yourself? ..... ☐ Yes ☐ No
53. Have you ever been physically, sexually, or emotionally abused? .... ☐ Yes ☐ No ☐ Not sure
54. When you get angry, do you do violent things? .... ☐ Yes ☐ No
55. Would you like to get counseling about something you have on your mind? .... ☐ Yes ☐ No ☐ Not sure

Special Circumstances

56. In the past year, have you been around someone with tuberculosis (TB)? .... ☐ Yes ☐ No ☐ Not sure
57. In the past year, have you stayed overnight in a homeless shelter, jail, or detention center? .... ☐ Yes ☐ No
58. Have you ever lived in foster care or a group home? .... ☐ Yes ☐ No

Self

59. What four words best describe you? _____
60. If you could change one thing about your life or yourself, what would it be? _____

61. What do you want to talk about today? _____

© 1997 American Medical Association   all rights reserved   97-802:1.2M:11/97

Appendix M
WHO Immunization Routine LifeSpan Vaccinations

Table 1: Summary of WHO Position Papers - Recommendations for Routine Immunization

(updated 15 November 2012)

Antigen	Children (see Table 2 for details)		Adolescents	Adults	Considerations (see footnotes for details)
Recommendations for all					
BCG[1]	1 dose				Exceptions HIV
Hepatitis B[2]	3-4 doses (see footnote for schedule options)		3 doses (for high-risk groups if not previously immunized) (see footnote)		Birth dose; Premature and low birth weight; Co-administration and combination vaccine; Definition high-risk
Polio[3]	3 doses, with DTP				OPV birth dose; Transmission and importation risk criteria; Type of vaccine
DTP[4]	3 doses	Booster (DTP) 1-6 years of age	Booster (Td) (see footnote)	Booster (Td) in early adulthood or pregnancy	Delayed/interrupted schedule; Combination vaccine
Haemophilus influenzae type b[5]	3 doses, with DTP				Single dose if 12-24 months of age; Delayed/interrupted schedule; Co-administration and combination vaccine
Pneumococcal (Conjugate)[6] Option 1	3 doses, with DTP				Vaccine options; Initiate before 6 months of age; Co-administration; HIV+ and preterm neonates booster
Option 2	2 doses before 6 months of age, plus booster dose at 9-15 months of age				
Rotavirus[7]	Rotarix: 2 doses with DTP; RotaTeq: 3 doses with DTP				Vaccine options
Measles[8]	2 doses				Combination vaccine; HIV early vaccination; Pregnancy
Rubella[9]	1 dose (see footnote)		1 dose (adolescent girls and/or child bearing aged women if not previously vaccinated; see footnote)		Achieve and sustain 80% coverage; Combination vaccine and Co-administration; Pregnancy
HPV[10]			3 doses (girls)		Vaccination of males for prevention of cervical cancer is not recommended at this time

Refer to http://www.who.int/immunization/documents/positionpapers/, for most recent version of this table and position papers.

This table summarizes the WHO child vaccination recommendations. It is designed to assist the development of country specific schedules and is not intended for direct use by health care workers. Country specific schedules should be based on local epidemiologic, programmatic, resource and policy considerations.

While vaccines are universally recommended, some children may have contraindications to particular vaccines.

Appendix M

Table 1: Summary of WHO Position Papers - Recommendations for Routine Immunization

(updated 15 November 2012)

Antigen	Children (see Table 2 for details)	Adolescents	Adults	Considerations (see footnotes for details)
Recommendations for certain regions				
Japanese Encephalitis[11]	Live attenuated vaccine: 1 dose Booster after 1 year Mouse brain-derived vaccine: 2 doses Booster after 1 year then every 3 years	Mouse brain-derived vaccine: booster every 3 years up to 10-15 years of age		Vaccine options
Yellow Fever[12]	1 dose, with measles containing vaccine			Co-administration
Tick-Borne Encephalitis[13]	3 doses (> 1 yr FSME-Immun and Encepur; > 3 yrs TBE-Moscow and EnceVir) with at least 1 booster dose (every 3 years for TBE-Moscow and EnceVir)			Definition of high-risk Vaccine options; Timing of booster
Recommendations for some high-risk populations				
Typhoid[14]	Vi polysaccharide vaccine: 1 dose; Ty21a live oral vaccine: 3-4 doses (see footnote). Booster dose 3-7 years after primary series			Definition of high-risk Vaccine options
Cholera[15]	Dukoral (WC-rBS): 3 doses ≥ 2-5 yrs, booster every 6 months; 2 doses adults/children > 6 yrs, booster every 2nd year; Shanchol & mORCVAX: 2 doses ≥1 yrs, booster dose after 2 yrs			Minimum age Definition of high-risk
Meningococcal[16] MenA conjugate / MenC conjugate / Quadrivalent conjugate	2 doses (2-11 months) with booster 1 year after 1 dose (≥12 months) 1 dose (1-29 years) 2 doses (9-23 months) 1 dose (≥2 years)			Definition of high-risk; Vaccine options
Hepatitis A[17]	At least 1 dose ≥ 1 year of age			Level of endemicity; Vaccine options; Definition of high risk groups
Rabies[18]	3 doses			Definition of high-risk; Booster
Recommendations for immunization programmes with certain characteristics				
Mumps[19]	2 doses, with measles containing vaccine			Coverage criteria > 80% Combination vaccine
Influenza (inactivated)[20]	First vaccine use: 2 doses Revaccinate annually: 1 dose only (see footnote)	1 dose from 9 yrs of age. Revaccinate annually (see footnote)		Priority targets Definition of high-risk Lower dosage for children

Summary Table 1 - Notes

- Refer to http://www.who.int/immunization/documents/positionpapers/ for the most recent version of the tables and position papers.
- The attached table summarizes the recommendations for vaccine administration found in the WHO position papers which are published in the Weekly Epidemiological Review. Its purpose is to assist planners to develop an appropriate immunization schedule. Health care workers should refer to their national immunization schedules. While vaccines are universally recommended, some children may have contraindications to particular vaccines.
- Vaccines can generally be co-administered (i.e. more than one vaccine given at different sites during the same visit). Recommendations that explicitly endorse co-administration are indicated in the table, however, lack of an explicit co-administration recommendation does not imply that the vaccine cannot be co-administered; further, there are no recommendations against co-administration.
- Doses administered by campaign may or may not contribute to a child's routine immunization schedule depending on type and purpose of campaign (e.g. supplemental versus routine/pulse campaign for access reasons).
- For some antigens, recommendations for the age of initiation of primary immunization series and/or booster doses are not available. Instead, the criteria for age at first dose must be determined from local epidemiologic data.
- If a catch-up schedule for interrupted immunization is available, it is noted in the footnotes.
- Other vaccines, such as varicella and pneumococcal polysaccharide vaccines, may be of individual benefit but are not recommended for routine immunization. See the specific position papers for more details.
- For further background on immunization schedules refer to "Immunological Basis for Immunization" series which is available at: http://www.who.int/immunization/documents/immunological_basis_series/en/index.html

1 BCG

- Position paper reference: Weekly Epid. Record (2004, 79: 27-38) [pdf 468kb]
- Recommended for children living in countries with a high-disease burden and for high-risk children living in countries with low-disease burden. See position paper for details.
- While BCG vaccination is especially important in countries with significant HIV prevalence, children who are HIV positive or unknown HIV status with symptoms consistent with HIV should not be vaccinated. Reference: Weekly Epid. Record (2007, 82: 193-196) [pdf 167kb]

2 Hepatitis B

- Position paper reference: Weekly Epid. Record (2009, 84: 405-420) [pdf 630kb]
- Since perinatal or early postnatal transmission is an important cause of chronic infections globally, all infants should receive their first dose of hepatitis B vaccine as soon as possible (<24 hours) after birth even in low-endemicity countries.
- The primary hepatitis B immunization series conventionally consists of 3 doses of vaccine (1 mono-valent birth dose followed by 2 monovalent or combined vaccine doses at the time of DTP1 and DTP3 vaccine doses). However, 4 doses may be given for programmatic reasons (e.g. 1 monovalent birth-dose followed by 3 monovalent or combined vaccine doses with DTP vaccine doses), according to the schedules of national routine immunization programmes.
- Premature low birth weight (<2000g) may not respond well to vaccination at birth. However, by 1 month of chronological age, premature infants, regardless of their initial weight or gestational age at birth, are likely to respond adequately. Therefore, doses given to infants <2000g should not be counted towards the primary series.
- Additional target groups for vaccination include people with risk factors for acquiring HBV infection, such as those who frequently require blood or blood products, dialysis patients, recipients of solid organ transplantations, people interned in prisons, injecting drug users, household and sexual contacts of people with chronic HBV infection, people with multiple sexual partners, as well as health-care workers and others who may be exposed to blood and blood products through their work.

Reference: Weekly Epid. Record (2010, 85: 213-228) [pdf 815.1kb]

3 Polio

- The primary series of 3 OPV vaccinations should be administered according to the respective national immunization schedule, for example at 6, 10 and 14 weeks, or 2, 4, and 6 months of age. The interval between doses should be at least 4 weeks.
- Where the potential for poliovirus importation is very high (i.e in countries bordering endemic countries or countries that have recurrent outbreaks) or high (i.e. country with a history of importation plus high traffic across the border), and the transmission potential high (e.g. <90% DTP3 coverage, low socio-economic status, majority of areas with open sewage) or moderate (e.g. <90% DTP3 coverage, all states/provinces with moderate socio-economic status, only secondary sewage treatment) an OPV birth dose should be given as soon as possible after birth.
- OPV alone, including a birth dose, is recommended in all polio-endemic countries and those at high risk for importation and subsequent spread. A birth dose is not considered necessary in countries where the risk of polio virus transmission is low, even if the potential for importation is high/very high.
- Where the risk of wild polio virus importation is high/very high, the transmission potential should be low (>90-95% DTP3 coverage, high socio-economic status, tertiary sewage treatment) before alternatives to OPV alone may be considered.
- In countries with very high risk of wild polio virus importation, a sequential IPV/OPV schedule should not be introduced unless immunization coverage is approximately 95%, or, with low importation risk, approximately 90%. Where sequential IPV/OPV is used, the initial administration of 1-2 doses of IPV should be followed by 2 or more doses of OPV to ensure both sufficient levels of protection in the intestinal mucosa and a decrease in the burden of vaccine-associated paralytic poliomyelitis (VAPP). For IPV/OPV sequential schedules, WHO recommends that IPV be administered at 2 months of age (e.g. an IPV-OPV-OPV schedule) or at 2 months and 3-4 months of age (e.g. a 4-dose schedule of IPV-IPV-OPV-OPV). Each dose of the primary series, whether IPV or OPV, should be separated by an interval of 4-8 weeks, depending on the risk of exposure to polio in early childhood.
- IPV alone can be considered as an alternative to OPV alone (or an IPV/OPV sequential schedule) only in countries with the lowest risk of both wild polio importation and WPV transmission. IPV may be offered as a component of combination vaccines. A primary series of 3 IPV doses should be administered beginning at 2 months of age. If the primary series begins earlier (e.g. with a 6, 10, and 14 week schedule) then a booster dose should be administered with an interval of at least 6 months (4 - dose IPV schedule).
- Switching from OPV to IPV for routine vaccination during the pre-eradication era is not cost-effective based on the existing economic analyses and current IPV costs.

4 DTP (Diphtheria, Tetanus and Pertussis)

- Position paper reference: Diphtheria - Weekly Epid. Record (2006, 81: 24-32) [pdf 214kb]; Tetanus - Weekly Epid. Record (2006, 81: 198-208) [pdf 229kb]; Pertussis - Weekly Epid. Record (2010, 85: 385-400) [pdf 320kb]
- Recommended for three doses during the first year of life. In areas where pertussis is of particular risk to young infants, DTP should be started at 6 weeks with 2 subsequent doses at intervals of 4-8 weeks each. The last dose of the primary series should be completed by the

Table 1: Recommended Routine Immunization (updated: 15 November 2012)

Appendix M

age of 6 months.

- The duration of immunological protection will be extended in many instances if an additional booster is given later.
- Diphtheria booster - to compensate for the loss of natural diphtheria boosting in some areas, childhood boosters should be given. The optimal timing of and number of diphtheria-containing booster doses should be based on epidemiological surveillance as well as on immunological and programmatic considerations.
- Tetanus toxoid containing booster - A childhood tetanus immunization schedule of 5 doses is recommended. Boosters are ideally administered in early childhood and during adolescence e.g. 12-15 years. Tetanus booster doses may use either DTP or Td vaccines depending on the child's age. Td should be used for tetanus and diphtheria booster doses after the age of 7 years.
- Pertussis vaccine: Neo-natal immunization, and vaccination of pregnant women and household contacts ("cocooning") against pertussis is not recommended by WHO.
- Both acellular (aP) and whole cell pertussis (wP) containing vaccines have excellent safety records, and protection against severe pertussis in infancy and early childhood can be obtained with wP or aP vaccine. Changing among or within the wP and aP vaccine groups is unlikely to interfere with the safety or immunogenicity of these vaccines.
- Only aP-containing vaccines should be used for vaccination of those >6 years.
- Pertussis containing booster - A booster dose is recommended for children age 1-6 years, preferably during the second year of life. The booster should be given > 6 months after the last primary dose. Completion of this schedule (primary series plus booster) is expected to ensure protection against pertussis for > 6 years.
- Delayed or interrupted DTP series - Children 1-7 years or older who have not previously been immunized should receive three doses of wP or aP vaccine, with an interval of 2 months between the first and second dose and an interval of 6-12 months between the second and third. Children whose vaccination series has been interrupted should have their series resumed, without repeating previous doses. For unvaccinated individuals 7 years of age and older, Td in combination vaccine can be administered, 2 doses 1-2 months apart and a third dose after 6-12 months can be used with subsequent boosters at least 1 year apart for a total of 5 appropriately spaced doses to obtain same long term protection. See position paper for details of interrupted immunization schedules.

5 Haemophilus influenzae type b (Hib)

- Position paper reference: Weekly Epid. Record (2006, 81; 210-220) [pdf 209kb]
- Immunization should start as early as possible after the age of 6 weeks.
- The 3-dose primary series is given at the same time as the DTP primary series often in combination vaccines.
- The vaccine is not generally offered to children aged >24 months owing to the limited burden of Hib disease among children older than that age.
- Delayed series- If a child 12-24 months of age has not received their primary vaccination series, a single dose of the vaccine is sufficient.
- Booster dose may be administered to children aged between 12 - 18 months although there is no WHO recommendation on this yet.

6 Pneumococcal (Conjugate)

- Position paper reference: Weekly Epid. Record (2012, 87; 129-143) [pdf 1.04 Mb]
- Pneumococcal conjugate vaccines (PCVs) are considered safe in all target groups for vaccination, also in immunocompromised individuals. The vaccines are not currently licensed for use in age

groups that include women of childbearing age. Although theoretically highly unlikely to be harmful, there is no information on the safety of PCV10 and PCV13 during pregnancy.

- Except for very rare anaphylactic reactions that may follow the administration of any medicine, there are no contraindications to the use of these vaccines. However, it is advisable to defer vaccination until after an acute infection with temperature >39 °C.
- When injected at different sites, PCVs can be administered concurrently with any other vaccines in infant immunization programmes.
- When primary immunization is initiated with one of these vaccines, it is recommended that remaining doses are administered with the same product. Interchangeability between PCV10 and PCV13 has not yet been documented. However, if it is not possible to complete the series with the same type of vaccine, the other PCV product should be used.
- For infants, 3 primary doses (the 3p+0 schedule) or, as an alternative, 2 primary doses plus a booster (the 2p+1 schedule).
- In choosing between the 3p+0 and 2p+1 schedules, countries should consider locally relevant factors including the epidemiology of pneumococcal disease, the likely coverage, and the timeliness of the vaccine doses.
- If disease incidence peaks in young infants (<32 weeks of age), a 2p+1 schedule might not offer optimal individual protection for certain serotypes (e.g. 6B, 23F) compared to a 3p+0 schedule, particularly in the absence of herd protection.
- In contrast, higher antibody levels are induced by the third (booster) dose in a 2p+1 schedule compared to the third dose in a 3p+0 schedule. This may be important for duration of protection or effectiveness against some serotypes.
- If the 3p+0 schedule is used, vaccination can be initiated as early as 6 weeks of age with an interval between doses of 4-8 weeks, depending on programmatic convenience.
- If the 2p+1 schedule is selected, the 2 primary doses should ideally be completed by six months of age, starting as early as 6 weeks of age with a minimum interval of 8 weeks or more between the two doses (for infants aged ≥7 months a minimum interval of 4 weeks between doses is possible). One booster dose should be given between 9-15 months of age.
- Previously unvaccinated or incompletely vaccinated children (including those who had laboratory confirmed invasive pneumococcal disease) should be vaccinated using the recommended age-appropriate regimens. Interrupted schedules should be resumed without repeating the previous dose.
- HIV-positive infants and pre-term neonates who have received their 3 primary vaccine doses before reaching 12 months of age may benefit from a booster dose in the second year of life.
- Catch-up vaccination as part of introduction will accelerate herd protection and therefore the PCV impact on disease and carriage. Maximized protection at the time of introduction of PCV10 or PCV13 can be achieved by providing 2 catch-up dose(s) at an interval of at least 8 weeks to unvaccinated children aged 12-24 months and to children aged 2-5 years who are at high risk of pneumococcal infection.
- Further data are needed from different epidemiological settings on the impact of large-scale PCV vaccination of individuals ≥50 years of age in order to establish the relative priority of immunization programmes in that age group. However, given the documented effects of herd protection in adult age groups following routine infant immunization with PCV7, higher priority should normally be given to introducing and maintaining high coverage of infants with PCVs.
- The use of pneumococcal vaccine should be seen as complementary to the use of other pneumonia control measures, such as appropriate case management, promotion of exclusive breastfeeding for first 6 months of life, and the reduction of known risk factors, such as indoor pollutants and tobacco smoke.
- For polysaccharide pneumococcal vaccine see position paper: Weekly Epid. Record (2008, 83; 373-384) [pdf 308kb]

Table 1: Recommended Routine Immunization (updated: 15 November 2012)

In resource-limited settings where there are many competing health priorities, evidence does not support routine immunization of the elderly and high-risk populations with PPV23. Also, because of the low level of evidence for benefit, routine PPV23 vaccination of HIV-infected adults is not recommended in such settings. In countries that do not routinely administer PPV23 to high-risk populations, data are insufficient to recommend introducing this vaccine to reduce the morbidity and mortality associated with influenza.

7 Rotavirus

- Position paper reference: Weekly Epid. Record (2009, 84: 533-560) [pdf 764kb] NOTE: This position paper is currently being revised in light of the vaccination schedule recommendations made by SAGE at their April 2012 meeting Weekly Epid. Record (2012, 87: 201-216) [pdf 1.11Mb]
- Recommended to be included in all national immunization programmes.
- Rotarix vaccine is administered orally in a 2-dose schedule with the first and second doses of DTP.
- RotaTeq requires an oral 3-dose schedule with DTP1, DTP2, and DTP3 with an interval of 4-10 weeks between doses.
- First dose of either RotaTeq or Rotarix be administered as soon as possible from 6 weeks of age.
- The interchangeability of the current rotavirus vaccines is unknown.
- In various settings, rotavirus vaccines have been found not to interfere significantly with the immunogenicity or safety of OPV or other childhood vaccines.
- The use of rotavirus vaccines should be part of a comprehensive strategy to control diarrhoeal diseases and should include, among other interventions, improvements in hygiene and sanitation, zinc supplementation, community-based administration of oral rehydration solution and overall improvements in case management.

8 Measles

- Position paper reference: Weekly Epid. Record (2009, 84: 349-360) [pdf 724kb]
- Reaching all children with two doses of measles containing vaccine (MCV) should be the standard for all national immunization programmes.
- Delivery of the second dose (MCV2) may occur either at a scheduled age through routine services or periodically through mass campaigns, depending on which strategy achieves the higher coverage. A MCV2 dose may be added to the routine immunization schedule in countries that have achieved > 80% coverage of measles first dose (MCV1) at the national level for 3 consecutive years as determined by the most accurate means available (e.g. survey or WHO/UNICEF estimates). In general, countries that do not meet this criterion should prioritize improving MCV1 coverage and conducting high-quality follow-up SIAs, rather than adding MCV2 to their routine schedule.
- In countries with ongoing transmission in which the risk of measles mortality remains high, MCV1 should be given at age 9 months. MCV2 should be given between 15-18 months, as providing MCV2 in the 2nd year of life reduces the rate of accumulation of susceptible children and the risk of an outbreak.
- In countries with low rates of measles transmission (that is, those that are near elimination) and where there is a low risk of measles infection among infants, the first dose may be administered at age 12 months to take advantage of the higher seroconversion rates achieved at this age (>90% seroconversion). In these countries the optimal age for delivering a routine 2nd dose of measles is based on programmatic considerations that achieve the highest coverage and hence the highest population immunity. Administration of the second dose at age 15-18 months ensures early protection of the individual, slows accumulation of susceptible young children

and may correspond with other routine immunizations (for example, DTP booster). If first dose coverage is high (>90%) and school enrolment is high (>95%), giving the second dose at school entry may be an effective strategy for achieving high coverage and preventing outbreaks in schools.
- Combined vaccines (Measles and Rubella or Measles, Mumps and Rubella) may not be optimal for use in countries where vaccine coverage for measles vaccine of at least 80% cannot be achieved or maintained.
- Measles vaccination should be routinely administered to potentially susceptible, asymptomatic HIV-positive children and adults. In areas where there is a high incidence of both HIV infection and measles, MCV1 may be offered as early as age 6 months. Two additional doses of measles vaccine should be administered to these children according to the national immunization schedule.
- Mild, concurrent infections are not considered a contraindication to vaccination, but it should be avoided if the patient has a high fever or other signs of serious disease. Theoretically, measles vaccine – alone or in combination with other vaccines – should also be avoided by pregnant women. Furthermore, measles vaccination is contraindicated in people who are severely immunocompromised due to congenital disease; severe HIV infection; advanced leukaemia or lymphoma, etc.

9 Rubella

- Position paper reference: Weekly Epid. Record (2011, 86: 301-316) [pdf 413kb]
- All countries that have not yet introduced rubella vaccine, and are providing 2 doses of measles vaccine using routine immunization, or SIAs, or both, should consider including rubella containing vaccines (RCVs) in their immunization programme. Countries planning to introduce RCVs should review the epidemiology of rubella, including the susceptibility profile of the population; assess the burden of CRS; and establish rubella and CRS prevention as a public health priority.
- There are two general approaches to the use of rubella vaccine: (i) exclusive focus on reducing CRS by immunizing adolescent girls or women of childbearing age, or both groups, to provide individual protection; (ii) focus on interrupting transmission of rubella virus and eliminating rubella and CRS, by introducing rubella vaccination into the routine childhood immunization schedule combined with the vaccination of older age groups who are susceptible to rubella.
- Because rubella is not as highly infectious as measles and because the effectiveness of 1 dose of an RCV is > 95% even at 9 months of age, only 1 dose of rubella vaccine is required to achieve rubella elimination if high coverage is achieved. However, when combined with measles vaccination, it may be easier to implement a second dose of RCVs using the same combined MR vaccine or MMR vaccine for both doses.
- To avoid the potential of an increased risk of CRS, countries should achieve and maintain immunization coverage of 80% or greater with at least 1 dose of an RCV delivered through routine services or regular campaigns, or both.
- The first dose of RCV can be delivered at 9 or 12 months depending on the measles vaccination schedule.
- RCVs can be administered concurrently with inactivated vaccines. As a general rule, live vaccines should be given either simultaneously with RCVs, or at least 4 weeks apart. An exception to this is oral polio vaccine, which can be given at any time before or after RCVs without interfering in the response to either vaccine. Interference may occur between MMR and yellow fever vaccines if they are simultaneously administered to children < 2 years of age.
- Because of a theoretical, but never demonstrated, teratogenic risk rubella vaccination in pregnant women should be avoided in principle, and those planning a pregnancy are advised to avoid pregnancy for 1 month following vaccination.

Table 1: Recommended Routine Immunization (updated: 15 November 2012)

Appendix M

- Administration of blood or blood products before or shortly after vaccination may interfere with vaccine efficacy. If using only rubella vaccines persons who received blood products should wait at least 3 months before vaccination and, if possible, blood products should be avoided for up to 2 weeks postvaccination. Vaccinated persons are not eligible to donate blood for 1 month after vaccination.

10 Human Papillomavirus (HPV)

- Position paper reference: Weekly Epid. Record (2009, 84: 118-131) [pdf 267kb]
- Two vaccines are currently available. Quadrivalent (HPV types 6,11,16 and 18) licensed for use in females as young as 9 years of age to prevent cervical precancers and cancers. In addition, the quadrivalent vaccine is licensed for prevention of vulvar and vaginal precancers and cancers as well as anogenital warts in females. In some countries, the vaccine is also licensed for the prevention of anogenital warts in males. Bivalent (HPV types 16 and 18) has been licensed for use in females as young as 10 years of age to prevent cervical precancers and cancers.
- Both vaccines are intended for females before the onset of sexual activity, i.e. before first exposure to HPV infection. A three-dose schedule is recommended. The quadrivalent is given at baseline and after 2 and 6 months. A minimum interval of 4 weeks between the first and second dose, and a minimum interval between the second and third doses of 12 weeks is recommended by the manufacturer. The bivalent vaccine is given at baseline and after 1 and 6 months. If flexibility in the schedule is necessary the manufacturer recommends that the second dose is administered between 1 and 2.5 months after the first dose.
- For both vaccines alternative schedules are being explored. Restarting the 3-dose series is not necessary if interrupted, but remaining doses should be administered as close to the schedule intervals as possible.
- Currently, the manufacturers do not recommend any booster dose following completion of the primary series.
- HPV vaccination of males for prevention of cervical cancer is not recommended at this time because vaccination strategies that achieve high coverage (>70%) in the primary target population of young adolescent girls are expected to be more cost-effective in reducing cervical cancer than including vaccination of males.

11 Japanese Encephalitis (JE)

- Position paper reference: Weekly Epid. Record (2006, 81: 331-340) [pdf 192kb]
- JE vaccine should be given in all areas where JE constitutes a public health problem.
- Vaccine options – Three types of vaccines are available: (1) a cell culture-based live attenuated, (2) a cell culture-based inactivated and (3) an inactivated mouse brain-derived. The WHO position paper provides recommendations for the mouse brain-derived and live attenuated vaccines.
- Booster: If administering cell-culture based live-attenuated vaccine, a booster dose is currently recommended after an interval of one year, even though observational studies suggest long-term protection after a single dose. If using mouse brain-derived vaccine, a booster dose should be administered after an interval of one year then every 3 years until 10-15 years of age.

12 Yellow Fever

- Position paper reference: Weekly Epid. Record (2003, 78: 349-359) [pdf 339kb]
- Recommended for use in countries at risk of Yellow Fever.
- For convenience and improved coverage, Yellow Fever vaccine should be administered simultaneously with the measles containing vaccine, but in a separate syringe and at a different injection site.
- Yellow Fever vaccine should be offered to all travellers to and from at-risk areas, unless they belong to the group of individuals for whom Yellow Fever vaccination is contraindicated.
- Interference may occur between MMR and yellow fever vaccines if they are simultaneously administered to children < 2 years of age
- In addition to the introduction of Yellow Fever vaccine for routine childhood vaccination, WHO recommends the implementation of mass preventive vaccination campaigns to protect susceptible older age groups. In the event of limited resources, assessment of the degree of risk can help prioritize areas for mass preventive campaigns.

13 Tick-Borne Encephalitis (TBE)

- Position paper reference: Weekly Epid. Record (2011, 86: 241-256) [pdf 318kb]
- Since the incidence of tick-borne encephalitis may vary considerably between and even within geographical regions, public immunization strategies should be based on risk assessments conducted at country, regional or district level, and they should be appropriate to the local endemic situation. Therefore, establishing case reporting of the disease is essential before deciding on the most appropriate preventive measures to be taken.
- In areas where the disease is highly endemic (that is, where the average prevaccination incidence of clinical disease is ≥5 cases/100 000 population per year), implying that there is a high individual risk of infection, WHO recommends that vaccination be offered to all age groups, including children.
- Because the disease tends to be more serious in individuals aged >50–60 years this age group constitutes an important target for immunization.
- Where the prevaccination incidence of the disease is moderate or low (that is, the annual average during a 5-year period is <5/100 000) or is limited to particular geographical locations or certain outdoor activities, immunization should target individuals in the most severely affected cohorts.
- People travelling from non-endemic areas to endemic areas should be offered vaccination if their visits will include extensive outdoor activities.
- Vaccination against the disease requires a primary series of 3 doses; those who will continue to be at risk should probably have ≥1 booster doses.
- Within the considerable range of acceptable dose intervals, the relevant national authorities should select the most national primary schedule for their national, regional or district immunization programmes.
- Although there is a strong indication that the spacing of doses could be expanded considerably from the intervals currently recommended by the manufacturers (every 3–5 years), the evidence is still insufficient for a definitive recommendation on the optimal frequency and number of booster doses. Countries should therefore continue to recommend the use of vaccines in accordance with local disease epidemiology and current schedules until more definitive information becomes available.
- For the vaccines manufactured in Austria and Germany (FSME-Immun and Encepur) that can be given starting from > 1year of age an interval of 1–3 months is recommended between the first 2 doses, and 5–12 months between the second and third doses. When rapid protection is required, for example for people who will be travelling to endemic areas, the interval between the first 2 doses may be reduced to 1–2 weeks.
- With the vaccines manufactured in the Russian Federation (TBE-Moscow and EnceVir) the recommended intervals are 1–7 months between the first 2 doses, and 12 months between the second and third doses. Booster doses are recommended every 3 years for those at continued risk of exposure.
- The currently recommended booster interval should be maintained until more data have been obtained on the duration of protection induced by the Russian vaccines.
- Regardless of the duration of the delay, interrupted schedules should be resumed without repeating previous doses.

Table 1: Recommended Routine Immunization (updated: 15 November 2012)

10 Human Papillomavirus (HPV)

- Position paper reference: Weekly Epid. Record (2009, 84: 118-131) [pdf 267kb]

- Two vaccines are currently available. Quadrivalent (HPV types 6,11,16 and 18) licensed for use in females as young as 9 years of age to prevent cervical precancers and cancers. In addition, the quadrivalent vaccine is licensed for prevention of vulvar and vaginal precancers and cancers as well as anogenital warts in females. In some countries, the vaccine is also licensed for the prevention of anogenital warts in males. Bivalent (HPV types 16 and 18) has been licensed for use in females as young as 10 years of age to prevent cervical precancers of males.

- Both vaccines are intended for females before the onset of sexual activity, i.e. before first exposure to HPV infection. A three-dose schedule is recommended. The quadrivalent is given at baseline and after 2 and 6 months. A minimum interval of 4 weeks between the first and second dose, and a minimum interval between the second and third dose of 12 weeks is recommended by the manufacturer. The bivalent vaccine is given at baseline and after 1 and 6 months. If flexibility in the schedule is necessary the manufacturer recommends that the second dose is administered between 1 and 2.5 months after the first dose.

- For both vaccines alternative schedules are being explored. Restarting the 3-dose series is not necessary if interrupted, but remaining doses should be administered as close to the schedule intervals as possible.

- Currently, the manufacturers do not recommend any booster dose following completion of the primary series.

- HPV vaccination of males for prevention of cervical cancer is not recommended at this time because vaccination strategies that achieve high coverage (>70%) in the primary target population of young adolescent girls are expected to be more cost-effective in reducing cervical cancer than including vaccination of males.

11 Japanese Encephalitis (JE)

- Position paper reference: Weekly Epid. Record (2006, 81: 331-340) [pdf 192kb]

- JE vaccine should be given in all areas where JE constitutes a public health problem.

- Vaccine options - Three types of vaccines are available: (1) a cell culture-based live attenuated, (2) a cell culture-based inactivated and (3) an inactivated mouse brain-derived. The WHO position paper provides recommendations for the mouse brain-derived and live attenuated vaccines.

- Booster - If administering cell-culture based live-attenuated vaccine, a booster dose is currently recommended after an interval of one year, even though observational studies suggest long-term protection after a single dose. If using mouse brain-derived vaccine, a booster dose should be administered after an interval of one year then every 3 years until 10-15 years of age.

12 Yellow Fever

- Position paper reference: Weekly Epid. Record (2003, 78: 349-359) [pdf 339kb]

- Recommended for use in countries at risk of Yellow Fever.

- For convenience and improved coverage, Yellow Fever vaccine should be administered simultaneously with the measles containing vaccine, but in a separate syringe and at a different injection site.

- Yellow Fever vaccine should be offered to all travellers to and from at-risk areas, unless they belong to the group of individuals for whom Yellow Fever vaccination is contraindicated.

- Interference may occur between MMR and yellow fever vaccines if they are simultaneously administered to children < 2 years of age

- In addition to the introduction of Yellow Fever vaccine for routine childhood vaccination, WHO recommends the implementation of mass preventive vaccination campaigns to protect susceptible older age groups. In the event of limited resources, assessment of the degree of risk can help prioritize areas for mass preventive campaigns.

13 Tick-Borne Encephalitis (TBE)

- Position paper reference: Weekly Epid. Record (2011, 86: 241-256) [pdf 318kb]

- Since the incidence of tick-borne encephalitis may vary considerably between and even within geographical regions, public immunization strategies should be based on risk assessments conducted at country, regional or district level, and they should be appropriate to the local endemic situation. Therefore, establishing case reporting of the disease is essential before deciding on the most appropriate preventive measures to be taken.

- In areas where the disease is highly endemic (that is, where the average prevaccination incidence of clinical disease is ≥5 cases/100 000 population per year), implying that there is a high individual risk of infection, WHO recommends that vaccination be offered to all age groups, including children.

- Because the disease tends to be more serious in individuals aged >50-60 years this age group constitutes an important target for immunization.

- Where the prevaccination incidence of the disease is moderate or low (that is, the annual average during a 5-year period is <5/100 000) or is limited to particular geographical locations or certain outdoor activities, immunization should target individuals in the most severely affected cohorts.

- People travelling from non-endemic areas to endemic areas should be offered vaccination if their visits will include extensive outdoor activities.

- Vaccination against the disease requires a primary series of 3 doses; those who will continue to be at risk should probably have ≥1 booster doses.

- Within the considerable range of acceptable dose intervals, the relevant national authorities should select the most national primary schedule for their national, regional or district immunization programmes.

- Although there is a strong indication that the spacing of boosters could be expanded considerably from the intervals currently recommended by the manufacturers (every 3-5 years), the evidence is still insufficient for a definitive recommendation on the optimal frequency and number of booster doses. Countries should therefore continue to recommend the use of vaccines in accordance with local disease epidemiology and current schedules until more definitive information becomes available.

- For the vaccines manufactured in Austria and Germany (FSME-Immun and Encepur) that can be given starting from > 1year of age an interval of 1-3 months is recommended between the first 2 doses, and 5-12 months between the second and third doses. When rapid protection is required, for example for people who will be travelling to endemic areas, the interval between the first 2 doses may be reduced to 1-2 weeks.

- With the vaccines manufactured in the Russian Federation (TBE-Moscow and EnceVir) the recommended intervals are 1-7 months between the first 2 doses, and 12 months between the second and third doses. Booster doses are recommended every 3 years for those at continued risk of exposure.

- The currently recommended booster interval should be maintained until more data have been obtained on the duration of protection induced by the Russian vaccines.

- Regardless of the duration of the delay, interrupted schedules should be resumed without repeating previous doses.

Table 1: *Recommended Routine Immunization (updated: 15 November 2012)*

Appendix M

14 Typhoid

- Position paper reference: Weekly Epid. Record (2008, 83: 49-59) [pdf 297kb]
- Recommended for school-age and/or preschool-age children in areas where typhoid fever in these age groups is shown to be a significant public health problem, particularly where antibiotic-resistant *S. Typhi* is prevalent.
- Vaccine options - Vi polysaccharide typhoid vaccine requires one parenterally administered dose which may be given after the age of 2 years; the liquid form of Ty21a live oral vaccine (for use in individuals from the age of 2 years) is no longer available; the capsule form of Ty21a (for use in individuals from the age of 5 years) requires 3 or 4 orally administered doses. See position paper for further details.
- Booster - In most endemic settings, a booster dose of the concerned vaccine 3 to 7 years after the primary immunization seems appropriate.

15 Cholera

- Position paper reference: Weekly Epid. Record (2010, 85: 117-128) [pdf 283kb]
- In cholera-endemic countries, vaccinating the entire population is not warranted. Rather, vaccination should be targeted at high-risk areas and population groups. The primary targets for cholera vaccination in many endemic areas are preschool-aged and school-aged children. Other groups that are especially vulnerable to severe disease and for which the vaccines are not contraindicated may also be targeted, such as pregnant women and HIV-infected individuals. Consider vaccinating older age groups if funding is available.
- Two types of oral cholera vaccines are available: (i) Dukoral (WC-rBS) and (ii) Shanchol and mORCVAX. The live attenuated single-dose vaccine (CVD 103-HgR) is no longer produced. The injectable vaccine is still manufactured in a few countries but its use is not recommended mainly because of its limited efficacy and short duration of protection.
- Dukoral is not licensed for children < 2 years. Children aged 2-5 years should receive 3 doses ≥7 days apart (but not more than 6 weeks). Intake of food and drink should be avoided for 1 hour before and after vaccination. If the interval between doses is delayed >6 weeks, primary vaccination should be restarted. One booster dose is recommended every 6 months, and if the interval between primary immunization, and the booster is >6 months, primary immunization must be restarted.
- Adults and children ≥6 years should receive 2 doses of Dukoral ≥ 7 days apart (but not more than 6 weeks). Intake of food and drink should be avoided for 1 hour before and after vaccination. If the interval between doses is delayed >6 weeks, primary vaccination should be restarted. A booster dose every 2 years is recommended. If the interval between the primary series and booster immunization is > 2 years, primary immunization must be repeated.
- Shanchol and mORCVAX: two liquid doses orally 14 days apart for individuals ≥1 year. A booster dose is recommended after 2 years.

16 Meningococcal

- Position paper reference: Weekly Epid. Record (2011, 86: 521-540) [pdf 1.1Mb] [Note: Updated position paper will be available in 2011).
- Conjugate vaccines are preferred over polysaccharide vaccines due to their potential for herd protection and their increased immunogenicity, particularly in children <2 years of age.
- Both conjugate and polysaccharide vaccines are efficacious and safe when used in pregnant women.
- Monovalent MenA conjugate vaccine should be given as one single intramuscular dose to individuals 1-29 years of age. The possible need for a booster is not yet established.
- For monovalent MenC conjugate vaccine one single intramuscular dose is recommended for children aged >12 months, teenagers and adults. Children 2-11 months require 2 doses administered at an interval of at least 2 months and a booster about 1 year after. If the primary series is interrupted, vaccination should be resumed without repeating the previous dose.
- Quadrivalent conjugate vaccines (A,C,W135,Y-D and A,C,W135,Y-CRM) should be administered as one single intramuscular dose to individuals ≥ 2 years. A,C,W135,Y-D is also licensed for children 9-23 months of age, and given as a 2-dose series, 3 months apart beginning at age 9 months. If the primary series is interrupted, vaccination should be resumed without repeating the previous dose.
- Meningococcal polysaccharide vaccines are less, or not, immunogenic in children under 2 years of age.
- Meningococcal polysaccharide vaccines can be used for those > 2 years of age to control outbreaks in countries where limited economic resources or insufficient supply restrict the use of meningococcal conjugate vaccines. Polysaccharide vaccines should be administered to individuals > 2 years old as one single dose. One booster 3-5 years after the primary dose may be given to persons considered to be at a continued high risk of exposure, including some health workers. See position paper for details.

17 Hepatitis A

- Position paper reference: Weekly Epid. Record (2012, 87: 261-276) [pdf 1.24 Mb]
- Hepatitis A vaccination is recommended for inclusion in the national immunization schedule for children ≥ 1 year if indicated on the basis of incidence of acute hepatitis A, change in the endemicity from high to intermediate, and consideration of cost-effectiveness.
- In highly endemic countries almost all persons are asymptomatically infected with HAV in childhood, which effectively prevents clinical hepatitis A in adolescents and adults. In these countries, large-scale vaccination programmes are not recommended.
- Countries with improving socioeconomic status may rapidly move from high to intermediate endemicity. In these countries, a relatively large proportion of the adult population is susceptible to HAV and large-scale hepatitis A vaccination is likely to be cost-effective and therefore is encouraged.
- For individual health benefit targeted vaccination of high-risk groups should be considered in low and very low endemicity settings. Those at increased risk of hepatitis A include travelers to areas of intermediate or high endemicity, those requiring life-long treatment with blood products, men who have sex with men, workers in contact with non-human primates, and injection drug users. In addition, patients with chronic liver disease are at increased risk for fulminant hepatitis A and should be vaccinated.
- Inactivated HAV vaccine is licensed for intramuscular administration in a 2-dose schedule with the first dose given at the age of 1 year or older. The interval between the first and second dose is flexible (from 6 months up to 4-5 years) but is usually 6-18 months. Countries may consider a 1-dose schedule as this option seems comparable in terms of effectiveness, and is less expensive and easier to implement. However, in individuals at substantial risk of contracting hepatitis A and in immunocompromised individuals, a 2-dose schedule is preferred. Inactivated HAV vaccines produced by different manufacturers, including combined hepatitis A vaccines, are interchangeable. Apart from severe allergic reaction to the previous dose, there is no contraindication to their use. These vaccines can be co-administered simultaneously with other routine childhood vaccines, and should be considered for use in pregnant women at definite risk of HAV infection.
- Live attenuated HAV vaccine is administered as a single subcutaneous dose to those ≥ 1 year of age. Severe allergy to components included in the live attenuated hepatitis A vaccine is a contraindication to their use. As a rule, live vaccines should not be used in pregnancy or in severely immunocompromised patients. There is no information available on co-administration of live attenuated hepatitis A vaccines with other routinely used vaccines.

Table 1: Recommended Routine Immunization (updated: 15 November 2012)

Appendix N
WHO Routine Immunization Children

Appendix N

Table 2: Summary of WHO Position Papers - Recommended Routine Immunizations for Children

(updated 15 November 2012)

Antigen		Age of 1st Dose	Doses in Primary Series	Interval Between Doses			Booster Dose	Considerations (see footnotes for details)
				1st to 2nd	2nd to 3rd	3rd to 4th		
Recommendations for all children								
BCG [1]		As soon as possible after birth	1					Exceptions HIV
Hepatitis B [2]	Option 1	As soon as possible after birth (<24h)	3	4 weeks (min) with DTP1	4 weeks (min) with DTP3			Premature and low birth weight; Co-administration and combination vaccine
	Option 2	As soon as possible after birth (<24h)	4	4 weeks (min) with DTP1	4 weeks (min) with DTP2	4 weeks (min) with DTP3		High risk groups
Polio [3]	OPV	6 weeks (see footnote for birth dose)	3	4 weeks (min) with DTP2	4 weeks (min) with DTP3			OPV birth dose; Transmission and importation risk criteria
	IPV / OPV Sequential	8 weeks (IPV 1st)	1-2 IPV 2 OPV	4-8 weeks	4-8 weeks	4-8 weeks		IPV booster needed for early schedule
	IPV	8 weeks	3	4-8 weeks	4-8 weeks		1-6 years of age (see footnote)	Delayed/ interrupted schedule; Combination vaccine
DTP 4		6 weeks (min)	3	4 weeks (min) - 8 weeks	4 weeks (min) - 8 weeks		(see footnote)	Single dose if >12 months of age; Delayed/ interrupted schedule; Co-administration and combination vaccine
Haemophilus Influenzae type b [5]		6 weeks (min) with DTP1, 24 months (max)	3	4 weeks (min) with DTP2	4 weeks (min) with DTP3			
Pneumococcal (Conjugate) [6]	Option 1	6 weeks (min)	3	4 weeks (min)	4 weeks		(see footnote)	Vaccine options; Initiate before 6 months of age; Co-administration
	Option 2	6 weeks (min)	2	8 weeks (min)			9-15 months	HIV+ and preterm neonates booster
Rotavirus [7]	Rotarix	6 weeks (min) with DTP1	2	4 weeks (min) with DTP2				Vaccine options
	Rota Teq	6 weeks (min) with DTP1	3	4 weeks (min) - 10 weeks with DTP2	4 weeks (min) with DTP3			
Measles [8]		9 or 12 months (6 months min, see footnote)	2	4 weeks (min) (see footnote)				Combination vaccine; HIV early vaccination; Pregnancy
Rubella [9]		9 or 12 months with measles containing vaccine	1					Achieve and sustain 80% coverage; Combination vaccine and Co-administration; Pregnancy
HPV [10]		Quadrivalent: 9-13 years of age; Bivalent: 10-13 years of age	3	Quadrivalent: 2 mos (min 4 wks); Bivalent: 1 mos (max 2.5 mos)	Quadrivalent: 4 mos (min 12 wks); Bivalent: 5 mos			Vaccination of males for prevention of cervical cancer not recommended currently

Refer to: http://www.who.int/immunization/documents/positionpapers/ for table & position updates.

This table summarizes the WHO vaccination recommendations for children. The ages/intervals cited are for the development of country specific schedules and are not for health workers. National schedules should be based on local epidemiologic, programmatic, resource & policy considerations. While vaccines are universally recommended, some children may have contraindications to particular vaccines.

P.1 / 8

Appendix N

(updated 15 November 2012)

Table 2: Summary of WHO Position Papers – Recommended Routine Immunizations for Children

Antigen		Age of 1st Dose	Doses in Primary Series	Interval Between Doses			Booster Dose	Considerations (see footnotes for details)
				1st to 2nd	2nd to 3rd	3rd to 4th		
Recommendations for children residing in certain regions								
Japanese Encephalitis 11	Mouse-brain derived	1 year	2	4 weeks (min)			After 1 year and every 3 years up to 10-15 years of age	Vaccine options
	Live attenuated	9-12 months	1					
Yellow Fever 12		9-12 months with measles containing vaccine	1					Co-administration
Tick-Borne Encephalitis 13		≥ 1 yr FSME-Immun and Encepur; ≥ 3 yrs TBE-Moscow and EnceVir	3	1-3 months FSME-Immun and Encepur; 1-7 months TBE-Moscow and EnceVir	5-12 months FSME-Immun and Encepur; 12 months TBE-Moscow and EnceVir		At least 1; Every 3 years (see notes)	Definition of high-risk; Vaccine options; Timing of booster
Recommendations for children in some high-risk populations								
Typhoid 14	Vi PS	2 years (min)	1				Every 3 years	Definition of high risk
	Ty21a	Capsules 5 years (min) (see footnote)	3 or 4 (see footnote)	1 day	1 day	1 day	Every 3-7 years	Definition of high risk
Cholera 15	Dukoral (WC-rBS)	2 years (min)	3 (2-5 years); 2 (≥6 years)	≥ 7 days (min) < 6 weeks (max)	≥ 7 days (min) < 6 weeks (max)		Every 6 months; Every 2 years	Minimum age; Definition of high risk
	Shanchol and mORCVAX	1 year (min)	2	14 days			After 2 years	
Meningococcal 16	MenA conjugate	1-29 years	1					Definition of high risk; Vaccine options
		2-11 months	2	8 weeks				Definition of high risk; Vaccine options
	MenC conjugate	≥12 months	1				After 1 year	
	Quadrivalent conjugate	9-23 months	2	12 weeks				Definition of high risk; Vaccine options
		≥2 years	1					
Hepatitis A 17		1 year	At least 1					Level of endemicity; Vaccine options; Definition of high risk groups
Rabies 18		As required	3	7 days	14-21 days		(see footnote)	Definition of high risk, booster
Recommendations for children receiving vaccinations from immunization programmes with certain characteristics								
Mumps 19		12-18 months with measles containing vaccine	2	1 month (min) to school entry				Coverage criteria > 80%; Combo vaccine
Influenza (Inactivated) 20		6 months (min)	2 (<9 years); 1 (≥9 years)	1 month				Revaccinate annually; 1 dose only; Priority targets

P.2 / 8

Summary Table 2 - Notes

Refer to http://www.who.int/immunization/documents/positionpapers/ for the most recent version of the tables and position papers.

- The attached table summarizes the recommendations for vaccine administration found in the WHO position papers which are published in the Weekly Epidemiological Review. Its purpose is to assist planners to develop an appropriate immunization schedule. Health care workers should refer to their national immunization schedules. While vaccines are universally recommended, some children may have contraindications to particular vaccines.

- Vaccines can generally be co-administered (i.e., more than one vaccine given at different sites during the same visit). Recommendations that explicitly endorse co-administration are indicated in the table, however, lack of an explicit co-administration recommendation does not imply that the vaccine cannot be co-administered; further, there are no recommendations against co-administration.

- Doses administered by campaign may or may not contribute to a child's routine immunization schedule depending on type and purpose of campaign (e.g. supplemental versus routine/pulse campaign for access reasons).

- For some antigens, recommendations for the age of initiation of primary immunization series and/or booster doses are not available. Instead, the criteria for age at first dose must be determined from local epidemiologic data.

- If a catch-up schedule for interrupted immunization is available, it is noted in the footnotes.

- Other vaccines, such as varicella and pneumococcal polysaccharide vaccines, may be of individual benefit but have not been generally recommended for routine immunization. See the specific position papers for more details.

- For further background on immunization schedules refer to "Immunological Basis for Immunization" series which is available at: http://www.who.int/immunization/documents/immunological_basis_series/en/index.html

¹ BCG

- Position paper reference: Weekly Epid. Record (2004, 79: 27-38) [pdf 468kb]
- Recommended for children living in countries with a high-disease burden and for high-risk children living in countries with low-disease burden. See position paper for details.
- While BCG vaccination is especially important in countries with significant HIV prevalence, children who are HIV positive or unknown HIV status with symptoms consistent with HIV should not be vaccinated. Reference: Weekly Epid. Record (2007, 82: 193-196) [pdf 167kb]

² Hepatitis B

- Position paper reference: Weekly Epid. Record (2009, 84: 405-420) [pdf 830kb]
- Since perinatal or early postnatal transmission is an important cause of chronic infections globally, all infants should receive their first dose of hepatitis B vaccine as soon as possible (<24 hours) after birth even in low-endemicity countries.
- The primary hepatitis B immunization series conventionally consists of 3 doses of vaccine (1 monovalent birth dose followed by 2 monovalent or combined vaccine doses at the time of DTP1 and DTP3 vaccine doses). However, 4 doses may be given for programmatic reasons (e.g. 1 monovalent birth-dose followed by 3 monovalent or combined vaccine doses with DTP vaccine doses), according to the schedules of national routine immunization programmes.
- Premature low birth weight (<2000g) infants may not respond well to vaccination at birth. However, by 1 month of chronological age, premature infants, regardless of their initial weight or gestational age at birth, are likely to respond adequately. Therefore, doses given to infants <2000g should not be counted towards the primary series.
- Additional target groups for vaccination include people with risk factors for acquiring HBV infection, such as those who frequently require blood or blood products, dialysis patients, recipients of solid organ transplantations, people interned in prisons, injecting drug users, household and sexual contacts of people with chronic HBV infection, people with multiple sexual partners, as well as health-care workers and others who may be exposed to blood and blood products through their work.

Reference: Weekly Epid. Record (2010, 85: 213-228) [pdf 815.1kb]

³ Polio

- The primary series of 3 OPV vaccinations should be administered according to the respective national immunization schedule, for example at 6, 10 and 14 weeks, or 2, 4, and 6 months of age. The interval between doses should be at least 4 weeks.

- Where the potential for poliovirus importation is very high (i.e. in countries bordering endemic countries or countries that have recurrent outbreaks) or high (i.e. country with a history of DTP3 coverage plus high traffic across the border), and the transmission potential high (e.g. <90% DTP3 coverage, low socio-economic status, majority of areas with open sewage) of moderate (e.g. <90% DTP3 coverage, all states/provinces with moderate socio-economic status, only secondary sewage treatment), an OPV birth dose should be given as soon as possible after birth.

- OPV alone, including a birth dose, is recommended in all polio-endemic countries and those at high risk for importation and subsequent spread. A birth dose is not considered necessary in countries where the risk of polio virus transmission is low, even if the potential for importation is high/very high.

- Where the risk of wild polio virus importation is high/very high, the transmission potential should be low (>90-95% DTP3 coverage, high socio-economic status, tertiary sewage treatment) before alternatives to OPV alone may be considered.

- In countries with very high risk of wild polio virus importation, a sequential IPV/OPV schedule should not be introduced unless immunization coverage is approximately 95%, or, with low importation risk, approximately 90%. Where sequential IPV/OPV is used, the initial administration of 1 or 2 doses of IPV should be followed by 2 or more doses of OPV to ensure both sufficient levels of protection in the intestinal mucosa and a decrease in the burden of vaccine-associated paralytic poliomyelitis (VAPP). For IPV/OPV sequential schedules, WHO recommends that IPV be administered at 2 months of age (e.g. an IPV-OPV-OPV schedule) or at 2 months and 3-4 months of age (e.g. a 4-dose schedule of IPV-IPV-OPV-OPV). Each dose of the primary series, whether IPV or OPV, should be separated by an interval of 4-8 weeks, depending on the risk of exposure to polio in early childhood.

- IPV alone can be considered as an alternative to OPV alone (or an IPV/OPV sequential schedule) only in countries with the lowest risk of both wild polio importation and WPV transmission. IPV may be offered as a component of combination vaccines. A primary series of 3 IPV doses should be administered beginning at 2 months of age. If the primary series begins earlier (e.g. with a 6, 10, and 14 week schedule), then a booster dose should be administered with an interval of at least 6 months (4-dose IPV schedule).

- Switching from OPV to IPV for routine vaccination during the pre-eradication era is not cost-effective based on the existing economic analyses and current IPV costs.

⁴ DTP (Diphtheria, Tetanus and Pertussis)

- Position paper reference: Diphtheria - Weekly Epid. Record (2006, 81: 24-32) [pdf 214kb]; Tetanus - Weekly Epid. Record (2006, 81: 198-208) [pdf 229kb]; Pertussis - Weekly Epid. Record (2010, 85: 385-400) [pdf 320kb]

- Recommended for three doses during the first year of life. In areas where pertussis is of particular risk to young infants, DTP should be started at 6 weeks with 2 subsequent doses at intervals of 4-8 weeks each. The last dose of the primary series should be completed by the

Table 2: Recommended Routine Immunization for Children (updated 15 November 2012)

Appendix N

age of 6 months.

- The duration of immunological protection will be extended in many instances if an additional booster is given later.
- Diphtheria booster – to compensate for the loss of natural diphtheria boosting in some areas, childhood boosters should be given. The optimal timing of and number of diphtheria-containing booster doses should be based on epidemiological surveillance as well as on immunological and programmatic considerations.
- Tetanus toxoid containing booster – A childhood tetanus immunization schedule of 5 doses is recommended. Boosters are ideally administered in early childhood and during adolescence e.g. 12–15 years. Tetanus booster doses may use either DTP or Td vaccines depending on the child's age. Td should be used for tetanus and diphtheria booster doses after the age of 7 years.
- Pertussis vaccine: Neo-natal immunization, and vaccination of pregnant women and household contacts ("cocooning") against pertussis is not recommended by WHO.
- Both acellular (aP) and whole cell pertussis (wP) containing vaccines have excellent safety records, and protection against severe pertussis in infancy and early childhood can be obtained with wP and aP vaccine. Changing among or within the wP and aP vaccine groups is unlikely to interfere with the safety or immunogenicity of these vaccines.
- Only aP-containing vaccines should be used for vaccination of those >6 years.
- Pertussis containing booster – A booster dose is recommended for children age 1-6 years, preferably during the second year of life. The booster should be given > 6 months after the last primary dose. Completion of this schedule (primary series plus booster) is expected to ensure protection against pertussis for > 6 years.
- Delayed or interrupted DTP series – Children 1–7 years or older who have not previously been immunized should receive three doses of wP or aP vaccine, with an interval of 2 months between the first and second dose and an interval of 6-12 months between the second and third. Children whose vaccination series has been interrupted should have their series resumed, without repeating previous doses. For unvaccinated individuals 7 years of age and older, Td combination vaccine can be administered, 2 doses 1-2 months apart and a third dose after 6-12 months can be used with subsequent boosters at least 1 year apart for a total of 5 appropriately spaced doses to obtain same long term protection. See position paper for details of interrupted immunization schedules.

⁵ *Haemophilus influenzae* type b (Hib)

- Position paper reference: Weekly Epid. Record (2006, 81: 210-520) [pdf 209kb]
- Immunization should start as early as possible after the age of 6 weeks.
- The 3-dose primary series is given at the same time as the DTP primary series often in combination vaccines.
- The vaccine is not generally offered to children aged >24 months owing to the limited burden of Hib disease among children older than that age.
- Delayed series – If a child 12-24 months of age has not received their primary vaccination series, a single dose of the vaccine is sufficient.
- Booster dose may be administered to children aged between 12-18 months although there is no WHO recommendation on this yet.

⁶ Pneumococcal (Conjugate)

- Position paper reference: Weekly Epid. Record (2012, 87: 129-143) [pdf 1.04 Mb]
- Pneumococcal conjugate vaccines (PCVs) are considered safe in all target groups for vaccination, also in immunocompromised individuals. The vaccines are not currently licensed for use in age groups that include women of childbearing age. Although theoretically highly unlikely to be harmful, there is no information on the safety of PCV10 and PCV13 during pregnancy.
- Except for very rare anaphylactic reactions that may follow the administration of any medicine, there are no contraindications to the use of these vaccines. However, it is advisable to defer vaccination until after an acute infection with temperature >39 °C.
- When injected at different sites, PCVs can be administered concurrently with any other vaccines in infant immunization programmes.
- When primary immunization is initiated with one of these vaccines, it is recommended that remaining doses are administered with the same product. Interchangeability between PCV10 and PCV13 has not yet been documented. However, if it is not possible to complete the series with the same type of vaccine, the other PCV product should be used.
- For infants, 3 primary doses (the 3p+0 schedule) or, as an alternative, 2 primary doses plus a booster (the 2p+1 schedule).
- In choosing between the 3p+0 and 2p+1 schedules, countries should consider locally relevant factors including the epidemiology of pneumococcal disease, the likely coverage, and the timeliness of the vaccine doses.
- If disease incidence peaks in young infants (<32 weeks of age), a 2p+1 schedule might not offer optimal individual protection for certain serotypes (e.g. 6B, 23F) compared to a 3p+0 schedule, particularly in the absence of herd protection.
- In contrast, higher antibody levels are induced by the third (booster) dose in a 2p+1 schedule compared to the third dose in a 3p+0 schedule. This may be important for duration of protection or effectiveness against some serotypes.
- If the 3p+0 schedule is used, vaccination can be initiated as early as 6 weeks of age with an interval between doses of 4–8 weeks, depending on programmatic convenience.
- If the 2p+1 schedule is selected, the 2 primary doses should ideally be completed by six months of age, starting as early as 6 weeks of age with a minimum interval of 8 weeks or more between the two doses (for infants aged ≥7 months a minimum interval of 4 weeks between doses is possible). One booster dose should be given between 9–15 months of age.
- Previously unvaccinated or incompletely vaccinated children (including those who had laboratory confirmed invasive pneumococcal disease) should be vaccinated using the recommended age-appropriate regimens. Interrupted schedules should be resumed without repeating the previous dose.
- HIV-positive infants and pre-term neonates who have received their 3 primary vaccine doses before reaching 12 months of age may benefit from a booster dose in the second year of life.
- Catch-up vaccination as part of introduction will accelerate herd protection and therefore the PCV impact on disease and carriage. Maximized protection at the time of introduction of PCV10 or PCV13 can be achieved by providing 2 catch-up dose(s) at an interval of at least 8 weeks to unvaccinated children aged 12–24 months and to children aged 2–5 years who are at high risk of pneumococcal infection.
- Further data are needed from different epidemiological settings on the impact of large-scale PCV vaccination of individuals >50 years of age in order to establish the relative priority of immunization programmes in that age group. However, given the documented effects of herd protection in adult age groups following routine infant immunization with PCV7, higher priority should normally be given to introducing and maintaining high coverage of infants with PCVs.
- The use of pneumococcal vaccine should be seen as complementary to the use of other

Table 2: Recommended Routine Immunization for Children (updated 15 November 2012)

pneumonia control measures, such as appropriate case management, promotion of exclusive breastfeeding for first 6 months of life, and the reduction of known risk factors, such as indoor pollutants and tobacco smoke.

- For polysaccharide pneumococcal vaccine see position paper: Weekly Epid. Record (2008, 83: 373-384) [pdf 308kb]

- In resource-limited settings where there are many competing health priorities, evidence does not support routine immunization of the elderly and high-risk populations with PPV23. Also, because of the low level of evidence for benefit, routine PPV23 vaccination of HIV-infected adults is not recommended in such settings. In countries that do not routinely administer PPV23 to high-risk populations, data are insufficient to recommend introducing this vaccine to reduce the morbidity and mortality associated with influenza.

7 Rotavirus

- Position paper reference: Weekly Epid. Record (2009, 84: 533-540) [pdf 764kb]] NOTE: This position paper is currently being revised in light of the vaccination schedule recommendations made by SAGE at their April 2012 meeting Weekly Epid. Record (2012, 87: 201-216) [pdf 1.11Mb]

- Recommended to be included in all national immunization programmes.

- Rotarix vaccine is administered orally in a 2-dose schedule with the first and second doses of DTP.

- RotaTeq requires an oral 3-dose schedule with DTP1, DTP2, and DTP3 with an interval of 4-10 weeks between doses.

- First dose of either RotaTeq or Rotarix be administered as soon as possible from 6 weeks of age.

- The interchangeability of the current rotavirus vaccines is unknown.

- In various settings, rotavirus vaccines have been found not to interfere significantly with the immunogenicity or safety of OPV or other childhood vaccines.

- The use of rotavirus vaccines should be part of a comprehensive strategy to control diarrhoeal diseases and should include, among other interventions, improvements in hygiene and sanitation, zinc supplementation, community-based administration of oral rehydration solution and overall improvements in case management.

8 Measles

- Position paper reference: Weekly Epid. Record (2009, 84: 349-360) [pdf 724kb]

- Reaching all children with two doses of measles containing vaccine (MCV) should be the standard for all national immunization programmes.

- Delivery of the second dose (MCV2) may occur either at a scheduled age through routine services or periodically through mass campaigns, depending on which strategy achieves the higher coverage. A MCV2 dose may be added to the routine immunization schedule in countries that have achieved > 80% coverage of measles first dose (MCV1) at the national level for 3 consecutive years as determined by the most accurate means available (e.g. survey or WHO/UNICEF estimates). In general, countries that do not meet this criterion should prioritize improving MCV1 coverage and conducting high-quality follow-up SIAs, rather than adding MCV2 to their routine schedule.

- In countries with ongoing transmission in which the risk of measles mortality remains high, MCV1 should be given at age 9 months. MCV2 should be given between 15-18 months, as providing MCV2 in the 2nd year of life reduces the rate of accumulation of susceptible children and the risk of an outbreak.

- In countries with low rates of measles transmission (that is, those that are near elimination) and where there is a low risk of measles infection among infants, the first dose may be administered at age 12 months to take advantage of the higher seroconversion rates achieved at this age (>90% seroconversion). In these countries the optimal age for delivering a routine 2nd dose of measles is based on programmatic considerations that achieve the highest coverage and hence the highest population immunity. Administration of the second dose at age 15-18 months ensures early protection of the individual, slows accumulation of susceptible young children and may correspond with other routine immunizations (for example, DTP booster). If first dose coverage is high (>90%) and school enrolment is high (>95%), giving the second dose at school entry may be an effective strategy for achieving high coverage and preventing outbreaks in schools.

- Combined vaccines (Measles and Rubella or Measles, Mumps and Rubella) may not be optimal for use in countries where vaccine coverage for measles vaccine of at least 80% cannot be achieved or maintained.

- Measles vaccination should be routinely administered to potentially susceptible, asymptomatic HIV-positive children and adults. In areas where there is a high incidence of both HIV infection and measles, MCV1 may be offered as early as age 6 months. Two additional doses of measles vaccine should be administered to these children according to the national immunization schedule.

- Mild, concurrent infections are not considered a contraindication to vaccination, but it should be avoided if the patient has a high fever or other signs of serious disease. Theoretically, measles vaccine – alone or in combination with other vaccines – should also be avoided by pregnant women. Furthermore, measles vaccination is contraindicated in people who are severely immunocompromised due to congenital disease; severe HIV infection; advanced leukaemia or lymphoma, etc.

9 Rubella

- Position paper reference: Weekly Epid. Record (2011, 86: 301-316) [pdf 413kb]

- All countries that have not yet introduced rubella vaccine, and are providing 2 doses of measles vaccine using routine immunization, or SIAs, or both, should consider including rubella containing vaccines (RCVs) in their immunization programme. Countries planning to introduce RCVs should review the epidemiology of rubella, including the susceptibility profile of the population; assess the burden of CRS; and establish rubella and CRS prevention as a public health priority.

- Because rubella is not as highly infectious as measles and because the effectiveness of 1 dose of an RCV is > 95%, even at 9 months of age, only 1 dose of rubella vaccine is required to achieve rubella elimination if high coverage is achieved. However, when combined with measles vaccination, it may be easier to implement a second dose of RCV's using the same combined MR vaccine or MMR vaccine for both doses.

- There are two general approaches to the use of rubella vaccine: (i) exclusive focus on reducing CRS by immunizing adolescent girls or women of childbearing age, or both groups, to provide individual protection; (ii) focus on interrupting transmission of rubella virus and eliminating rubella and CRS, by introducing rubella vaccination into the routine childhood immunization schedule combined with the vaccination of older age groups who are susceptible to rubella.

- To avoid the potential of an increased risk of CRS, countries should achieve and maintain immunization coverage of 80% or greater with at least 1 dose of an RCV delivered through routine services or regular campaigns, or both.

- The first dose of RCV can be delivered at 9 or 12 months depending on the measles vaccination schedule.

- RCVs can be administered concurrently with inactivated vaccines. As a general rule, live vaccines should be given either simultaneously with RCV's, or at least 4 weeks apart. An exception to this is oral polio vaccine, which can be given at any time before or after RCV's without interfering in the response to either vaccine. Interference may occur between MMR and yellow fever vaccines

Table 2: Recommended Routine Immunization for Children (updated 15 November 2012)

Appendix N

- If they are simultaneously administered to children < 2 years of age.
- Because of a theoretical, but never demonstrated, teratogenic risk rubella vaccination in pregnant women should be avoided in principle, and those planning a pregnancy are advised to avoid pregnancy for 1 month following vaccination.
- Administration of blood or blood products before or shortly after vaccination may interfere with vaccine efficacy. If using only rubella vaccines persons who received blood products should wait at least 3 months before vaccination and, if possible, blood products should be avoided for up to 2 weeks postvaccination. Vaccinated persons are not eligible to donate blood for 1 month after vaccination.

10 Human Papillomavirus (HPV)

- Position paper reference: Weekly Epid. Record (2009, 84: 118-131) [pdf 267kb]
- Two vaccines are currently available. Quadrivalent (HPV types 6,11,16 and 18) licensed for use in females as young as 9 years of age to prevent cervical precancers and cancers. In addition, the quadrivalent vaccine is licensed for prevention of vulvar and vaginal precancers and cancers as well as anogenital warts in females. In some countries, the vaccine is also licensed for the prevention of anogenital warts in males. Bivalent (HPV types 16 and 18) has been licensed for use in females as young as 10 years of age to prevent cervical precancers and cancers.
- Both vaccines are intended for females before the onset of sexual activity, i.e. before first exposure to HPV infection. A three-dose schedule is recommended. The quadrivalent is given at baseline and after 2 and 6 months. A minimum interval of 4 weeks between the first and second dose, and a minimum interval between the second and third doses of 12 weeks is recommended by the manufacturer. The bivalent vaccine is given at baseline and after 1 and 6 months. If flexibility in the schedule is necessary the manufacturer recommends that the second dose is administered between 1 and 2.5 months after the first dose.
- For both vaccines alternative schedules are being explored. Restarting the 3-dose series is not necessary if interrupted, but remaining doses should be administered as close to the schedule intervals as possible.
- Currently, the manufacturers do not recommend any booster dose following completion of the primary series.
- HPV vaccination of males for prevention of cervical cancer is not recommended at this time because vaccination strategies that achieve high coverage (>70%) in the primary target population of young adolescent girls are expected to be more cost-effective in reducing cervical cancer than including vaccination of males.

11 Japanese Encephalitis (JE)

- Position paper reference: Weekly Epid. Record (2006, 81: 331-340) [pdf 192kb]
- JE vaccine should be given in all areas where JE constitutes a public health problem.
- Vaccine options – Three types of vaccines are available: (1) a cell culture-based live attenuated, (2) a cell culture-based inactivated and (3) an inactivated mouse brain-derived. The WHO position paper provides recommendations for the mouse brain-derived and live attenuated vaccines.
- Booster - If administering cell culture-based live-attenuated vaccine, a booster dose is currently recommended after a single dose. If using mouse brain-derived vaccine, a booster dose should be administered after an interval of one year then every 3 years until 10-15 years of age.

12 Yellow Fever

- Position paper reference: Weekly Epid. Record (2003, 78: 349-359) [pdf 339kb]
- Recommended for use in countries at risk of Yellow Fever.
- For convenience and improved coverage, Yellow Fever vaccine should be administered simultaneously with the measles containing vaccine, but in a separate syringe and at a different injection site.
- Yellow Fever vaccine should be offered to all travellers to and from at-risk areas, unless they belong to the group of individuals for whom Yellow Fever vaccination is contraindicated.
- Interference may occur between MMR and yellow fever vaccines if they are simultaneously administered to children < 2 years of age
- In addition to the introduction of Yellow Fever vaccine for routine childhood vaccination, WHO recommends the implementation of mass preventive vaccination campaigns to protect susceptible older age groups. In the event of limited resources, assessment of the degree of risk can help prioritize areas for mass preventive campaigns.

13 Tick-Borne Encephalitis (TBE)

- Position paper reference: Weekly Epid. Record (2011, 86: 241-256) [pdf 318kb]
- Since the incidence of tick-borne encephalitis may vary considerably between and even within geographical regions, public immunization strategies should be based on risk assessments conducted at country, regional or district level, and they should be appropriate to the local endemic situation. Therefore, establishing case reporting of the disease is essential before deciding on the most appropriate preventive measures to be taken.
- In areas where the disease is highly endemic (that is, where the average prevaccination incidence of clinical disease is ≥5 cases/100 000 population per year), implying that there is a high individual risk of infection, WHO recommends that vaccination be offered to all age groups, including children.
- Because the disease tends to be more serious in individuals aged >50–60 years this age group constitutes an important target for immunization.
- Where the prevaccination incidence of the disease is moderate or low (that is, the annual average during a 5-year period is <5/100 000) or is limited to particular geographical locations or certain outdoor activities, immunization should target individuals in the most severely affected cohorts.
- People travelling from non-endemic areas to endemic areas should be offered vaccination if their visits will include extensive outdoor activities.
- Vaccination against the disease requires a primary series of 3 doses; those who will continue to be at risk should probably have ≥1 booster doses.
- Within the considerable range of acceptable dose intervals, the relevant national authorities should select the most rational primary schedule for their national, regional or district immunization programmes.
- Although there is a strong indication that the spacing of boosters could be expanded considerably from the intervals currently recommended by the manufacturers (every 3–5 years), the evidence is still insufficient for a definitive recommendation on the optimal frequency and number of booster doses. Countries should therefore continue to recommend the use of vaccines in accordance with local disease epidemiology and current schedules until more definitive information becomes available.
- For the vaccines manufactured in Austria and Germany (FSME-Immun and Encepur) that can be given starting from > 1year of age an interval of 1–3 months is recommended between the first 2 doses, and 5–12 months between the second and third doses. When rapid protection is required, for example for people who will be travelling to endemic areas, the interval between the first 2 doses may be reduced to 1–2 weeks.
- With the vaccines manufactured in the Russian Federation (TBE-Moscow and EnceVir) the recommended intervals are 1–7 months between the first 2 doses, and 12 months between the second and third doses. Booster doses are recommended every 3 years for those at continued risk of exposure.

Table 2: Recommended Routine Immunization for Children (updated 15 November 2012)

- The currently recommended booster interval should be maintained until more data have been obtained on the duration of protection induced by the Russian vaccines.
- Regardless of the duration of the delay, interrupted schedules should be resumed without repeating previous doses.

14 Typhoid

Position paper reference: Weekly Epid. Record (2008, 83: 49-59) [pdf 297kb]

- Recommended for school-age and/or preschool-age children in areas where typhoid fever in these age groups is shown to be a significant public health problem, particularly where antibiotic-resistant *S. Typhi* is prevalent.
- Vaccine options - Vi polysaccharide typhoid vaccine requires one parenterally administered dose which may be given after the age of 2 years; the liquid form of Ty21a live oral vaccine (for use in individuals from the age of 5 years) is no longer available; the capsule form of Ty21a (for use in individuals from the age of 5 years) requires 3 or 4 orally administered doses. See position paper for further details.
- Booster - In most endemic settings, a booster dose of the concerned vaccine 3 to 7 years after the primary immunization seems appropriate.

15 Cholera

Position paper reference: Weekly Epid. Record (2010, 85, 117-128) [pdf 283kb]

- In cholera-endemic countries, vaccinating the entire population is not warranted. Rather, vaccination should be targeted at high-risk areas and population groups. The primary targets for cholera vaccination in many endemic areas are preschool-aged and school aged children. Other groups that are especially vulnerable to severe disease and for which the vaccines are not contraindicated may also be targeted, such as pregnant women and HIV-infected individuals. Consider vaccinating older age groups if funding is available.
- Two types of oral cholera vaccines are available: (i) Dukoral (WC-rBS) and (ii) Shanchol and mORCVAX. The live attenuated single-dose vaccine (CVD 103-HgR) is no longer produced. The injectable vaccine is still manufactured in a few countries but its use is not recommended mainly because of its limited efficacy and short duration of protection.
- Dukoral is not licensed for children < 2 years. Children aged 2-5 years should receive 3 doses ≥7 days apart (but not more than 6 weeks). Intake of food and drink should be avoided for 1 hour before and after vaccination. If the interval between doses is delayed >6 weeks, primary vaccination should be restarted. One booster dose is recommended every 6 months, and if the interval between primary immunization, and the booster dose is >6 months, primary immunization must be restarted.
- Adults and children ≥6 years should receive 2 doses of Dukoral ≥7 days apart (but not more than 6 weeks). Intake of food and drink should be avoided for 1 hour before and after vaccination. If the interval between doses is delayed >6 weeks, primary vaccination should be restarted. A booster dose every 2 years is recommended. If the interval between the primary series and booster immunization is > 2 years, primary immunization must be repeated.
- Shanchol and mORCVAX: two liquid doses orally 14 days apart for individuals ≥1 year. A booster dose is recommended after 2 years.

16 Meningococcal

Position paper reference: Weekly Epid. Record (2011, 86: 521-540) [pdf 1.1Mb] (Note: Updated position paper will be available in 2011).

- Conjugate vaccines are preferred over polysaccharide vaccines due to their potential for herd protection and their increased immunogenicity, particularly in children <2 years of age.
- Both conjugate and polysaccharide vaccines are efficacious and safe when used in pregnant women.
- Monovalent MenA conjugate vaccine should be given as one single intramuscular dose to individuals 1-29 years of age. The possible need for a booster is not yet established.
- For monovalent MenC conjugate vaccine one single intramuscular dose is recommended for children aged >12 months, teenagers and adults. Children 2-11 months require 2 doses administered at an interval of at least 2 months and a booster about 1 year after. If the primary series is interrupted, vaccination should be resumed without repeating the previous dose.
- Quadrivalent conjugate vaccines (A,C,W135,Y-D and A,C,W135,Y-CRM) should be administered as one single intramuscular dose to individuals > 2 years. A,C,W135,Y-D is also licensed for children 9-23 months of age, and given as a 2-dose series, 3 months apart beginning at age 9 months. If the primary series is interrupted, vaccination should be resumed without repeating the previous dose.
- Meningococcal polysaccharide vaccines are less, or not, immunogenic in children under 2 years of age.
- Meningococcal polysaccharide vaccines can be used for those > 2 years of age to control outbreaks in countries where limited economic resources or insufficient supply restrict the use of meningococcal conjugate vaccines. Polysaccharide vaccines should be administered to individuals ≥ 2 years old as one single dose. One booster 3-5 years after the primary dose may be given to persons considered to be at continued high risk of exposure, including some health workers. See position paper for details.

17 Hepatitis A

Position paper reference: Weekly Epid. Record (2012, 87: 261-276) [pdf 1.24 Mb]

- Hepatitis A vaccination is recommended for inclusion in the national immunization schedule for children ≥ 1 year if indicated on the basis of incidence of acute hepatitis A, change in the endemicity from high to intermediate, and consideration of cost-effectiveness.
- In highly endemic countries almost all persons are asymptomatically infected with HAV in childhood, which effectively prevents clinical hepatitis A in adolescents and adults. In these countries, large-scale vaccination programmes are not recommended.
- Countries with improving socioeconomic status may rapidly move from high to intermediate endemicity. In these countries, a relatively large proportion of the adult population is susceptible to HAV and large-scale hepatitis A vaccination is likely to be cost-effective and therefore is encouraged.
- For individual health benefit targeted vaccination of high-risk groups should be considered in low and very low endemicity settings. Those at increased risk of hepatitis A include travelers to areas of intermediate or high endemicity, those requiring life-long treatment with blood products, men who have sex with men, workers in contact with non-human primates, and injection drug users. In addition, patients with chronic liver disease are at increased risk for fulminant hepatitis A and should be vaccinated.
- Inactivated HAV vaccine is licensed for intramuscular administration in a 2-dose schedule with the first dose given at the age of 1 year or older. The interval between the first and second dose is flexible (from 6 months up to 4-5 years) but is usually 6-18 months. Countries may consider a 1-dose schedule as this option seems comparable in terms of effectiveness, and is less expensive and easier to implement. However, in individuals at substantial risk of contracting hepatitis A and in immunocompromised individuals, a 2-dose schedule is preferred. Inactivated HAV vaccines produced by different manufacturers, including combined hepatitis A vaccines, are interchangeable. Apart from severe allergic reaction to the previous dose, there is no contraindication to their use. These vaccines can be co-administered simultaneously with other routine childhood vaccines, and should be considered for use in pregnant women at definite risk

Table 2: Recommended Routine Immunization for Children (updated 15 November 2012)

of HAV infection.

- Live attenuated HAV vaccine is administered as a single subcutaneous dose to those ≥ 1 year of age. Severe allergy to components included in the live attenuated hepatitis A vaccine is a contraindication to their use. As a rule, live vaccines should not be used in pregnancy or in severely immunocompromised patients. There is no information available on co-administration of live attenuated hepatitis A vaccines with other routinely used vaccines.
- Vaccination against hepatitis A should be part of a comprehensive plan for the prevention and control of viral hepatitis, including measures to improve hygiene and sanitation and measures for outbreak control.

18 Rabies

- Position paper reference: Weekly Epid. Record (2010, 85: 309-320) [pdf 370]
- Production and use of nerve-tissue rabies vaccines should be discontinued and replaced with cell-culture-based vaccines (CCVs).
- Recommended for anyone who will be at continual, frequent or increased risk of exposure to the rabies virus, either as a result of their residence or occupation. Travellers with extensive outdoor exposure in rural high-risk areas where immediate access to appropriate medical care may be limited should also be vaccinated regardless of the duration of stay. Where canine rabies is a public health problem, WHO encourages studies on the feasibility, cost-effectiveness, and long-term impact of incorporating rabies vaccination into the immunization programme for infants and children.
- The series is given by intramuscular or intradermal injection at 0, 7 and 21 or 28 days.
- Intramuscular administration: For adults and children aged ≥2 years, the vaccine should always be administered in the deltoid area of the arm; for children aged < 2 years, the anterolateral area of the thigh is recommended. Rabies vaccine should not be administered in the gluteal area, as the induction of an adequate immune response may be less reliable.
- Booster doses of rabies vaccines are not required for individuals living in or travelling to high-risk areas who have received a complete primary series of pre-exposure or post-exposure prophylaxis with a cell-culture-based rabies vaccine (CCV).
- Periodic booster injections are recommended only for people whose occupation puts them at continual or frequent risk of exposure. If available, antibody monitoring is preferred to the administration of routine boosters.
- Because vaccine-induced immunity persists in most cases for years, a booster is recommended only if rabies-virus neutralizing antibody titres fall to <0.5 IU/ml.
- Antibody testing should be done every 6 months for people at risk of laboratory exposure to high concentrations of live rabies virus, and every 2 years for professionals who are not at continual risk of exposure through their activities, such as certain categories of veterinarians and animal health officers.

19 Mumps

- Position paper reference: Weekly Epid. Record (2007, 82: 49-60) [pdf 311kb]
- Recommended for use in high performing immunization programs with the capacity to maintain coverage over 80% and where mumps reduction is a public health priority.
- If implemented, a combination vaccine of measles, mumps and rubella is recommended.

20 Seasonal Influenza (Inactivated Vaccine)

- Position paper reference: Weekly Epid. Record (2005, 33: 279-287) [pdf 220kb]
- The World Health Assembly recommended increased immunization coverage of high-risk groups including the elderly, in those countries where influenza vaccination policies exist (Reference: WHA56.19, 2003). See position paper for detailed description of high-risk groups.
- Dose - If a child under 9 years of age requires vaccination and has not previously received influenza vaccine, a two-dose series with doses one-month apart should be administered. Annual re-vaccination in all individuals and initial vaccination in individuals 9 years of age or older require only a single dose. Children aged 6-36 months should receive half the adult dose.

Table 2: Recommended Routine Immunization for Children (updated 15 November 2012)

Appendix O
WHO Delayed Routine Immunization

Table 3: Recommendations* for Interrupted or Delayed Routine Immunization – Summary of WHO Position Papers

(Updated 15 November 2012)

Antigen	Age of 1st Dose	Doses in Primary Series (min interval between doses)**	Interrupted primary series***	Doses for those who start vaccination late — If ≤ 12 months of age	Doses for those who start vaccination late — If > 12 months of age	Booster
Recommendations for all						
BCG [1]	As soon as possible after birth	1 dose	NA	1 dose	Not recommended	Not recommended
Hepatitis B [2]	As soon as possible after birth (<24h)	Birth dose <24 hrs plus 2-3 doses with DTP (4 weeks)	Resume without repeating previous dose	3 doses	3 doses	Not recommended
Polio [3] — OPV	6 weeks (see footnote for birth dose)	3 doses with DTP (4 weeks)	Resume without repeating previous dose	3 doses	3 doses	Not recommended
Polio [3] — IPV / OPV Sequential	8 weeks (IPV 1st)	1-2 doses IPV and 2 doses OPV (4 weeks)	Resume without repeating previous dose	1-2 doses IPV and 2 doses OPV	1-2 doses IPV and 2 doses OPV	If the primary series begins < 2 months of age, booster to be given at least 6 months after the last dose
Polio [3] — IPV	8 weeks	3 doses (4 weeks)	Resume without repeating previous dose	3 doses	3 doses	
DTP [4]	6 weeks (min)	3 doses (4 weeks)	Resume without repeating previous dose	3 doses	3 doses with interval of 2 months between 1st & 2nd dose, and 6-12 months between 2nd & 3rd dose (If > 5 yrs use only a P-containing vaccine; if > 7 yrs of age use Td containing vaccine)	DTP booster at 1-6 yrs of age (preferable in 2nd yr of life). Use DTaP if > 6 yrs and dTap if > 7 yrs. To booster in adolescence, and another in adulthood or pregnancy (for total of 6 doses if primary series started in childhood).
Haemophilus influenzae type b [5]	6 weeks (min)	3 doses with DTP (4 weeks)	Resume without repeating previous dose	3 doses	1-2 yrs: 1 dose >2 yrs: Not recommended	Not recommended
Pneumococcal (Conjugate) [6]	6 weeks (min)	3 doses with DTP (4 weeks) or 2 doses (8 weeks)	Resume without repeating previous dose	2-3 doses	1-2 yrs: 2 doses 2-5 yrs at high-risk: 2 doses	Booster at 9-15 months if following 2 dose schedule. Another booster if HIV+ or preterm neonate
Rotavirus [7] — Rotarix	6 weeks (min)	2 doses with DTP (4 weeks)	Resume without repeating previous dose	2 doses	> 24 months limited benefits	Not recommended
Rotavirus [7] — Rota Teq	6 weeks (min)	3 doses with DTP (4 weeks)	Resume without repeating previous dose	3 doses	> 24 months limited benefits	Not recommended
Measles [8]	9 or 12 months (6 months min, see footnote)	2 doses (4 weeks)	Resume without repeating previous dose	2 doses	2 doses	Not recommended
Rubella [9]	9 or 12 months	1 dose with measles containing vaccine	NA	1 dose	1 dose	Not recommended
HPV 10	9 or 10 years	3 doses (1st to 2nd 4 weeks; 2nd to 3rd 3 months for quadrivalent and 5 months for bivalent)	Resume without repeating previous dose	NA	Girls: 9-13 yrs: 3 doses	Not recommended

* For some antigens the WHO position paper does not provide a recommendation on interrupted or delayed schedules at this present time. When the position paper is next revised this will be included. In the meantime, some of the recommendations are based on expert opinion.
** See Table 2: Summary of WHO Position Papers - Recommended Routine Immunizations for Children for full details (www.who.int/immunization/documents/positionpapers/).
*** Same interval as primary series unless otherwise specified.

Appendix O

Table 3: Recommendations* for Interrupted or Delayed Routine Immunization Summary of WHO Position Papers
(Updated 15 November 2013)

Antigen		Age of 1st Dose	Dose in Primary Series (min interval between doses)**	Interrupted primary series***	Doses for those who start vaccination late — If ≤ 12 months of age	Doses for those who start vaccination late — If > 12 months of age	Booster Dose
Recommendations for children residing in certain regions							
Japanese Encephalitis 11	Mouse-brain derived	1 year	2 (4 weeks)	Resume without repeating previous dose	2 dose	2 dose	After 1 year and every 3 years up to 10-15 years of age
	Live attenuated	9-12 months	1 dose	NA		1 dose	After 1 year
Yellow Fever 12		9-12 months	1 dose with measles containing vaccine	NA		1 dose	Not recommended
Tick-Borne Encephalitis 13	FSME-Immun & Encepur	≥ 1 yr	3 doses (1st to 2nd 1-3 mos; 2nd to 3rd 12 mos)	Resume without repeating previous dose		3 doses	At least 1 booster
	TBE_Moscow & EnceVir	≥ 3 yr	3 doses (1st to 2nd 1-7 mos; 2nd to 3rd 12 mos)	Resume without repeating previous dose		3 doses	Every 3 years
Recommendations for children in some high-risk populations							
Typhoid 14	Vi PS	2 years (min)	1 dose	NA	Not recommended	1 dose	Every 3 years
	Ty21a	Capsules 5 years (min) (see footnote)	3-4 doses (1 day) (see footnote)	NA. If interruption between doses is ≤ 21 days resume without repeating previous dose. If > 21 days restart primary series	Not recommended	> 5 yrs: 3-4 doses	Every 3-7 years
Cholera 15	Dukoral (WC-rBS)	2 years (min)	2-5 yrs: 3 doses (≥ 6 yrs: 2 doses (≥ 7 days)	If interval since last dose ≥ 6 weeks restart primary series	Not recommended	2-5 yrs: 3 doses > 6 yrs: 2 doses	2-5 yrs: every 6 months. If booster is delayed > 6 months the primary series must be repeated. > 6 yrs: every 2 years. If booster is delayed > 2 yrs the primary series must be repeated.
	Shanchol and mORCVAX	1 year (min)	2 doses (2 weeks)	Resume without repeating previous dose	Not recommended	2 doses	After 2 years
Meningococcal 16	MenA conjugate	1-29 months	1	NA	Not recommended	1 dose	
	MenC conjugate	2-11 months	2 (8 weeks min)	Resume without repeating previous dose	2 doses	1 dose	2-11 months of age after 1 year
		>12 months	1	NA			
	Quadrivalent conjugate	9-23 months	2 (12 weeks min)	Resume without repeating previous dose	2 doses	1 dose	
		≥ 2 years	1	NA			
Hepatitis A 17		1 year (min)	At least 1 dose		Not recommended	At least 1 dose	Not recommended
Rabies 18		As required	3 doses (1st to 2nd 7 days; 2nd to 3rd 14-21 days)	Resume without repeating previous dose; interval between last two doses should be 14 days minimum	3 doses	3 doses	Only if occupation puts a frequent or continual risk of exposure
Recommendations for children receiving vaccinations from immunization programmes with certain characteristics							
Mumps 19		12-18 months	2 doses with measles containing vaccine (4 weeks)	Resume without repeating previous dose	Not recommended	2 doses	Not recommended
Influenza (Inactivated) 20		6 months (min)	< 9 yrs: 2 doses ≥ 9 yrs: 1 dose	Resume without repeating previous dose	2 doses	< 9 yrs: 2 doses > 9 yrs: 1 dose	Revaccinate annual 1 dose only

Summary Table 3 - Notes

- The attached table summarizes the WHO recommendations for interrupted or delayed routine vaccination. Its purpose is to assist national decision-makers and programme managers to develop appropriate policy guidance in relation to their national immunization schedule.

- This table is designed to be used together with two other summary tables - Table 1: Summary of WHO Position Papers - Recommendations for Routine Immunization; and Table 2: Summary of WHO Position Papers - Recommended Routine Immunization for Children.

- Vaccines can generally be co-administered (i.e. more than one vaccine given at different sites during the same visit). Recommendations that explicitly endorse co-administration are indicated in the footnotes. Lack of an explicit co-administration recommendation is often due to a lack of evidence and does not necessarily imply that the vaccine cannot be co-administered. Exceptions to co-administration are stated.

- Refer to http://www.who.int/immunization/positionpapers/ for the most recent version of this table (and Tables 1 and 2) and position papers.

1 BCG

- Position paper reference: Weekly Epid. Record (2004, 79: 22-38) [pdf 468kb]

- Expert opinion indicates that vaccination of children older than 12 months of age is usually of limited benefit (although it is not harmful or contraindicated).

- BCG vaccination of adolescents and adults has shown variation in protective efficacy with geographical region, possibly as a consequence of differences in previous exposure to environmental mycobacteria. See position paper for details.

- Infants who are HIV positive or unknown HIV status with symptoms consistent with HIV should not be vaccinated. Reference: Weekly Epid. Record (2007, 82: 193-196) [pdf 167kb]

2 Hepatitis B

- Position paper reference: Weekly Epid. Record (2009, 84: 405-420) [pdf 830kb]

- In general, the dose for infants and children (aged < 15 years) is half the recommended adult dose.

- Co-administration of HepB vaccine does not interfere with the immune response to any other vaccine and vice versa.

- Data on immunogenicity suggest that in any age group, interruption of the vaccination schedule does not require restarting the primary series. If the primary series is interrupted after the first dose, the second dose should be administered as soon as possible and the second and third doses separated by a minimum interval of 4 weeks; if only the third dose is delayed, it should be administered as soon as possible.

3 Polio

- Reference: Weekly Epid. Record (2010, 85: 213-228) [pdf 815.1kb]

- The primary series of 3 OPV vaccinations should be administered according to the respective national immunization schedule, for example at 6, 10 and 14 weeks, or 2, 4, and 6 months of age. The interval between doses should be at least 4 weeks.

- Where the potential for poliovirus importation is very high (i.e. countries bordering endemic countries, or in countries with recurrent outbreaks) or high (i.e. countries with a history of importation plus high traffic across the border), and the transmission potential high (e.g. <90% DTP3 coverage, low socio-economic status, majority of areas with open sewage) or moderate (e.g. <90% DTP3 coverage, all states/provinces with moderate socio-economic status, only secondary sewage treatment) an OPV birth dose should be given as soon as possible after birth.

- OPV alone, including a birth dose, is recommended in all polio-endemic countries and those at high risk for importation and subsequent spread. A birth dose is not considered necessary in countries where the risk of polio virus transmission is low, even if the potential for importation is high/very high.

- Where the risk of wild polio virus importation is high/very high, the transmission potential should be low (>90-95% DTP3 coverage, high socio-economic status, tertiary sewage treatment) before alternatives to OPV alone may be considered.

- In countries with very high risk of wild polio virus importation, a sequential IPV/OPV schedule should not be introduced unless immunization coverage is approximately 95%, or, with low importation risk, approximately 90%. Where sequential IPV/OPV is used, the initial administration of 1 or 2 doses of IPV should be followed by 2 or more doses of OPV to ensure both sufficient levels of protection in the intestinal mucosa and a decrease in the burden of VAPP. For IPV/OPV sequential schedules WHO recommends that IPV be administered at 2 months of age (e.g. an IPV-OPV-OPV schedule) or at 2 months and 3-4 months of age (e.g. a 4-dose schedule of IPV-IPV-OPV-OPV). Each dose of the primary series, whether IPV or OPV, should be separated by an interval of 4-8 weeks, depending on the risk of exposure to polio in early childhood.

- IPV alone can be considered as an alternative to OPV alone (or an IPV/OPV sequential schedule) only in countries with the lowest risk of both wild polio importation and WPV transmission. IPV may be offered as a component of combination vaccines. A primary series of 3 IPV doses should be administered beginning at 2 months of age. If the primary series begins earlier (e.g. with a 6, 10, and 14 week schedule) then a booster dose should be administered with an interval of at least 6 months (4- dose IPV schedule).

- Switching from OPV to IPV for routine vaccination during the pre-eradication era is not cost-effective based on the existing economic analyses and current IPV costs.

- Both IPV and OPV may be administered simultaneously with other vaccines in national childhood immunization programmes

4 DTP (Diphtheria, Tetanus and Pertussis)

- Position paper reference: Diphtheria - Weekly Epid. Record (2006, 81: 24-32) [pdf 214kb]; Tetanus - Weekly Epid. Record (2006, 81: 198-208) [pdf 229kb]; Pertussis - Weekly Epid. Record (2010, 85: 385-400) [pdf 320kb]

- WHO recommends that the primary series of 3 doses should be given in infancy (aged < 1 year). The exact timing of the booster should be flexible to take account of the most appropriate health service contacts in different countries. Ideally a DTP booster should be provided at 1-6 years of age. A Td booster should be provided in adolescence, and another in adulthood to further assure life-long protection against tetanus (a total of 6 doses when DTP primary series is given in infancy).

- Delayed or interrupted DTP series - For children 1-7 years or older who have not previously been immunized should receive three doses of wP or aP vaccine, with an interval of 2 months between the first and second dose and an interval of 6-12 months between the second and third. Children whose vaccination series has been interrupted should have their series resumed, without repeating previous doses. For unvaccinated individuals 7 years of age and older, Td combination vaccine can be administered, 2 doses 1-2 months apart and a third dose after 6-12 months can be used with subsequent boosters at least 1 year apart for a total of 5 appropriately spaced doses to obtain same long term protection. See position paper for details of interrupted immunization schedules.

- For previously non-immunized adolescents and adults, the recommended tetanus schedule is 2 doses administered at least 4 weeks apart followed by a third dose administered at least 6 months after the second dose, and subsequent boosters at least 1 year apart. Those who receive their first tetanus vaccine doses as adolescents or adults require a total of only 5 appropriately spaced doses to obtain long-term protection. See position paper for details.

Table 3: Recommendations for Interrupted or Delayed Routine Immunization (Updated 15 November 2012)

5 Haemophilus influenzae type b (Hib)

- Position paper reference: Weekly Epid. Record (2006, 81: 210–220) [pdf 209kb]
- Immunization should start as early as possible after the age of 6 weeks
- The 3-dose primary series is given at the same time as the DTP primary series often in combination vaccines.
- Delayed series: If a child 12–24 months of age has not received their primary vaccination series, a single dose of the vaccine is sufficient.
- Booster dose may be administered to children aged between 12–18 months although there is no WHO recommendation on this yet.
- The vaccine is not generally offered to children aged >24 months owing to the limited burden of Hib disease among children older than that age.

6 Pneumococcal (Conjugate)

- Position paper reference: Weekly Epid. Record (2012, 87: 129–143) [pdf 1.04 Mb]
- Pneumococcal conjugate vaccines (PCVs) are considered safe in all target groups for vaccination, also in immunocompromised individuals. The vaccines are not currently licensed for use in age groups that include women of childbearing age. Although theoretically highly unlikely to be harmful, there is no information on the safety of PCV10 and PCV13 during pregnancy.
- Except for very rare anaphylactic reactions that may follow the administration of any medicine, there are no contraindications to the use of these vaccines. However, it is advisable to defer vaccination until after an acute infection with temperature >39 °C.
- When injected at different sites, PCVs can be administered concurrently with any other vaccines in infant immunization programmes.
- When primary immunization is initiated with one of these vaccines, it is recommended that remaining doses are administered with the same product. Interchangeability between PCV10 and PCV13 has not yet been documented. However, if it is not possible to complete the series with the same type of vaccine, the other PCV product should be used.
- For infants, 3 primary doses (the 3p+0 schedule) or, as an alternative, 2 primary doses plus a booster (the 2p+1 schedule).
- In choosing between the 3p+0 and 2p+1 schedules, countries should consider locally relevant factors including the epidemiology of pneumococcal disease, the likely coverage, and the timeliness of the vaccine doses.
- If disease incidence peaks in young infants (<32 weeks of age), a 2p+1 schedule might not offer optimal individual protection for certain serotypes (e.g. 6B, 23F) compared to a 3p+0 schedule, particularly in the absence of herd protection.
- In contrast, higher antibody levels are induced by the third (booster) dose in a 2p+1 schedule compared to the third dose in a 3p+0 schedule. This may be important for duration of protection or effectiveness against some serotypes.
- If the 3p+0 schedule is used, vaccination can be initiated as early as 6 weeks of age with an interval between doses of 4–8 weeks, depending on programmatic convenience.
- If the 2p+1 schedule is selected, the 2 primary doses should ideally be completed by six months of age, starting as early as 6 weeks of age with a minimum interval of 8 weeks or more between the two doses (for infants aged ≥7 months a minimum interval of 4 weeks between doses is possible). One booster dose should be given between 9–15 months of age.
- Previously unvaccinated or incompletely vaccinated children (including those who had laboratory confirmed invasive pneumococcal disease) should be vaccinated using the recommended age-appropriate regimens. Interrupted schedules should be resumed without repeating the previous dose.
- HIV-positive infants and pre-term neonates who have received their 3 primary vaccine doses before reaching 12 months of age may benefit from a booster dose in the second year of life.
- Catch-up vaccination as part of introduction will accelerate herd protection and therefore the PCV impact on disease and carriage. Maximized protection at the time of introduction of PCV10 or PCV13 can be achieved by providing 2 catch-up dose(s) at an interval of at least 8 weeks to unvaccinated children aged 12–24 months and to children aged 2–5 years who are at high risk of pneumococcal infection.
- Further data are needed from different epidemiological settings on the impact of large-scale PCV vaccination of individuals >50 years of age in order to establish the relative priority of immunization programmes in that age group. However, given the documented effects of herd protection in adult age groups following routine infant immunization with PCV7, higher priority should normally be given to introducing and maintaining high coverage of infants with PCVs.
- The use of pneumococcal vaccine should be seen as complementary to the use of other pneumonia control measures, such as appropriate case management, promotion of exclusive breastfeeding for first 6 months of life, and the reduction of known risk factors, such as indoor pollutants and tobacco smoke.
- For polysaccharide pneumococcal vaccine see position paper: Weekly Epid. Record (2008, 83: 373–380) [pdf 308kb]
- In resource-limited settings where there are many competing health priorities, evidence does not support routine immunization of the elderly and high-risk populations with PPV23. Also, because of the low level of evidence for benefit, routine PPV23 vaccination of HIV-infected adults is not recommended in such settings. In countries that do not routinely administer PPV23 to high-risk populations, data are insufficient to recommend introducing this vaccine to reduce the morbidity and mortality associated with influenza.

7 Rotavirus

- Position paper reference: Weekly Epid. Record (2009, 84: 533–540) [pdf 764kb]] NOTE: This position paper is currently being revised in light of the vaccination schedule recommendations made by SAGE at their April 2012 meeting Weekly Epid. Record (2012, 87: 201–216) [pdf 1.11Mb]
- Recommended to be included in all national immunization programmes.
- Rotarix vaccine is administered orally in a 2-dose schedule with the first and second doses of DTP.
- RotaTeq requires an oral 3-dose schedule with DTP1, DTP2, and DTP3 with an interval of 4–10 weeks between doses.
- First dose of either RotaTeq or Rotarix be administered as soon as possible from 6 weeks of age.
- The interchangeability of the current rotavirus vaccines is unknown.
- In various settings, rotavirus vaccines have been found not to interfere significantly with the immunogenicity or safety of OPV or other childhood vaccines.
- The use of rotavirus vaccines should be part of a comprehensive strategy to control diarrhoeal diseases and should include, among other interventions, improvements in hygiene and sanitation, zinc supplementation, community-based administration of oral rehydration solution and overall improvements in case management.

Table 3: Recommendations for Interrupted or Delayed Routine Immunization (Updated 15 November 2012)

8 Measles

- Position paper reference: Weekly Epid. Record (2009, 84: 349-360) [pdf 724kb]

- Reaching all children with two doses of measles containing vaccine (MCV) should be the standard for all national immunization programmes.

- Delivery of the second dose (MCV2) may occur either at a scheduled age through routine services or periodically through mass campaigns, depending on which strategy achieves the higher coverage. A MCV2 dose may be added to the routine immunization schedule in countries that have achieved > 80% coverage of measles first dose (MCV1) at the national level for 3 consecutive years as determined by the most accurate means available (e.g. survey or WHO/UNICEF estimates). In general, countries that do not meet this criterion should prioritize improving MCV1 coverage and conducting high-quality follow-up SIAs, rather than adding MCV2 to their routine schedule.

- In countries with ongoing transmission in which the risk of measles mortality remains high, MCV1 should be given at age 9 months. MCV2 should be given between 12-18 months, as providing MCV2 in the 2nd year of life reduces the rate of accumulation of susceptible children and the risk of an outbreak.

- In countries with low rates of measles transmission (that is, those that are near elimination) and where there is a low risk of measles infection among infants, the first dose may be administered at age 12 months to take advantage of the higher seroconversion rates achieved at this age (>90% seroconversion). In these countries the optimal age for delivering a routine 2nd dose of measles is based on programmatic considerations that achieve the highest coverage and hence ensures early protection of the individual, slows accumulation of susceptible young children and may correspond with other routine immunizations (for example, DTP booster). If first dose coverage is high (>95%) and school enrolment is high (>95%), giving the second dose at school entry may be an effective strategy for achieving high coverage and preventing outbreaks in schools.

- Combined vaccines (Measles and Rubella or Measles, Mumps and Rubella) may not be optimal for use in countries where vaccine coverage for measles vaccine of at least 80% cannot be achieved or maintained.

- In areas where there is a high incidence of both HIV infection and measles, MCV1 may be offered as early as age 6 months. Two additional doses of measles vaccine should be administered to these children according to the national immunization schedule.

- As a general rule, live vaccines should be given either simultaneously, or at intervals of 4 weeks. An exception to this rule is OPV, which can be given at any time before or after measles vaccination, without interference in the response to either vaccine.

- Available data suggest that vaccines against measles, yellow fever, and Japanese encephalitis may be administered at the same time at different injection sites. Interference may occur between MMR and yellow fever vaccines if they are simultaneously administered to children < 2 years of age.

9 Rubella

- Position paper reference: Weekly Epid. Record (2011, 86: 301-316) [pdf 413kb]

- All countries that have not yet introduced rubella vaccine, and are providing 2 doses of measles vaccine using routine immunization, or SIAs, or both, should consider including rubella containing vaccines (RCVs) in their immunization programme. Countries planning gto introduce RCVs should review the epidemiology of rubella, including the susceptibility profile of the population; assess the burden of CRS; and establish rubella and CRS prevention as a public health priority.

- Because rubella is not as highly infectious as measles and because the effectiveness of 1 dose of an RCV is > 95% even at 9 months of age, only 1 dose of rubella vaccine is required to achieve rubella elimination if high coverage is achieved. However, when combined with measles vaccination, it may be easier to implement a second dose of RCV's using the same combined MR vaccine or MMR vaccine for both doses.

- RCVs can be administered concurrently with inactivated vaccines. As a general rule, live vaccines should be given either simultaneously with RCVs, or at least 4 weeks apart. An exception to this is oral polio vaccine, which can be given at any time before or after RCVs without interfering in the response to either vaccine.

- Interference may occur between MMR and yellow fever vaccines if they are simultaneously administered to children < 2 years of age.

- Because of a theoretical, but never demonstrated, teratogenic risk rubella vaccination in pregnant women should be avoided in principle, and those planning a pregnancy are advised to avoid pregnancy for 1 month following vaccination.

- Administration of blood or blood products before or shortly after vaccination may interfere with vaccine efficacy. If using only rubella vaccines persons who received blood products should wait at least 3 months before vaccination and, if possible, blood products should be avoided for up to 2 weeks post-vaccination. Vaccinated persons are not eligible to donate blood for 1 month after vaccination.

10 Human Papillomavirus (HPV)

- Position paper reference: Weekly Epid. Record (2009, 84: 118-131) [pdf 267kb]

- HPV vaccines are most efficacious in females who are naïve to vaccine-related HPV types. Programmes should initially prioritize high coverage in the primary target population of young adolescent girls 9-10 through to 13 years of age prior to sexual debut. Vaccination of secondary target populations of older adolescent females or young women is recommended only if this is feasible, affordable, cost-effective.

- Alternative schedules for HPV vaccines are being explored.

- Restarting the 3-dose series is not necessary if interrupted, but remaining doses should be administered as close to the schedule intervals as possible.

- Currently, the manufacturers do not recommend any booster dose following completion of the primary series.

- HPV vaccination of males for prevention of cervical cancer is not recommended at this time because vaccination strategies that achieve high coverage (>70%) in the primary target population of young adolescent girls are expected to be more cost-effective in reducing cervical cancer than including vaccination of males.

11 Japanese Encephalitis (JE)

- Position paper reference: Weekly Epid. Record (2006, 81: 331-340) [pdf 192kb]

- JE vaccine should be given in all areas where JE constitutes a public health problem.

- Vaccine options- Three types of vaccines are available: (1) a cell-culture based live attenuated, (2) a cell-culture-based inactivated and (3) an inactivated mouse brain-derived. The WHO position paper provides recommendations for the mouse brain-derived and live attenuated vaccines.

- Booster - If administering cell-culture based live-attenuated vaccine, a booster dose is currently not recommended after an interval of one year, even though observational data studies suggest long-term protection after a single dose. If using mouse brain-derived vaccine, a booster dose should be administered after an interval of one year then every 3 years until 10-15 years of age.

- As a general rule, live vaccines should be given either simultaneously, or at intervals of 4 weeks.

Table 3: Recommendations for Interrupted or Delayed Routine Immunization (Updated 15 November 2012)

Appendix O

- Available data suggest that vaccines against measles, yellow fever, and Japanese encephalitis may be administered at the same time at different injection sites. Interference may occur between MMR and yellow fever vaccines if they are simultaneously administered to children < 2 years of age.

12 Yellow Fever

- Position paper reference: Weekly Epid. Record (2003, 78: 349-359) [pdf 339kb]
- Recommended for use in countries at risk of Yellow Fever.
- For convenience and improved coverage, Yellow Fever vaccine should be administered simultaneously with the measles containing vaccine, but in a separate syringe and at a different injection site.
- Yellow Fever vaccine should be offered to all travellers to and from at-risk areas, unless they belong to the group of individuals for whom Yellow Fever vaccines is contraindicated.
- Interference may occur between MMR and yellow fever vaccines if they are simultaneously administered to children < 2 years of age
- In addition to the introduction of Yellow Fever vaccine for routine childhood vaccination, WHO recommends the implementation of mass preventive vaccination campaigns to protect susceptible older age groups. In the event of limited resources, assessment of the degree of risk can help prioritize areas for mass preventive campaigns.

13 Tick-Borne Encephalitis (TBE)

- Position paper reference: Weekly Epid. Record (2011, 86: 241-256) [pdf 318kb]
- Since the incidence of tick-borne encephalitis may vary considerably between and even within geographical regions, public immunization strategies should be based on risk assessments conducted at country, regional or district level, and they should be appropriate to the local endemic situation. Therefore, establishing case reporting of the disease is essential before deciding on the most appropriate preventive measures to be taken.
- In areas where the disease is highly endemic (that is, where the average prevaccination incidence of clinical disease is ≥5 cases/100 000 population per year), implying that there is a high individual risk of infection, WHO recommends that vaccination be offered to all age groups, including children.
- Because the disease tends to be more serious in individuals aged >50–60 years this age group constitutes an important target for immunization.
- Where the prevaccination incidence of the disease is moderate or low (that is, the annual average during a 5-year period is <5/100 000) or is limited to particular geographical locations or certain outdoor activities, immunization should target individuals in the most severely affected cohorts.
- People travelling from non-endemic areas to endemic areas should be offered vaccination if their visits will include extensive outdoor activities.
- Vaccination against the disease requires a primary series of 3 doses; those who will continue to be at risk should probably have ≥1 booster doses.
- Within the considerable range of acceptable dose intervals, the relevant national authorities should select the most rational primary schedule for their national, regional or district immunization programmes.
- For the vaccines manufactured in Austria and Germany (FSME-Immun and Encepur) that can be given starting from > 1 year of age an interval of 1-3 months is recommended between the first 2 doses, and 5-12 months between the second and third doses. When rapid protection is required, for example for people who will be travelling to endemic areas, the interval between the first 2 doses may be reduced to 1-2 weeks.

- With the vaccines manufactured in the Russian Federation (TBE-Moscow and EnceVir) the recommended intervals are 1-7 months between the first 2 doses, and 12 months between the second and third doses. Booster doses are recommended every 3 years for those at continued risk of exposure.
- The currently recommended booster interval should be maintained until more data have been obtained on the duration of protection induced by the Russian vaccines.
- Regardless of the duration of the delay, interrupted schedules should be resumed without repeating previous doses.

14 Typhoid

- Position paper reference: Weekly Epid. Record (2008, 83: 49-59) [pdf 297kb]
- Recommended for school-age and/or preschool-age children in areas where typhoid fever in these age groups is shown to be a significant public health problem, particularly where antibiotic-resistant S. Typhi is prevalent.
- Vaccine option– Vi polysaccharide typhoid vaccine requires one parenterally administered dose which maybe given after the age of 2 years; the liquid form of Ty21a live oral vaccine (for use in individuals from the age of 2 years) is no longer available; the capsule form of Ty21a (for use in individuals from the age of 5 years) requires 3 or 4 orally administered doses. See position paper for further details.
- If the schedule for Ty21a is interrupted by an interval longer than 21 days, expert opinion indicates that the series should be restarted from the beginning. If the interruption is less than 21 days, resume vaccination without repeating the previous dose.
- Booster- In most endemic settings, a booster dose of the concerned vaccine 3 to 7 years after the primary immunization seems appropriate.

15 Cholera

- Position paper reference: Weekly Epid. Record (2010, 85: 117-128) [pdf 283kb]
- In cholera-endemic countries, vaccinating the entire population is not warranted. Rather, vaccination should be targeted at high-risk areas and population groups. The primary targets for cholera vaccination in many endemic areas are preschool-aged and school aged children. Other groups that are especially vulnerable to severe disease and for which the vaccines are not contraindicated may also be targeted, such as pregnant women and HIV-infected individuals. Consider vaccinating older age groups if funding is available.
- Two types of oral cholera vaccines are available: (i) Dukoral (WC–rBS) and (ii) Shanchol and mORCVAX. The live attenuated single-dose vaccine (CVD 103-HgR) is no longer produced. The injectable vaccine is still manufactured in a few countries but its use is not recommended mainly because of its limited efficacy and short duration of protection.
- Dukoral is not licensed for children < 2 years. Children aged 2-5 years should receive 3 doses > 7 days apart (but not more than 6 weeks). Intake of food and drink should be avoided for 1 hour before and after vaccination. If the interval between doses is delayed >6 weeks, primary vaccination should be restarted. One booster dose is recommended every 6 months, and if the interval between primary immunization, and the booster is >5 months, primary immunization must be restarted.
- Adults and children > 6 years should receive 2 doses of Dukoral > 7 days apart (but not more than 6 weeks). Intake of food and drink should be avoided for 1 hour before and after vaccination. If the interval between doses is delayed >6 weeks, primary vaccination should be restarted. A booster dose every 2 years is recommended. If the interval between the primary series and booster immunization is > 2 years, primary immunization must be repeated.
- Shanchol and mORCVAX: two liquid doses orally 14 days apart for individuals > 1 year. A booster dose is recommended after 2 years.

Table 3: Recommendations for Interrupted or Delayed Routine Immunization (Updated 15 November 2012)

16 Meningococcal

- Position paper reference: Weekly Epid. Record (2011, 86: 521-540) [pdf 1.01mb].

- Conjugate vaccines are preferred over polysaccharide vaccines due to their potential for herd protection and their increased immunogenicity, particularly in children <2 years of age.

- Both conjugate and polysaccharide vaccines are efficacious and safe when used in pregnant women.

- Monovalent MenA conjugate vaccine should be given as one single intramuscular dose to individuals 1-29 years of age. The possible need for a booster is not yet established.

- For monovalent MenC conjugate vaccine one single intramuscular dose is recommended for children aged >12 months, teenagers and adults. Children 2-11 months require 2 doses administered at an interval of at least 2 months and a booster about 1 year after. If the primary series is interrupted, vaccination should be resumed without repeating the previous dose.

- Quadrivalent conjugate vaccines (A,C,W135,Y-D and A,C,W135,Y-CRM) should be administered as one single intramuscular dose to individuals > 2 years. A,C,W135,Y-D is also licensed for children 9-23 months of age, and given as a 2-dose series, 3 months apart beginning at age 9 months. If the primary series is interrupted, vaccination should be resumed without repeating the previous dose.

- Meningococcal polysaccharide vaccines are less, or not, immunogenic in children under 2 years of age.

- Meningococcal polysaccharide vaccines can be used for those > 2 years of age to control outbreaks in countries where limited economic resources or insufficient supply restrict the use of meningococcal conjugate vaccines. Polysaccharide vaccines should be administered to individuals ≥ 2 years old as one single dose. One booster 3-5 years after the primary dose may be given to persons considered to be a continued high risk of exposure, including some health workers. See position paper for details.

17 Hepatitis A

- Position paper reference: Weekly Epid. Record (2012, 87: 261-276) [pdf 1.24 Mb]

- Hepatitis A vaccination is recommended for inclusion in the national immunization schedule for children ≥ 1 year if indicated on the basis of incidence of acute hepatitis A, change in the endemicity from high to intermediate, and consideration of cost-effectiveness.

- In highly endemic countries almost all persons are asymptomatically infected with HAV in childhood, which effectively prevents clinical hepatitis A in adolescents and adults. In these countries, large-scale vaccination programmes are not recommended.

- Countries with improving socioeconomic status may rapidly move from high to intermediate endemicity. In these countries, a relatively large proportion of the adult population is susceptible to HAV and large-scale hepatitis A vaccination is likely to be cost-effective and therefore is encouraged.

- For individual health benefit targeted vaccination of high-risk groups should be considered in low and very low endemicity settings. Those at increased risk of hepatitis A include travelers to areas of intermediate or high endemicity, those requiring life-long treatment with blood products, men who have sex with men, workers in contact with non-human primates, and injection drug users. In addition, patients with chronic liver disease are at increased risk for fulminant hepatitis A and should be vaccinated.

- Inactivated HAV vaccine is licensed for intramuscular administration in a 2-dose schedule with the first dose given at the age of 1 year or older. The interval between the first and second dose is flexible (from 6 months up to 4-5 years) but is usually 6-18 months. Countries may consider a 1-dose schedule as this option seems comparable in terms of effectiveness, and is less expensive and easier to implement. However, in individuals at substantial risk of contracting hepatitis A and in immunocompromised individuals, a 2-dose schedule is preferred. Inactivated HAV vaccines produced by different manufacturers, including combined hepatitis A vaccines, are interchangeable. Apart from severe allergic reaction to the previous dose, there is no contraindication to their use. These vaccines can be co-administered simultaneously with other routine childhood vaccines, and should be considered for use in pregnant women at definite risk of HAV infection.

- Live attenuated HAV vaccine is administered as a single subcutaneous dose to those ≥ 1 year of age. Severe allergy to components included in the live attenuated hepatitis A vaccine is a contraindication to their use. As a rule, live vaccines should not be used in pregnancy or in severely immunocompromised patients. There is no information available on co-administration of live attenuated hepatitis A vaccines with other routinely used vaccines.

- Vaccination against hepatitis A should be part of a comprehensive plan for the prevention and control of viral hepatitis, including measures to improve hygiene and sanitation and measures for outbreak control.

18 Rabies

- Position paper reference: Weekly Epid. Record (2010, 85: 309-320) [pdf 370]

- Production and use of nerve-tissue rabies vaccines should be discontinued and replaced with cell-culture-based vaccines (CCVs).

- Recommended for anyone who will be at continual, frequent or increased risk of exposure to the rabies virus, either as a result of their residence or occupation. Travellers with extensive outdoor exposure in rural high-risk areas where immediate access to appropriate medical care may be limited should also be vaccinated regardless of the duration of stay. Where canine rabies is a public health problem, WHO encourages studies on the feasibility, cost-effectiveness, and long-term impact of incorporating rabies vaccination into the immunization programme for infants and children.

- The series is given by intramuscular or intradermal injection at 0, 7, and 21 or 28 days.

- Intramuscular administration: For adults and children aged ≥2 years, the vaccine should always be administered in the deltoid area of the arm; for children aged < 2 years, the anterolateral area of the thigh is recommended. Rabies vaccine should never be administered in the gluteal area, as the induction of an adequate immune response may be less reliable.

- Booster doses of rabies vaccines are not required for individuals living in or travelling to high-risk areas who have received a complete primary series of pre-exposure or post-exposure prophylaxis with a cell-culture-based rabies vaccine (CCV).

- Periodic booster injections are recommended only for people whose occupation puts them at continual or frequent risk of exposure. If available, antibody monitoring is preferred to the administration of routine boosters.

- Because vaccine-induced immunity persists in most cases for years, a booster is recommended only if rabies-virus neutralizing antibody titres fall to <0.5 IU/ml.

- Antibody testing should be done every 6 months for people at risk of laboratory exposure to high concentrations of live rabies virus, and every 2 years for professionals who are not at continual risk of exposure through their activities, such as certain categories of veterinarians and animal health officers.

Appendix O

19 Mumps

- Position paper references: Weekly Epid. Record (2007, 82: 49-60) [pdf 311kb]
- Recommended for use in high performing immunization programs with the capacity to maintain coverage over 80% and where mumps reduction is a public health priority.
- If implemented, a combination vaccine of measles, mumps and rubella is recommended.
- As a general rule, live vaccines should be given either simultaneously, or at intervals of 4 weeks.
- Interference may occur between MMR and yellow fever vaccines if they are simultaneously administered to children < 2 years of age.

20 Seasonal Influenza (Inactivated Vaccine)

- Position paper reference: Weekly Epid. Record (2005, 33: 275-287) [pdf 220kb]
- The World Health Assembly recommended increased immunization coverage of high-risk groups including the elderly, in those countries where influenza vaccination policies exist. (Reference: WHA56.19, 2003). See position paper for detailed description of high-risk groups.
- Dose- If a child under 9 years of age requires vaccination and has not previously received influenza vaccine, a two-dose series with doses one-month apart should be administered. Annual re-vaccination in all individuals and initial vaccination in individuals 9 years of age or older require only a single dose. For children aged 6-36 months should receive half the adult dose.

Index

A

Acute disseminated encephalomyelitis (ADEM), 247
Acute respiratory infections
  asthma, 201–202
  bronchospasm, 201
  clinical assessment
    etiology and differential diagnosis, 196, 197
    physical examination and chest radiography, 195, 197
    pulse oximetry, 197
    severity of illness, 195
  epidemiology, 194
  pneumonia (*see* Pneumonia)
  risk factors, 194
  stridor, 202
Adolescence
  adult disease effects, 140
  anemia, 128, 134
  child health gains, 140
  communicable diseases, 128, 131
  contraception (*see* Contraception)
  definition, 122
  disability-adjusted life years (DALYs), 128, 129
  disease spectrum, 127
  early childbirth, 122
  injuries, 128
  mental health, 122
  millennium development goals (MDG), 131, 135–136
  mortality rates, 126, 127
  neuropsychiatric disorders, 128
  nutritional issues, 128, 133
  population, 122, 123
  pregnancy and childbirth, 128, 130
  preventative care
    abuse, 145
    counseling, 146–147
    depressive disorders, 142
    economic status, social determinants, 146
    education, social determinants, 146
    ethnicity and race, social determinants, 146
    family situation, social determinants, 146
    food security, social determinants, 146
    gender issues, social determinants, 146
    hypertension, 145
    immunization, 148
    infectious disease, 141–142
    nutritional issues, 141
    psychiatric illness, 142
    refractive errors, 146
    reproductive health needs, 144–145
    SIGECAPS screening tool, 142, 143
    substance use, 143–144
    suicidal ideation, 142
    TV and social media use, 146
    violence, 144
  primary prevention, 140–141
  sexually transmitted infections, 122
    bacterial vaginosis, 155, 165
    behavioral risk factors, 152
    biological risk factors, 152
    candida vaginal discharge, 156, 167
    chancroid, 157, 168
    chlamydia cervicitis, 154, 163
    clue cells and saline prep, vaginal fluid, 155, 164
    cognitive risk factors, 153
    genital herpes, 157, 167

Adolescence (cont.)
  genital warts and buboes, 160–161, 171
  gonococcal urethritis, 156, 162
  gram negative intracellular diplococci, 154, 163
  granuloma inguinale, 159, 170
  in HIV transmission, 171
  lymphogranuloma venereum, 164, 170
  mucopurulent cervicitis, 156, 162
  non-gonococcal urethritis, 156, 165, 166
  prevalence of, 151–152
  primary measures, 176
  primary syphilis, 158, 168
  secondary measures, 177
  secondary syphilis, 153, 168–169
  special adolescent populations, 177
  strawberry cervix, 155, 164
  syndromic management, 172–174
  tertiary measures, 177
  vaginal and penile ulcers, 154, 157–159
  vaginal/urethral/penile discharge, 154–156
  yeast KOH prep, 156, 166
 as social determinant of health
  brain volume, 122, 124
  decision-making, 124
  digital age, 124
  limbic system, 124
  proximal determinants, 125–126
  social movements, 124
  structural determinants, 125
 tobacco and alcohol use, 128, 132
 underweight prevalence, 128, 133
American trypanosomiasis
 clinical presentation, 297
 diagnosis, 297–298
 differential diagnosis, 297
 prevention, 298
 treatment, 298
Antenatal care
 anemia, 76
 birth and emergency plan, 76
 deworming, 77
 due date estimation, 75
 family planning, 77
 HIV testing, 76
 malaria, intermittent preventive treatment, 77
 nutrition and self-care, 77
 overview of, 74, 75
 preeclampsia, 76
 pregnancy, basic assessment, 74–75
 signs and symptoms, 75
 syphilis testing, 76
 tetanus toxoid, 77
 vitamin supplementation, 77
Asthma, 201–202

B
Bitot's spots, 247
Bronchospasm, 201

C
Child mortality
 disparities, 10, 11
 infant, 6
 millennium development goal 4 (MDG4), 4
 neonatal mortality rate (NMR), 4, 6
 survival improvement, 11
 under-five mortality rate (U5MR)
  disproportionate mortality rates, 6, 7
  levels and trends in, 4, 5
  malaria, 8
  in middle-income countries, 6, 9
  pneumonia, 6
  preventable infectious diseases, 10
  in sub-Saharan Africa, 6, 8
  undernutrition, 8
Contraception
 history, 179–180
 hormonal
  emergency contraception, 184
  injectable, 183–188
  oral contraceptive pill, 180–182
  transdermal, 182
  vaginal ring, 182–183
 nonhormonal IUD, 188–189
 traditional methods
  fertility awareness methods, 189
  lactational amenorrhea (LAM), 189–190
  withdrawal or coitus interruptus, 189
 tubal ligation, 192
 vasectomy, 192
Convention on the Rights of the Child (CRC)
 AAA-Q criteria, 385–386
 challenges and gross violations, 382
 declarations, 383
 general comments, 386
 interests of the child, 384
 International human rights treaties, 383
 nondiscrimination, 384
 principle of participation, 384
 survival rights, 384
 vulnerability analysis, 387–388

Index 561

D

Dental caries (cavities)
  clinical presentation, 393
  diagnosis, 392
  etiology, 392
  patient management, 393–394
  prevalence, 392
  prevention, 392
Diarrhea
  characterization, 206
  comorbid conditions, 207
  definitions, 206
  gastroenteritis, 207
  hydration status, 207
  hypertonic dehydration, 207
  hypotonic dehydration, 207
  isotonic dehydration, 207
  malnutrition, clinical signs, 207
  syndromic presentations
    acute watery diarrhea, 208, 209
    invasive (bloody) diarrhea
      (*see* Dysentery)
    with malnutrition, 214–215
    persistent diarrheal illness, 213–214
  warning signs, 207
Dysentery
  complications, 208, 210–211
  infectious etiology, 208, 210–211
  symptoms, 208, 210–211
  transmission, 208, 210–211
  treatment
    antibiotics, 212–213
    early refeeding, 213
    follow-up recommendations, 213
    ORT, 208, 212
    supportive care, 208
    zinc supplementation, 213

E

Emergency contraception (EC)
  copper IUD, 187
  efficacy, 187–188
  indications, 186
  POPs, 187
  side effects, 188
  ulipristal acetate, 187
  Yuzpe regime, 187
Emergency pediatric care
  animal bite management, 357–358
  black widow, 359
  head trauma, 348–351
  with laceration/abrasion, 351

  near-drowning, 357
  orthopedic injury, 352–354
  pain control, 354–356
  poisoning, 356–357
  primary survey of, injured child, 348, 349
  scorpion stings, 359
  snake bite, 358
Encephalitis, 247
Epilepsy
  antiepileptic drugs
    dosing of, 412, 413
    education, 414
    efficacy, 414
    follow-up, 414
    principles of, 413–414
    side effects of, 412, 413
  clinical history/presentation, 410, 411
  definitions, 410
  diagnostic testing, 411
  epidemiology, 410
  physical examination, 411

G

Global health system
  building blocks of
    financing, 28–29
    health workforce, 27–28
    information, 28
    leadership/governance, 29
    medical products, vaccines, and
      technologies, 28
    service delivery, 27
  ethical engagement, 32–33
  failures, 26
  primary health care (*see* Primary
    health care)

H

Head trauma
  minor head injury, 348–349
  significant head injury
    patient management, 349–351
    physical exam findings, 349
Human immunodeficiency virus (HIV)
  adolescents and, 268, 277
  global burden of, 252
  HIV-positive adolescents, 279
  modes of transmission, 252
  mother-to-child transmission, 252
  opportunistic infections (OIs),
    258, 269–276

Human immunodeficiency virus (HIV) (*cont.*)
    prevention strategies
        early maternal diagnosis, 253
        early maternal diagnosis and diagnostic studies, 253
        infant feeding options, 253–255
        infant prophylaxis, 253
        infant testing, 257
        maternal antiretroviral treatment, 253, 254
    staging and treatment of
        adverse reactions, 256, 262–266
        antiretroviral formulations, 256, 262–266
        ARV treatment, 256
        dosing, 256, 262–266
        health visits, 256
        immunization of, 256
        rationale and criteria for, 256, 260
        side effect profiles, 256, 262–266
        TMP/SMZ dosing recommendations, 256, 268
        WHO recommendations antiretroviral treatment regimen, 256, 261
    uninfected infants/children, 260
    WHO clinical staging
        for adolescents and adults, 256, 259
        for infants and children, 256–258
Human rights
    advocacy, 386–387
    CRC (*see* Convention on the Rights of the Child)
    human rights-based approach to programming, 387
    legal mechanisms, 387
    Right to health
        AAA-Q criteria, 385–386
        CRC general comments, 386
        vulnerability analysis, 387–388
Hydrocephalus, 414–415
Hypervulnerability, 38, 39

I
Immigrants
    history of, 420–421
    immunizations, 422
    physical examination, 421
    psychosocial assessment, 422
    screening tests, 422–425
Injectable contraception, progestin-only contraception
    depot medroxyprogesterone acetate (DMPA), 184
    levonorgestrel-releasing intrauterine contraceptive system (LNG-IUS), 185–186
    progestin-only pills (POP), 184
    subcutaneous DMPA formulation, 185
    subdermal contraceptive implant, 185
International Nongovernmental Organizations (INGOS), 18
Iron deficiency
    diagnostic testing, 340
    etiology/pathogenesis, 339
    International Public Health Programs, 340, 341
    prognosis, 340

K
Kwashiorkor, 328, 329

L
Lymphatic filariasis (LF)
    clinical presentation, 289–290
    differential diagnosis, 290
    drug treatment, 291, 292
    microfilariae identification, 290
    prevention, 291
Lymphoid interstitial pneumonitis, 262

M
Malaria
    blood smears
        false negatives, 224
        parasite density determination, 224
        parasite ring forms, 224, 225
        thin and thick, 224
    clinical diagnosis, 224
    clinical manifestations, 222–223
    epidemiology, 218
    modes of acquisition, 219
    parasites, 218
    prevention
        household protection, 236
        intermittent preventive treatment (IPT), 236–237
        personal protection, 235
        for travelers, 237–240
        vector control, 236

Index 563

rapid diagnostic tests (RDTs), 224–225
treatment
   adjunctive measures, 226
   antimalarial drug, 235
   antimalarial resistance and regional variation, 226
   endemic regions and dosing guidelines, United States, 226–234
   high-grade parasitemia, 235
vector and host characteristics, 221
vulnerable groups, 221–222

Malnutrition
anthropometric evaluation
   age-appropriate techniques, 324
   kwashiorkor, 328, 329
   marasmic kwashiorkor, 328
   marasmus, 328, 329
   mid-upper arm circumference (MUAC), 326–328
   protein energy malnutrition, 326, 328
   stunting, 326
   wasting, 326–327
   weight, 326
growth and nutritional status assessment
   clinical assessment, 324, 325
   by history, 322, 324
nutritional interventions
   classification of, 330, 331
   eating habits, 330
   edema classification, 330, 331
   food choices, 330
   inpatient treatment, 332–334
   Plumpy'nut©, 331, 332
   ready to-usetherapeutic foods (RUTF), 330–331
prevalence of, 322, 323

Marasmus, 328, 329

Maternal health
antenatal care essentials (*see* Antenatal care)
pregnancy, contraindicated medications, 85
risks, and interventions, 77–84

Measles
clinical presentation
   desquamation, 246
   Koplik spots, 245
   maculopapular and erythematous rash, 245
complications
   acute disseminated encephalomyelitis, 247
   Bitot's spots, 247
   encephalitis, 247
   pneumonia, 247
   subacute sclerosing panencephalitis (SSPE), 247
diagnosis, 246–247
epidemiology, 244
management of
   acetaminophen, 248
   conjunctivitis, 248
   measles croup, 249
   mouth ulcers, 249
   pneumonia, 248
   vitamin A dosing, 248
vaccination, 249–250

Mental health
anxiety disorders, 362
attention deficit hyperactivity disorder (ADHD)
   clinical presentation, 374
   diagnosis and differential diagnosis, 374
   epidemiology, 374
   oppositional defiant and conduct problems, 374–376
   patient management, 374
   prognosis, 374
   screening, 374
care and management
   communication, 365
   medication, 366–367
   psychotherapy, 365–366
eating disorders, 378–379
internalizing problems
   anxiety, 368–370
   depression, 370–371
   psychosomatic illness, 373
   safety/violence, 372–373
   self-harm/suicide, 372
neuropsychiatric disorders, 362
psychosocial evaluation
   bio-psycho-social approach, 362
   DSM 4 classification, 363
   family history, 363–364
   functional impairment, 364
   interviewing, 363
   medical history, 363
   11 mental health action signs, 363
   screening, 363
   stigma, 362–363
psychotic disorders, 377–378
substance use disorders, 376–377
suicide, 362

Micronutrient deficiency
　etiology and causes, 338
　folic acid, 344
　iodine, 343
　iron deficiency
　　clinical signs and symptoms, 339
　　diagnostic testing, 340
　　etiology/pathogenesis, 339
　　International Public Health Programs, 340, 341
　　prognosis, 340
　long-term consequences, 339
　niacin (Pellagra), 346
　prevalence, 338
　short-term consequences, 339
　vitamin A, 341–342
　vitamin B1 (Beriberi), 345
　vitamin B2 (Riboflavin), 345
　vitamin B12, 346
　vitamin C, 345
　vitamin D, 344
　zinc, 343–344
Motor deficits, 415–417

N

Neglected tropical diseases (NTDs)
　American trypanosomiasis
　　clinical presentation, 297
　　diagnosis, 297–298
　　differential diagnosis, 297
　　prevention, 298
　　treatment, 298
　global burden of, 288
　lymphatic filariasis
　　clinical presentation, 289–290
　　differential diagnosis, 290
　　drug treatment, 291, 292
　　microfilariae identification, 290
　　prevention, 291
　onchocerciasis
　　clinical presentation, 291, 293
　　diagnosis, 293
　　differential diagnosis, 293
　　prevention, 294
　　treatment, 294
　schistosomiasis
　　clinical presentation, 294
　　diagnosis, 295–296
　　differential diagnosis, 295
　　prevention, 296
　　treatment, 295
　visceral leishmaniasis
　　clinical presentation, 299

　　diagnosis, 299, 300
　　differential diagnosis, 299
　　prevention, 300
　　treatment, 299–300
Neonatal infections
　bacterial sepsis and meningitis, 109
　cytomegalovirus (CMV), 116
　epidemiology, 106–108
　gonococcal infection, 111, 112
　hepatitis B virus (HBV), 114
　herpes simplex virus (HSV), 116, 117
　pneumonia, 106
　prevention, 117–118
　rubella, 115
　skin infections, 112
　syphilis, 113–114
　tetanus, 110, 111
　toxoplasmosis, 114–115
　tuberculosis, 109–110
　umbilical infections, 112–113
Newborn health
　deaths, direct causes of, 88
　guidelines for
　　immediate newborn, 91–92
　　immediate postpartum, 90–91
　　intrapartum/birth history, 90
　　maternal history, 90
　　neonatal period, 92–93
　interventions
　　asphyxia-related newborn deaths, 89
　　early breastfeeding, 90
　　emergency preparedness, 88
　　essential newborn care, 88
　　extra newborn care, 88
　　hand hygiene, 90
　　maternal vaccinations, 89
　　skin-to-skin care, 90
　　umbilical cord care, 90
　progress in, 93–94
　resuscitation
　　asphyxia, 96
　　breathing assessment, 100
　　chest compressions, 102
　　in developing countries, 96–97
　　drying process, 99
　　environment, 97–98
　　epinephrine, 102–103
　　global advances in, 97
　　head position, 100
　　intrapartum-related hypoxic events, 96
　　intubation, 102
　　meconium, 99
　　routine care, 99
　　skilled birth attendants, 98

Index 565

sniffing position, 100
stimulation, 100
supplemental oxygen, 102
supplies and equipment, 98
ventilation, 100–101

O

Onchocerciasis
    clinical presentation, 291, 293
    diagnosis, 293
    differential diagnosis, 293
    prevention, 294
    treatment, 294
Oral health care
    anatomy, 390–392
    cleft lip/cleft palate, 399–400
    dental caries (cavities)
        clinical presentation, 393
        diagnosis, 392
        etiology, 392
        patient management, 393–394
        prevalence, 392
        prevention, 392
    fluoride varnish (FV) application, 402, 403
    gingivitis, 394
    herpes simplex, 397–398
    with HIV/ AIDS, 400–401
    noma, 400
    oral candidiasis/oral thrush, 398–399
    oral hygiene
        dentist visits, 402
        healthy diet, 401–402
        tooth brushing, 402
    primary teeth extraction
        elevation, 403, 405, 406
        forceps position, 405, 407
        hand positioning, 403, 405, 406
        inferior alveolar block, 403, 404
        instruments, 403, 405
        periodontal ligament injection, 403, 404
        postoperative instructions, 406–407
    pulpitis, 394–396
    retained primary tooth, 396
    trauma, 396–397
Oral rehydration therapy (ORT), 208, 212, 305
Orthopedic injury
    amputations, 353–354
    dislocated (Nursemaid's) elbow, 353
    dislocated shoulder, 352
    lower extremity, 353
    overview of, 352
    upper extremity fractures, 353

P

Pain control
    burns
        body surface area (BSA), 354
        degree of, 354, 355
        minor burn management, 355–356
        severe burn management, 356
        tertiary center, 356
    WHO pain management pyramid, 354, 355
Parasitic diseases. *See* Neglected tropical diseases (NTDs)
Pediatric care
    child abuse
        diagnosis of, 68
        history and physical examination, 67–68
        WHO definition, 67
    resource-limited settings (*see* Resource-limited settings)
    resource-poor settings
        evidence-based medicine, 44–45
        family, 44
        health care workers, 45–46
        limitations in, 44–45
    WHO essential drug list, 50
Pneumonia, 247
    in children 2 months to 5 years, 198, 199
    empyema, 199
    with HIV/AIDS, 199–200
    lung abscess, 199
    malnutrition, 200–201
    necrotizing, 199
    parapneumonic effusion, 199
    under-five mortality rate (U5MR), 6
Preventative care, adolescence
    counseling, 146–147
    immunization, 148
    screen for
        abuse, 145
        depressive disorders, 142
        hypertension, 145
        infectious disease, 141–142
        nutritional issues, 141
        psychiatric illness, 142
        refractive errors, 146
        reproductive health needs, 144–145
        SIGECAPS screening tool, 142, 143
        substance use, 143–144
        suicidal ideation, 142
        TV and social media use, 146
        violence, 144
    social determinants
        economic status, 146
        education, 146
        ethnicity and race, 146

Preventative care, adolescence (*cont.*)
    family situation, 146
    food security, 146
    gender issues, 146
Primary health care
    history of, 29
    leadership reforms, 32
    public policy reforms, 32
    service delivery reforms, 31
    universal coverage reforms, 30–31
Primary teeth extraction
    elevation, 403, 405, 406
    forceps position, 405, 407
    hand positioning, 403, 405, 406
    inferior alveolar block, 403, 404
    instruments, 403, 405
    periodontal ligament injection, 403, 404
    postoperative instructions, 406–407

R

Resource-limited settings
    abdominal ultrasound, 66
    emergency pediatric care
        animal bite management, 357–358
        black widow, 359
        head trauma, 348–351
        with laceration/abrasion, 351
        near-drowning, 357
        orthopedic injury, 352–354
        pain control, 354–356
        poisoning, 356–357
        primary survey of, injured child, 348, 351
        scorpion stings, 359
        snake bite, 358
    microscopy, 61, 66
    newborn head ultrasound, 66
    sick child
        coma, 57, 58–59
        dehydration estimation, 60
        fluids maintenance, 61–66
        IMCI guidelines, 52–53
        laboratory investigations, 53–54
        lower airway obstruction, 55–56
        malnourished child, 60
        medical history, 52
        moderate dehydration, 60
        seizures, 57, 58–59
        severe dehydration, 61
        triaging, 51
        unconsciousness, 57, 58–59
        upper airway obstruction, 54–55
        WHO danger signs, 51
        WHO priority signs, 51–52
    well child
        anemia, 48
        anthropometric measurements, 47
        anticipatory guidance, 49, 50
        history, 46
        hydration status, 49
        infants and toddlers, 47, 48
        malnutrition, 48
        psychosocial health, 47
        routine assessment, 48
        routine screenings, 49
Right to health, Convention on the Rights of the Child (CRC)
    AAA-Q criteria, 385–386
    general comments, 386
    vulnerability analysis, 387–388

S

Schistosomiasis
    clinical presentation, 294
    diagnosis, 295–296
    differential diagnosis, 295
    prevention, 296
    treatment, 295
Schizophrenia, 377–378
Sexually transmitted infections (STIs)
    behavioral risk factors, 152
    biological risk factors, 152
    candida vaginal discharge, 156, 167
    cognitive risk factors, 153
    genital warts and buboes, 160–161, 171
    in HIV transmission, 171
    prevalence of, 151–152
    prevention and control
        primary measures, 176
        secondary measures, 177
        special adolescent populations, 168–169
        tertiary measures, 177
    syndromic management
        abdominal pain, 173, 176
        vs. etiologic management, 172
        evaluation and treatment, limited factors, 172
        genital ulcers, 171, 173
        risk assessment approach, 172
        syndromic modules, 172
        urethral discharge evaluation, 172, 173

Index 567

vaginal discharge evaluation, 173, 174
vaginal and penile ulcers, 154, 157–159
  chancroid, 157, 168
  genital herpes, 157, 167
  granuloma inguinale, 159, 170
  lymphogranuloma venereum, 164, 170
  primary syphilis, 158, 168
  secondary syphilis, 153, 168–169
vaginal/urethral/penile discharge, 154–156
  bacterial vaginosis, 155, 165
  chlamydia cervicitis, 154, 163
  clue cells and saline prep, vaginal fluid, 155, 164
  gonococcal urethritis, 156, 162
  gram negative intracellular diplococci, 154, 163
  mucopurulent cervicitis, 156, 162
  non-gonococcal urethritis, 156, 165, 166
  strawberry cervix, 155, 164
  yeast KOH prep, 156, 166
Stakeholders, child health programs
  agencies types
    bilateral aid and development organizations, 18
    International Nongovernmental Organizations (INGOS), 18
    largest funders, 19, 20
    mega-donors, 19
    multinational agencies, 16–17
    official development assistance, 15–16
  factors affecting
    financial constraints, 14–15
    human resource, 15
    natural disasters and civil unrest, 15
  global access to vaccines initiative (GAVI), 19–20
  IMCI, guidelines, 20–21
  millennium development goals, 21–23
Stridor, 202
Subacute sclerosing panencephalitis (SSPE), 247

T

Traumatic brain injury, 417–418
Tuberculosis
  clinical presentation, 280–281
  diagnosis
    clinical diagnosis, 284
    imaging modalities, 283
    immunologic diagnostic modalities, 283–284
    mycobacteriologic modalities, 283
  differential diagnosis, 282
  epidemiology, 280
  prevention, 286
  treatment
    antiretroviral therapy, 285
    drug-resistant, 286
    first-line anti-TB medications, 285
    immune reconstitution inflammatory syndrome (IRIS), 285
    TB meningitis, 285

U

Under-five mortality rate (U5MR)
  causes of
    malaria, 8
    pneumonia, 6
    preventable infectious diseases, 10
    undernutrition, 8
  disproportionate mortality rates, 6, 7
  levels and trends in, 4, 5
  in middle-income countries, 6, 9
  in sub-Saharan Africa, 6, 8

V

Vaccine-preventable diseases
  anthrax, 304–305
  diphtheria, 305–306
  global burden of, 304
  haemophilus influenzae B (Hib), 308
  hepatitis A, 306
  hepatitis B, 306–307
  immunizations
    administration, 317
    routinely recommended vaccines, 316
    WHO vaccine schedule, 315–316
  Japanese encephalitis, 308–309
  meningococcal, 309
  mumps, 309–310
  pertussis, 310
  pneumococcal, 310–311
  polio, 311–313
  rabies, 312
  rubella, 312–313
  tetanus, 313
  typhoid/enteric fever, 314
  varicella, 314–315
  yellow fever, 315

Visceral leishmaniasis
  clinical presentation, 299
  diagnosis, 299, 300
  differential diagnosis, 299
  prevention, 300
  treatment, 299–300
Vulnerability
  in humanitarian crisis settings, 36–37
  hypervulnerability, 38, 39
  steps to
    education/economic security, 40
    family/connection, 40
    health care assessment and physiological needs, 40
    SAFE Child Impact Assessment (SCIA), 38
    safety/protection, 40

The manufacturer's authorised representative in the EU is Springer Nature Customer Service Centre GmbH, Europaplatz 3, 69115 Heidelberg, Germany. If you have any concerns regarding our products, please contact ProductSafety@springernature.com

Printed and bound by CPI Group (UK) Ltd, Croydon, CR0 4YY

23/03/2026

02076657-0002